Cognitive–Behavioral Psychology in the Schools

Cognitive-Behavioral Psychology in the Schools
A COMPREHENSIVE HANDBOOK

Edited by
JAN N. HUGHES
ROBERT J. HALL
Texas A&M University

THE GUILFORD PRESS
New York   London

© 1989 The Guilford Press
A Division of Guilford Publications, Inc.
72 Spring Street, New York, NY   10012

Printed in the United States of America

Last digit is print number: 9 8 7 6 5 4 3 2

Library of Congress Cataloging-in-Publication Data

Cognitive-behavioral psychology in the schools:
   a comprehensive handbook/edited by Jan N. Hughes, Robert J. Hall.
        p.   cm.
   Includes bibliographies and index.
   ISBN 0-89862-736-2
   1. Behavior modification.   2. Behavioral assessment of children.
3. Cognitive therapy.   I. Hughes, Jan N., 1949–   II. Hall,
Robert J. (Robert James), 1948–
LB1060.2.H37 1989
370.15′3—dc 19   88-23598
                                                          CIP

CONTRIBUTORS

Patricia A. Alexander, Department of Educational Curriculum and Instruction, Texas A&M University, College Station, Texas.

Kathryn M. Benes, Department of Educational Psychology, University of Nebraska–Lincoln, Lincoln, Nebraska.

A. Jerry Benson, College of Education and Human Services, James Madison University, Harrisonburg, Virginia.

Leslie R. Best, Department of Educational Psychology, University of Texas at Austin, Austin, Texas.

Robert Cohen, Department of Psychology, Memphis State University, Memphis, Tennessee.

Jane Close Conoley, Department of Educational Psychology, University of Nebraska–Lincoln, Lincoln, Nebraska.

Thomas G. Fetsco, Department of Psychology, Dickinson State University, Dickinson, North Dakota.

Michael M. Gerber, Department of Special Education, University of California, Santa Barbara, Santa Barbara, California.

Ernest T. Goetz, Department of Educational Psychology, Texas A&M University, College Station, Texas.

Steve Graham, Department of Special Education, University of Maryland, College Park, Maryland.

Robert J. Hall, Department of Educational Psychology, Texas A&M University, College Station, Texas.

Virginia Chou Hare, College of Education, University of Illinois at Chicago, Chicago, Illinois.

Karen R. Harris, Department of Special Education, University of Maryland, College Park, Maryland.

Jan N. Hughes, Department of Educational Psychology, Texas A&M University, College Station, Texas.

Clayton E. Keller, University of Minnesota at Duluth, Duluth, Minnesota.

Jack J. Kramer, Department of Educational Psychology, University of Nebraska–Lincoln, Lincoln, Nebraska.

Thomas R. Kratochwill, Department of Educational Psychology, University of Wisconsin–Madison, Madison, Wisconsin.

John Wills Lloyd, Curriculum, Instruction, and Special Education, University of Virginia, Charlottesville, Virginia.

Rebecca A. McReynolds, Private practice, Tucson, Arizona, and Department of Educational Psychology, University of Arizona, Tucson, Arizona.

Andrew W. Meyers, Department of Psychology, Memphis State University, Memphis, Tennessee.

Joel Meyers, School Psychology Program, Education, State University of New York at Albany, Albany, New York.

Richard J. Morris, Department of Educational Psychology, University of Arizona, Tucson, Arizona.

Douglas J. Palmer, Department of Educational Psychology, Texas A&M University, College Station, Texas.

Jack H. Presbury, College of Education and Human Services, James Madison University, Harrisonburg, Virginia.

William S. Rholes, Department of Psychology, Texas A&M University, College Station, Texas.

Paula Savage, Licensed Consulting Psychologist, Minnetonka, Minnesota.

Robert Schleser, Lewis College of Arts and Letters, Illinois Institute of Technology, Chicago, Illinois.

Eric A. Sellstrom, Department of Educational Psychology, University of Texas at Austin, Austin, Texas.

Kevin D. Stark, Department of Educational Psychology, University of Texas at Austin, Austin, Texas.

Andrew G. Stricker, Behavioral Sciences and Leadership, United States Air Force Academy, Colorado Springs, Colorado.

Eugene S. Urbain, Wilder Foundation, Wilder Child Guidance Clinic, St. Paul, Minnesota.

Bernice Y. L. Wong, Education, Simon Fraser University, Burnaby, British Columbia, Canada.

Glenn Yelich, School Psychology Program, Education, State University of New York at Albany, Albany, New York.

Sydney S. Zentall, Department of Special Education, Purdue University, West Lafayette, Indiana.

CONTENTS

1
COGNITIVE-BEHAVIORAL APPROACHES IN THE SCHOOLS: AN OVERVIEW

ROBERT J. HALL
JAN N. HUGHES
Texas A&M University

The terms "cognitive-behavior modification" (CBM) and "cognitive-behavior therapy" (CBT) identify a diverse assemblage of models and strategies. They share, however, three primary assumptions. First, cognitive mediating events affect behavior. Second, individuals are active participants in their own learning. And third, validity of theoretical constructs and practice recommendations has been subjected to empirical inquiry. Underlying these assumptions is the general notion that because outcome behaviors are mediated by internal thought processes, models of cognitive processing, and hence interpretation of cognitions, may lead to more individualized strategies or interventions for effecting predictable behavior change.

As the chapters in this book illustrate, cognitive behaviorism is not a unified theory. Rather, it represents a set of models and strategies loosely tied together by these three assumptions. We would remind the reader and ourselves, however, that although the controversy of the 1960s and 1970s between cognitivists and behaviorists has abated, allowing a merging of these perspectives in both research and clinical practice, there is still concern that psychology, because of its quest for understanding internal determiners, cannot be viewed as a science of behavior (Skinner, 1987).

ISSUES RELATED TO COGNITIVE-BEHAVIOR MODIFICATION

The terms "cognitive-behavior modification" (CBM), "cognitive-behavior therapy" (CBT), and "cognitive training" are often used interchangeably in the literature. Technically, however, these terms do differ in ways that are important to the layout and design of this book. CBM, the broadest term, refers to educational and clinical applications involving mediational theories of learning and behavior. Cognitive training refers to instructional efforts designed specifically to help learners improve their academic problem-solving ability via the use of cognitive mediational strategies. CBT, in contrast, refers to clinical applications of mediational models of behavior. Chapters in this book, though classified under the term CBM, are separated into those that focus primarily on cognitive training in academic areas and those that are directed toward the development of therapeutic training programs dealing with social/emotional problems. Both cognitive training and CBT represent emerging practice domains, and, as we will attempt to articulate, each is developing its own set of issues and concerns.

Cognitive Training

Cognitive-training programs seek to generate and develop mediating "thinking" skills for the purpose of enhancing children's overt problem-solving behaviors. These procedures, though orderly, systematic, and strategy-based, are often static. Practically, this means that most cognitive-training programs are not designed to accommodate subtle but crucial individual differences. Variables such as prior knowledge, partial automatization of component skills, and language competence are all likely to affect how children understand and at what level they are motivated to respond to the ordered parameters characteristic of most cognitive-training programs. Once training efforts have begun, knowledge base, automatization, language competence, motivation, and the corresponding information-processing network links begin to change, rendering static training programs ineffective or less effective at fostering the development of competent academic skills.

In most instances it is not the presence or absence of a specific strategy that accounts for the relatively poor performance of an individual or a group. Instead, breakdowns in complex strategic functions govern how well individuals will perform in given contexts. These organizational functions are thought to be determined by (1) an individual's breadth of information; (2) the degree of automaticity associated with relevant, acquired cognitive skills; (3) the repertoire of relevant, specific strategies; and (4) the ability to access those strategies efficiently (Keogh & Hall, 1984).

Cognitive-Behavior Therapy

Although CBT has been successfully applied to a wide range of emotional and behavioral disorders in children, evidence of its superiority over alternative treatments is generally lacking. For CBT to achieve the results its proponents envision, researchers in this area must attend to several important issues.

First, many of the clinical applications of CBT with children are derived from treatment models formulated for and tested with adults. Child practitioners must carefully consider the cognitive and linguistic demands these programs place on the child and modify treatment models to match children's abilities and social-developmental levels. That is, the theory on which the treatment is based may be more applicable to adults than to children.

Chapter 15 in this volume by Stark, Best, and Sellstrom, on a school-based model for the treatment of depression in children, illustrates the sensitivity to differences between children and adults that is required to modify adult-derived theories and treatment models for use with children. The authors review and extend an interpretation of research findings that demonstrates how adult models of depression can be used with children. For example, depressed children appear to have the same negative perceptual biases, attributional biases, and self-critical thinking patterns as depressed adults. Thus, Stark and his colleagues have adapted adult-derived treatment approaches to take into account the social and emotional characteristics of children and the natural settings in which children are typically found (i.e., the school).

A second issue in cognitive-behavior therapy with children is durability and generalizability of the skills taught. The greater investment of time and effort that CBT interventions require, relative to contingency management interventions, must be justified by attaining evidence of greater generalizability and durability using CBT approaches. To date, evidence favoring CBT approaches over strict behavioral interventions is promising but far from conclusive. We believe that, rather than representing a panacea for children's social/emotional problems, CBT represents a valuable addition to the therapist's available treatment approaches. Often intervention approaches combining reinforcement contingencies with CBT will result in optimal treatment results (e.g., Bierman, Miller, & Stabb, 1987).

Third, CBT practitioners need to determine child characteristics that interact with treatments to produce differential results. Important characteristics to consider include age, sex, cognitive level, cognitive style, and ethnicity. Additionally, subtle child variables such as attributional style, interest in peer interaction, perceptual biases, or expectations for treatment may interact with interventions. The accurate identification of subtle child characteristics that come to interact with treatment interventions requires assessment techniques that are both sensitive to individual differences and technically valid.

In this book, Palmer and Rholes (Chapter 8) present an extensive review of attributional studies that highlight important assessment questions. In their view, attributions are important because they describe the texture that summarizes the interaction between person and environment. Thus, identification and evaluation of these interactional elements can alert us to situations that tend to support or disrupt development by focusing our attention on the interplay between attributions and interventions. Their message is one of caution, however, as they outline methodological issues that impede the measurement of attributional styles or situation-specific attributions.

In Chapter 13, Zentall deals directly with issues related to self-control training with hyperactive and impulsive children. Her work nicely illustrates subtle differences that exist among treatments, components, and philosophies that are a part of the self-control literature. Moreover, by infusing her own work in the discussion, she has effectively established her presence in this area and has provided some direction for practitioners attempting to deal with the difficult problems associated with modifying hyperactive behavior.

Finally, an important issue confronting cognitive-behavior therapy is the appropriate target for the intervention. We believe that an exclusive focus on child variables (i.e., behaviors, cognitions, feelings) will be less effective than a focus on child, setting, and agent variables. This ecological perspective is further articulated in Chapter 4 in this volume by Meyers, Cohen, and Schleser and in Chapter 19 by Conoley. In Chapter 4 on the history and future of cognitive-behavior therapy, Meyers, Cohen, and Schleser review research findings on cognitive-behavioral approaches and offer support for the notion that CBT programs should be designed with consideration for ecological constraints. In general agreement, Conoley argues convincingly (in Chapter 19, on prevention) that by considering child, setting, and agent variables, the interventionist is most likely to achieve the prevention of learning and emotional/behavioral disorders.

PURPOSE AND SCOPE OF THIS BOOK

We believe that the emergence of cognitive-behavioral approaches in schools will do more to realize William James's vision of psychology applied to teaching than will any single development in psychology. Although the behaviorist paradigm did find its way into educational practice, creating opportunities for psychologists in schools, strict behavioral applications have tended to be in areas peripheral to teaching children new problem-solving or content mastery skills. Instead, reinforcement programs have been designed to modify children's academically relevant behaviors (e.g., completing assignments, staying in one's seat, and complying with teacher directives). Recent advances in CBM procedures, along with careful consideration of learner characteristics and task requirements, have aided our ability to improve performance effectively in areas such as social problem solving, reading comprehension, spelling, and mathematics. Teaching these process and content skills, we would argue, is the central goal of education.

Virtually every survey on the role of school psychologists has documented their desire to broaden their professional scope beyond testing and assessment (Benson & Hughes, 1985; Hughes, 1979; Meacham & Peckham, 1978). Questions concerning how best to measure cognitive skill and how to interpret children's performance are beginning to be addressed by researchers with backgrounds outside school psychology and psychometrics. The result is a perspective on performance that emphasizes careful documentation of learner skill, task and strategic requirements, and setting demands. Although this change in perspective does not eliminate or even minimize the role of assessment, it fundamentally changes its nature. Thus, for school psychologists to become more involved with the process of schooling, they will need to become aware of how data can be used to inform teaching. Cognitive-behavior therapies and academic interventions may serve to enhance and expand the knowledge base of school psychologists to the extent that they are designed to promote efficient transitions from teaching to learning in educational settings.

The type of teaching that occurs with the application of CBM procedures differs from the type of teaching evident in most classrooms. Teachers using CBM programs attempt to engender competence in pupils by teaching students *how* to think rather than *what* to think. In this book, chapters focus on different aspects of competence—academic, personal, and social. Together, the chapters cover a variety of techniques for instilling in children general self-control and problem-solving strategies. As is evident in the work represented in this book, CBM procedures have a strong preventive thrust. Thus, the emphasis is on helping individuals to develop skills and strategies for adapting to and dealing with current and future stressors.

We believe that school psychologists who apply a broadened behavioral model to developing child competencies will secure for themselves a more central role in schooling. For the past decade, the role of the school psychologist has been restricted to determining qualification for special education placement or to formulating behavioral management plans for use with disruptive students. As Goetz, Hall, and Fetsco argue in Chapters 5 and 6 of this volume, the school psychologist, functioning as gatekeeper, is able to offer few instructionally relevant recommendations to teachers. Moreover, as behavior management planners, school psychologists contribute only tangentially to the main purpose of schooling: teaching.

APPROACH

To facilitate the integration of cognitive-behavioral theories and research into educational practice, the bulk of this book is organized according to the three primary levels of service offered by school psychology: assessment, teaching and direct intervention, and indirect intervention. The first section of the text provides a historical and conceptual context for these three levels of service.

In Chapter 2, Benes and Kramer present a brief historical overview on how behavior modification, the "science of behavior," has affected education, and suggest directions for future research in applied behavior analysis. We have included this chapter because it offers a point of view that otherwise would not be represented. We want the reader to evaluate critically the position held by some behaviorists that cognitive psychology has contributed little to our understanding of human behavior or to improving educational processes. Thus, Benes and Kramer's chapter provides a counterpoint for the rest of this book. Although we take issue with their conclusions, we are in general agreement with their concern about inferences far removed from observable behavior, and we encourage readers to evaluate critically the evidence, or lack of evidence, that Benes and Kramer provide for their assertions.

Benes and Kramer have invented an interesting metaphor to represent "what is missing" from behavioral psychology. In critiquing their field, they argue that contemporary behavioral psychology lacks (1) a unified theory, (2) an understanding that humans are biological organisms derived from an evolutionary process, and (3) a recognition of the interaction effects that are part of an individual's ecosystem. They liken behavioral psychology to an environmental landscape and suggest that cognitive psychology is an ill-chosen substitute for the aforementioned missing elements in the landscape. We would argue that if the techniques of behavior modification had demonstrated functional adaptiveness across "landscapes," thereby fulfilling their intended functions of understanding and modifying behavior, then the emergence of cognitive psychology would have been suppressed. Behavior modification works best, however, in settings where there is a high level of external control over behavior. When the environmental landscape changes (i.e., when a high degree of environmental control is absent), behavior modification falls far short of its goal of effecting durable and generalizable behavior change. Cognitive-behavior modification is a functional adaptation of neobehaviorist techniques in the sense that individuals engaged in these interventions are taught to monitor their own behaviors for the purpose of structuring their own environments. General question-asking procedures common to many CBM programs are designed to help individuals to select and apply the environmental constraints that will foster the ongoing modification of behavioral responses. We believe that a joint cognitive and behavioral approach deals more effectively with children's educationally relevant problems (i.e., is more functional) than a strictly behavioral approach. The reader may find, however, that Chapters 3 through 19 provide the best counterpoint to Benes and Kramer's assertion that cognitive psychology has contributed little to improving educational processes. Our hope is that the reader will reach his or her own conclusions via careful consideration of the evidence presented by Benes and Kramer and critical evaluation of the empirical base associated with recommended assessment and intervention practices that are presented throughout this book.

In Chapter 3, Benson and Presbury remind us that educators have always been concerned with what goes on in the minds of children. Their view of how cognition has affected both psychology and education makes for informative and entertaining reading. They encourage psychologists and educators to reexamine philosophical issues left relatively unattended to during the reign of behaviorism. These issues include the nature of reality, consciousness, and the mind.

In Chapter 4, the last chapter in this first part, Meyers, Cohen, and Schleser trace the evolution of cognitive-behavior modification and articulate their developmental cognitive-behavioral model. In emphasizing the importance of complex interactions among factors such as cognitive status of the learner, nature of the learning materials, procedures used during learning, and tasks used to assess learning outcomes, these authors provide a useful framework for understanding and critically evaluating subsequent chapters.

Part Two begins with Chapters 5 and 6 by Goetz, Hall, and Fetsco. Chapter 5 opens with an in-depth look at a child's written composition. This story is then used to illustrate how an information-processing analysis of performance might differ from a more traditional quantitative analysis. In Chapter 6, the authors discuss the role of school psychologists relative to the needs of classroom teachers, arguing ultimately for the emergence of scientist/practitioners. Along the way, they (1) present a brief overview of the development of the current cognitive approach and some of its major theoretical constructs; (2) outline a cognitive-instructional approach to guide application of theory; (3) present interpretive examples of student performance on standardized ability tests; and (4) present an alternative, cognitive approach to assessment.

Chapter 7 by Hughes proposes an information-processing model for the assessment of children's social skills and social competence. In this chapter, she elaborates on a model previously offered by Hughes and Hall (1987), extending our understanding of that earlier work by showing how the model might serve as a guide for developing CBT interventions in the area of social competence. An important feature of this chapter is the way in which Hughes demonstrates, through use of a case study, how to collect increasingly more specific assessment information to establish the exact nature of underlying inefficient problem-solving performance. She goes on to illustrate how this information is contextually relevant to the proposed theoretical model and how it can be used to inform the development of precise training programs in the area of social competence.

The final chapter in this section, Chapter 8 by Palmer and Rholes, provides truly comprehensive coverage of issues related to the assessment of children's attributions. Their scholarly treatment of the literature makes this chapter a good reference article for the rest of the book. The assessment issues discussed, including talk-aloud approaches, verbal reports, and the use of hypothetical versus real-life situations, are relevant to each chapter in this book. In addition, they have developed two unique and detailed tables summarizing (1) the methodologies used in the literature for attributional assessment and (2) internal consistency information for selected measures of attributional style. For comparative and research purposes, these tables are of enormous value.

Part Three of the book begins with a short chapter by Bernice Wong (Chapter 9). In a departure from the format of other chapters, Wong was asked to provide a brief overview of issues related to cognitive training and then to review Chapter 10 by Alexander and Hare, Chapter 11 by Graham and Harris, Chapter 12 by Keller and Lloyd, and Chapter 13 by Zentall. Thus, her chapter serves as a guide to other chapters on cognitive training with handicapped learners and as a preview for Zentall's insightful theoretical conceptualization linking Berlyne's optimal stimulation theory to problems associated with hyperactivity. Of note in Wong's chapter is her comment that the concept of "inactive learner," despite its having spawned much research in the area of learning disabilities, is "too loose to serve as a research-engendering frame-work." She argues, instead, that a cognitive-training approach, though not a theory in itself, can be of great use if paired with an academic or social/emotional process theory. Wong's familiarity with research in the fields of metacognition, cognitive training, and learning disabilities leads her to suggest that, for learning-disabled children, cognitive-strategy training must be concurrent with training that teaches learners to define their own problem-solving difficulties. The reader is encouraged to read her work carefully before delving into other chapters in this section.

In Chapter 10, Alexander and Hare look at cognitive training relative to reading instruction. Consistent with the comments of Wong, they begin their work by reviewing theoretical constructs that serve to constrain not only the reading process but also cognitive-training programs that might be developed to improve reading comprehension. Their review of extant cognitive-training programs is highlighted by an in-depth look at the work of Paris and of Palinscar and Brown. Interestingly, statements made by Alexander and Hare with regard to the importance of assessment and motivation for the development of effective cognitive-training programs in reading are consistent with those raised in Chapters 5 and 6 by Goetz, Hall, and Fetsco and in Chapter 8 by Palmer and Rholes. Finally, Alexander and Hare illustrate how Alexander's current research, training and evaluating analogical reasoning skills in young children, can serve as a guide to setting up academic skill–based training programs in other areas.

Chapter 11, by Graham and Harris, provides a good theoretical discussion of the writing process and its associated cognitive-processing demands. This is followed by specific illustrations of CBM programs used to develop writing skills for learning-disabled students. Graham and Harris critically evaluate each of the presented programs, followed by a comprehensive presentation of their own work with learning-disabled children in the area of training written language skills. Like Wong, these authors are concerned with issues related to the generalizability of training effects, and see the need to try to ensure that children, who do not have well-developed writing skills, learn first to define where in the process they are uncertain and then to be strategic in response to the identified problem.

Keller and Lloyd begin Chapter 12 with a brief review of cognitive and behavioral factors important to mathematics instruction. Like other chapters in this section, they focus our attention on research and theoretical frameworks for understanding individual differences. Unlike the other chapter authors, however, they provide a more in-depth review of variables important for establishing effective instruction, such as modeling, reinforcement, and combinations of teaching behaviors. Keller and Lloyd also take a detailed look at the development and use of addition strategies. Not only is this section illustrative from a program design standpoint, but their review of research also raises questions about the role that metacognitive processes play in the solution of basic addition facts. This point seems particularly important given the concerns expressed by Goetz, Hall, and Fetsco (Chapters 5 and 6) and by Hall, Gerber, and Stricker (Chapter 14) about overtraining information-processing components that are already well established for the learner. The chapter then elaborates on how blending curriculum-based assessment of component skills in mathematics with principles of effective teaching can lead instructional designers to develop interventions that will have a more durable and generalizable impact on mathematics performance.

Also included in this section is the very long chapter by Hall, Gerber, and Stricker on cognitive training and spelling (Chapter 14). This chapter was not ready in time to be sent to Bernice Wong for review, so mention of this work does not appear in Chapter 9. As in the other chapters in this section, Hall, Gerber, and Stricker have emphasized background information—where the spelling system comes from, how spelling is taught, and how spelling skill develops. In two ways, however, this chapter differs from others in this section. First, the authors describe, through the use of case studies, how careful observation, analysis, and interpretation of students' attempts to spell can lead to instructionally useful developmental models of students' ability to solve spelling problems. This discussion is also relevant to the design of cognitive-behavioral interventions. Second, the authors use extant intelligent computer-assisted instructional (ICAI) software to outline the components of effective teaching in the area of spelling. These programs serve to inform teachers about the sequence and pace of instruction and to extend the dialogue in this book to include suggestions for how microcomputer technology might be linked with CBT intervention strategies to produce ICAI programs in spelling. As in the Goetz, Hall, and Fetsco chapters, the real message in this work is how important it is for school psychologists and teachers to understand that complex information processing does not easily reduce to simple statements of cause and effect. Rather, to be a professional means making a commitment to developing expert knowledge across a number of theoretical, academic, and affective domains.

Zentall's chapter, already reviewed, serves as a nice bridge between chapters on CBM with academic problems and those on CBM with social/emotional problems, the topic for Part Four.

In Chapter 15, Stark, Best, and Sellstrom provide a conceptual overview of childhood depression. In their overview, they summarize the major cognitive and behavioral theories of depression and evaluate empirical evidence supportive of each theory. They then describe, on the basis of their own work, how a school-based treatment program for childhood depression can be implemented and evaluated. Of particular value to the research practitioner is their sensitive discussion of the "gentle balance" involved in conducting clinical research in schools.

In Chapter 16, McReynolds, Morris, and Kratochwill present the reader with a comprehensive review of the literature on children's fears and anxieties, emphasizing cognitive-behavioral approaches to assessment and intervention. Certainly, instructors who use this text will appreciate the authors' broad coverage of the topic and their systematic, organized approach. Frequent cautions regarding extrapolations from the extant research to practice are much appreciated, given the scarcity of methodologically adequate treatment-outcome studies researching fearful children.

In Chapter 17, the last chapter in the direct intervention section, Urbain and Savage summarize and critically evaluate the expanding literature on interpersonal cognitive problem-solving (ICPS) training. Because their recommendations for future research and practice are based on their extensive personal experience in teaching ICPS skills to children and adolescents, their suggestions seem especially relevant. Interpersonal cognitive problem-solving training attempts to teach children general problem-solving skills that will enable them to deal more effectively with current and future stressors. Thus, the Urbain and Savage chapter is an excellent introduction to the final section of this book.

The final two chapters of the book are addressed to psychologists and educational specialists involved in promoting systemwide changes in schools. In Chapter 18 on cognitive-behavioral approaches in school consultation, Meyers and Yelich make an important distinction between consultation content and consultation process. Appropriately, they focus their chapter on the application of cognitive-behavioral principles used in the consultation process. Their discussion of how processes such as social power, attributions, and dissonance apply to consultation interactions is both insightful and integrative.

Finally, Conoley, in Chapter 19, focuses on applications of cognitive-behavioral principles to prevention of mental health problems in the schools. Conoley's breadth of coverage, scholarly approach, and conceptualization of the field of prevention make this an essential chapter for anyone hoping to have an impact on children's mental health. She begins her chapter by providing an overview of what is known about prevention in general and about cognitive-behavioral approaches to prevention, in particular. Next she critically reviews the research data on three cognitive-behavioral approaches to prevention (social problem solving, social skills training, and rational emotive therapy). Finally, she shows how these and other approaches are relevant to specific prevention programs (e.g., teenage pregnancy, children of divorced parents, and drug abuse). Although these three scaffolded levels constitute the major organizational structure for Conoley's work, several subthemes are introduced early in the chapter and further developed throughout the chapter. She examines in detail the need to teach skills in a specific context, the importance of demonstrating Type II change, to consider nonskill characteristics of the host, and to develop a generative base for prevention programming.

In summary, this book is written for school psychologists, child clinical psychologists, and special educators. As editors, we have encouraged authors (1) to review critically the theoretical and empirical bases used to support suggested applications, (2) to note limitations of applications, and (3) to delineate important areas for future inquiry. Thus, the book is targeted at professional school and child clinical psychologists and special educators, as well as advanced graduate students in these disciplines. We see the book as an appropriate text for graduate courses in psychological assessment, child behavior therapy and counseling, school consultation, and (as an overview) for courses in special-education instructional methods. Our hope is that these chapters will promote more substantive dialogue between school psychologists and classroom teachers, enabling both to develop more detailed and empirically informed "clinical" judgments about children's academic, social, and emotional competencies and to generate hypotheses about what program works best with which child.

REFERENCES

Benson, A. J., & Hughes, J. N. (1985). Perceptions of role processes in school psychology: A national survey. *School Psychology Review, 14,* 64–74.

Bierman, K. L., Miller, C. L., & Stabb, S. D. (1987). Improving the social behavior and peer acceptance of rejected boys: Effect of social skill training with instructions and prohibitions. *Journal of Consulting and Clinical Psychology, 55,* 194–200.

Hughes, J. N. (1979). Consistency of administrators' and psychologists' actual and ideal perceptions of school psychologists' activities. *Psychology in the Schools, 16,* 234–239.

Hughes, J. N., & Hall, R. J. (1987). A proposed model for the assessment of children's social competence. *Professional School Psychology, 2,* 247–260.

Keogh, B K., & Hall, R. J. (1984). Cognitive training with learning-disabled pupils. In A. W. Meyers & W. E. Craighead (Eds.), *Cognitive behavior therapy with children* (pp. 163–191). New York: Plenum Press.

Meacham, M. L., & Peckham, P. D. (1978). School psychologists at three-quarters century: Congruence between training, practice, preferred role and competence. *Journal of School Psychology, 16,* 195–206.

Skinner, B. F. (1987). Whatever happened to psychology as the science of behavior? *American Psychologist, 42,* 780–786.

PART ONE
Historical and Conceptual Overview

2
THE BEHAVIORAL TRADITION IN SCHOOLS (AND MILES TO GO BEFORE WE SLEEP)

KATHRYN M. BENES
JACK J. KRAMER
University of Nebraska–Lincoln

When a science of behavior had once rid itself of psychic fictions, it faced these alternatives: either it might leave their places empty and proceed to deal with its data directly, or it might make replacements. The altogether too obvious alternative to a mental science was a natural science, and that was the choice made by a non-mentalistic psychology. The possibility of a directly-descriptive science of behavior and its peculiar advantages have received little attention. (Skinner, 1938, p. 4)

It no longer can be said that the directly descriptive science of behavior referred to by Skinner (1938) above has gone unattended. The impact of the science of behavior on education has been both remarkable and disappointing—remarkable in the extent to which this analysis has been productive in the development of effective assessment and treatment methodologies, and disappointing in the extent to which this technology has been adopted by school systems and individual teachers. We intend to trace the behavioral tradition in the schools, from the early speculations of behaviorists to the more recent analyses of academic ecologies. An analysis of the importance of a behavioral psychology for education and future considerations for the experimental analysis of behavior are also provided. Our analysis is not "cognitive," as one might suspect based on the title of this book; but, like some "cognitive-behaviorists," we foresee a need for an expanding behavioral psychology.

LEARNING THEORY—FROM WHENCE IT CAME

The Egyptian pyramids and the Great Wall of China serve as lasting evidence that over the centuries individuals have had some knowledge of human behavior and how to modify it effectively (sometimes by inhumane methods). In this introductory section, we will briefly trace the evolution of thought regarding a behavioral, learning-oriented psychology and discuss some of the primary contributors to that line of thought. This history provides but an overview in order to set the stage for the material that follows; for an in-depth historical review, the reader is referred to other sources (Borin, 1950; Hilgard, 1987; Kendler, 1987).

Historical Roots

Behaviorism's "official" birth can be traced to John B. Watson's article entitled "Psychology as the Behaviorist Views It":

> Psychology as the behaviorist views it is a purely objective experimental branch of natural science. Its theoretical goal is the prediction and control of behavior. Introspection forms no essential part of its methods, nor is the scientific value of its data dependent upon the readiness with which they lend themselves to interpretation in terms of consciousness. The behaviorist, in his efforts to get a unitary scheme of animal response, recognized no dividing line between man and brute. The behavior of man, with all its refinement and complexity, forms only a part of the behaviorist's total scheme of investigation. (Watson, 1913, p. 158)

The preceding description represented (and continues to represent) the cornerstone on which behaviorism was built. The primary position posed by Watson was that psychology is a science of behavior rather than of mind. Although the behavioral position was quite radical for the day, the groundwork for such a science had been initiated at least two hundred years before (Kendler, 1987).

Julian Offray de La Mettrie (1709–1751), a French philosopher, wrote a book entitled *L'Homme Machine* ("Man a Machine") (1960/1748). La Mettrie postulated that the most effective way to study human psychology was to view the human in a detached manner, as a sort of machine, the characteristics of which one could examine and analyze objectively. This historical "brick" was present in Watson's initial definition of behaviorism and remains a primary factor constituting modern behaviorism.

Charles Darwin's (1809–1882) theory of evolution, establishing a continuity between animal and human, also paved the way for behaviorism to become a discipline. Behaviorists would eventually take this principle as a rationale for using infrahuman subjects in their experimentation.

C. Lloyd Morgan (1852–1936) also contributed to the historical roots and philisophical underpinnings of behaviorism. He made the proposition that came to be known as Lloyd Morgan's canon: "In no case may we interpret an action as the outcome of the exercise of a higher psychical activity, if it can be interpreted as the outcome of the exercise of one which stands lower in the psychological scale" (Morgan, 1894, p. 288).

Jacques Loeb (1859–1924), a German physiologist and zoologist, was an influential force on behaviorism. Loeb, who taught at the University of Chicago while Watson was a student there, developed a theory of animal behavior based on *tropism*, the involuntary motor response to a stimulus. He maintained that much of animal behavior could be explained by tropism and did not require conscious processes. Loeb did not deny the existence of conscious processes; he simply believed they were not necessary to explain animal behavior.

In the same physiological vein as Loeb, Russian physiologists such as Ivan Sechenov (1829–1905), Vladimir Bekhterev (1857–1927), and Ivan Pavlov (1849–1936) had a great impact on behavioral psychology. Pavlov, in particular, provided the empirical structure that later supported behavior methodology.

Edward L. Thorndike also contributed greatly to the emerging new discipline of behaviorism. The central theme of Thorndike's work was that learning was a trial-and-error process with "accidental success" (Thorndike, 1898). The unsuccessful behaviors were "stamped out" while the successful behaviors, those that were "satisfying," were repeated.

Although each of the aforementioned individuals contributed to behaviorism, without question it was John B. Watson who synthesized the research and "marketed" the approach so effectively that even neobehaviorism rests firmly on Watsonian principles.

Neobehaviorism encompasses a variety of behavioral variations, including Clark Hull's (1884–1952) stimulus–response reinforcement theory and Donald Hebb's (1904–1985) neurophysiological theory. But the most popular and most widely used of the neobehavioral mechanisms are those posed by B. F. Skinner, who was born in 1904.

Like Watson's, Skinner's principles of radical behaviorism have maintained an approach that strictly attends to overt behavior, objective discriptions, and functional quality of behavior. Psychology, from a Skinnerian perspective, is focused on prediction and control of behavior. Skinner (1953) states:

> We are concerned with the causes of behavior. We want to know why men behave as they do. Any condition or event which can be shown to have an effect upon behavior must be taken into account. By discovering and analyzing these causes we can predict behavior; to the extent that we can manipulate them, we can control behavior. (p. 23)

Summary

Each of the individuals mentioned in this section has helped to define behaviorism. Collectively, they have developed subtle norms and mores that extend far beyond any one person's contributions. In essence, these individuals have created an independent psychological culture. Behaviorism, however, should be viewed as a never-ending process that encourages the examination and reexamination of the science of human behavior.

APPLIED BEHAVIOR ANALYSIS: EARLY APPLICATIONS

As indicated in the material presented earlier, the experimental analysis of behavior was built on the principles of objective description, experimental measurement, functional relationships, and single-subject designs. Early attempts to research the basic principles of behavior analysis involved investigations of laboratory phenomena, primarily with infrahuman species.

During the 1950s, behavioral research began to take an applied bent. Spurred by Skinner's laboratory work on operant conditioning, researchers began to move out of the laboratory and into schools, clinics, and hospitals. "Humans were included as subjects, socially meaningful responses were studied, and much discussion ensued regarding the practical significance of the experimental results" of these applied efforts (Kratochwill & Bijou, 1987).

The basic principles of operant conditioning used in these early investigations were reinforcement, punishment, and stimulus control. Some of the earliest demonstrations of the potential of these principles in an applied context involved teaching machines (e.g., Skinner, 1954), programmed instruction (e.g., Keller, 1968), and operant conditioning with severely impaired populations (e.g., Kazdin, 1978). The success of these investigations and the excitement generated by these discoveries led to a desire to examine the application of basic learning principles in educational settings. The variables mentioned in Table 2-1, which had been investigated in more controlled laboratory and applied settings, were now ready for examination in educational contexts. Next we examine examples of early research studies documenting the efficacy of the use of procedures derived from the principles cited above.

TABLE 2-1. Basic Principles of Operant Conditioning

Basic Principle	Definition and Examples
Reinforcement	May involve either the application of a positive stimulus or the removal of a negative stimulus following the response of the organism. Specific reinforcement procedures include, for example, shaping, chaining, fading, and token economies.
Punishment	May involve either the application of a negative stimulus or the removal of a positive stimulus following the response of the organism. Specific punishment procedures include response cost, overcorrection, extinction (which includes time out), and systematic desensitization.
Stimulus control	Procedures designed to teach the organism that different stimuli within the environment serve as "signals" regarding the likelihood that a particular response will be reinforced or punished. Specific procedures derived from stimulus control include prompting, discrimination training, and stimulus generalization.

Reinforcement: Developing, Maintaining, and Increasing Behavior

Two of the most frequently cited early experimental applications of behavioral technology in the schools are Hall, Lund, and Jackson's (1968) investigation of study behavior and Madsen, Becker, and Thomas's (1968) analysis of classroom management practices.

The Hall *et al.* (1968) study demonstrated that systematic alteration of teacher behavior affected children's attention in the classroom. An observer seated in the class would hold up a small piece of colored paper when a particular child was attending to a task. Signals were presented unobtrusively to prevent disrupting the class and were followed by the teacher's verbal reinforcement directed at the target child. Not only did this procedure result in an increase in children's on-task behavior, but this was accomplished with no increase in the total amount of time that teachers were attending to children. Instead, it was demonstrated that *how* teacher attention was delivered was more important than *how much* teacher attention was available. This study was also important in demonstrating that teachers with no previous training in behavior analysis were capable of carrying out reinforcement procedures with a minimum of in-class supervision.

The Madsen *et al.* (1968) study is important because it was an attempt to evaluate all three of the basic principles of operant conditioning cited in Table 2-2 on classroom management practices (or, as the authors of this article referred to them, rules, praise, and ignoring). Simply stated, this study suggested that (1) rules alone were relatively ineffective in changing students' behavior within a class; (2) approval for appropriate behavior and ignoring of inappropriate behavior, used in combination, were very effective in classroom management; and (3) approval for appropriate behavior was probably the single most important factor in improving classroom behavior.

As a result of the studies cited here and many others completed during the following decade, it became clear that the principles derived from laboratory analysis and the procedures derived from these principles could be used to increase the frequency of desired behavior in school settings.

Punishment: Decreasing Behavior

Most of the early applied behavior analysis studies in education involved demonstration of the utility of reinforcement principles. Some studies, however, clearly demonstrated the efficacy of punishment procedures. Most of the punishment studies were examinations of the effects of the denial of previously reinforcing stimuli (i.e., extinction) rather than the application of aversive stimuli. For example, Sachs (1973) used time out (from reinforcement) to reduce the activity level and acting-out behavior of a 10-year-old boy who had been diagnosed as hyperactive. The time-out room was specially designed to be devoid of any stimulation and included a microphone to monitor the boy's verbalizations. The child was informed that he would be placed in the room for 5 minutes whenever he engaged in inappropriate behavior (he was provided with descriptions of specific behaviors) and that if he made noise in the room, his stay there would be extended until he was quiet for 5 minutes. This procedure was effective in dramatically reducing the child's disruptive behavior and was accomplished in a relatively short period of time.

One exception to the preponderance of investigations examining the effects of denial of reinforcing stimuli on behavior was a study by Kircher, Pear, and Martin (1971). In this study the effects of the verbal response "no" and of shock (9–15 Ma lasting for approximately 25 msec) on inattentiveness and incorrect responses in a picture-naming task were assessed. The subjects were two severely retarded children, 5 and 6 years of age, living in a hospital setting. Though undertaken in a hospital rather than a school setting, the task was educational in nature and the study actually took place in a classroom within the hospital setting. The authors found that both procedures ("no" and shock) were effective at decreasing incorrect responses, but that shock was more efficient in decreasing the number of errors and the amount of inattentiveness. It should also be noted that these subjects were reinforced for correct responses during the course of this experiment.

As the result of studies of this type, completed under a variety of conditions with varied subject populations, the efficacy of punishment procedures in the management of educationally relevant behavior was documented in a clear and irrefutable manner.

Stimulus Control: Alerting the Organism

Lovitt and Curtiss (1968) reported a study in which an 11-year-old boy exhibited a great deal of variability in his mathematics performance. After initially establishing a baseline, the boy was simply instructed to verbalize his math problems before completing them (e.g., "Some number minus 20 equals 20"). Numbers of problems solved correctly increased during the experimental phase, with numbers of incorrect problems approaching zero. Interestingly, the subject's error rate remained low even after he was instructed to stop verbalizing the problem. Today such a study might be described as cognitive behavior modification. Whatever label one attaches to such a study, it appears that by altering antecedent stimuli, behavior can be changed. In some cases simply altering these antecedent events would allow for subsequent environmental control (i.e., reinforcement) such that the desired behavior would continue to exist even when the prompt was removed.

In a similar manner, Risley and Reynolds (1970) have shown that by a teacher stressing (or emphasizing) certain words as she read a sentence, children's ability to imitate the words emphasized could be influenced. Although emphasis could be used as a prompt to increase imitation, this effect was only apparent when relatively few words were emphasized. That is, prompts proved to be effective, but only when not used too often. In a study with broader implications, Van Houten and Sullivan (1975) demonstrated that audio cues were effective at increasing rates of teacher praise and that teacher praise resulted in improved behavior in the classroom.

These studies were but a few examples of the many conducted during the early years of behavioral analysis documenting the effectiveness of prompts (or signals that indicated the availability of reinforcers/punishers) in the behavior change process. These studies made clear the importance of understanding and analyzing antecedent events in the assessment, design, and evaluation of remedial activities in educational settings.

Summary

The impact of these early investigations of behavioral analysis in the schools was not a result of their technological sophistication or their magnitude of outcome. Rather, it was that simply by defining behavior in precise, observable terms, and by arranging stimuli in a specified manner, behaviors of importance could be altered so as to increase the likelihood of learning. The focus in these early investigations was on the management of classroom behavior. We acknowledge that our simple representation of the use of reinforcement, punishment, and stimulus control does not do justice to the complexity of many of the early applications of behavior analysis. For example, we do not mean to imply that punishment should be used exclusively when developing strategies for decreasing behavior. We have, however, attempted to show how the simple procedures described in Table 2–1 could be used to develop technologies for behavior change.

Blackham and Silberman (1980) have summarized the findings of this line of early research as suggesting these seven ingredients for successful classroom management:

1. Specify in positive terms the desired classroom behavior.
2. Individualize learning tasks so that every student can succeed.
3. Specify consequences for both desirable and undesirable behavior.
4. Determine when and how reinforcement will be delivered.
5. Develop an individual and a group reinforcement system.
6. Model the behavior students should emulate.
7. Develop your reinforcement properties as a teacher.

During the 1960s and 1970s, applications of behavioral technology to educational concerns flourished. Journals were established, many additional studies were completed, and the relationship between environmental events and learning was well established. In some areas, such as special education, behavioral analysis had taken hold. The total picture, however, was not so promising. Although the efficiency of the technologies derived from behavioral analysis were well documented, the philosophy and methods of behavioral analysis were not summarily embraced by all areas of the educational establishment.

The failure to generalize effective methods may be a function of the failure of behaviorists to apply appropriate contingencies, or may be due to the fact that behaviorists have not controlled the contingencies. The situation described here has led some to suggest that a more global form of analysis, a concern for the larger environment in which the organism is behaving, would be necessary in order for behaviorists to understand how to generalize the technology and devise strategies for influencing social behavior in a more pervasive manner.

APPLIED BEHAVIOR ANALYSIS IN SCHOOLS: CURRENT APPLICATIONS

Current trends in behavioral analysis in education are diverse and complex. Next we examine three specific applications that have emerged within the past decade and consider the contributions of each to education and the schools. Other promising approaches, such as the stimulus control literature with the severely handicapped (Browder & D'Huyetters, 1988) and direct instruction (Becker & Carnine, 1980), are not examined here but warrant the attention of educational psychologists. Each approach discussed here represents an attempt to apply behavioral analysis in a broader, more comprehensive way than that illustrated by the early contingency management studies cited earlier.

Behavioral Consultation

Many different models of consultation have been proposed, all generally involving the development of a voluntary, egalitarian, and collegial relationship between a consultee and a consultant, with the goal of promoting change in individual behavior and/or systems (Gutkin & Curtis, 1982). All models tend to involve a method of providing indirect services to a client (e.g., a child) who is served through a consultee (e.g., a teacher) by a consultant (e.g., a school psychologist). As suggested in its name, behavioral consultation is a form of consultation based on the principles of behavioral analysis. The most widely cited model of behavioral consultation for school practitioners is Bergan's (1977) four-stage problem-solving approach: (1) problem identification, (2) problem analysis, (3) plan implementation, and (4) plan evaluation. Advocates of this model suggest that this approach is effective because:

> Use of the behavioral knowledge base in plan design has the obvious advantage of producing plans based on principles that have been found to be effective in controlled studies. Plans based on research findings should have a greater likelihood of success than plans derived from informal sources of knowledge such as clinical experience. (Bergan, 1977, p. 22)

The Bergan model described here has been shown to be effective in assisting consultants and consultees in defining problems within school contexts (e.g.,

Bergan & Tombari, 1976; Kratochwill & Bergan, 1978). In general, the behavioral consultation model has more empirical support than any other model of consultation (Gutkin & Curtis, 1982; Medway, 1979). More important than the amount of support for the behavioral consultation model is the fact that the evidence supporting this model helps us to understand the types of behaviors in which consultants should engage if they are to maximize the effectiveness of the consultation process. In general, this model emphasizes the specific types of interview skills (i.e., verbal behavior) needed during problem identification and analysis. More specific information on this model and its effectiveness can be found in Bergan (1977) and Kratochwill (1982).

Direct Measurement of Academic Behavior

Many criticisms have been advanced regarding shortcomings in traditional approaches for assessing academic achievement in the schools, not the least of which is that the current assessment process does not adequately measure change in skills (Carver, 1974). The model most recently and repeatedly suggested as an alternative to the traditional approach has involved direct and repeated assessment of a student's skills within his or her curriculum—what has come to be called curriculum-based assessment (CBA). According to Gickling and Thompson (1985), this approach is "a procedure for determining the instructional needs of students based upon the student's ongoing performance in existing course content" (p. 206).

Although defined in a broad manner by Gickling, the work by Stanley Deno and his colleagues at the University of Minnesota has shown specifically how such a system can be designed and implemented. For example, Deno (1985) has provided evidence showing that the number of words read correctly from a third-grade reading passage is a reliable indicator of growth in reading skills across elementary school ages. Similar results have been obtained in CBA of spelling and written expression skills (e.g., Deno, Marston, & Mirken, 1982; Deno, Mirken, Lowrey, & Kuehnle, 1980).

Shapiro (1987) has suggested that curriculum-based assessment has two major advantages over norm-referenced and criterion-referenced assessment. These advantages include test–text overlap and direct linkage to instruction. This failure to master skills cannot be the result of a poor test–curriculum match, since testing takes place with material from the curriculum, and CBA allows for a direct assessment of the skills that have not been mastered and the point where instruction should begin.

The documented advantages and the potential of curriculum-based assessment are many and varied. Some of these advantages have been discussed herein. The future of academic assessment will undoubtedly be both norm- and curriculum-based, but we clearly believe that the importance of the latter will continue to grow for some time to come. Galagan (1985) writes in his analysis of the past and future of academic assessment, "Psychoeducational Testing: Turn Out the Lights, the Party's Over." To that we would add: It's about time.

Assessment of the Learning Environment

The research cited herein and the many additional studies completed since the late 1960s provide empirical support for the direct relationship between academic performance and certain classroom variables. According to Lentz and Shapiro (1986), these classroom variables can be considered an academic ecology,

> conceptualized as a network of relationships among student and classroom environmental variables as they affect acquisition of new skills and student engagement in appropriate academic work. Teacher behaviors such as goal setting and progress monitoring, direct questioning about academic work, providing performance feedback, appropriate instructional pacing, attending contingently to appropriate work, praising, prompting, contacting pattern during individual seatwork, and arranging contingencies for desirable academic engagement are related directly to student progress and performance. Other environmental variables such as time allotted for academic work, instructions, peer attention, and post-work contingencies are likewise important. (p. 350)

These authors go on to suggest three strategies for assessing the relationship among these classroom variables: teacher interview (see the previous discussion of behavioral consultation, direct observation (see the previous discussion of direct measurement), and permanent products (e.g., worksheets, tests, homework assignments). The manner in which these assessment approaches can be used to provide functional data on the classroom environment is reproduced in Table 2-2.

Observational schedules such as The State–Event Classroom Environment Scale (Saudargas & Lentz, 1982), the Code for Instructional Structure and Student Academic Response (Stanley & Greenwood, 1981), and the Instructional Environment Scale (Ysseldyke & Christensen, 1987) all provide for the type of assessment suggested in Table 2-2. This approach to assessment assumes a direct, causal relationship between teacher and pupil behavior. Perhaps most important of all, this approach makes no assumptions about either student (e.g., lazy, unmotivated) or teacher (incompetent, unmotivated) characteristics, and instead attempts to elucidate the functional relationship between teacher and student behavior. (We realize, of course, that the ability to use information gained during the type of assessment described above in a manner that is helpful to both teachers and students is yet another skill not necessarily taught as part of the assessment process described above.)

Summary

If it is not already clear, the three applications of behavioral analysis cited have in common an emphasis on assessment. The assessment process described is very different, however, from that normally practiced by psychologists working in the schools. All three approaches have in common an emphasis on

TABLE 2-2. Classroom Ecological Variables and Related Assessment Methods

Variables	Behavior Interview	Direct Observation	Permanent Product
Immediately impinging environment			
Engagement			
Scheduled time	X		
Allotted time	X	X	
On-task		X	
Opportunities to respond	X	X	X
Response rate	X		X
Events concurrent with engagement			
Instruction	X	X	
Models	X	X	
Prompts		X	
Pacing		X	
Praise		X	
Error correction		X	
Contingencies			
Teacher attention		X	
Peer attention		X	
Accuracy feedback	X	X	
Class structure			
Grouping	X	X	
Pattern of contacts	X	X	
Competing behaviors	X	X	
Pre- or postwork events			
Instructions	X	X	
Contingencies for completion			
Accuracy	X	X	
Performance feedback	X	X	
Teacher planning/evaluation	X	X	

functional analysis, repeated measurement, and operational definition of variables (e.g., problems). For that reason, these approaches seem to fulfill most of the basic requirements of a behavioral-assessment approach (Haynes, 1978).

Whereas most of the early research in behavioral application focused on development of treatment technologies, especially as related to classroom management, most recent research has focused on strategies for response definition and assessment. The importance of a strong assessment–treatment link (see Fuchs & Fuchs, 1986, for a special journal issue on this topic) has been emphasized throughout the work reviewed here.

Perhaps, however, there may be more to advances in education than just the development of effective assessment and remediation strategies. Perhaps in their zeal to reduce educational processes and concepts to operational definitions and reinforcement technologies, behaviorists have failed to take a good look at the big picture, the human ecology that is our education system. The assessment strategies cited here are definitely steps in the right direction; but there is much yet to be accomplished—miles to go before we sleep. In the section that follows, we examine some of the shortcomings of current applications of behavioral analysis and provide some suggestions for change.

FUTURE DIRECTIONS FOR BEHAVIOR ANALYSIS

In the early 1800s a young naturalist journeyed to South America to observe and document the natural history of the area. As he rode across the Argentine pampas, this keen observer was troubled. He could not put his finger on anything specific that was out of the ordinary, but still he felt something was wrong with the countryside. Being an avid hunter, he soon realized that what was wrong was rabbits. The pampas, with its lush grasses, bushes in which to hide, and dirt in which to dig, did not have a single rabbit. The young naturalist wondered why an apparently perfect environment for rabbits had none. A strange long-legged, long-eared animal resembling a guinea pig lived in the pampas and appeared to fulfill many of the same functions as the rabbit, but clearly was not a rabbit. This minor incident may have been the catalyst that sparked young Charles Darwin's interest in what would later be known as evolution (Wallace, King, & Sanders, 1981).

A parallel can be drawn between the Argentine pampas of the 1800s and behavioral psychology of today. As we assess the current position of behavioral psychology in education, there seems to be something lacking—something that is troubling to practitioner and scientist alike. That is, everything seems to be in place (and to have been in place for some time) for the emergence of a behaviorally based technology within education. The relationship between the environment and behavior is clear, assessment and treatment techniques have been developed, but still the technology moves only slowly into the school system. Just as Darwin noticed that rabbits were missing from the pampas, so we suggest that there are some "rabbits" missing from the behavioral landscape. What are these "rabbits" of behavioral psychology, and how does their absence influence the future of behavioral psychology in education?

Rabbits and Other Varmints

There are a number of features—"rabbits and other varmints"—missing from the countryside of behavioral psychology. Three will be addressed in this chapter: theory, humans as biological organisms, and individual behavior existing within a larger ecosystem.

Theory

The creation of a theory is a complex process that begins with the scientific method. Wallace, King, and Sanders (1981) contend that the scientific process begins and ends with observations and facts about the real world. It is not well documented exactly what the intervening behaviors between the beginning and ending observations are, but it is believed that they may simply be a process of considering the phenomenon and asking why it exists—what its functional purpose is. The initial stages of the scientific process give rise to speculations that are untestable in nature. Speculation, in turn, provides fuel for the generation of hypotheses or predictions that can potentially be supported, typically through experimentation. Experiments can be conducted in a laboratory or in a naturalistic setting such as a classroom. Hypotheses can also be tested without experimentation. The researcher might make a prediction that can be tested by reviewing existing records. The important point is that proposals are made in ways that can be supported or rejected through some systematic means.

Observation of facts, speculation, hypothesis generation, and subsequent experimentation are all important components of science, but they are not science, nor do they naturally result in the composition of a theory. What the scientific method does is provide a vehicle for the identification of scientific mechanisms. Mechanisms can be defined as the means by which a particular phenomenon is produced or an objective accomplished. Mechanisms do not explain *why* the phenomenon occurred, but *how* it occurred. An example is the principle of reinforcement. Much research exists that supports the effectiveness of reinforcement in increasing the probability of a future behavioral occurrence, but the research does not indicate *why* reinforcement works. A behavior recurs because it is reinforced in the environment, and reinforcement increases the likelihood that a behavior will recur. The limitation of operant conditioning is that it explains *how* particular principles function, but not *why* they function. The various components of operant conditioning constitute mechanisms, rather than fulfilling the qualifications necessary for a theory.

A theory is composed of a coherent group of general principles that explain a class of phenomena. A theory provides a synthesis of the mechanisms of a known body of facts. The behavioral psychology literature abounds with research addressing the "hows," or the mechanisms, of operant conditioning, but little is postulated about the "whys" of its effectiveness or the systematic synthesis of the independent mechanisms. Many behaviorists would say that to focus on the "whys" is unproductive and leads the field of study to untestable speculation; however, organizing the existing research information into a theory may have some value. Such theorizing may help us better understand how to go about influencing the educational process, in terms of both educational programs and educational process.

It is not accidental that the experimental analysis of human behavior is a discipline without a theory. It was Skinner's intent that behavioral science be built in an inductive manner rather than a deductive manner (Kratochwill & Bijou, 1987). Skinner believed that research generated from a faulty theory would yield little understanding of an organism's behavior. Therefore, he and many other behaviorists have spent their lives building a massive data base of discrete, well-designed experiments examining the functional relationship between behavior and environmental events.

The inductive approach to constructing a scientific theory about behavior has not been without its drawbacks, especially when taken from the laboratory to an applied setting such as a classroom. Kratochwill and Bijou (1987) point out that behavioral analysis has come under fire as being simplistic and improperly implemented. We suspect that some of the misunderstanding that exists is in part due to the large number of behavioral mechanisms or techniques that exist without a uniform framework or contextual organization. Further, we believe that the preponderance of techniques, in the absence of an understanding of the complexity of a functional analytic approach, leads many to view behavioral psychology as a simplistic technology, of value only when specific techniques are needed to solve discrete problems. The value of functional analysis in understanding all human interaction and behavior is simply not apparent.

The future of behavioral analysis must include a synthesizing of existing research data. It is necessary not so much to explain *why* operant conditioning is effective—for that may ultimately be answered through anthropological or sociobiological studies—but, rather, to provide a uniform and consistent framework from which to operate. In addition to providing an operational context, a systematic examination of who we are and where we've been may also provide information on how we can facilitate the growth of behavioral science. Nowhere is the need greater for such an understanding than in school systems.

Biological Organism

Another "rabbit" that is absent (or at least hiding) from the behavioral psychology countryside is the concept that humans are biological organisms derived from an evolutionary process. The topography of behaviors, like that of physical features, is subject to laws of natural selection. Those behaviors that increase the likelihood of survival will be selected for and passed on to subsequent generations, and those that are not adaptive to the environment will die out.

Skinner (1984) maintains that humans "behave in a given way both because we are members of a given species and because we live in a world in which certain contingencies of reinforcement prevail" (p. 220). In essence, there exist two types of behavioral development, that which is a result of phylogenic evolution (occurring over thousands of years) and that which can be attributed to ontogenic development (occurring within an organism's lifetime).

The phylogenic process that has occurred through natural selection has resulted in the human organism being more susceptible to certain stimuli associated with survival, while responding in a neutral manner or not responding at all to noncritical stimuli. Although we are not aware of any empirical evidence to support the contention advanced here, one example of this phylogenic process may be a mother's response to a crying infant. The mother responds to the child by holding or feeding it, resulting in the reduction of the infant's crying; the response increases the probability of the child's survival. In addition, this interaction serves as the first form of communication between mother and child. These innate (admittedly presumed) traces from our past may play a major role in the likelihood of success or failure of behavioral interventions, and may also serve as possible confounding variables in behavioral research.

Let us consider the importance of assessing the role of phylogenic evolution when planning a behavioral intervention. To continue the crying infant scenario, after the birth of a child to one of the authors (K. M. B.), the infant was awakening a number of times during the night. When she responded to the child, she found that the child was not hungry, wet, or ill, but simply wanted to play. The author was not getting enough sleep and was becoming increasingly impatient with the nighttime antics of her infant. One intervention that immediately came to mind was that of ignoring the child's nighttime cries, since to respond to the cries would reinforce the behavior and thus increase the probability of its future occurrence; however, she found this intervention very difficult to implement. When discussing the issue with her colleagues, she found them divided into two camps, male and female. The male colleagues with children indicated that they experienced little difficulty in allowing their infants to cry, while female colleagues with children found it extremely hard to ignore the cries of their infants. Although not meant to represent a scientific study, when viewed in an evolutionary sense, the probability of success of the "ignoring" intervention may be much lower for mothers of infants than for fathers. Historically, the mother's response has increased the likelihood of the species' survival and contributed to the genetic propensity of such behaviors. This phylogenic influence does not mean that any intervention should be abandoned, but simply that it should be designed in such a manner as to capitalize on tendencies of the organism to be reinforced (i.e., susceptibility to reinforcement) by certain behaviors rather than to combat them with interventions that fly in the face of the history of the species. For example, an alternative intervention to ignoring the crying of an infant may be to have the mother out of earshot of the cries and let the father remain to ensure the child's safety.

Phylogenic evolution, in essence, provides the framework for ontogenic conditioning. Although Skinner (1987) attributes the strengthening effect of an operant reinforcer to its survival value in the species, he also contends that processes exist that subject individuals of the species to specific environmental contingencies. Moreover, Skinner (1984) maintains that "In the human species, operant conditioning has very largely replaced natural selection. A long infancy gives the ontogenic process greater scope, and its role in adapting to very unstable environments is a great advantage" (p. 220). This behavioral plasticity allows individuals to survive extreme social stresses in a manner that at least superficially appears to be maladaptive and counterproductive to the survival of the species as a whole. However, the complexity of the human organism and the ecosystems within which humans live make it difficult to discern which behaviors are a result of cultural adaptation and which represents phylogenic traces (Wilson, 1975).

The importance of understanding human behavior in a biological context with regard to education may simply be that we must be aware that human behavior exists for a reason, and that, as with other oganisms, human behavior exists as a result of its functional value. The functional value may be related to either species or individual survival. When analyzing behavior, we must ask, "What functional value is the current behavior to the individual, and how do we go about designing an environment that produces behavior consistent with our current goals and objectives for that individual?"

Human Ecosystem

The final "rabbit" missing from the behavioral countryside discussed in this chapter is that of the human ecosystem. Unfortunately, the reductionistic methodology that has been so productive in our understanding of operant-conditioning principles does not transfer well to analysis of "multiple contemporaneous stimuli" (Russo & Budd, 1987). Although the environment plays a paramount role in behavioral technology, behavioral interventions have traditionally been individually focused and have downplayed possible interaction effects or unanticipated effects within the individual's ecosystem.

The human ecosystem, like any life support ecology, can be defined in the same way as all external factors, both living and nonliving, that affect the target organism (Wallace, King, & Sanders, 1981). The study of human ecosystems examines the interaction between organisms and their environments, with the emphasis on interaction.

Edwin Willems (1974, 1977) outlined the ecological gap in behavioral technology that resulted in a conference examining the ecological perspectives in behavior analysis. After more than a decade, however, behavioral science has remained slow to respond to Willem's prod.

Willems (1977) outlined seven central themes that underlie a behavioral-ecological view:

1. Human behavior must be conceptualized and studied at levels of complexity that are quite atypical in behavioral science.
2. The complexity lies in systems of relationships that link person, behavior, social environment, and physical environment.
3. Such systems cannot be understood piecemeal.
4. Such behavior–environment systems have important properties that change, unfold, and become clear only over long periods of time.

5. Tampering with any part of such a system will probably affect the other parts and alter the whole.

6. We must develop an ecological grasp of the many ways in which
   a) simple intrusions can produce unintended effects,
   b) indirect harm may follow from narrowly defined good, and
   c) long-term harm may follow from short-term good.

7. The focal challenge is to achieve enough understanding of such systems so that the effect of interventions and planned changes can be anticipated in comprehensive fashion. (Willems, 1977, pp. 42–43)

Although some of Willems's central themes imply (incorrectly) that behavioral scientists have been negligent in recognizing the complexity of human behavior and haphazardly "tampering" with environmental systems, he does make some very important points. Operant-conditioning principles must be examined beyond the singular focus of main effects to interactional analysis. The complexity of such a task may, in part, be responsible for the failure of scientists to respond in any systematic fashion to the analysis of ecological interactions (Risley, 1977). It is not easy to identify response covariations consistently, much less understand their ramifications within the environment. The problems that arise from analyzing behaviors within an ecological context pose a challenge to the new generation of behaviorists. A shift in behavioral analysis, akin to the paradigm shift that occurred in physics (from Newtonian to Einsteinian) (Kuhn, 1970), may be necessary to accommodate an ecobehavioral perspective. The principles of operant conditioning will have to be evaluated through novel means in order to test their applicability within human ecosystems.

Advanced technology is likely to aid in the complex task of identifying significant variance within the environment. Currently, wildlife ecologists have compiled data bases and developed programs that allow them to analyze the effects of changes within the environment. For example, via a computer terminal, the wildlife ecologist can ascertain the effects that extinction of a particular predator would have on an ecosystem. Concomitantly, human behavioral ecologists could collect a myriad of data concerning biological, environmental, and behavioral factors and conduct experimental manipulations that would otherwise be impossible. These studies, though extremely enlightening, may never provide definitive predictions of human behavior within various ecosystems. Predictions of behavioral change throughout the environment would be based on probabilities; as more precise, discrete data accumulate within the data base, however, the predictions would become more reliable.

It seems reasonable to suggest that the large number of inductively oriented research studies that have been done in the area of human behavior analysis provide for the beginnings of such data bases. It should be possible for those data to be compiled systematically to determine whether they can be utilized effectively to make ecobehavioral predictions. Work of this type has already begun in classrooms (Stanley & Greenwood, 1981) and with families (Wahler & Dumas, 1984). Future applications await the combined efforts of skilled practitioners and behavioral scientists.

Summary

Behaviorism has historically provided a systematic, inductive means for analyzing behavior that has advanced an emerging science in immeasurable ways. This adherence to scientific rigor, however, has not been without tradeoffs. Perusal of major behavioral journals over the past few years indicates that we have reached a point of stagnation in our field, with numerous replications and minor variations yielding limited new information. The time has come to move forward, using the vast stores of existing information as a firm platform to continue to analyze human behavior within the environment. As stated earlier, this move will require novel ways of thinking about the effects of operants, new data collection techniques, and new means of analyzing those data. Such a paradigm shift seems necessary now, however, if we are to continue to unravel the complex issue of the human organism within its environment.

So, what do rabbits have to do with future directions in behavioral applications in education, and what is that "long-legged, long-eared, strange guinea pig–type animal" that is serving the function of the rabbit? We believe that the "missing rabbits" cited in this section must be recognized and brought out into the open if behavioral psychology has any hope of maximizing its impact on education and schools. Examination of the "rabbits" discussed in this chapter will help behavioral scientists chart a course for the future of psychology. Furthermore, we suggest that there *is* an "animal" that serves in the place of a behavioral psychology in education, and that this animal impedes the progress of behavioral applications in education, with little concomitant value of its own.

Now, what is that long-legged, long-eared, guinea pig–type animal that is functioning as a rabbit in the psychological countryside? That is, what has evolved in the place of behavioral psychology applications in education, and what currently serves the organizing role that we suggest needs to filled by behavioral psychology? We are suggesting that the guinea pig–type animal of the psychological countryside is cognitive psychology. Cognitive psychology serves primarily as untestable speculation. Hypothetical concepts (e.g., schemata) and models (e.g., information processing) are developed, tests are contrived to examine the hypothetical concepts and models, and finally we start believing that what is being examined actually exists. The danger of psychology following this "internal" line of research lies in the fact that most internal questions can be answered only by neurophysiological means, rather than psychological techniques. Wilson (1975) predicts that

> Cognition will be translated into circuitry. Learning and creativeness will be defined as the alteration of specific portions of the cognitive machinery regulated

by input from the emotive centers. Having cannibalized psychology, the new neurobiology will yield an enduring set of first principles for sociology. (p. 575)

Skinner (1987) has made similar points in regard to both the cognitive psychology–neuropsychology connection and the negative influence of cognitive psychology on our understanding of human behavior.

Perhaps we would feel differently if there were evidence that cognitive psychology had contributed much of merit to educational processes or educational technology. In the midst of the current cognitive revolution within educational psychology, the procedures and techniques that have been developed and validated for improving schools and schooling have stemmed largely from a behavioral perspective. The evidence cited in this chapter indicates that behavioral psychology has made significant, valid, and clearly demonstrable contributions to our understanding of how to influence learning. Where are the contributions of cognitive psychology?

The study of cognitive processes may indeed be an important function of a scientific process; it seems, however, that the science it will serve is not psychology, but neuropsychology. To avoid future cannibalization, and in order to contribute objective information to the understanding of human organisms, psychology must go about examining behavior and the impact of the environment on the organism. Throughout this book, different authors discuss the impact of cognitive behavioral psychology on education. Much has been accomplished in this area during the past decade. The evidence is clear, however, that the progress has flowed from a focus on the manner in which environmental events (e.g., modeling and coaching) influence intraverbal and overt behavior, and not as a result of studying cognitive processing (e.g., metacognition, simultaneous or successive processing) in the absence of environmental influence or ecologically valid behavior.

FINAL CONSIDERATIONS

The behavioral tradition in the schools has clearly been a productive one. Much, however, remains to be accomplished. We have not, for example, been very successful in influencing teacher education. A perusal of current texts used in undergraduate educational psychology courses reveals a definite bias toward cognitive psychology, despite the meager contributions that traditional cognitive approaches have made to education. As outlined previously, we believe that the behavioral approach has much to offer to an ecological model of human behavior, even if such a synthesis has not proved to be widely understood to date.

In a piece written two decades ago, Bijou (1970) stated that:

a small but rapidly growing group of psychologists can now offer educators (1) a set of concepts and principles derived entirely from the experimental analysis of behavior, (2) a methodology for the practical application of these concepts and principles, (3) a research method that deals with changes in individual behavior, and (4) a philosophy of science that says, "Look carefully to the relationships between observable events and their changes." (p. 70)

In the years since the appearance of this article, the small band of psychologists referred to has grown slowly, but inexorably. Furthermore, we have come to understand that individual behavior exists in a broader context than just that defined by the individual's personal learning history. Further experimental analysis of the ecosystem in which an individual exists, and of the interplay between individual behavior and the ecology, must be undertaken if we are to expand our ability to influence individual children, educational programs, school systems, and public policy. The time for ecobehavioral analysis is at hand.

ACKNOWLEDGMENT

We gratefully acknowledge the contributions of all our UNL friends who took the time to comment on earlier versions of this chapter, including Scott Brase, Jane Close Conoley, Terry Gutkin, Dave Moshman, and Royce Ronning. A special thank you is offered to Francis E. Lentz of the University of Cincinnati for his thoughtful critique of our work.

REFERENCES

Becker, W. C., & Carnine, D. W. (1980). Direct instruction: An effective approach to educational intervention with the disadvantaged and low performers. In B. B. Lahey & A. E. Kazdin (Eds.), *Advances in clinical child psychology* (Vol. 3, pp. 429–473). New York: Plenum Press.

Bergan, J. R. (1977). Behavioral consultation. Columbus, OH: Charles Merrill.

Bergan, J. R., & Tombari, M. L. (1976). Consultant skill and efficiency and the implementation and outcomes of consultation. *Journal of School Psychology, 14*, 3–14.

Bijou, S. W. (1970). What psychology has to offer education—now. *Journal of Applied Behavior Analysis, 3*, 65–71.

Blackham, G. J., & Silberman, A. (1980). *Modification of child and adolescent behavior* (3rd ed.). Belmont, CA: Wadsworth.

Boring, E. G. (1950). *A history of experimental psychology* (2nd ed.). New York: Appleton-Century-Crofts.

Browder & D'Huyetters (1988). An evaluation of transfer of stimulus control and of comprehension in sight word reading for children with mental retardation and emotional disturbance. *School Psychology Review, 17*, 331–342.

Carver, R. P. (1974). Two dimensions of tests: Psychometric and edumetric. *American Psychologist, 29*, 512–518.

Deno, S. L. (1985). Curriculum-based assessment: The emerging alternative. *Exceptional Children, 52*, 219–232.

Deno, S. L., Marston, D., & Mirken, P. (1982). Valid measurement procedures for continuous evaluation of written expression. *Exceptional Children, 48,* 368–371.

Deno, S. L., Mirken, P. K., Lowery, L., & Kuehnle, K. (1980). *Relationships among simple measures of spelling and performance on standardized achievement tests.* Research Report No. 21. Minneapolis: University of Minnesota, Institute for Research on Learning Disabilities. ERIC Document Reproduction Service No. ED 197 508.

Fuchs, L. S., & Fuchs, D. (Eds.). (1986). Linking assessment to intervention [miniseries]. *School Psychology Review, 15* (Whole No. 3).

Galagan, J. E. (1985). Psychoeducational testing: Turn out the lights, the party's over. *Exceptional Children, 52,* 288–299.

Gickling, E. E., & Thompson, V. P. (1985). A personal view of curriculum-based assessment. *Exceptional Children, 52,* 205–218.

Gutkin, T. B., & Curtis, M. J. (1982). School-based consultation: Theory and techniques. In C. R. Reynolds & T. B. Gutkin (Eds.), *The handbook of school psychology* (pp. 796–828). New York: Wiley.

Hall, R. V., Lund, D., & Jackson, D. (1968). Effects of teacher attention on study behavior. *Journal of Applied Behavior Analysis, 4,* 1–12.

Haynes, S. N. (1978). *Principles of behavioral assessment.* New York: Gardner Press.

Hilgard, E. R. (1987). *Psychology in America: A historical survey.* San Diego, CA: Harcourt Brace Jovanovich.

Kazdin, A. E. (1978). *History of behavior modification: Experimental foundations of contemporary research.* Baltimore, MD: University Park Press.

Keller, F. S. (1968). Goodbye teacher . . . *Journal of Applied Behavior Analysis, 1,* 79–89.

Kendler, H. H. (1987). *Historical foundations of modern psychology.* Philadelphia: Temple University Press.

Kircher, A. S., Pear, J. J., & Martin, G. L. (1971). Shock as punishment in a picture naming task with retarded children. *Journal of Applied Behavior Analysis, 4,* 227–233.

Kratochwill, T. R. (1982). Advances in behavioral assessment. In C. R. Reynolds & T. B. Gutkin (Eds.), *The handbook of school psychology* (pp. 314–350). New York: Wiley.

Kratochwill, T. R., & Bergan, J. R. (1978). Evaluating programs in applied settings through behavioral consultation. *Journal of School Psychology, 16,* 375–378.

Kratochwill, T. R., & Bijou, S. W. (1987). The impact of behaviorism on educational psychology. In J. A. Glover & R. R. Ronning (Eds.), *A history of educational psychology* (pp. 151–187). New York: Plenum Press.

Kuhn, T. S. (1970). *The structure of scientific revolutions* (2nd ed.). Chicago: University of Chicago Press.

La Mettrie, J. de (1960/1748). *L'homme machine: A study in the origins of an idea.* Princeton, NJ: Princeton University Press.

Lentz, F. E., & Shapiro, E. S. (1986). Functional assessment of the academic environment. *School Psychology Review, 15,* 346–357.

Lovitt, T. C., & Curtiss, K. A. (1968). Effects of manipulating an antecedent event on mathematics response rate. *Journal of Applied Behavior Analysis, 1,* 329–333.

Madsen, C. H., Jr., Becker, W. C., & Thomas, D. R. (1968). Rules, praise and ignoring: Elements of elementary classroom control. *Journal of Applied Behavior Analysis, 1,* 139–150.

Medway, F. J. (1979). How effective is school consultation research? *Journal of School Psychology, 17,* 275–282.

Morgan, C. L. (1894). *Introduction to comparative psychology*. London: W. Scott Ltd.

Risley, T. R. (1977). The ecology of applied behavior analysis. In A. Rogers-Warren & S. F. Warren (Eds.), *Ecological perspectives in behavior analysis* (pp. 149–163). Baltimore, MD: University Park Press.

Risley, T. R., & Reynolds, N. J. (1970). Emphasis as a prompt for verbal imitation. *Journal of Applied Behavior Analysis, 3*, 185–190.

Russo, D. C., & Budd, K. S. (1987). Limitations of operant practice in the study of disease. *Behavior Modification, 11*, 264–285.

Sachs, D. A. (1973). The efficacy of time-out procedures in a variety of behavior problems. *Journal of Behavior Therapy and Experimental Psychiatry, 4*, 237–242.

Saudargas, R., & Lentz, F. (1982). *State–event classroom observation system*. Knoxville: University of Tennessee.

Shapiro, E. S. (1987). *Behavioral assessment in school psychology*. Hillsdale, NJ: Lawrence Erlbaum.

Skinner, B. F. (1938). *The behavior of organisms: An experimental analysis*. New York: Appleton-Century.

Skinner, B. F. (1953). *Science and human behavior*. New York: Macmillan.

Skinner, B. F. (1954). The science of learning and the art of teaching. *Harvard Educational Review, 24*, 86–97.

Skinner, B. F. (1984). The evolution of behavior. *Journal of the Experimental Analysis of Behavior, 41*, 217–221.

Skinner, B. F. (1987). Whatever happened to psychology as the science of behavior? *American Psychologist, 42*, 780–786.

Stanley, S. O., & Greenwood, C. R. (1981). *CISSAR: Code for Instructional Structure and Student Academic Response*. Kansas City: Juniper Gardens Children's Project, Bureau of Child Research, University of Kansas.

Thorndike, E. L. (1898). *Animal intelligence: An experimental study of the associative processes in animals*. Psychological Monographs, Vol. 2, No. 8.

Van Houten, R. V., & Sullivan, K. (1975). Effects of an audio cueing system on the rate of teacher praise. *Journal of Applied Behavior Analysis, 8*, 197–201.

Wahler, R. E., & Dumas, J. E. (1984). Changing the observational coding styles of insular and noninsular mothers: A step towards maintenance of parent training effects. In R. F. Dangel & R. A. Polster (Eds.), *Parent training: Foundations of research and practice* (pp. 379–416). New York: Guilford Press.

Wallace, R. A., King, J. L., & Sanders, G. P. (1981). *Biology: The science of life*. Glenview, IL: Scott, Foresman.

Watson, J. B. (1913). Psychology as the behaviorist views it. *Psychological Review, 20*, 158–177.

Willems, E. P. (1974). Behavioral technology and behavioral ecology. *Journal of Applied Behavior Analysis, 7*, 151–165.

Willems, E. P. (1977). Steps toward an ecobehavioral technology. In A. Rogers-Warren & S. F. Warren (Eds.), *Ecological perspectives in behavior analysis* (pp. 39–61). Baltimore, MD: University Park Press.

Wilson, E. O. (1975). *Sociobiology: The new synthesis*. Cambridge, MA: Belknap Press.

Ysseldyke, J. E., & Christenson, S. L. (1987). *The instructional environment scale*. Austin, TX: PRO-ED.

3
THE COGNITIVE TRADITION IN SCHOOLS

A. JERRY BENSON
JACK H. PRESBURY
James Madison University

Writing in 1966, William Kessen suggested that the term "cognition" had become nearly obsolete. "You may go searching, if you like, in textbooks of psychology, and you will find that the place in the index between 'cochlea' and 'cold spots', or between 'coefficient of correlation' and 'coition' is usually unmarked by 'cognition'" (p. 55). Furthermore, he stated that even to employ the term "cognition" in psychological company of that day was to create the uneasy feeling of fear and daring one felt when first speaking the word "damn" in front of Mother. Such was the status of cognitive psychology in the mid-1960s after the nearly 50-year reign of behaviorism. But, like the sperm whale, the snail darter, and the bald eagle, cognition as an area of study in psychology has made a robust recovery from near extinction. Only the most radical behaviorist would suggest that the study of how the mind works (cognition) is not a legitimate focus for psychologists. The old debate as to whether psychology is a science of mind or a science of behavior turned out to be a category mistake. Most psychologists would agree that it is both.

Kessen (1966), Neisser (1967), and others signaled the renewed emphasis on the examination of one of our most ancient psychological and educational puzzles—knowledge. Mahoney (1977) noted that "very few clinical cases were as simple or as straightforward as those traditionally portrayed by the behavioral journals . . . the awesome and intimate complexities of real-life human problems are often humbling reminders of our relative ignorance . . ." (p. 6). Psychologists were beginning to wonder whether they were as free of entanglements with philosophical presuppositions as the behaviorist movement had led them to believe. The zeitgeist in the late 1960s and early 1970s was one of the behaviorists and cognitive psychologists cautiously easing into the same theoretical bed, that is, the cognitive-learning trend (Mahoney, 1977).

Cognitive psychology was never completely absent from psychology or education, even during the reign of behaviorism. Reviewing the period of time from Watson's 1913 article outlining the behaviorist's principles to the renewal of emphasis on cognition, Bruner (1985) speculated that the reemphasis on cognitive psychology was aided by two primary sociocultural factors. First, the development of the computer freed us from the radical behavioral notions, such as the "black box" representations, and placed an emphasis on the mind in mental activities. As had happened so many times before, our technological advancements had provided an impetus and structuring metaphor for theoretical reconceptualization. Second, the postindustrial revolution began to place a premium on the skills of the generalist and the problem solver.

A comprehensive and exhaustive review of cognitive psychology goes beyond the limitations and purpose of this chapter. The chapter will, however, review some of the history and major underpinnings of cognitive psychology so that the reader may have some perspective on how the cognitive tradition relates to the behavioral tradition presented in the preceding chapter and the cognitive-behavioral framework of the following chapter. This chapter initially provides a brief overview of where cognitive psychology has been in the general field of psychology and discusses some of the important issues that cognitive psychology addresses but that are absent from the radical behavioral tradition. Second, the cognitive tradition in education will be reflected through a discussion of the various movements in American education and selected aspects of educational practice. The chapter concludes with a synthesis of the cognitive tradition to aid the practitioner in formulating an overall framework for making decisions as to when to employ a strategem or intervention. It is the purpose of this presentation to provide a framework to aid the reader in organizing the practices reviewed later in this text with a sense of direction, purpose, and coherence.

THE COGNITIVE TRADITION IN PSYCHOLOGY

The saga of the estrangement of the cognitive and behavioral approaches in psychology—and their eventual reconciliation—is an interesting story, beginning with the origins of psychology itself. The scientific study of human thought and behavior is relatively new, having its beginnings in the second half of the nineteenth century (Hayes, 1978). Before 1850, the study of human cognition was the province of philosophers, and there was little agreement as to how thought and behavior were related or how they could be controlled and predicted. The method of these philosophers had become known as "armchair speculation." This pejorative term suggests that the conclusions of armchair speculators would be *erroneous* because their ideas were not tied to a method of verification in the real world and *useless* because they had no utility in concrete, everyday experience. Science, a method of inquiry originating during the Enlightenment, was the way in which "natural" philosophers went about studying the physical universe. This method consisted of carefully observing what could be experienced concretely and then drawing general conclusions (called "facts") from these observations (Ray & Ravizza, 1985). Many psychologists believed that if they hoped to be as successful as the physicists and biologists had been, the methods of science would have to be adopted, and that only carefully conducted experiments could begin to reveal the mysteries of the mind.

In Europe, the study of mental mechanisms remained the focus of psychology. Wilhelm Wundt, in 1879, established the first laboratory for studying the facts of human experience under controlled conditions (Watson, 1968). He combined these facts with the laws of "associationism," a theory that consisted of three basic ideas: atomism, connectionism, and empiricism. "Atomism" is the belief that everything consists of basic elements and that the best way to understand anything is to know the parts or elements from which it is constructed. "Connectionism" is the theory that all events or elements are connected to one another by bonds of associations. In other words, certain happenings or things tend to occur together, and to know their connections is to begin to develop principles regarding such occurrences. Finally, "empiricism" is the doctrine that everything we know is learned through personal experience with the world (Hayes, 1978). The reader will no doubt recognize that the laws of associationism have come to be regarded as fundamental to the science of psychology.

The difference between Wundt's science of psychology and the American variety, later to be known as behaviorism, was that Wundt believed the proper subject matter to be studied was immediate conscious experience rather than merely behavior (Hayes, 1978). The method employed in Wundt's laboratory was systematic introspection. Subjects in controlled conditions reported their experience, which would be broken down into its elements—sensations, images, feelings, and acts of will. Through this process, Wundt hoped to generate laws of perception and association that would eventually explain the complex experiences of judgment, belief, illusion, problem solving, and creativity. This method became known as "introspectionism" and was popular from about 1875 to 1910.

In 1913, John Watson, who coined the label "behaviorism" which was to identify his way of doing science in psychology, published his classic article, "Psychology as the Behaviorist Views It." In the article, Watson stated that psychology was a natural science and that "introspection forms no essential part of its methods" (p. 158). Introspection was criticized as "mentalism," an unreliable and unscientific vestige of a superstitious past. The subject matter of psychology became behavior rather than mind, and it became unfashionable in the United States to speak as a scientist of such things as cognition and consciousness. Not until the later 1960s (some say with the publication of Neisser's *Cognitive Psychology* in 1967) was it generally acceptable once again to turn our attention to the study of mental events and processes. Thus was born the new era of cognitive psychology. The difference was to be that, unlike introspectionism, which employed subjective methods such as self-report, cognitive psychology would use objective methods; that is, mental events would be inferred from observed behavior (Martindale, 1981).

Although most people place the emergence of cognitive psychology in the 1960s, many scholars who studied cognitive processes were at work long before

that time attempting to understand memory, perception, cognitive development, concept formation, and the like. The popularity of behaviorism in the
United States never influenced the Europeans, who favored a tradition that
Kessen (1966) called *verstehen*. Loosely translated, the word means
understanding and represents a point of view that retained an emphasis on the
human mind. In the early 1930s people in remote areas of the Soviet Union
were studied by Luria (1966) and Vygotsky (1962) regarding their ability to
generalize and abstract information, their style of deduction and inference, and
their ability to problem-solve and self-analyze. Werner (1948) conducted a
comparative analysis of the thought processes of children, primitive peoples,
and schizophrenics. Psychoanalysis and *Dasein*analysis continued to explore
the thought patterns involved in mental illness.

Even in the United States, the "New Look" psychologists (Bruner & Postman,
1949; McGinnes, 1949) at Harvard University were interested in unconscious
inference in the act of perception and were publishing articles on the subject 20
years before the "birth" of cognitive psychology. The testing movement in the
United States, spawned about the time of World War I, enjoyed increasing
popularity from that time and implied much about the workings of the mind as
related to general intelligence, personality styles, vocational interest, and achievement. All these movements or areas of study have influenced psychology and
education in both dramatic and subtle ways. They were the foundation for the
cognitive revolution, and the insights achieved by these pioneers are apparent in
our current school curriculum and educational practices.

With the reemergence of "mind" as a legitimate subject matter of psychology, it became necessary to reexamine some areas of scholarly debate that had
remained dormant during the era of behaviorism. First, the metaphysical
question of reality became much more complicated with the cognitive revolution. Specifically, a theory that deals with a participating consciousness—or
mind—must take a position as to how much "reality" a mind is capable of
apprehending and how much of what is considered to be real is constructed by
the mind itself. The second issue is one of individual differences, or style. Do
individuals differ in the ways they experience and know things and do preferences for certain ways of knowing ("traynes" of thought) exist? Finally, we
must ask whether a technology of mind, equal or superior to the technology of
behavior that now exists, can be developed. Do mental events consist of
elements that can be analyzed and combined into a predictable and controllable pattern—that is, artificial intelligence? The next three sections—on the
question of reality, on "traynes" (trains) of thought, and on the information-
processing approach, respectively—will discuss these issues.

The Question of Reality

The relationship between reality and human representation of reality is a
crucial point in our understanding of the process of knowing. The "science" of
psychology, whether of mind or of behavior, adopted the same posture relative

to the nature of reality as did the physical scientists. This position, simply stated, is that reality exists—it is out there—and we perceive it by making copies of it. According to this position, our experiences are veridical images of an independently existing external reality (Martindale, 1981). It is likely that if the reader is an American, this belief about reality does not seem very controversial. American psychology has generally adopted this paradigm of positivism or realism.

There are others, however, who take a different view (Martindale, 1981; Watzlawick, 1984). They suggest there is no reason to believe that the universe is actually organized in the way in which we receive it, which instead may simply be the structure that we impose on it. The philosophical argument, usually attributed to Kant (1963/1781), is difficult to consider. A simple and obvious aspect of our limited ability to perceive reality is illustrated by the following:

> Common sense tells us that our senses are windows on the world that serve to bring us as much information as possible into consciousness. But it turns out that it is more profitable to take just the opposite viewpoint. Our sensory receptors really serve to reduce, filter, and exclude as much data as possible. . . . The electromagnetic spectrum ranges in wavelength from a billionth of a meter up to more than a thousand meters . . . of this spectrum we see only the tiny portion between 400 and 700 billionths of a meter. Our eyes are completely insensitive to everything else. (Martindale, 1981, p. 8)

The fact that we cannot see other phenomena on this spectrum, such as ultraviolet light, infrared radiation, X-rays, and radar, is well known and suggests that our apprehension of reality is limited at best. This argument, however, does not reduce our belief in the existence of reality, but only in our unaided ability to apprehend it.

Another argument regarding the variable nature of reality is that we must learn to see what we see. A dramatic study by Senden (1960) illustrates this point. The study involved people who had been cataract victims from birth and who later had their vision restored by surgery after they had acquired language. Before the operation, their visual world was an amorphous blur, and none of them could distinguish form. After the surgery, with their sight restored, they were given objects of different geometric forms. When asked which one was a triangle, a shape they knew by touch, even the most motivated and intelligent subjects had to search painstakingly for the corners in order to be sure of what they were seeing.

Perhaps the best example of how "reality" needs us to experience it before it comes into existence is what is known as the "phi phenomenon." In 1910 Max Wertheimer was traveling by train from Vienna to the Rhineland on vacation when he was struck by such a compelling insight that he abandoned his vacation plans and left the train at Frankfurt (Watson, 1968). Wertheimer bought a toy stroboscope and took it to his hotel room to verify his hypothesis.

A stroboscope is a device that allows still pictures to be exposed at a constant rate of speed, so that movement is perceived—the same principle as motion pictures. If the pictures are exposed at the correct rate, they "move." What Wertheimer realized is that the pictures do not move, we perceive them as moving. If there is too long a time between exposures, the pictures do not move. When the exposure time is precisely in sync with our perceptual apparatus, the pictures flow in a smooth manner so as to be indistinguishable from our experience of any other type of movement. In a very strict sense, it could be argued that *we* move the pictures.

With each example cited, it appears that reality becomes more dependent on the perceiver for its existence in the form we know it. The ultimate argument along this line is the philosophy of solipsism. Solipsism, or idealism, is the point of view that suggests that reality, rather than impressing itself on our senses so that we copy it, is a construction of our experience and may have no independent existence at all. In the extreme, this is the old argument: "If a tree fell in the forest, and no one heard it fall, would it make a sound?"

Recently, a point of view known as "constructivism" has been influencing much of the thinking in psychology and has become a competing paradigm to the old ways of thinking about science (Watzlawick, 1984). Constructivism retains the subjective quality of solipsism while suggesting that an independent reality does exist. The constructivist would hold that the cognition–reality relationship is more like a "fit" than a "match" (Watzlawick, 1984). The human organism thus responds primarily to cognitive representations of its environment rather than to that environment per se. Mahoney (1977), in outlining the fundamentals of the cognitive-learning trend, noted that "when there is a discrepancy between a person's cognitions and reality (as externally defined), the former should account for more of his 'experiential variance' (i.e., behaviors, feelings, etc.) . . . phenomenology is a better predictor than external reality . . ." (p. 8).

The cognitive-behavioral approaches acknowledge such cognitive mediation of behavior. Albert Ellis (1962) was the first modern cognitive therapist to address this issue. He did so by resurrecting a statement of Epictetus (born about A.D. 50), who said, "What disturbs men's minds is not events, but their judgment of events" (Thompson & Rudolph, 1983). Thus, as the focus moved from changing behaviors to changing mental representations of events, "it soon became apparent that naive realism (or the doctrine of 'immaculate perception') was functionally untenable in human behavior. An individual responds—not to some *real* environment—but to a *perceived* environment" (Mahoney, 1974, pp. 4, 5; emphasis in original).

Two "Traynes" (Trains) of Thought

The active participation of individuals in the knowing process not only involves one's definition of reality, but also involves how that which is perceived is processed and organized. Long before education and psychology experienced their dalliance with the left-brain/right-brain phenomenon, it had already been clearly articulated by philosophers that people seem to operate in two opposing modes of thought. The philosopher Hobbes, in 1642, wrote that the "trayne" of thoughts, or mental discourse, was of two sorts: "the first is unguided, without Designe, and inconstant . . . as in a dream . . . the second is more constant, as being regulated by some desire, and designe" (quoted in Martindale, 1981, p. 307).

Harry Stack Sullivan (1953) described these two modes as "parataxic" and "syntaxic," the former being a primitive type of thinking and the latter more modern and organized. Joseph Bogen (1969), noted for his reports of the consequences of "split-brain" operations, collected a list of descriptions by 39 authors of two opposing modes of thought, which he attributed to the differences in brain hemisphere processing. Included were such examples as: digital–analogic (Kolb & Whishaw, 1980), secondary process–primary process (Freud, 1900), analytic–holistic (Ornstein, 1972), and successive–simultaneous (Luria, 1966). Some people insist that these two general modes inhere in the brain hemispheres and compete for dominance. Invoking the brain in this argument is an attempt to dignify the notions of philosophers and psychologists who have noted these differences, but such an argument sometimes serves only to confuse the issue. Keeping to the realm of cognitive process, it is more useful to state that there does seem to be a continuum of human thought with positivistic, realistic, taxonomic, organized thinking at one end and holistic, idealistic, associational, less organized thinking at the other.

According to Geschwind (1974), the brain develops simultaneously along three dimensions: bottom to top, back to front, and side to side (right to left). The lower regions of the brain are vital to the automatic functioning of the body and to the establishment of primary affect. The "newer" parts of the brain are responsible for what we commonly refer to as "thinking." The frontal lobes, called by Wilke (1981) "the brain of last resort," seem to have developed the ability to override some of the functioning of the older parts of the brain. We often control our emotions, ignore our hunger, demand ourselves to stay awake, inhibit our desires, and "watch our tongues." We can also alter seemingly independent bodily processes such as blood flow and the secretion of hormones by controlling our mental state.

The fundamental assumption of cognitive-behavioral therapy is that inefficient or dysfunctional thinking, governed by emotion or fuzziness, can be brought under control (Mahoney, 1974; Meichenbaum, 1977). The metaphor is one of the newest parts of the brain controlling the lower, older regions through methods such as self-monitoring, positive self-talk, metastrategies, and cognitive restructuring. We might say that, through rehearsal, the new program becomes automatic and "sinks" into the lower regions of the brain, where it takes the place of a formerly dysfunctional program. Since the brain is a system in which all parts participate, it is not useful to separate it into localized areas of cognitive functioning. Likewise, it is not productive to consider scientific thought as the only truly cognitive mode. Emotion also is a way of cognizing, albeit more primitive and amorphous (Minsky, 1985). Since the human body, the emotions, and the more recent modes of thinking all work together as a system, it may be more useful to consider that this is all cognition.

The Information-Processing Approach

Martindale (1981) pointed out that the models psychologists develop to think about how the mind works are often a reflection of current technology. Today, nothing fascinates us more than the computer and its ability to perform complex tasks with incredible speed and accuracy. The circuitry of a digital computer is based on a very simple principle: binary operation. Each logic gate is either on or off, one or zero. Each neuron in the human brain works the same way. If its energy level reaches a certain threshold, it will "fire" and transmit its information to adjacent neurons; if not, it is quiescent. Since the digital computer and the human nervous system work on the same principle in processing information, it was predictable that a branch of computer science would develop bearing the label "artificial intelligence" and that cognitive psychology would develop a model known as "information-processing" theory using the computer as its metaphor.

The input into the computer through keyboard or disk drive is seen as analogous to human sensory inputs (Thorndike, 1984). These inputs are encoded by the computer as patterns of binary choices. A certain amount of computer input may be held for immediate processing just as the human problem solver has a short-term working memory held in consciousness. For extended storage, large amounts of information may be held on tapes or disks in a way similar to the storage of human long-term memory. The computer has a host of executive programs or strategies, and these are processed by a read-only memory (ROM), which may be seen in humans as an innate potential to learn ways of using learned facts and acquired experiences. Thorndike (1984) points out that the heart of the enterprise in a computer is the central processor. The central processor can translate the input we send it into its own working language, carry out large numbers of routines or simple decisions, and in general run the whole show with faultless speed. The central processor is as mysterious to a computer novice as intelligence is to everyone.

Thorndike (1984) further distinguishes between executive systems and production systems within the central processor. Production systems are like automatized learned human behavior, which is carried out without much conscious monitoring: "much of human behavior runs off relatively automatically in the form of wired-in reflex responses or of well-learned habits. And practice and feedback serve to reinforce and shape such habitual behavior" (p. 28). In various texts this automatic running of established routines is called "habituation," "automatization," or "executive ignorance." In the parlance of education, this may come about as the result of drill, overlearning, or incidental learning. Two important points are worthy of emphasis when considering the production systems:

1. What might be the subject of deliberate and concentrated learning at one point in time becomes, upon repeated use and practice, more routine and automatic.
2. As Brown (1978) points out, conscious control of one's own activities is *not* essential for all forms of knowing.

Much of the current emphasis in cognitive theory and research, and a central emphasis within cognitive behavioral approaches, is on the executive systems. Thorndike (1984) characterized the executive system by contrasting it with the production systems:

> . . . as situations arise for which established patterns of habitual response do not provide an automatic pattern of action, strategies of search and attack upon the problem are activated. And some overall control directs the form that this search takes. . . . (p. 28)

Brown (1978) emphasizes that in the domain of deliberate learning and problem-solving situations, "conscious executive control of the routines available to the system is the essence of intelligent activity" (p. 79). This executive control has been labeled "metacognition" or "metacognitive process" by various theorists of cognition, for example, Brown (1978), Flavell (1976), and Sternberg (1985). "Metacognition" refers to "one's knowledge concerning one's own cognitive processes and products or anything related to them" (Flavell, 1976, p. 232) and includes the ability to: (1) predict the system's capacity limitations, (2) be aware of its repertoire of routines and their appropriate domain of utility, (3) identify and characterize the problem at hand, (4) relate this to the application of appropriate routines, (5) monitor and supervise the effectiveness of the routines called into service, and (6) evaluate the operations (Brown, 1978). It is here, at the executive system level, that many cognitive theorists see the computer analogy beginning to break down. Although the quest for artificial intelligence reflects computer programs that are claimed to be progressively more capable of "running" the abilities listed here (Rose, 1984), others contend that computers are not conscious of any level of their own functioning—and we presume humans are.

This distinction between production systems (conceptualized as overlearned facts, routines, and habits) and executive systems (whose emphasis on the ability to reflect about one's cognitive processes and performance implies a dimension of cognitive functions on which intentional and automatic processes compete for control) underlies much of the methodology of cognitive behavioral approaches. The reader will recognize the differences in the systems in his or her own experience of driving an automobile without consciousness of doing so until an emergency arises, whereupon consciousness is raised to a metalevel of executive control.

Rourke (1982) further illustrates this distinction of the systems and their working together through an analysis of the initial learning-to-read process. He suggests that initially reading is a novel task requiring the application and relation of an existing descriptive system (i.e., natural language) to the printed text. The next stage involves taking the letter, syllable, word, and word chunk processes and having them routinized. Finally, when faced with the demands of comprehension, the learner must do two things at once: decode and comprehend (analyze, organize, synthesize). Rourke proposes that the most efficient method of comprehending text is to have the initial decoding processes become automatized, thereby "freeing" one to concentrate on and emphasize the unique role the executive system plays in dealing with novelty, informational complexity, and intermodel integration—that is, comprehension.

Another area of cognitive functioning in which the digital computer is not quite like the human being is the distinction between the problem-solving strategies of algorithms and heuristics (Hunt, 1982; Thorndike, 1984). An algorithm can be defined as a rule or as a set of rules or procedures that are fixed. An algorithm is often expressed as a formula that can be uniformly applied to give an exact answer. It is a soundly logical procedure that does not vary. A heuristic, on the other hand, is a strategy based on accumulated experience, which is chosen on the basis of a probable outcome. Computers are very good at algorithms. They never forget a formula, nor do they make errors in its application. People often do.

Humans are rarely logical in their problem solving but are often plausible in their use of heuristic methods (Hunt, 1982). It seems that sometimes humans reason according to their prejudices: ". . . we're not just frequently incompetent, we're also willfully and skillfully illogical. When a piece of deductive reasoning leads to a conclusion we don't like, we often rebut it with irrelevancies and sophistries of which, instead of being ashamed, we act proud" (Hunt, 1982, p. 128). Human reasoning and problem solving are often guided by emotions, distortions, and avoidances.

It would seem, then, that a computer, with its use of exact algorithms for problem solving, would have the edge over humans, and that artificial intelligence represents a significant advance over the natural variety of intelligence. Hofstadter (1985) depicts this notion of advanced problem solving as a pyramid in which the more precise cognitive events are near the top, "and as you move down the hierarchy of lower-level functions, you get increasingly everdumber subroutines, until you bottom out in a myriad of trivial, subcognitive ones" (p. 452). Decision making based on feelings and other forms of illogic would be, in this view, a "dumb" method of thinking. At the heart of the issue seems to be whether precision is superior to "fuzziness" in decision making, and whether cognition is nothing more than computation.

In 1854, when George Boole published his *Laws of Thought*, he was constructing the "mathematics of the human intellect" (Rose, 1984). It was Boole's belief that human thought could be expressed in a series of unambiguous mathematical symbols, and that all logic could be presented in a series of yes-or-no responses. This type of thought was taken to be a superior evolutionary step above the fuzzy, contaminated thought of human sense. Recently, however, studies of human expertise have revealed that it is this aspect of fuzziness or fluidity in common sense that makes the expert adaptable. "Common sense is not an 'area of expertise,' but a general—that is, domain-independent—capacity that has to do with fluidity in representation of concepts, an ability to sift what is important from what is not, an ability to find unanticipated analogical similarities between totally different concepts . . ." (Hofstadter, 1985, p. 640). Cantor and Kihlstrom (1987) believe that it is this fuzziness or fluidity of concept formation that allows humans to function well in social situations. Zadeh, in a 1965 paper entitled "Fuzzy Sets" (cited in Rose, 1984), suggested that zero-or-one cannot include all the possibilities of real situations, and he suggested that the logic of digital computers was inadequate to be called "intelligence." Although computers are "intelligent" in certain domains, such as medical diagnosis, geological consultation, and designing experiments in molecular biology, there is at this time no computer "program that has common sense; no program that learns things that it has not been explicitly taught to learn; no program that can recover gracefully from its own errors. The 'artificial expertise' programs that do exist are rigid, brittle, inflexible" (Hofstadter, 1985, p. 636).

Bruner (1985) cautions that the computer-based model for problem solving is designed for the land of the well defined. Everyday problem solving, on the other hand, does not reduce so easily and readily to rational, algorithmic strategies. Instead, we are faced with poorly defined problems with multiple goals and shifting standards. Bruner points out that the multiple goals may, in fact, be in a nested relationship to each other, and that this relationship shifts with the course of the attempted solution. In other words, we cannot set a target and plot a path because the target changes, as does the path, as we transcend the path.

In summary, the cognitive-behavioral approaches stress executive systems and oftentimes assume an algorithmic approach to problem solving. Many of the cognitive-behavioral approaches to psychotherapy seem to come down in favor of the logic-over-emotion view. This helps one develop expertise or mastery over certain aspects of life. Similarly, the critical-thinking movement current in education is a further expression of this belief in the superiority of algorithmic logic. Although the information-processing model and computer metaphor are useful in planning and implementing some instructional, assessment, and indirect intervention practices in school settings, cognition appears to be much more than computation. Taking Hofstadter's pyramid analogy, to have an apex (i.e., the more precise cognitive processes), one must have a solid base (i.e., the recognition of feelings and automatized subroutines in the decision-making process). And it is the base and the apex *together* that form the pyramid.

THE COGNITIVE TRADITION IN EDUCATION

Many of the issues raised by cognitive psychology can be related to various practices in education. It is helpful to have some general framework for understanding changes in education as they have influenced specific practices. As any student of education can attest, the tradition of education is a dizzying array of "isms," "movements," and "pronouncements." First, there are the "isms": philosophical points of view based on such issues as metaphysics, ethics, aesthetics, epistemology, and the like. These include such viewpoints as idealism, realism, pragmatism, existentialism, progressivism, and humanism. Such philosophical points of view are studied by educators, but often without an emphasis on how they influence the day-to-day educational practice at any point in time.

"Movements" and "pronouncements" in education seem to have varying influence on the schooling process. Some amount to mere dalliances, brief fads that seem to come and go with increasing speed. Some modern examples are open education, critical thinking, perceptual-motor training, and left-brain/ right-brain. Just about the time teachers have developed a partial concept of the movement and have learned its attendant lingo, they are dismayed to hear that it is passé. Some movements or pronouncements that have the force of law (such as Public Law 94-142) or represent a true paradigm shift seem to persist and slowly change the face of education.

Jerome Bruner (1983) has said that one must know what sort of map to use when trying to negotiate the territory. This is especially true in reviewing the cognitive tradition in education. To chart the course of education over long periods of time, one needs a macroscopic view—or a topographic map. With such a map, one can disregard the vagaries of atmospheric comings and goings—educational movements that blow hard but are soon gone—and can concentrate on long-term or topographic movements, as if charting mountain ranges of the earth. Our topographic map suggests that the educational tradition has always been *cognitive* in nature. Schools have never really abandoned the notion that something is going on in the human mind when education takes place. Armed with our topographical map, we might also assert that the great land mass of educational thought has gone through three major stages of evolution—all of which still exist today. Although the different stages of evolution may appear, paradoxically, both overlapping and antithetical to each other, they have existed in a dialectic—a dynamic tension—in education for centuries. Schools must always choose how much of their efforts will be allocated to one or the other stages.

The first stage was education as *indoctrination*: designed to cultivate an individual's responsibility to his or her reference group, to know its laws, its technology, and its world view. The goal of such a process is compliance or "appropriate" thought and behavior. This stage was heavily influenced by the cultural–political–theological context of the church. Early educational practice was based on the premise that the only road to salvation was through knowledge of the Bible and adherence to its teachings (Lee, 1973). Thus, the universal assumption was that learning is based on reading, and that all people must be able to read so they might "know the truth." This theological tradition was the source of such school practices as teacher-centered instruction, with all students doing the same thing at the same time, as well as the traditional structured layout of the classroom and the use of the textbook—that is, literally, the book of texts, Book of Truth (Foshay, 1973). This "absolutist" perspective, stressing authoritarianism, self-denial, and glorification of work, implies that there is essential knowledge that must be passed from generation to generation (Lee, 1973). The idea of the mind as passive and receptive has developed from Locke's *tabula rasa* through J. F. Herbart's designation of a formal method of instruction involving a core curriculum and lesson plans, E. L. Thorndike's laws of learning (exercise, law of effect), and the behaviorist practices of Watson and later Skinner (Lee, 1973). This wedding of empiricism, positivism, and determinism is captured in L. A. White's (1948) observation that "it is not the people who control their culture through education, it is rather the other way around: Education is what culture is doing to people, namely, equipping them with ideas, beliefs, ideals, codes of conduct, tools, utensils, machines, and the like—in short, determining how they shall think, feel and behave" (p. 240). The role of cognition, in this view, was one of acquiring and retaining facts.

The *individuation* stage, with its emphasis on the inherent goodness of man and the belief that human actions are the result of seeking to meet basic needs, was the second major stage of evolution and has served as the primary dialectic to indoctrination. While Locke expounded his empiricism in England, Leibnitz, during the same time period in Germany, offered an alternative concept of man as the source of his acts and behavior as purposive (Lee, 1973). The "relativist" perspective implies that values and knowledge must be constantly reassessed and that the role of education is to develop such inquiry and experimentation (Lee, 1973). The "tender-minded" philosophies of idealism, rationalism, and existentialism emphasized the importance of human values and the qualitative aspects of experience (Smith, 1973). The role of cognition, in terms of values and needs, was central to educational practices.

Perhaps the major pioneer of the importance of the qualitative aspects of experience in learning was John Dewey (1859–1952). Dewey's "pupil-purposing"—that is, the idea that pupils achieve their purpose through their own planning—and project method placed an emphasis on thinking, not doing: Dewey (1910) was most concerned with the insight at which a child arrived by considering some action the child had taken or observed. The developmental theorists also influenced the individuation stage by changing the way teachers regarded learners. The stage theorists of development saw the child as a developing being reaching various levels of growth in a systematic order, though at different rates. The stage theorists, exemplifed in the work of Piaget, held that each level enables the learner to perceive in certain ways and to accomplish certain kinds of tasks, which he or she was unable to perceive or do previously. The uniqueness of each child's perceptions, the personal quality of all of his knowing, and the belief that knowing is the result of process were emphasized. Educational practices that involve the learner both physically and affectively with learning tasks have their roots in individuation.

Although the *remediation* attitude, the third major stage, did not infiltrate the schools until fairly recently, its origins date back to the psychotherapy movement (Ornstein & Levine, 1985). The focus of childhood academic and mental health problems in the United States is reflected in the establishment of a psychological clinic at the University of Pennsylvania in 1896 (Craighead, 1982). Through the work of Binet in the early 1900s in France and that of Gesell in the 1930s in the United States, attention was called to levels of development and readiness in learning (Sattler, 1982). Later, during the Great Depression, education began to recognize that environmental influences affected school learning. Out of such a climate, schools began to think about providing special education for the educationally handicapped and compensatory education for the culturally different student. In addition, several new positions grew: that of school social worker, to help families and school coordinate their efforts around the education of children; school counselor, whose original job it was to help students toward the best match of their potentials and interests with the world of work; and, to some degree, school psychologist, to deal with academic and mental health dysfunctions.

Later events that served to institutionalize further the notion of remediation as an educational process were: (1) the Sputnik crisis of 1957, which caused us to believe that our science and math courses needed to be "beefed up"; (2) the civil rights movement of the 1960s and the passage of Public Law 94-142 in 1975; and (3) reports published in the 1980s by a number of commissions studying education, most of which expressed concern about "excellence" in the academic curriculum. More recently, increases in drug use among children, childhood suicide, child abuse, AIDS (acquired immune deficiency syndrome), and other issues have brought more pressure on the schools to provide education as remediation in those social/emotional areas formerly thought to be outside the school's purview.

Given the dynamic and continuous interplay among the indoctrination–individuation–remediation stages, one can begin to distinguish among various educational practices along a conforming–becoming–coping continuum. Additionally, many educational theorists and researchers (e.g., Bloom, 1964; Fenstermacher & Soltis, 1986; McNeil, 1985) characterize educational interventions according to the focus of the intervention: teaching style, learning style, and learning environment (Bloom, 1964).

The focus on teaching style emphasizes *what the teacher does* as the crux of the learning process. This approach holds the teacher as the executive and is grounded in behaviorism and positivism (Fenstermacher & Soltis, 1986). The purpose of learning within this approach is the acquiring of specific knowledge communicated by the teacher. In general, this focus may be represented by movements such as measurable competencies, accountability, and behavioral objectives.

The focus on the individual learner's style, grounded in existentialism and humanism, emphasizes *who the student is* as the focal point of the learning process. Here the purpose of learning is to enable the learner to become an authentic human being capable of making choices and accepting responsibility for choices made (Fenstermacher & Soltis, 1986). In general, this focus may be represented by approaches such as individual differences/learning styles, open schools, and alternative schools.

The final aspect, focusing on the learning process, emphasizes learning as freeing the student's mind from the limits of convention and developing a coherent conceptual system that is the foundation of any subject (Bruner, 1960; Chomsky, 1968; Hirst, 1974). In general, this focus emphasizes the teacher as modeling the process, the manner of instruction reflecting the cognitive structures associated with the content, and the approaches of executive control or metastrategies discussed earlier. Learning and intervention thus relate to developing a system applicable to various content- or situation-specific settings.

The reader has now been presented with two dimensions for highlighting the differences among various educational practices, that is, the dialectic tension of the evolutionary stages (intent) and the emphasis placed by a practice on one of the components of the learning process (focus). A matrix combining these two approaches is presented in Figure 3-1. The matrix is far from an exact representation or categorization, as the dimensions offered are *not* orthogonal and the categories along each dimension are *not* mutually exclusive. The matrix is offered rather as a means of stimulating the reader's analysis of a specific educational practice, assessment approach, or intervention strategy with respect to its assumptions and intended purposes. In trying to place a practice or strategy on the matrix, the reader will likely encounter the problem of practices "bleeding" across more than one cell, depending on the specific situation. Some examples of practices have been depicted in the matrix to illustrate the general variation of practices from the more radical behaviorist approaches to the more cognitive, especially metacognitive, approaches.

For example, the reader might trace the history of individual differences and cognitive processes across the matrix. The early psychometricians, such as Binet and Spearman, were cognitive psychologists as they sought to describe the cognitive processes underlying intelligence—for example, attention, memory, apprehension of experience, judgment, self-criticism, and the like (Kirby, 1980). Although the ultimate end of their work was to enhance the learner's confirmation to societal values and store of knowledge, the focus was more on the learner's style. With the radical behaviorist's ascent and the use of tests as means of categorization during World War I, constructs of individual differences (e.g., intelligence, abilities, etc.) and of cognitive processes (e.g., attention, memory, coding, etc.) were presumed to be separate. As the technology of testing increased, the push was on identifying the factor construction of abilities, with no concern for how such factors came about or what they were (Kirby, 1980). Today, cognitive processes are being used to construct theories of intelligence (e.g., Gardner, 1983; Sternberg, 1985), are being seen as essential

	Indoctrination (Conforming)	Individuation (Becoming)	Remediation (Coping)
Teaching Style (Intervenor as Authority)	Radical behaviorism Lecture, textbooks Standardized assessment to measure mastery of facts Locke—tabula rasa Error analysis—Prescriptive teaching	Psychoanalysis Guidance movement	Drill, repeated practice Behavioral contracts Psychometrically oriented assessment for categorization and placement
Learner's Style (Intervenor as Facilitator)	CAI Cognitive style assessment Binet, Spearman	Rogerian therapy Leibnitz Dewey A. S. Neil Self-actualization	Self-esteem Personality style assessment Headstart
Process (Intervenor as Consultant)	Critical thinking Sequenced curriculum	Discovery learning Piagetian-developmental assessment Bruner	Cognitive restructuring Self-management (e.g., self-talk) Developing skills of learning Protocol analysis assessment Simulation as assessment

FIGURE 3-1. Instructional, assessment, intervention matrix with illustrative examples.

in academic or instructional approaches (e.g., Brown, 1978; Flavell, 1976), and are highlighted in the increased literature of cognitive development, thinking skills, and neuropsychology.

With the limitations of radical behavioral approaches and in an age where the storage of facts is less needed than strategies to deal with an overabundance of information, current educational movements are stressing the content and structure of knowledge. Looking at the effects of formal schooling, Brown (1977) noted that "without the intervention of formal schooling, differences between adults and children reflect the increasing richness and diversity of human experience across the life span rather than fundamentally different modes of thought" (p. 251). What we regard as intelligence, in this light, is very much an outcome of societal values. "It is not that unschooled populations don't think, it is just that they don't think like we do" (Brown, 1977, p. 248). Brown sees schooling as dealing with knowledge as decontextualized; that is, the student develops by adding to the context derived knowledge of experience and spatial–temporal systems to gain context-free, or more logically derived, knowledge. The control, under one's own volition, of the repertoire of strategies for acquiring, accessing, and using information is the goal of education (the reader will recognize this as an emphasis on executive control and metacognition).

Cognitive-behavioral approaches in education, then, seem to follow along this current emphasis on metacontrol while maintaining strategies based in the research findings of behaviorism. These approaches recognize and appreciate the individual learner's style while transferring the control of initial learning and remediation from the external source of the teacher or intervenor to self-control. These approaches also emphasize the structure of knowledge and attempt to give to the learner (through directed instruction) the structure underlying the processing of information, transferable across content areas.

THE DIMENSIONS OF COGNITION

Attempting to understand the cognitive tradition can be a complex task. The history of psychology and education is steeped in theories regarding human cognition, leaving us with a confusing array of terms, notions, and assertions regarding the mind and its workings. In 1748 the philosopher David Hume was optimistic that during his lifetime the "secret springs and principles" of the mind would become known. At present, however, there exists no unifying theory of the psychology of mind (Flavell, 1979; Hunt, 1982; Lucas, 1985; von Bertalanffy, 1981). Cognitive science, as some call it, appears to exist as areas of special interest rather than a unified field. New discoveries in the study of neuropsychology, human and artificial intelligence, human memory, and the like have contributed to the interest of educators in cognitive styles in learning, creative and critical thinking, visual imagery, intuition, and metacognition. There is much excitement and there is also much confusion. The danger is that those who wish to apply recent findings will proceed in a willy-nilly and half-baked manner, such as has been evident in the development of the so-called left/right brain curricula.

The cognitive-behavioral approach to the mind and its workings could be characterized as a conservative one. Whereas many others may enthusiastically invoke processes of the mind as causal in the events they witness, the cognitive-behaviorist remembers the law of parsimony. This law, sometimes known as Occam's razor, suggests that one should avoid unnecessary inferences and inessential complexities in explaining behavior (Mahoney, 1974). This law was essentially the basis for behaviorism in the first place. Since behavior is apparent to the observer, whereas mind must be inferred, radical behaviorists considered mind to be unparsimonious and unnecessary. Cognitive-behaviorists consider that the mind is essential to our understanding of behavior. Although reinstating the mind has certainly added complexity and made it necessary for psychologists to infer rather than simply observe, it was a necessary step. Perhaps Bannister (cited in Mahoney, 1974) said it best: "Oc-cam's Razor should be used to sharpen our wits, not to whittle away our imaginations" (p. 22). The cognitive-behaviorist attempts to be parsimonious while also realizing that the mind is complex and that Mother Nature does not owe us simplicity (Mahoney, 1974).

The focus of this book is cognitive-behavioral intervention in schools. Such a focus is not so grandiose as the quest of cognitive science to understand the workings of the mind and its substrate—the brain. Nevertheless, those who seek to understand and apply the techniques of cognitive-behaviorism might profit from a general understanding of the mind. At the risk of oversimplifica-tion, but in the spirit of parsimony, we offer a three-dimensional "scaffold" for the organization of what is known about the workings of the mind.

> What can we do when things are hard to describe? We start by sketching out the roughest shapes to serve as scaffolds. . . . that's what we do in real life, with puzzles that seem very hard. It's much the same for shattered pots as for the cogs of great machines. Until you've seen some of the rest, you can't make sense of any part. (Minsky, 1985, p. 17)

The reader may find it useful to think of the mind as existing and function-ing along three dimensions: prehension, paradigm, and purview. Thinking, or the processing of information, always exists at some level of abstraction—*prehension* (Kolb, 1984). Likewise, this thinking is either conceptually precise or "fuzzy" along a dimension of personal *paradigm*. The paradigm of science is precise and algorithmic in its logic, but, as pointed out previously, people also tend to think in a more prototypical or heuristic manner. Finally, all thinking appears to exist along a dimension of control, or *purview*. Intentional, or metaconscious, control is self-reflexive (Brown, 1978; Flavell, 1979; Sternberg, 1985), whereas automatic, or paraconscious, control often runs off without our awareness (Lozanov, 1984; Schneider & Shiffrin, 1986).

One way to characterize the cognitive-behavioral approaches is to say that they: (1) recognize that abstract thinking can affect concrete responses along the prehension dimension, (2) favor the movement from fuzzy concepts to more precise thinking along the paradigm dimension, and (3) emphasize the intentional control of formerly automatic processing along the purview dimen-sion. For instance, whereas most theorists consider the experience of creative thinking to be concrete (prehension), metaphorical (paradigm), and automatic (purview), one cognitive-behavioral theorist, Meichenbaum (1977), emphasizes problem analysis (abstract prehension), precision of thought (paradigm), and positive self-talk and metaconscious self-direction (purview) in creativity.

The Prehension Dimension

John Dewey (1910) said that we know in two major ways: direct understand-ing, which he called "apprehension," and mediated understanding, which he called "comprehension." Kolb (1984) called these ways of knowing concrete and abstract and asserted that everything we know can be located on the "prehension" dimension. Prehension—the dynamic of grasping information—exists along a ladder of abstraction (Hayakawa, 1964) ranging from the actual existence of what is experienced to our most ideal conceptions, having no physical or actual referents. This hierarchical way of knowing can transform an actual cow—Bessie, for instance—into "livestock" or, at even higher levels of abstraction, "farm asset" or "wealth." Through such a transformation, Bessie's uniqueness can be virtually abstracted out of existence. This is the level of knowing that Karl Popper called "world three," where "intentions and thoughts become linked to ideas, issues, and institutions that have long had a reality of their own . . . where ideas and paradigms and truths live independently of their origins" (Bruner, 1983, p. 56).

Most cognitive-development theories emphasize this dimension of mind and view cognitive abilities as becoming more abstract with increasing age and experience.

The Paradigm Dimension

Most psychologists would agree that a "concept" is a method by which humans classify or categorize a vast array of experience. Since, however, no two individuals have the same experience, the concepts people form will differ (Rosser & Nicholson, 1984). The term paradigm is defined as: "a pattern, example, or model" (Guralnik, 1972). A paradigm is the habit of conceptually representing one's experience in a certain way. Concepts could be said to differ along a dimension from the vaguest and most loosely organized to the most precise and binary. A binary or logical concept is based on Aristotle's laws of: (1) identity (A equals A); (2) the excluded middle (everything is either A or not-A); and (3) noncontradiction (nothing is both A and not-A) (Hayakawa, 1964). This produces a "two-valued logic," which is the language of digital computers and positivistic science. Critical thinking is associated with this type of logic. A concept in this form would be attained by identifying the critical attributes of the objects of experience and classifying together all objects that share those attributes. All others would be excluded from the class.

For instance, *Webster's New World Dictionary* defines a "bird" as "1. any of a class (Aves) of warmblooded, two-legged, egg-laying vertebrates with feathers and wings . . ." (Guralnik, 1972, p. 143). In a binary concept, anything not matching these defining attributes is a "not-bird." Rosch (1977), however, stated that most conceptual thinking is not of this type, but is "prototypical." In other words, there are birds and then there are birds. A robin, for instance, is usually considered to be a very birdy bird. A kiwi, however, with its underdeveloped wings, hairlike feathers, and lack of a tail is a not-so-birdy bird. Rosch's point is that we often classify by the use of a prototype or idealized image of the category, and membership in the category is on a more-or-less rather than an either–or basis. Cantor and Kihlstrom (1987) insisted that the use of such "fuzzy" concepts in construing social situations is preferable to more precise processing. As Hayakawa (1964) said:

> The belief that logic will substantially reduce misunderstanding is widely and uncritically held, although, as a matter of common experience, we all know that people who pride themselves on their logic are usually . . . the hardest to get along with. (p. 241)

Werner (1948) went even further with this line of thinking by identifying "quasi-class concepts." This type of concept is often expressed using the suffix "-like" or "-ish." Werner stated that, "when we speak of pot-like hats, we do not mean that these hats belong to the class of pots, but that the impression made by such hats is approximately equivalent to that made by a pot" (p. 245). With this type of concept, the subjectivity of the observer becomes more obvious. This is what Berman (1981) called "participant-observation" in which the distance between the thing observed and the perceiver is decreased to the point of fusion. Concepts then become metaphorical, and how a thing is viewed is dependent on the individual perspective. Through the use of birdlike attributes, "spirits can soar," someone's "feathers can be ruffled," or a person can be referred to as a "birdbrain." As concepts become less logical and are no longer binary, they possess a richness that Arieti (1976) considered to be the foundation of creative thinking.

The Purview Dimension

The word "purview" is defined by *Webster's* as "2. the extent or range of control, activity, or concern; province 3. range of sight or understanding" (Guralnik, 1972). The purview dimension concerns itself with levels of control. Polar aspects of the dimension are metaconscious and paraconscious. When information is grasped at some level of abstraction on the prehension dimension and conceptualized through some model on the paradigm dimension, it also falls under the purview of some level of control.

Paraconscious mental activity was described by Lozanov (1984) as "more or less unconscious."

> The term "paraconsciousness" covers . . . all automatic or secondary automated activities; unconscious automated elements in the field of conscious mental activity; subsensory (subliminal) stimuli; peripheral (marginal) perceptions; most of the emotional stimuli; intuitive creativity; the second plane of the communicative process; a considerable part of the processed information in the process of conditioning, associating, coding and symbolizing; and a number of unconscious interrelations which have informational, algorithmical and reprogramming effects on the personality. (p. 74)

Writers on the evolution of the brain (MacLean, 1973; Sagan, 1977; Taylor, 1979) have suggested that as the human brain developed over millions of years from bottom to top, certain stratified functions were laid down that still exist today. At the area of the pons and below exist the vegetative functions. In the limbic system, such functions are elaborated and are accompanied by memory and emotion. Finally, the cerebral cortex appears responsible for higher mental processes. At the lowest level, "wired-in" instinctive knowing may never become conscious. Some knowing runs off without intent—the way a spider "knows" how to spin a web (Galloway, 1976). Other types of paraconscious knowing enter into awareness or become conscious objects of our experience. The tip-of-the-tongue or "felt sense" (Gendlin, 1962) experience appears to dwell just out of our grasp, but we know it is there. Other experiences such as "tacit" knowing (Polanyi, 1958; Sternberg, 1985) are those in which we know something without knowing how we know. Additional instances of knowing in the paraconscious purview are: (1) unconscious motivation (Freud, 1900); (2) incubation (Mackinnon, 1978; Patrick, 1955); (3) automatized information (Sternberg, 1985); (4) executive ignorance (Martindale, 1981); (5) "knowing by heart" (Ryle, 1949); and (6) the storage of long-term memory contents and "archaic material," which emerges in dreams and projective techniques (Klopfer, Ainsworth, Klopfer, & Holt, 1954).

At the other end of the purview dimension is reflective consciousness, or metacognition. Schneider and Shiffrin (1986) distinguish between "controlled" (metacognition) and "automatic" processing. Controlled processing is: (1) comparatively slow, (2) sequential in nature, (3) effortful, (4) under conscious control, and (5) limited by short-term memory. Automatic processing is (1) relatively fast, (2) executed in parallel (multiple operations done at once), (3) almost effortless, (4) not limited by short-term memory capacity, and (5) for the most part subconscious.

Through controlled processing, humans can become their own executives, able to control their emotions, behaviors, and—to a large extent—their destinies. The ability to plan and execute intentionally is considered a major component of intelligence (Brown, 1978; Sternberg, 1985).

It has been traditional to consider thinking as "cognitive" and feeling as something else; this is the cognitive–affective distinction. Emotions, however, are varieties or types of thoughts (Minsky, 1985). Feeling, or affect, *is* a cognitive process. According to Klopfer and co-workers (1954),

> we are able to test the reality of an emotional situation without the benefit of intellectual processes . . . Jung includes this assumption in his thinking when he describes feeling along with thinking as a rational function. (pp. 570–571)

Zajonc (1980) meant something similar to this when he stated that preferences need no inferences. Wilke (1981) held that the lower portions of the brain make decisions constantly and that this process becomes conscious only when it breaks down.

Cognitive-behaviorists (Mahoney, 1977) have argued that thinking about a situation creates the feeling reaction to it. Zajonc (1980) made a strong case for the primacy of feeling. Goodyear and Bradley (1981) suggest that in some situations feelings come first, in others thinking. This certainly makes sense when one considers that the frontal lobes of the brain have many connections to the limbic system and can inhibit emotional responses, whereas "archaic" areas of the brain may react emotionally without intellective decision making (Zajonc, 1980).

CONCLUSION

Cognitive-behavioral processes, like all other cognitive processes, lend themselves to analysis along the prehension, paradigm, and purview dimensions of mind. Although these dimensions are merely a scaffold, we hope they will serve the practitioner as a mnemonic device or quick mental reference for thinking about cognitive processes. The outstanding feature of cognitive-behavioral approaches, for instance, is the aspect of self-monitoring and self-control. Brown (1978) speaks of "meta" knowing as being in control of one's knowledge. If someone should *not know* what he or she knows, this is referred to as "secondary ignorance." If such knowledge were to be used, it would run off automatically in what Lozanov (1984) calls a "para" fashion. This is the purview dimension of mind. On this same dimension, Meichenbaum (1977) speaks of "self-regulatory deficits," and Mahoney (1974) gives clients "self-monitoring assignments" to improve their metacontrol. Closely akin to this, but on the prehension dimension of mind, is the cognitive-behavioral belief that people become dysfunctional because of an inadequate or faulty representation system. Their ideas do not prove to be useful in concrete situations. Meichenbaum (1977) speaks of "unhealthy" self-talk and the need for cognitive restructuring. Through this process, abstractions of the situation are brought into line with the evidence. Finally, on the paradigm dimension, the emphasis is on clearer thinking or a more logical paradigm. Emotions appear to be regarded as something to be either intentionally controlled, overcome, or ignored.

Mahoney (1974) views the cognitive-behaviorist as the "thinking behaviorist" who employs the mind as a mediational step to behavior. He also uses the term "humanistic empiricist" to describe the attitude of a scientific approach to human behavior. The use of metacontrol, the alignment of abstract representations with concrete evidence, and the shaping of greater clarity in thinking all reflect the strong foothold of cognitive-behaviorists in the theories and findings of the cognitive tradition.

REFERENCES

Arieti, S. (1976). *Creativity: The magic synthesis.* New York: Basic Books.
Berman, M. (1981). *The reenchantment of the world.* Ithaca, NY: Cornell University Press.

Bloom, B. S. (1964). *Stability and change in human characteristics.* New York: Wiley.

Bogen, J. E. (1969). The other side of the brain: An appositional mind. *Bulletin of Los Angeles Neurological Societies, 34,* 135–162.

Brown, A. L. (1977). Development, schooling and the acquisition of knowledge about knowledge. In R. C. Anderson, R. J. Spiro, & W. E. Montague (Eds.), *Schooling and the acquisition of knowledge* (pp. 241–255). Hillsdale, NJ: Lawrence Erlbaum.

Brown, A. L. (1978). Knowing when, where, and how to remember: A problem of metacognition. In R. Glaser (Ed.), *Advances in instructional psychology* (Vol. 1, pp. 77–165). Hillsdale, NJ: Lawrence Erlbaum.

Bruner, J. S. (1960). *The process of education.* Cambridge, MA: Harvard University Press.

Bruner, J. S. (1983). *In search of mind: Essays in autobiography.* New York: Harper & Row.

Bruner, J. S. (1985). On teaching thinking: An afterthought. In J. W. Segal, S. F. Chipman, & R. Glaser (Eds.), *Thinking and learning skills: Vol. 2, Research and open question* (pp. 597–608). Hillsdale, NJ: Lawrence Erlbaum.

Bruner, J. S., & Postman, L. (1949). On the perception of incongruity: A paradigm. *Journal of Personality, 18,* 206–223.

Cantor, N., & Kihlstrom, J. F. (1987). *Personality and social intelligence.* Englewood Cliffs, NJ: Prentice-Hall.

Chomsky, N. (1968). *Language and mind.* New York: Harcourt Brace Jovanovich.

Craighead, W. E. (1982). A brief clinical history of cognitive-behavioral therapy with children. *School Psychology Review, 11*(1), 5–13.

Dewey, J. (1910). *How we think.* New York. D. C. Heath.

Ellis, A. (1962). *Reason and emotion in psychotherapy.* New York: Lyle Stuart.

Fenstermacher, G., & Soltis, J. (1986). *Approaches to teaching.* New York: Teacher's College Press.

Flavell, J. H. (1976). Metacognitive aspects of problem solving. In L. B. Resnick (Ed.), *The nature of intelligence* (pp. 231–296). Hillsdale, NJ: Lawrence Erlbaum.

Flavell, J. H. (1979). Metacognition and cognitive monitoring. *American Psychologist, 34,* 906–911.

Foshay, A. W. (1973). Sources of school practice. In J. I. Goodlad & H. G. Shane (Eds.), *The elementary school in the United States* (pp. 173–197). Chicago: University of Chicago Press.

Freud, S. (1900). *The interpretation of dreams.* New York: Modern Library.

Galloway, C. (1976). *Psychology for learning and teaching.* New York: McGraw-Hill.

Gardner, H. (1983). *Frames of mind: The theory of multiple intelligences.* New York: Basic Books.

Gendlin, E. T. (1962). *Experiencing and the creation of meaning.* New York: Macmillan.

Geschwind, N. (1974). *Selected papers on language and the brain.* Dordrecht: Reidel.

Goodyear, R. K., & Bradley, F. O. (1981). Cognition and feeling states: Unraveling the issues. *Personnel and Guidance Journal, 59*(5), 314–317.

Guralnik, D. B. (Ed.). (1972). *Webster's New World Dictionary of the American Language* (2nd college ed.). New York: World.

Hayakawa, S. I. (1964). *Language in thought and action.* New York: Harcourt Brace & World.

Hayes, J. R. (1978). *Cognitive psychology: Thinking and creating.* Homewood, IL: Dorsey.

Hirst, P. H. (1974). *Knowledge and the curriculum.* London: Routledge & Kegan Paul.

Hofstadter, D. R. (1985). *Metamagical themas: Questing for the essence of mind and pattern.* New York: Basic Books.

Hunt, M. (1982). *The universe within: A new science explores the human mind.* New York: Simon & Schuster.

Kant, I. (1963). *Critique of pure reason.* London: Macmillan. (Original work published 1781.)

Kessen, W. (1966). Questions for a theory of cognitive development. In J. Stevenson (Ed.), *Concept of development.* Monographs of the Society for Research in Child Development, *31*, 55–70.

Kirby, J. R. (1980). Individual differences and cognitive processes: Instructional application and methodological difficulties. In J. R. Kirby & J. B. Biggs (Eds.), *Cognition, development and instruction* (pp. 119–144). New York: Academic Press.

Klopfer, B., Ainsworth, M. D., Klopfer, W. G., & Holt, R. R. (1954). *Developments in the Rorschach technique: Technique and theory* (Vol. 1). New York: Harcourt Brace Jovanovich.

Kolb, B., & Whishaw, I. Q. (1980). *Foundations of human neuropsychology.* San Francisco: Freeman.

Kolb, D. A. (1984). *Experiential learning: Experience as the source of learning and development.* Englewood Cliffs, NJ: Prentice-Hall.

Lee, D. M. (1973). Views of the child. In J. I. Goodlad & H. G. Shane (Eds.), *The elementary school in the United States* (pp. 138–172). Chicago: University of Chicago Press.

Lozanov, G. (1984). *Suggestology and outlines of suggestopedy.* New York: Gordon and Breach Science Publishers.

Lucas, C. (1985). Out at the edge: Notes on a paradigm shift. *Journal of Counseling and Development, 65,* 165–172.

Luria, A. R. (1966). *Higher cortical functions in man.* London: Tavistock.

Mackinnon, D. (1978). *In search of human effectiveness.* Buffalo, NY: Creative Education Foundation.

MacLean, P. D. (1973). *A triune concept of brain and behavior.* Toronto: University of Toronto Press.

Mahoney, M. J. (1974). *Cognition and behavior modification.* Cambridge, MA: Ballinger.

Mahoney, M. J. (1977). Reflections on the cognitive-learning trend in psychotherapy. *American Psychologist, 32*(1), 5–13.

Martindale, C. (1981). *Cognition and consciousness.* Homewood, IL: Dorsey.

McGinnes, E. (1949). Discussion of Howe's and Solomon's note on "Emotionality and perceptual defense." *Psychological Review, 56,* 244–251.

McNeil, J. D. (1985). *Curriculum: A comprehensive introduction.* Boston: Little, Brown.

Meichenbaum, D. (1977). *Cognitive-behavior modification: An integrative approach.* New York: Plenum Press.

Minsky, M. (1985). *The society of mind.* New York: Simon & Schuster.

Neisser, U. (1967). *Cognitive psychology.* New York: Appleton-Century-Crofts.

Ornstein, R. E. (1972). *The psychology of consciousness.* New York: Viking.

Ornstein, A., & Levine, D. (1985). *An introduction to the foundations of education* (3rd ed.). Boston: Houghton Mifflin.

Patrick, D. (1955). *What is creative thinking?* New York: Philosophical Library.

Polanyi, M. (1958). *Personal knowledge.* Chicago: University of Chicago Press.

Ray, W., & Ravizza, R. (1985). *Methods toward a science of behavior and experience* (2nd ed.). Belmont, CA: Wadsworth.

Rosch, E. (1977). Classification of real-world objects: Origins and representations in cognition. In P. N. Johnson-Laird & P. C. Wason (Eds.), *Thinking: Readings in cognitive science* (pp. 212–222). New York: Cambridge University Press.

Rose, F. (1984). *Into the heart of mind: An American quest for artificial intelligence.* New York: Harper & Row.

Rosser, R. A., & Nicholson, G. I. (1984). *Educational psychology.* Boston: Little, Brown.

Rourke, B. P. (1982). Central processing deficiencies in children: Toward a developmental neuropsychological model. *Journal of Clinical Neuropsychology, 4*(1), 1–18.

Ryle, G. (1949). *The concept of mind.* New York: Barnes and Noble.

Sagan, C. (1977). *The dragons of Eden: Speculations on the evolution of human intelligence.* New York: Random House.

Sattler, J. M. (1982). *Assessment of children's intelligence and special abilities* (2nd ed.). Boston: Allyn and Bacon.

Schneider, W., & Shiffrin, R. (1986). Controlled and automated human information processing: I. Detection, search and attention. *Psychological Review, 84,* 1–66.

Senden, M. V. (1960). *Space and sight.* Glencoe, IL: Free Press.

Smith, P. G. (1973). The philosophical context. In J. I. Goodlad & H. G. Shane (Eds.), *The elementary school in the United States* (pp. 109–127). Chicago: University of Chicago Press.

Steinberg, R. J. (1985). *Beyond IQ: A triarchic theory of human intelligence.* Cambridge: Cambridge University Press.

Sullivan, H. S. (1953). *Conceptions of modern psychiatry.* New York: Norton.

Taylor, G. R. (1979). *The natural history of the mind.* New York: Dutton.

Thompson, C. L., & Rudolph, L. B. (1983). *Counseling Children.* Monterey, CA: Brooks/Cole.

Thorndike, R. L. (1984). *Intelligence as information processing: The mind and the computer.* A CEDR Monograph. Bloomington, IN: Phi Delta Kappa.

von Bertalanffy, L. (1981). *A systems view of man.* Boulder, CO: Westview Press.

Vygotsky, L. S. (1962). *Thought and language.* New York: Wiley.

Watson, J. B. (1913). Psychology as the behaviorist views it. *Psychological Review, 20,* 158–177.

Watson, R. I. (1968). *The great psychologists: From Aristotle to Freud* (2nd ed.). Philadelphia: Lippincott.

Watzlawick, P. (1984). *The invented reality.* New York: Norton.

Werner, H. (1948). *Comparative psychology of mental development* (rev. ed.). Chicago: Follett.

White, L. A. (1948). Man's control over civilization. *Scientific Monthly, 66,* 235–242.

Wilke, J. T. (1981). *A neuro-psychological model of knowing.* Washington, DC: University Press.

Zajonc, R. B. (1980). Feeling and thinking: Preferences need no inferences. *American Psychologist, 35,* 151–175.

4

A COGNITIVE-BEHAVIORAL APPROACH TO EDUCATION: ADOPTING A BROAD-BASED PERSPECTIVE

ANDREW W. MEYERS
ROBERT COHEN
Memphis State University

ROBERT SCHLESER
Illinois Institute of Technology

The philosopher Nelson Goodman (1978) tells the story of the woman shopping for fabric to recover her overstuffed chair and sofa. At her favorite textile shop she studies the 2″ by 3″ zigzag-edged fabric swatches in the upholsterer's sample book. She makes her selection and orders enough material to complete the job, with the stipulation that the material be exactly like the sample. When the fabric is delivered, the woman opens the bundle and, to her chagrin, finds hundreds of 2″ by 3″ swatches exactly like the one in the sample book. She calls the textile shop and complains bitterly. The frustrated proprietor reminds her that she demanded that the material be exactly like the sample, and that he and his assistants worked through the night cutting it just so.

Several months later, after the woman has painstakingly sewed the fabric pieces together and recovered her furniture, she decides to give a party. She travels to the local bakery and selects a chocolate cupcake from the display case. She orders enough for 50 guests and requests delivery in 2 weeks. As the guests arrive, the bakery truck appears and the driver unloads one huge cupcake. Upon receiving the woman's complaint, the proprietress of the bakery pleads to the customer concerning the trouble that she and her staff went to in order to produce the giant cupcake. The bake shop owner says, "My husband runs the textile shop and he warned me that your order would have to be placed all in one piece" (Goodman, 1978, pp. 63–64).

Goodman's tale pleasantly awakens us to the fact that we perceive and understand the world in our own unique ways—indeed, that through our perceptual and cognitive processes, we may be actively creating our own world. In this chapter we argue that children are, perhaps even more than adults, active creators of their worlds. And for a comprehensive understanding of child behavior, one must examine the cognitive processes in which they engage in. We begin by building and illustrating a cognitive-behavioral model of child behavior. We then explicate this model and adopt a critical perspective which, we hope, will enable the model to continue to respond to conceptual and empirical challenges. We label our critical reevaluation a developmental-cognitive view. This perspective recognizes the role in child behavior of developmental variables, affect, and family and social systems. We conclude with a discussion of the issues surrounding the application of our model in the classroom.

A COGNITIVE-BEHAVIORAL MODEL

During the last three decades, behaviorism has had a major and positive impact on our understanding of children's behavior. Recent developments in behavior therapy have moved beyond the study of observable behavior and encouraged the inclusion of the child's cognitive mediational processes (Kazdin, 1978). This addition, away from—but at the same time encompassing—operant- and classical-conditioning-based models of behavior, has led to the acknowledgement of the active role of the individual in perceiving, interpreting, and understanding the world. Rather than assume that the individual reacts passively to a real environment, we now hypothesize that the individual responds constructively to a perceived world. This creates a dynamic and reciprocal interaction among the child's behavior, cognitive processes (including beliefs, rules, and expectations), and the environment. Each of these factors—behavioral, intrapersonal, and environmental—requires our attention if the dysfunctional child is to be understood and helped (Bandura, 1985).

Since Bandura's (1973) early work on children's observational learning and Meichenbaum's (1974) description of self-instruction training with children, mediational approaches to children's behavior have flourished. Cognitive-behavioral intervention strategies for aiding learning-disabled children, the mentally retarded, psychotic children, and social isolates, as well as children manifesting anxiety, attention deficits, aggression, delinquency, and academic problems, have all received empirical support (Meyers & Cohen, 1982; Meyers & Craighead, 1984a). Although later in this chapter we summarize our self-instruction work with children, it is beyond the scope of the present effort to review child cognitive-behavioral interventions (see Meyers & Craighead, 1984a, for a review of a broad range of relevant intervention areas). To illustrate this cognitive-behavioral paradigm, we present a prototypic example of the development and implementation of a cognitive-behavioral intervention program with a population of dysfunctional children.

The Think Aloud program (Camp, Blom, Hebert, & van Doornick, 1977) was an attempt to apply a mediational model to decrease the inappropriately aggressive behavior and increase the prosocial behavior of aggressive boys.

Camp and her colleagues at the University of Colorado Medical School demonstrated that young, aggressive boys showed deficient nonverbal problem-solving performance, more impulsivity, and more task-irrelevant speech when compared to nonaggressive boys (Camp, 1977). From this assessment work, Camp's group concluded that interventions with this population must inhibit aggressive behavior and guide the dysfunctional child to alternative desirable performances.

To meet these goals, Camp designed a psychoeducational training program conducted by teachers. Teachers were employed to facilitate the dissemination of the program, and to allow it to serve both treatment and prevention goals. The cognitive-behavioral intervention strategy for aggressive boys was delivered over approximately 40 sessions, with teachers working from prepared training manuals. The lessons began with a game called Copy Cat, which prepared the child to imitate the teacher while he or she proceeded through the development and application of relevant problem-solving strategies. In subsequent lessons, the teacher used the Copy Cat game across a broad range of tasks to model the problem-solving approach and strategies for coping with errors.

Once presented the adult problem-solving model, the child was prompted to employ overt verbalizations to guide task performance. The child's use of overt guiding verbalizations and the participation of the teacher were gradually faded to covert levels. Finally, the child was required to apply the problem-solving strategy in a variety of contexts to promote generalization both within and beyond the training program. Toward this end, training began with simple cognitive problems such as mazes and puzzles and progressed to increasingly complex cognitive and social problems.

The initial goals of the Think Aloud program included enabling the aggressive child to inhibit first responses to a problem situation and to develop an overarching, organized approach to problem solving. The program was directed toward improving the child's understanding of the concepts of cause and effect and increasing his or her repertoire of alternative response solutions and evaluation skills. The child was prepared to apply these skills to both cognitive/impersonal problems and social/interpersonal problems (Camp & Ray, 1984).

The Think Aloud program has been subjected to several experimentally controlled evaluations (Camp, 1977, 1980; Camp & Bash, 1981). Typically, measures of the child's cognitive change and teacher ratings of child behavior have been taken. On occasion, observation of the child's classroom behavior also was included. A summary of these studies (Camp & Ray, 1984) suggested that the Think Aloud program produced more desirable cognitive change and, on cognitive problem-solving measures, was more likely to return aggressive boys to normal levels than were no-treatment control groups or attention placebo groups. Teacher ratings of child behavior indicated that Think Aloud prompted significant improvements in those ratings when compared to no-treatment controls. The use of the program also was associated with less deviant aggressive behavior in class, although other forms of disruptive behavior continued to occur. Camp proposed that boys using the Think Aloud principles in the school situation channeled aggressive impulses into less socially disruptive acts.

Camp's intervention program for aggressive boys illustrates the cognitive-behavioral approach to dysfunctional child populations. In the next section, we review the historical development of this model.

THE TRANSITION TO A COGNITIVE-BEHAVIORAL MODEL

Behavioral interventions with children had their roots in Watson's work on the development and extinction of children's fear behavior and Skinner's influential research on operant conditioning. The first clinical applications of learning theory and other research in experimental psychology in the 1950s and early 1960s were dominated by these classical- and operant-conditioning approaches. At that time, behavior therapy with children centered around operant interventions with autistic children, the retarded, and children with motor deficits and conduct disorders (Meyers & Craighead, 1984b). Increasing success with these child populations permitted behaviorists greater involvement with less severely disabled children in less restrictive outpatient settings. The goals of this clinical work also shifted from children's disruptive and self-injurious behavior to educational and self-management tasks that required attention to the child's cognitive skills. Work with a more intact client population forced behavior therapists to consider the child's internal thought processes both as a target and as a mechanism of change.

The growth of a mediationally based behavioral model was fueled not only by these social changes but also by increasingly apparent empirical and theoretical deficiencies in behavior therapy. Although the conditioning-based model had generated a wide range of applications, Kazdin (1978) noted that, by the late 1970s, there was a growing conceptual stagnation. Advances in behavioral research had been limited largely to extensions to new populations, problems, and settings. At the applied level, the failure to find consistent generalization of behavior change to new responses and settings was extremely disappointing.

However, theorists and practitioners in behavior therapy were beginning to respond to a broader social science paradigm shift, one that Dember (1974) labeled, "the cognitive revolution." Kazdin (1978) singled out several information-processing research areas for their influence on this conceptual shift in behavior therapy. Experimentation in semantic condtioning, symbolic self-stimulation and imagery, the role of awareness in learning, observational learning or modeling, and the impact of perceived contingencies has served to complicate traditional behavioral assumptions.

Subjects' expectancies, self-delivered instructions, or awareness of contingency relationships all affect the acquisition and extinction of behavior. Evidence of this is found in research indicating that inaccurate instructions or beliefs may exert more control over behavior than the actual response–reinforcement relationships (Dulany, 1974). Other investigators have argued that operant consequences are effective behavior change strategies to the extent that they communicate information and instructions to the subject rather than through the direct operation of reinforcement contingencies (Murray & Jacobson, 1971). Often reinforcement consequences have little or no effect on behavior until the subject is informed of the contingency relationship. Typically, such instructions by the experimenter immediately modify the subject's response to conditioning trials.

Craighead (1982) identified three factors as instrumental in the shift from conditioning-based models of behavior to a cognitive-behavior therapy. These three factors are: (1) cognitive psychology and the information-processing perspective mentioned previously; (2) research in self-control; and (3) the development of cognitive therapy. Bandura (1969), working within the context of an information-processing model, laid the cornerstone for the construction of a cognitive-behavior therapy with his description of modeling or observational learning. Explanations of learning by the observation of a model emphasize the involvement of verbal and imaginal encoding of the modeled behavior. Symbolic encodings drawn from the model can then be used by the learner to structure performance and experience.

Bandura's research on observational learning was a central component of his social learning theory (Bandura, 1977). This position asserts that an individual's behavior, cognitive processes, and the environment are involved in a reciprocally deterministic relationship, each affecting and being affected by the other two sets of variables. Whereas conditioning models view the individual as a passive responder to environmental effects, social learning theory assumes that the individual plays an active role in manipulating the environment and controlling behavior.

A body of research that exemplifies the impact that Bandura's theory has had on behavior therapy is self-instruction. Meichenbaum's (1977) self-instruction training was based, in part, on the cognitive developmental psychology of Luria (1961) and Vygotsky (1962). These Soviet psychologists suggested that control of a child's behavior shifts during development from verbal control by adults in the child's social environment, to the child's own overt speech, and finally to the child's covert speech. From this position, Meichenbaum constructed a training program to teach impulsive children to control their own behavior more effectively by using self-delivered, task-guiding, first-person statements. The child first imitated an adult model who performed the target task while presenting relevant self-instructions. Eventually, the child imitated the behavior while self-instructing aloud, then while whispering, and finally while covertly rehearsing or "thinking" the instructions. In the past 15 years, self-instruction interventions have been used successfully with a variety of childhood problems, including hyperactivity, aggression, anxiety, social competence, and academic deficiencies (Craighead, Wilcoxon-Craighead, & Meyers, 1978). We shall return to the topic of self-instruction in a later section.

The second major factor identified by Craighead as influential in the development of a cognitive behavior therapy was research in self-control. Prior to 1965, the behavioral explanation for self-control behavior relied on Skinner's (1953) operant view that external consequences determined behavior. In that year, Homme offered the notion of "coverants" or operants of the mind. Homme (1965) argued that thoughts could serve to reinforce and thereby to modify behavior. Though still flirting with an operant theme, this work broached the role of internal factors in self-directed behavior. Homme's papers were followed in the early 1970s by Kanfer's (Kanfer & Karoly, 1972) analysis of self-control. Kanfer conceptualized the self-control process as being divisible into three components: self-monitoring, self-evaluation, and self-reinforcement. Applications of this model to clinical problems such as obesity, smoking, and impulsivity have come to play a major role in contemporary behavior therapy. Although it is plausible to argue for a causal role for external factors in the self-control process, Bandura's (1977) reciprocal determinism and other systemic perspectives encourage us to acknowledge the interaction of intrapersonal cognitive activity and environmental contributions to self-directed behavior.

Craighead's (1982) third and final influence on the growth of cognitive behavior therapy was the development, in the 1960s and 1970s, of cognitive therapy. Beginning with Ellis's (1962) *Reason and Emotion in Psychotherapy*, and reinforced by Beck's (1976) writings, a body of clinical approaches and procedures, developed in the clinic rather than the laboratory, gained popularity. These schools of intervention shared two basic assumptions: (1) that dysfunctional behavior was produced by inappropriate cognitive processes and (2) that successful intervention must modify those self-statements, expectancies, or beliefs. Research examining cognitive therapies has placed in doubt both of these basic assumptions and has supported more comprehensive causal models (Zeiss, Lewinsohn, & Munoz, 1979); these approaches, however, have continued to have an impact on remedial and preventive work with children.

This brief historical overview of cognitive-behavior therapy has outlined the social, theoretical, and experimental forces that have moved behavior therapy to a cognitive-mediational position. These influences have enabled educational and clinical psychologists to offer a more comprehensive model of childhood behavioral disorders and, in some situations, more effective intervention strategies. However, the cognitive-behavioral view has not flourished without critical comment from its' own adherents. In the next secion we examine some of this commentary.

CRITICAL ISSUES IN THE COGNITIVE-BEHAVIORAL MODEL

Bandura's social learning theory and its causal model, reciprocal determinism, have strongly influenced child cognitive-behavior therapy. As mentioned earlier, reciprocal determinism assumes that the child's behavior, intrapersonal variables, and environmental contexts interact to affect all factors in the interaction. Whereas Bandura argued for an attention to a wide range of systemic influences in the study of behavior, cognitive behaviorists often have emphasized cognition to the exclusion of other person variables, and typically have conceptualized context as linear antecedent and consequent events (Craighead, Meyers, & Wilcoxon-Craighead, 1985).

Cognitive positions have traditionally assumed that emotion is a product of cognition. Zajonc (1980) and others, however, have called for a new recognition of the primary role of emotion in human behavior. Rather than argue over the primacy of cognition versus affect, Craighead (1982) has suggested that we be concerned with the pattern of interaction of these variables. Mahoney (1985) has gone so far as to argue that distinctions such as cognition, affect, and behavior may not be helpful, and that these constructs, as communicative interactions with our world, would better be sujugated to notions of personal order and personal meaning. Clearly, a comprehensive cognitive-behavioral model must encompass the child's emotional responses.

A second person variable that is crucial to an understanding of children's behavior, but one that has received surprisingly little attention in the cognitive-behavioral literature, is the child's developmental status. Without an awareness of normal developmental sequences, it is difficult to assess the appropriateness of children's behavior or their response to educational and therapeutic interventions (Meyers & Cohen, 1982). The analysis of cognitive functioning in children within the field of child clinical psychology has been dominated by adult-derived, nondevelopmental models (Achenbach, 1978; Cohen & Meyers, 1984). That is, there is an assumed quantitative continuity between childhood conditions (behavior) and adult behavior. Analyses of childhood problems and of the etiology of adult problems, then, conceptualize the child's state as deficient. The child's behavior is typically viewed in terms of adult states minus some level of sophistication, and the age of the child is used as an index of functioning. An alternative approach to these issues, termed here a developmental cognitive perspective, is to view the child as progressing through qualitatively distinct stages of development. At each stage, the child has a complete system for interacting within his or her environment, with each stage building upon the accomplishments of previous stages but not simply reducible to the previous stage. Rather than the child being considered deficient, the child's functioning is considered different from adult states. This approach is *not* a denial of a continuity in a pathological process; rather, it is an assertion that this process may be exhibited in different forms at different developmental periods.

The significance of developmental variables is apparent when one finds age-dependent child performance on tests of conceptual style and concept learning, response to instructions and models, use of memory rehearsal and hypothesis-testing strategies, and measures of planfulness (Craighead, Meyers, Wilcoxon-Craighead, & McHale, 1983). Even more interesting, as we shall discuss at length later, is evidence that same-aged children at different Piagetian cognitive levels manifest discriminative cognitive task performance. This research illuminates the contrast between a "deficit" model and a "developmental" model of child behavior.

Finally, we turn to environmental variables. Traditionally, behavior therapy has concentrated on immediate antecedent and consequent events. Obversely, contemporary models of child development (Bronfenbrenner, 1979) and child psychopathology (Henggeler, 1982) have emphasized an integration of wide-ranging systems influences. These latter perspectives encompass reinforcement contingencies, but view the child as embedded in and interacting reciprocally with several social and familial systems (e.g., family dyads, the school, socio-economic conditions). Although these interactional perspectives have recently had impact on behavior therapy (Glenwick & Jason, 1984; Turkewitz, 1984) an increased awareness of systemic influences would benefit the child cognitive-behavioral model. For example, Panella, Cooper, and Henggeler (1982) found that teenagers who received consistently supportive discipline from parents or guardians were more resistant to the influences of delinquent peers.

That such broad environmental models mesh well with cognitive positions can be seen in both cognitive and developmental perspectives that argue for an inseparability of cognition and action. Piaget's concepts of accommodation and assimilation tied the child's cognitive development to interaction with the environment (Flavell, 1963). Weimer (1977), in a comment on "motor theories" of cognition, stated that cognition must be understood "from the outside inward." In a recent evaluation of cognitive theories of depression, Coyne (1982) argued against assigning causality to cognitive variables on the grounds that depressed adults were both perceiving and creating depressing environments.

Whether we choose to focus on the systemic interaction of the child's behavior, cognitive and emotional processes, and environment, or on the inherent inseparability of these constructs, recognition of a more comprehensive mediational model should present us with a framework for greater understanding of child behavior. In the following section we take advantage of this framework to build a developmental and systems-based child cognitive-behavioral perspective.

A DEVELOPMENTAL COGNITIVE-BEHAVIORAL VIEW

Our work has suggested that previous research into the use of cognitive behavior strategy training with children is deficient in one very important respect: little attention has been given to extant differences in the child's developmental status and functioning. The traditional educational and clinical perspective on the child is to ignore qualitative differences in the child's functioning in favor of quantifying the deficits of the child relative to older or "normal" children. Much is to be gained in changing this perspective. Rather than treating the child's behavior as deficient relative to some standard, we suggest that the child's behavior be considered as different and distinct yet complete unto itself. A discussion of our research over the past 8 years will serve as an example of specific applications of this developmental perspective.

From a developmental perspective, the age of the child is certainly an inexact index of developmental functioning. We selected same-aged children who differed in Piagetian-defined level of cognitive development. Specifically, we studied preoperational and concrete-operational children as determined by performance on two conservation tasks: conservation of number and conservation of continuous quantity (see Flavell, 1963). The thought of preoperational children is dominated by the evaluation of present circumstances, with little integration of past experiences with current affairs. Thus, perceptual and immediate circumstances are the focus of attention rather than more stable, conceptual analyses. In addition, physical consequences of actions are considered over social norms. Concrete-operational children assume exact answers to problems, are aware of irrelevant variants in problems, and understand and are responsive to the social demands of others. In short, preoperational children live in a here-and-now reality, influenced by their perceptions of their immediate environment. Their thought is characterized as often being egocentric, that is, being unable to take others' perspectives. The thinking of concrete-operational children is not tied to their immediate perceptions. These children can integrate past with present experiences and are not misled by state-changing transformations, such as rolling out a ball of clay, when making judgments about invariant properties such as quantity. It is important to reiterate that we selected children who varied in cognitive level while matching them on chronological age.

For this research we adapted a model of learning context from Bransford (1979). A full explication of this model may be found in Cohen and Meyers (1984). Virtually all learning situations can be conceptualized within this model, whether the behavior/thinking of interest is academic work, peer relations, or parent–child socialization situations. We conceptualized the outcome of any learning situation to be the product of a complex interaction among four factors: (1) cognitive status of the learner; (2) nature of learning materials; (3) procedures used during learning; and (4) criterial tasks for assessing learning, maintenance, and generalization.

We applied this model in a series of studies, defining cognitive status of the learner in terms of Piagetian stage membership, using the Matching Familiar Figures Test (MFFT; Kagan, Rossman, Day, Albert, & Phillips, 1964) as a training task and a perceptual perspective-taking task as a measure of generalization. Across the studies we investigated the role of various "nature of materials" and "procedures" issues for the training and generalization of self-instruction. Our goal has been to elucidate the specific interplay of the aforementioned four factors, with the focal point being the cognitive status of the child.

In each of the studies, children were assessed for Piagetian level and then served in two experimental sessions. In session 1, the child was pretested on the

MFFT and perspective-taking tasks and received self-instruction training according to assigned condition. In the second session, held 1 to 3 days after the first, the child received a second exposure to a self-instruction regimen, followed by a posttest on the two tasks.

In our first study (Schleser, Meyers, & Cohen, 1981), we manipulated the nature-of-materials component of the learning context by providing the child with either a self-instruction package designed specifically for use with the MFFT or a general problem-solving package that was applicable to a range of problem-solving situations. Children performed better on the MFFT training task following exposure to the specific content instructions, but it is important to note that only those children exposed to the general content instructions showed significant generalization effects to an untrained problem-solving task. Although concrete-operational children outperformed preoperational children overall (i.e., a main effect for cognitive level on both tasks), there were no differential training effects as a function of cognitive level in this first experiment.

Keeping nature of materials constant in our second experiment, using only the specific content instructions, we varied the learning procedures (Schleser, Cohen, Meyers, & Rodick, 1984). One group of children received the traditional fading of instructions procedures, whereby they rehearsed the self-guiding statements through a series of progressively less elaborated prompts. Another group of children was led to "discover" the same set of self-guiding statements through a Socratic dialogue procedure with the experimenter. We felt that this procedure not only demonstrated an efficient strategy for the child, but also put on display the process of strategy generation and application. Again, both preoperational and concrete-operational children benefited from training in the same fashion, with both the fading and the directed-discovery groups outperforming the control groups. It is noteworthy that only the concrete-operational children in the directed-discovery group significantly improved on the generalization task following training.

Given that both cognitive-level groups demonstrated significant generalization from a general-content, fading self-instruction procedure, while only the concrete-operational children generalized from a specific-content, directed-discovery procedure, the next logical experiment assessed the effects of fading versus directed discovery when the content of the instructions was general in nature (Nichol, Cohen, Meyers, & Schleser, 1982). As in the second experiment, only the concrete-operational children demonstrated significant generalization.

This set of studies, along with our other research on self-instructions (Brown, Meyers, & Cohen, 1984; Cohen, Schleser, & Meyers, 1981; Goodnight, Cohen, & Meyers, 1984; Meyers & Cohen, 1984; Schleser, Meyers, Cohen, & Thackwray, 1983; Thackwray, Meyers, Schleser, & Cohen, 1985), led us to propose the notion of optimal discrepancy as a general principle for structuring intervention settings (Cohen & Meyers, 1984). Piaget suggested that cognitive growth is best facilitated under conditions of moderate disequilibrium, that is, conditions that are new to the individual, thus requiring accommodation, yet not so novel as to be devoid of meaning.

As an extension of this notion to generalization of behavior change from training, optimal discrepancy is proposed as a principle dictating that generalization is best facilitated when the cognitive involvement of the individual is maximally captured. Involvement will be determined by the cognitive demands of the intervention setting and thus may be manipulated by the materials and procedures used, but will ultimately be determined by the cognitive status of the child.

For the problem-solving situations used in our work, preoperational children are optimally involved when the learning procedures are kept simple and the materials used require cognitive integration and effort, as in the case of the general-content instructions. Directed-discovery procedures, in contrast, are cognitively difficult for the child, requiring a tremendous investment in generating responses as well as in acquiring the strategy. When the procedures are difficult, as is the case with directed discovery, the preoperational child is overloaded in a cognitive sense. The child can perform the discovery operations (and, in fact, shows training effects as a result), but is unable to extract a strategy that can be carried to other tasks and into other situations.

The concrete-operational child is optimally engaged by the directed-discovery procedure, whether the content of the strategy is specific or general in nature. The procedure puts on display for this child a general plan not only for how to solve a problem, but also for how to go about solving problems. The concrete-operational child can understand this strategy generation procedure (separating form from content), whereas the preoperational child cannot.

We were interested in applying what we had learned from the above studies in an efficient manner to large groups of children. To this end, all first- and second-graders at a public elementary school were involved in a study where self-instructions were delivered in the class and/or at home (Cohen, Nichol, Cohen, & Meyers, 1985). Specifically, children served in one of four experimental conditions: classroom training, parent consultation training, classroom plus parent consultation training, or a no-training control group. Each child was individually pre- and posttested on the following measures of cognitive ability: Piagetian level; cognitive tempo (MFFT); Tower of Hanoi; metacognition (i.e., the child's awareness and control of cognitive processes); tests devised to assess abilities in following directions, self-monitoring, and coping with errors; and tests of math skills. Peer and teacher sociometric measures of academic competence, perceptions of self-control, and locus of control also were assessed. Teachers and parents gave sociometric ratings of the child and perceptions of the child's self-control.

Training consisted of 8 weeks of biweekly lessons. The classroom self-instruction regimen was embedded within regularly scheduled math lessons and was delivered by a female graduate student. Problem identification, planfulness, self-monitoring, and coping with errors were taught in the first 4 weeks (one component per week, cumulatively rehearsed). During the last 4 weeks these components were further integrated, and the children were encouraged to apply their "plans" to both academic and social situations. The format and materials for the parent consultation groups directly paralleled those of the classroom groups, with home visits made to help the parents before the first week of training and prior to the fifth week.

The most pervasive finding was the advantage of concrete-operational children over preoperational children across nearly all the measures (e.g., more reflective in style, more efficient on several cognitive tasks, better metacognitive awareness, better in math, more often nominated by peers and by teachers as academically competent, more internal attributions for behavior). In terms of training, the classroom presentation led to numerous improvements on the cognitive measures (e.g., Tower of Hanoi, cognitive tempo, metacognition, math skills). In sum, delivery of self-instruction strategies in the classroom appeared to be an efficient way to improve behavior, particularly on cognitive tasks. Although the classroom approach, where more control could be exerted over the manner of delivery, was superior to delivery by parents on the cognitive tasks and on sociometric measures by peers and teachers, parents involved in the home presentations reported that their children exhibited a greater degree of self-control at home by posttest than did children in the other groups.

Before a reevaluation of our developmental perspective, consider a recently completed doctoral dissertation by Craig Brown (1986), comparing self-report of depressive symptoms by 443 children (6 to 14-year-olds) with parent and teacher ratings of the child's depressive symptoms using a 57-item questionnaire. Factor analysis of the data revealed the following factors:

Child scale: Self-criticism, anxiety, somatic complaints, alienation, aggression, and self-esteem

Parent scale: School performance, social interaction, somatic complaints, anxiety, alienation, guilt, withdrawal, and self-criticism

Teacher scale: Aggression, somatic complaints, withdrawal, school performance, hopelessness, self-esteem, and self-criticism.

Discriminant analyses were performed using the factor-analytically derived dimensions from each set of raters to discriminate Piagetian stage membership (preoperational, transitional, concrete-operational). From the parents' scale, symptoms associated with school performance, social interaction, and somatic complaints were significantly higher for transitional children; symptoms associated with alienation were positively related to cognitive status (preoperational children low, concrete-operational children high); symptoms associated with anxiety were negatively associated with cognitive status (preoperational children high, concrete-operational children low); and symptoms associated with withdrawal were associated in a curvilinear fashion (i.e., lower for transitional than for preoperational or concrete-operational children). Predicting chronological age, somatic complaints on the child scale decreased with age, and aggression and self-criticism on the teacher scale increased with age. Predicting mental age, school performance and alienation on the teacher scale significantly increased with mental age. In short, developmental status of child, whether defined as Piagetian level, chronological age, or mental age, led to differential predictions of normative levels of depressive symptomotology as a function of who was rating the child's symptoms.

As related findings in Brown's project, the mean base rates for items on the depression scale varied as a function of rater, and the correlations between child–teacher and the child–parent ratings, though statistically significant, were low ($r = .22$ and $r = .28$, respectively). Parent–teacher ratings were not significantly correlated ($r = .12$). Although some of this discrepancy in responses from raters may be due to differences in how children and different adults conceptualized the items or response alternatives, the factor analyses in this study suggest an additional explanation. For the children, the self-criticism factor accounted for a substantial amount of variance (41.3%); for parents, the prominent factors were school performance and social interaction (37.9%); for teachers, aggression was the leading factor (44.7%). Not surprisingly, children are focusing on internal factors, while adults are concentrating on observable behavior relative to the social contexts in which they see the child. In short, Brown's data suggest to us that children, teachers, and parents do not always share the same conceptualization of dysfunction and, furthermore, that the child's conceptualization of psychological problems, such as depression, varies with the developmental status of the child.

Brown's (1986) research is consistent with the other research presented in this section in demonstrating the importance of tailoring interventions to the needs and abilities of the individual child—needs and abilities that vary with the child's developmental level. Also evident in these data is the recognition that distal as well as proximal social systems may perceive dysfunctioning differently than the child does. Thus, the need exists to examine these additional social systems when designing interventions, a point that is elaborated in the next section.

ELABORATING THE DEVELOPMENTAL PERSPECTIVE

We began this research program as a collaborative effort to integrate a developmental perspective with traditional child clinical concerns, a view we have termed a developmental clinical perspective (Cohen & Schleser, 1984). We feel that we have adequately demonstrated the utility of such an approach, showing that an assessment of a child's extant cognitive functioning can lead to differential predictions of intervention outcome. While focusing on the cognitive level of the child, we adapted the model of learning context from Bransford, as described previously. This also has proved quite useful, giving us conceptual tags for understanding variations in intervention materials and procedures and their relationship to variations in cognitive functioning. What we wish to propose in this section is a further elaboration of our position, particularly in terms of examining the role of systemic influences and of affect in understanding a child's behavior.

A growing number of researchers are beginning to examine behaviors as a function of physical and social dimensions of settings. For example, environmental psychologists emphasize that the physical environment is not simply a stage for the performance of behaviors (see Cohen, 1985). Rather, there are complex individual–environment transactions whereby the physical setting in conjunction with the psychological characteristics of individuals serve to determine the nature of behavior. A related position can be found in Bandura's (1977) reciprocal determinism, which hypothesizes an interdependence among behavior, environment, and person characteristics. Family therapists are also interested in the reciprocal interactions among family members (e.g., Minuchin, 1985) and how both proximal and distal social systems have an impact on an individual in a given context (e.g., Henggeler, 1982). In developmental psychology, Bronfenbrenner (1979) described the child's development as being influenced by four spheres of social exchange, from direct and immediate influences in the current environment, to more indirect influences such as social relations not immediately present, mother–father marital relations, and cultural mores.

There is no unifying theory to date on the role of context. Yet each of these positions shares a concern for an examination of an individual's behavior in relation to relevant characteristics of the setting in which the behavior is exhibited. This is not simply a call for naturalistic research. Rather, it is an acknowledgment of the complex, multidimensional nature of factors that influence and are influenced by an individual.

What does this mean for a cognitive-behavioral perspective? We believe that the basic premise of these positions—that an individual's cognitive functioning can and should serve as the focus for assessment and intervention—should remain as the focal point. The influence of settings, whether defined in terms of the physical and/or of the social characteristics of the environment, will be known to the individual in relation to that individual's level of cognitive functioning. What is needed is an expansion of this position to include a variety of additional variables. This expansion will be proposed next with reference to our research on self-instruction.

The case can be made that all knowledge has social origins, a position particularly emphasized by Vygotsky (1962). Parents, teachers, peers, and therapists transmit information and strategies to children through social discourse. This is, of course, a two-way street, with the giver of the information varying the message as a function of the abilities and behaviors of the learner. In the vast majority of research on clinical and educational interventions with children, we ignore these social exchanges and focus instead on the content, or the procedures, or the tasks of interest.

Recall the research cited previously where we presented self-instructions to classes of children and/or had parents deliver the strategy. It is interesting that the strategy training in the classroom resulted in cognitive gains on cognitive tasks, whereas the parent consultation groups led to little change in these assessments. Clearly, the parents were engaged in a different set of relationships with their children than we were in the classroom. Parents reported a change in self-control in their children. Thus, the parents may not have produced cognitive task changes in their children, but the self-instructions they presented to their children did lead to some change in the child's behavior at home (or at least a change in the parents' perceptions of that behavior).

Similarly, the research reported on the child, teacher, and parents as raters on a depression questionnaire led to findings of differences as a function of rater. The agenda of teachers, children, and parents are certainly not identical. The lack of relationship among the raters should not be viewed as "error variance" but, rather, as an assessment of different conceptualizations of the child's everyday contexts.

Significantly, in both these projects, the cognitive-developmental level of the child strongly influenced the findings. Although we are expressing a belief that cognitive interventions with children must examine more fully the dimensions that relate to the contexts of interest, again we urge that this study be performed in relation to the developmental status of the child. Piagetian stage membership is an excellent predictor of behavior, as shown in our research. It may not be the best construct in other work. Individual assessments of the understanding of peer relationships or family functioning, or the child's understanding of the power and control of authority figures, may be more appropriate indices of functioning in other projects. For example, a recent monograph by Dodge, Pettit, McClaskey, and Brown (1986) reported a domain-specific relationship between social cognition and social behavior. Specifically, social cognitive measures of group entry predicted group entry behavior, social cognitive measures of response to provocation predicted response to provocation. Group entry processing did not predict response to provocation behavior, nor did response to provocation processing predict group entry behavior. Importantly as well, the child's social behavior predicted peers' behavior in response.

One aspect of individual, developmental functioning that has received little empirical attention in the developmental, systemic expansion of cognitive behavior therapy with children is the role of affect in the child's behavior. Emotional processing of stimuli may proceed at a faster rate than cognitive processing, and thus emotion may influence cognition at least as much as cognition influences emotion. There is some evidence, reported in Anooshian and Siegel (1985) that the emotional "tags" related to events and situations are particularly more important for young children with less robust representation abilities than older children.

Regardless of the position one assumes on the relationship of affect and thought, the influence of affect can and should be included in analyses, assessment, and implementation of intervention strategies. We suggest that the development of affect, like that of cognitive development, follows a sequential qualitative pattern—that affect serves the child in communication with the environment and must be considered in an understanding of the child as a unified whole rather than as a miniature adult.

We remain aligned with the more traditional cognitive-behavioral position in terms of focusing on the cognitive processes of the individual. We expand on this basic premise by urging the consideration of the child in terms of a developmental perspective, viewing the child as an organism different rather than deficient relative to adult functioning and in terms of the context of the child's behavior. We also urge for the inclusion of the child's social and emotional status in both assessment and intervention considerations. Whether one chooses to intervene on an individual child, a classroom, or a family from a cognitive-behavioral perspective, we argue for the consideration of both direct and indirect, both proximal and distal, sets of variables. The final section examines the issues surrounding the application of cognitive-behavioral interventions in educational settings.

ECOLOGICAL UTILITY OF COGNITIVE-BEHAVIOR THERAPY

Despite strong evidence for the utility of cognitive-behavioral approaches to child dysfunction, evidence for generalization of treatment gains to the classroom (Meichenbaum & Asarnow, 1979) remains equivocal. Further, despite evidence of potential utility, there are few applications of cognitive-behavioral procedures to prevent the development of problem behaviors or to enhance the problem-solving skills of normal children. Finally, there is little indication that cognitive-behavioral technology is being adopted by relevant professionals in naturalistic settings. The following section will identify a number of potential explanations for the limited success and utilization of cognitive-behavioral interventions in applied settings. An alternative approach to encouraging children to employ appropriate self-instruction and cognitive-behavioral strategies will be presented.

Several investigators have suggested that the disappointing performance of self-instruction approaches could be attributed to the brevity of training, the narrow content of the self-instruction strategy, the questionable relevance of the training tasks, and the failure to train children to apply their new strategy or to understand the utility of using their new skills in novel situations and with different types of problems (Meichenbaum, 1977; Meichenbaum & Asarnow, 1979). Solutions to these problems included increasing the number of training sessions, using academic materials as training tasks, varying training locations and situations, using self-directed mastery trials, and employing booster sessions.

Few professionals have challenged the basic assumption that some form of self-instruction training would induce children actually to employ verbal mediators to direct their behavior in applied settings. Thus, the bulk of self-instruction applications continue to focus on relatively minor variations in the standard self-instruction procedure in an attempt to remediate children's cognitive deficits. An ecological analysis of the typical self-instruction program would suggest that these efforts are not practical, nor are they likely to greatly enhance intervention outcome.

Siegel (1982) presented a model to investigate the role of adult teaching strategies in the development of internalized speech in normal children. He argued that teaching does not necessarily involve a particular set of techniques or strategies. Rather, he suggested, teaching is a communicative act that is designed to achieve an educational goal.

Siegel identified a specific class of adult communication acts that have a particularly important influence on the development of children's ability to anticipate and plan. He termed these styles "distancing strategies." Distancing strategies are communicative acts that activate the child's cognitive processes and require the child to represent symbolically a relationship between objects or events. These strategies vary in form but generally involve the presentation of a question to which the child must respond.

Siegel conceptualized distancing strategies as social events, which occur through the child's interactions with affectively significant adults. These interactions are generally informal and embedded within the ongoing child–adult relationship. Siegel noted that, over time, children develop the ability to represent these social interactions internally. Once internalized, they serve as the basis for the child to generate his or her own metacognitive strategies.

Siegel's (1982) model raises interesting implications for future self-instruction programs. The concept of distancing strategies is similar in some respects to our directed-discovery procedure. Specifically, both distancing and directed discovery rely on conflict-inducing questions as a mechanism to prompt children to engage in adaptive self-guidance. Siegel, however, conceived of distancing strategies as a continuous series of informal training experiences.

Siegel (1982) reported a positive relationship between parental use of distancing strategies and 4-year-old children's performance on teaching tasks requiring anticipation, sequencing, classification, and conservation skills. These results suggest that very young children can benefit from sophisticated teaching strategies if they are embedded in an ongoing series of interactions with an affectively significant adult.

The high incidence of academic and conduct problems in the classroom suggests that not all children develop appropriate self-control skills through their interactions with adults. Siegel (1982) noted that adult caretakers were not always systematic in their use of distancing strategies with children, often relying on intrusive, diadactic commands to get children to complete an assigned task. Our own work (Schleser, Cohen, Meyers, & Rodick, 1984; Schleser, Meyers, & Cohen, 1981) suggested that these teaching styles do not facilitate the internalization of self-control strategies.

Previous self-instruction programs targeted the child as the focus of intervention. In essence, they attempted to "fit" the child to the environment.

Siegel's (1982) analysis of the ecological development of self-control, our developmental cognitive model presented previously, and the limited success of standard self-instruction programs suggest the need to alter the teaching environment to fit the needs of the child.

ECOLOGICAL APPLICATIONS OF SELF-INSTRUCTION IN THE CLASSROOM

Our recent work (Cohen, Nichol, Cohen, & Meyers, 1985) represented a departure from the standard self-instruction program. The results suggested that it is possible to successfully train large groups of children in naturalistic settings, that teachers and nonprofessional trainers such as parents can facilitate positive change in children, and that nondysfunctional children can benefit from self-instruction training.

Classroom teachers are a particularly important aspect of a child's environment. Yet, they have been relegated to a minor role in previous self-instruction programs. Teachers exert a powerful influence on the development of a child's cognitive skills through modeling, direct instruction, and the consequation of the child's behavior. They are also a powerful affective and motivational focus for the child, either administering or withholding social and material resources. Further, teachers constitute a valuable ongoing natural resource for the child. The nature of these teacher-pupil interactions facilitates or inhibits the course of the child's social and cognitive development.

Teachers have the relevant expert knowledge concerning the nature and content of the material that they teach. Cognitive-behavioral programs in education take these facts into consideration. Teachers should be included not only in the identification of problem children, but as active participants in the prevention or remediation of the problems they observe in the classroom.

Recently, we completed a series of clinical interventions in which teachers were the target of training (Schleser, Allen, & Asher, 1987). Three teachers, who had referred children for academic and classroom conduct problems, participated in a cognitive-behavioral training program. Each referred child had been diagnosed previously as attentional deficit disordered (DSM-III) by a pediatrician. Children were referred for reevaluation for stimulant medication.

Training consisted of 4 initial sessions and 12 weekly consultation sessions. During the first 4 sessions, teachers were taught to monitor specific behaviors that they wished to change, presented with a rationale for using self-instruction procedures, instructed in the development of specific strategies, and coached in the use of faded rehearsal and directed-discovery procedures. During the 12 consultation sessions, a research assistant observed the teachers' interactions with the children and provided additional feedback.

A variety of measures were used to assess the ecological utility of the training program. The measures included: children's class grades, teachers' ratings of child behavior problems, ratings of children's performance in two other classes (math and reading), teachers' interactions with targeted as well as nontargeted children, and teachers' perception of the efficacy of self-instruction procedures.

The results indicated that after 16 weeks, children's academic performance and classroom behavior had improved moderately in all three classes. Teacher reports indicated that they attributed these positive gains to their use of the self-instruction procedures. Observer ratings of teachers' interactions suggested that they relied increasingly on the use of directed-discovery or distancing strategies to correct problem behaviors in untargeted as well as targeted children. More important, all teachers reported that the targeted children were within "normal" academic and behavioral limits, and expressed the belief that continued use of the self-instructions would resolve the remaining problems without further clinical or medical intervention.

The results of these clinical interventions must be interpreted cautiously. Only a small number of teachers were trained, the assessment measures were not standardized, and the gains made by children were modest. However, they suggest the potentially fruitful outcome of enlisting teachers as colleagues in training children to employ adaptive self-instruction and self-control strategies.

We began by arguing for a consideration of the cognitive-mediational activities of the child. But our argument asserts that these cognitive processes are inseparable from the systemic contexts in which they occur. These systems include the child's processes of cognitive, emotional, and social development, as well as the complex environmental contexts that surround the child. A comprehensive understanding of child behavior and any model of education and intervention must consider these broad-ranging intrapersonal and environmental factors.

The child's world contains numerous interrelated social systems in addition to the ongoing, dynamic internal, developmental variables. Goodman's account of the lady shopper hints at these multidimensional influences. She fell victim first to an individual who, in a preoperational manner, followed her instructions to the letter. Next, she experienced the consequences of distal, interrelated social systems. It is our hope that researchers and practitioners can avoid both pitfalls by acknowledging and using both proximal and distal influences in their work.

REFERENCES

Achenbach, T. M. (1978). Psychopathology of childhood: Research problems and issues. *Journal of Consulting and Clinical Psychology, 46,* 759–776.

Anooshian, L. J., & Siegel, A. W. (1985). From cognitive to procedural mapping. In C. J. Brainerd & M. Pressley (Eds.), *Basic processes in memory development: Progress in cognitive development research* (pp. 47–102). New York: Springer-Verlag.

Bandura, A. (1969). *Principles of behavior modification.* New York: Holt, Rinehart & Winston.

Bandura, A. (1973). *Aggression: A social learning analysis.* Englewood Cliffs, NJ: Prentice-Hall.

Bandura, A. (1977). *Social learning theory.* Englewood Cliffs, NJ: Prentice-Hall.

Bandura, A. (1985). Model of causality in social learning theory. In M. J. Mahoney & A. Freeman (Eds.), *Cognition and psychotherapy* (pp. 81–99). New York: Plenum Press.

Beck, A. T. (1976). *Cognitive therapy and the emotional disorders.* New York: International Universities Press.

Bransford, J. D. (1979). *Human cognition: Learning, understanding, and remembering.* Belmont, CA: Wadsworth.

Bronfenbrenner, U. (1979). *The ecology of human development.* Cambridge, MA: Harvard University Press.

Brown, C. M. (1986). *Developmental contributions to the assessment of childhood depression.* Unpublished doctoral dissertation, Memphis State University.

Brown, C., Meyers, A. W., & Cohen, R. (1984). Long-term self-instruction training: Generalization to proximal and distal problem solving tasks with preschoolers. *Cognitive Therapy and Research, 8,* 427–438.

Camp, B. W. (1977). Verbal mediation in young aggressive boys. *Journal of Abnormal Psychology, 86,* 145–153.

Camp, B. W. (1980). Two psychoeducational treatment programs for young aggressive boys. In C. K. Whalen & B. Henker (Eds.), *Hyperactive children—The social ecology of identification and treatment* (pp. 191–220). New York: Academic Press.

Camp, B. W., & Bash, M. A. S. (1981). *Think aloud: Increasing social and cognitive skills—A problem-solving program for children (Primary level).* Champaign, IL: Research Press.

Camp, B. W., Blom, G. E., Hebert, F., & van Doorninck, W. J. (1977). "Think aloud": A program for developing self-control in young aggressive boys. *Journal of Abnormal Child Psychology, 5,* 157–169.

Camp, B. W., & Ray, R. S. (1984). Aggression. In A. W. Meyers & W. C. Craighead (Eds.), *Cognitive behavior therapy with children* (pp. 315–350). New York: Plenum Press.

Cohen, R. (Ed.). (1985). *The development of spatial cognition.* Hillsdale, NJ: Lawrence Erlbaum.

Cohen, R., & Meyers, A. W. (1984). The generalization of self-instructions. In B. Gholson & T. L. Rosenthal (Eds.), *Applications of cognitive-developmental theory* (pp. 95–112). New York: Academic Press.

Cohen, S. L., Nichol, G. T., Cohen, R., & Meyers, A. W. (1985). *Self-instruction learning at home and at school.* Paper presented at the biennial meeting of the Society for Research in Child Development, Toronto, April.

Cohen, R., & Schleser, R. (1984). Cognitive development and clinical interventions. In A. W. Meyers & W. E. Craighead (Eds.), *Cognitive behavior therapies with children* (pp. 45–68). New York: Plenum Press.

Cohen, R., Schleser, R., & Meyers, A. W. (1981). Self-instructions: Effects of cognitive level and active rehearsal. *Journal of Experimental Child Psychology, 32,* 65–76.

Coyne, J. (1982). A critique of cognitions as causal entities with particular reference to depression. *Cognitive Therapy and Research, 6,* 3–13.

Craighead, W. E. (1982). A brief clinical history of cognitive-behavior therapy with children. *School Psychology Review, 11,* 5–13.

Craighead, W. E., Meyers, A. W., & Wilcoxon-Craighead, L. (1985). A conceptual model for cognitive-behavior therapy with children. *Journal of Abnormal Child Psychology, 13*, 331–342.

Craighead, W. E., Meyers, A. W., Wilcoxon-Craighead, L. & McHale, S. (1983). Issues in cognitive behavior therapy with children. In M. Rosenbaum, C. Franks, & Y. Jaffe (Eds.), Perspectives on behavior therapy in the 80's (pp. 234–261). New York: Springer.

Craighead, W. E., Wilcoxon-Craighead, L., & Meyers, A. W. (1978). New directions in behavior modification with children. In M. Hersen, R. M. Eisler, & P. M. Miller (Eds.), *Progress in behavior modification* (Vol. 6, pp. 159–201). New York: Academic Press.

Dember, W. N. (1974). Motivation and the cognitive revolution. *American Psychologist, 29*, 161–168.

Dodge, K. A., Pettit, G. S., McClaskey, C. L., & Brown, M. M. (1986). *Social competence in children.* Monographs of the Society for Research in Child Development, *51* (2, Serial No. 213).

Dulany, D. E. (1974). On the support of cognitive theory in opposition to behavior theory: A methodological problem. In W. B. Weimer & D. S. Palermo (Eds.), *Cognition and the symbolic processes* (pp. 43–56). Hillsdale, NJ: Lawrence Erlbaum.

Ellis, A. (1962). *Reason and emotion in psychotherapy.* New York: Lyle Stuart.

Flavell, J. H. (1963). *The developmental psychology of Jean Piaget.* New York: Van Nostrand.

Glenwick, D. S., & Jason, L. A. (1984). Locus of intervention in child cognitive behavior therapy: Implications of a behavioral community perspective. In A. W. Meyers & W. C. Craighead (Eds.), *Cognitive behavior therapy with children* (pp. 129–162). New York: Plenum Press.

Goodman, N. (1978). *Ways of worldmaking.* Indianapolis, IN: Hackett.

Goodnight, J. A., Cohen, R., & Meyers, A. W. (1984). Generalization of self-instructions. The effect of strategy adaptation training. *Journal of Applied Developmental Psychology, 5*, 35–44.

Henggeler, S. (Ed.). (1982). *Delinquency and adolescent psychopathology.* Boston: John Wright-PSG.

Homme, L. (1965). Perspectives in psychology: Control of coverants, the operants of the mind. *Psychological Record*, 15, 501–511.

Kagan, J., Rossman, B. L., Day, D., Albert, J., & Phillips, W. (1964). *Information processing in the child: Significance of analytic and reflective attitudes.* Monographs of the Society for Research in Child Development, *41* (5).

Kanfer, F. H., & Karoly, P. (1972). Self-control: A behavioristic excursion into the lion's den. *Behavior Therapy, 3*, 398–416.

Kazdin, A. E. (1978). *History of behavior modification: Experimental foundations of contemporary research.* Baltimore, MD: University Park Press.

Luria, A. R. (1961). *The role of speech in the regulation of normal and abnormal behaviors.* New York: Liverwright.

Mahoney, M. J. (1985). Psychotherapy and human change processes. In M. J. Mahoney & A. Freeman (Eds.), *Cognition and psychotherapy* (pp. 3–48). New York: Plenum Press.

Meichenbaum, D. (1974). *Cognitive behavior modification.* Morristown, NJ: General Learning Press.

Meichenbaum, D. (1977). *Cognitive behavior modification: An integrative approach.* New York: Plenum Press.

Meichenbaum, D., & Asarnow, J. (1979). Cognitive-behavior modification and meta-cognitive development. In P. Kendall & S. Hollon (Eds.), *Cognitive-behavioral interventions: Theory, research, and procedures* (pp. 11-35). New York: Academic Press.

Meyers, A. W., & Cohen, R. (1982). The role of adolescent cognition in a family-ecological model. In S. Henggeler (Ed.), *Delinquency and adolescent psychopathology* (pp. 187-203). Boston: John Wright-PSG.

Meyers, A. W., & Cohen, R. (1984). Cognitive-behavioral interventions in educational settings. In P. C. Kendall (Ed.), *Advances in cognitive-behavioral research and therapy* (Vol. 3, pp. 131-166). New York: Academic Press.

Meyers, A. W., & Craighead, W. C. (Eds.). (1984a). *Cognitive behavior therapy with children.* New York: Plenum Press.

Meyers, A. W., & Craighead, W. C. (1984b). Cognitive behavior therapy with children: A historical, conceptual, and organizational overview. In A. W. Meyers & W. E. Craighead (Eds.), *Cognitive behavior therapy with children* (pp. 1-17). New York: Plenum Press.

Minuchin, S. (1985). Families and individual development: Provocations from the field of family therapy. *Child Development, 56,* 289-302.

Murray, E. J., & Jacobson, L. I. (1971). The nature of learning in traditional and behavioral psychotherapy. In A. E. Bergin & S. L. Garfield (Eds.), *Handbook of psychotherapy and behavior change: An empirical analysis* (pp. 709-747). New York: Wiley.

Nichol, G., Cohen, R., Meyers, A. W., & Schleser, R. (1982). Generalization of self-instruction training. *Journal of Applied Developmental Psychology, 3,* 205-215

Panclla, D., Cooper, P., & Henggeler, S. (1982). Peer relations in adolescents. In S. Henggeler (Ed.), *Delinquency and adolescent psychopathology* (pp. 139-161). Boston: John Wright-PSG.

Schleser, R., Allen, A., & Asher, M. (1987). *The utility of teachers as self-instruction trainers.* Unpublished manuscript, Department of Psychology, Illinois Institute of Technology, Chicago.

Schleser, R., Cohen, R., Meyers, A. W., & Rodick, J. D. (1984). The effects of cognitive level and training procedures on the generalization of self-instructions. *Cognitive Therapy and Research, 8,* 187-200.

Schleser, R., Meyers, A. W., & Cohen, R. (1981). Generalization of self-instructions: Effects of general versus specific content, active rehearsal, and cognitive level. *Child Development, 52,* 335-340.

Schleser, R., Meyers, A. W., Cohen, R., & Thackwray, D. (1983). Generalization of self-instructions by impulsive children: Effects of discovery versus faded rehearsal. *Journal of Consulting and Clinical Psychology, 51,* 954-955.

Siegel, I. E. (1982). The relationship between parental distancing strategies and the child's cognitive behavior. In L. M. Laosa & I. E. Siegel (Eds.), *Families as learning environments for children* (pp. 47-86). New York: Plenum Press.

Skinner, B. F. (1953). *Science and human behavior.* New York: Free Press.

Thackwray, D., Meyers, A. W., Schleser, R., & Cohen, R. (1985). Achieving generalization with general versus specific self-instructions: Effects on academically deficient children. *Cognitive Therapy and Research, 9,* 297-308.

Turkewitz, H. (1984). Family systems: Conceptualizing child problems within the family context. In A. W. Meyers & W. E. Craighead (Eds.), *Cognitive behavior therapy with children* (pp. 66-98). New York: Plenum Press.

Vygotsky, L. S. (1962). *Thought and language.* New York: Wiley.

Weimer, W. B. (1977). A conceptual framework for cognitive psychology: Motor theories of the mind. In R. Shaw & J. Bransford (Eds.), *Perceiving, acting, and knowing* (pp. 267–311). Hillsdale, NJ: Lawrence Erlbaum.

Zajonc, R. B. (1980). Feeling and thinking: Preferences need no inferences. *American Psychologist, 35,* 151–175.

Zeiss, A. M., Lewinsohn, P. M., & Munoz, R. F. (1979). Nonspecific improvement effects in depression using interpersonal skills training, pleasant activity schedules or cognitive training. *Journal of Consulting and Clinical Psychology, 47,* 427–439.

PART TWO
Assessment Practices

5

INFORMATION PROCESSING AND COGNITIVE ASSESSMENT I: BACKGROUND AND OVERVIEW

ERNEST T. GOETZ
ROBERT J. HALL
Texas A&M University
THOMAS G. FETSCO
Dickinson State University

JONATHAN'S STORY

Once upon a time, in the not too distant past, a boy complained to his father that there was nothing to do. The boy, a second-grader, was home from school with a malady thought to be contagious but not debilitating. The father, husband to a working wife, was working at home, trying to write a chapter that looked remarkably similar to the one you are reading. It was decreed, therefore, in these days of enlightened fatherhood, shared responsibility for child care, and Bill Cosby, that the father should look after the son. Not wanting to be tethered by this responsibility, but conscious that being a good parent (according to Doonesbury) means providing meaningful and instructive activities for one's children, the father responded to his son's complaints of boredom with, "Why don't you write a story?"

Much to the father's surprise, the son responded, "Yeah, that sounds like a great idea." With no further ado (Shakespeare, 1600), prompting, or instruction other than a request for paper (five sheets of unlined, continuous-feed computer paper complete with holed edges), the son embarked on his first-ever story-writing assignment.

And so begins our quest for mind. Jonathan, beginning the third month of the second grade, produced the following unedited story. In Figure 5-1, we have attempted to present the story exactly as Jonathan produced it on paper, preserving the number of lines, number of words used on each line, spelling, and punctuation. Page numbers are ours.

FIGURE 5-1. Reproduction of Jonathan's first story attempt.

Once upon a time
there were two
Elf's but they were
big Elf's not small
ones so they hid
in the forest of Darkness
no body ever go's
there because
a bad king lives
there.   infact this
king hates Elf's
he would kill the
Princess of every-
thing that's how bad   1

of the other Elf
the tracks lead him
right to the Bad
king's casttle so from
that Point on he tip-e-
toed to the draw-
bridge and maid
a mimic of the king's
reporter so the king's
men let the Drawbridge
Down and the Elf
ran in the casttle   4

he really is but
these Elf's were
brave they still
went in to the
forest of Darkness
in the forest of Darkness
       one day
the king sent two
of his men to
hunt for food and
on that very day
one Elf was going
to hunt for food to   2

he hid in a safe
Place when the king
saw people running
wich is a rule he ran
after them and the other
Elf ran into the foretresses
on his way he saw
some ropes he loerd
it between the two
bars and pulled him
up and they lived
happely ever after
     the End   The End   5

so that night the
the Elf had been capsherd
by the Bad king's
men the other
Elf was looking for
him and all of
the sudden he
saw two things
that the other Elf
was wearing and
he found some tracks   3

What can we make of Jonathan's story writing? We might note that there are a number of different ways to evaluate Jonathan's performance. From a quantitative perspective, we might be interested in the total number of words used, the number of words spelled correctly, the number of multisyllabic words, the number of words with six or more letters, the number of punctuation errors, the number of capitalization errors, and so on. From the qualitative side, we might be interested in the texture of the story itself. Are the events portrayed in an orderly fashion? Does the story make sense? Is the story complete? How many characters appear in the story, and is there any character development? Is the language used in the story roughly equivalent to the level of the child's language development? What kinds of errors does the child make? Is there a pattern to the child's errors?

It seems reasonable to suggest that by blending quantitative and qualitative information, a relatively cogent picture of a child's level of functioning in a given academic area can be developed. What, then, might Jonathan's story reveal to us about his level of skill development in spelling and written composition?

To summarize Jonathan's performance quantitatively, his story contained 242 words, of which 224 (93%) were spelled correctly. He used one period, 24 capital letters, 10 apostrophes, and one hyphenated word. In addition, two words that were carried over to the next line were hyphenated at the appropriate syllabic breaks. Thirty (12%) of the words used in the story contained six or more letters. Of those, 23 were spelled correctly. Obviously, we cannot evaluate Jonathan's writing skill relative to other students his age without normative data or at least quantitative information about comparable efforts by his peers. Nevertheless, we might ask if there is anything that stands out or is impressive about these numbers. Given the data presented, can we generate hypotheses about Jonathan's skill in language arts?

In reviewing Jonathan's performance from a correct versus an incorrect perspective, we're immediately struck by the fact that there is little in his work to indicate that he understands how or when to use capital letters or periods. Moreover, when he does use capital letters, they appear to be linked to what he thinks are proper nouns. We suspect that he is currently being taught about proper nouns in school but has not yet mastered their use in exercises that require him to create rather than to recognize. We know, however, that he does well on assignments requiring that he recognize correct forms of punctuation given a number of alternatives. We might also be alarmed at the number of misspelled words, but considering his age and the fact that he is attempting to use words that are somewhat complex or tricky ("because," "drawbridge," "darkness," "night," "princess"), we're inclined to be pleased with his overall spelling ability.

From a quantitative perspective, then, Jonathan has written a fairly lengthy story given that he has, to date, not been asked to write more than individual sentences or short paragraphs. The fact that his story contains little punctuation and that much of it is inaccurate (e.g., capital letters in the middle of sentences) makes us think that his understanding of how to punctuate sentences appropriately lags considerably behind what he should be able to do. Since Jonathan has accomplished much academically over the past two years, it is somewhat alarming that he does not spontaneously apply the rules of punctuation that he has been taught. At this point, the teacher or psychologist reviewing Jonathan's work would be faced with questions such as: Can I make an informed judgment about the kind of instructional program that will best address Jonathan's strengths and weaknesses as a developing writer and speller? Are Jonathan's errors predictable given the level of instruction that he currently receives? Is the instructional program sufficiently elaborated to promote a full range of skill development in composition?

If his current instructional program was limited in scope, Jonathan's understanding of punctuation might be anchored to the ditto sheet exercises used to illustrate rules. If the teacher did not plan transfer activities properly or has yet to teach children how worksheet exercises map onto creative writing assignments, then rule application becomes a function of an individual child's ability to bridge cognitive gaps in instruction. It might also be the case that the parental instructions to write a story were too open-ended, obscuring Jonathan's ability to produce more sophisticated work. For whatever reason, he seems to have interpreted his father's instructions as emphasizing content over form; thus, his literal response was to produce ideas, to get his thoughts on paper.

From a qualitative perspective, we might be very pleased with Jonathan's story. The story, though untitled, has a clear beginning, character introduction and development, a logical story line, and a conclusion. We would also note that he has attempted to put images into words even though he apparently lacks the more conventional or most efficient words for describing his image. For example, on page 4, when Jonathan writes, "maid a mimic of the king's reporter so the king's men let the Drawbridge Down," the reader smiles and thinks, "Oh, he must mean that the elf is attempting to disguise himself so that he can gain access to the castle and rescue his friend." Thus, we see in Jonathan's work evidence of good problem-solving skills, along with an ability to generate a logical progression of ideas in story form. We might also appreciate the richness in descriptive language used to support and elaborate his theme. Finally, although the story ends rather abruptly, our inclination is to think that this was more a function of the lack of paper, precipitating a need to end the story, than of not knowing how to close out the elves' adventure. In sum, from a qualitative perspective, Jonathan's work, given his age and the amount of time spent learning how to write, is most impressive.

Combining the two analyses, then, our initial thoughts are that an instructional program for Jonathan need not place a great deal of emphasis on teaching him how to sequence events. He does not appear to have any difficulty remembering or following the episodic train of thought characteristic of story telling. He manages to communicate his ideas on paper, but his technical writing skill appears somewhat underdeveloped for his age and experience. We might therefore recommend that an instructional program be designed along the lines suggested in the work of Graham and Harris (Chapter 11, this volume). Their work in written language emphasizes systematic instruction, teaching children how to be strategic in approaching problem-solving tasks such as composition writing. Fundamental to this type of instruction is the use of mnemonic devices such as COPS (Capitalization, Overall appearance, Punctuation, and Spelling) that remind children to carry out specific actions in a certain order. Thus, using such a program, children learn that certain rules and conventions appropriate to one setting or assignment are equally important across a number of different but related task environments.

Do we have enough information and have we done enough analysis to match Jonathan to an instructional program and move on to the next child? Maybe. Current thinking in the area of assessment (see Goetz & Hall, 1984; Goetz, Hall, & Fetsco, in press) emphasizes the dynamic nature of information processing characteristic of all individuals. This means that how questions are asked of children and how children are prompted to provide answers greatly influences the quality and quantity of work produced. Thus, before we would feel comfortable with the claim that Jonathan's technical writing skills are inadequate or underdeveloped, it is necessary to return to his story and ask him to respond to a different set of questions.

The father's first reaction to Jonathan's handwritten presentation was neither alarm at what wasn't there nor elation at what was there. Rather, the data-gathering process was viewed as incomplete. The father's response was to give Jonathan another assignment, related to the first, that would provide a clearer understanding of what Jonathan knew or did not know. His father suggested that he type his story into the computer. Although Jonathan does not know how to type, he is, like many children his age, fascinated with the computer. Hence, this suggestion was welcomed as a new and exciting adventure. Before he got started, however, his father mentioned that it might be a good idea to begin the story with a title and that the story might need some changes and additions in capitalization, punctuation, and spelling. The father also remarked that editorial changes could be made following entry of the story into the computer. Jonathan, anxious to get started, was given an illustration of how editorial changes might affect his original work by reviewing the first four lines plus one word of his story. Following this explanation, Jonathan asked a question about how to spell the word *captured* and told his father that at the end of his story he couldn't think of the word that was used to describe a jail in castles. The correct spelling for the word *captured* was discussed, and the word *dungeon* was suggested as a synonym for a castle's jail, to which Jonathan replied, "Yeah, that's it." Finally, possible titles for his story were reviewed, some pointers about how to use the word-processing program on the computer were given, and Jonathan embarked on his adventure. After about two hours of work, spread over three sessions, he produced a typed version of his orginal story. Figure 5-2 presents that version exactly as it was typed by Jonathan. Upon finishing, Jonathan announced that he had already "edited" his story and was ready to add some graphic illustrations and print it out.

FIGURE 5-2. Edited version of Jonathan's story typed into computer.

The Elves' Adventure
Once upon a time, there were two elves. They were big elves not
small ones. So they hid in the forest of darkness. Nobody ever went
there because a bad king lived there. In fact this king hated elves. He
would kill the princess of everything that's how bad he really was.
These elves were brave. One day the king sent two of his men to hunt
for food. And on that night the elf had been captured by the king's men.
The other elf was looking for him and all of the sudden he saw two
thing's that the other elf was wearing and he found some tracks of the
other elf. The tracks lead him right to the bad king's castle so from that
point on he tip-e-toed to the drawbridge and made a mimic of the
king's reporter. So the king's men let the drawbridge down and the elf
ran in the the castle! He hid in a safe place. When the king saw people
running, which they were not supposed to do, he ran after them. The elf
ran to the dungeon to free his friend. On his way to the dungeon, he
saw some ropes. He lowered it between the two bars. And pulled the elf
up and lived happily ever after   The End

The most notable thing about Jonathan's edited version is that it truly is
edited. Each of his sentences begins with a capital letter, and except for the last
sentence, all end with periods. The story has gone from one sentence to 18
sentences. Moreover, Jonathan has removed inappropriate capital letters that
were in the middle of sentences, corrected misspelled words, tried to use
commas, experimented with complex sentence structure, and added one excla-
mation point! And, while some of Jonathan's sentences are fragments, those
like "And on that night the elf had been captured by the king's men," would be
perfectly acceptable if appropriate punctuation had been used. On balance,
Jonathan's editing efforts are excellent and well informed.

What can be learned from this second effort? First, Jonathan clearly had
more technical information about writing than was reflected in his initial draft.
The combination of instruction, being able and willing to read, and a creative
mind have resulted in sophisticated and intricate information processing in this
7-year-old boy. Even his misspelled words reflect a substantial understanding
of English orthography (see Hall, Gerber, & Stricker, Chapter 14, this volume). Second, we are impressed with Jonathan's response to the opportunity
to edit. With very little prompting, we found that he had available much
additional information that could be used to improve the quality and clarity of
his own work. This illustrates how prompting can influence information gathering during the assessment process. Later in this chapter, we will discuss
Vygotsky's zone of proximal development and how contemporary thought on
assessment is beginning to stress that dynamic interactions between individual,

task, environment, and instructions need to be represented in ability and achievement evaluations. As we will point out, it is important, from an instructional standpoint, to match the content of instruction accurately to the level of already acquired skill. Third, when asked why he didn't captialize and punctuate in his first draft, Jonathan's response was that he was concentrating on content and couldn't think too hard about where to put commas, capitals, and periods. This is consistent with his verbal reports when, as a preschooler, he was asked why he sometimes reversed letters while spelling difficult words. Apparently, Jonathan is sensitive to his own level of skill development and recognizes that limitations in his information-processing capacity require that essential and inessential information be separated and prioritized. His response also reminds us that, when used cautiously, verbal report data can enrich interpretations of child behavior. We will illustrate how verbal report data has been used to improve our understanding of strategic behavior later in the chapter.

OF TEACHERS AND STUDENTS— THE TEACHER'S DILEMMA: WHERE TO TURN?

In examining Jonathan's story, we have had the luxury of three academics painstakingly analyzing a single child's performance at their leisure, not to mention the special attention bestowed by one of the authors, as befits his role as proud parent. But what happens in classrooms where 20 to 35 students and multiple programs confront the teacher daily? Although Jonathan does not appear to require any special attention or major revision of instruction, many students do. In view of the challenges inherent in interpreting and guiding students' academic performance, and given the other challenges facing the teacher (e.g., controlling student conduct, dealing with parents, responding to the mandates of school boards and state legislatures), teachers certainly seem in need of professional assistance. But to whom can teachers turn?

In reviewing what constitutes effective teaching, Mastropieri and Scruggs (1987) cite numerous studies to support the general notion that special educators can increase student achievement in special education by "(a) actively engaging students on task during instruction, (b) presenting information in clear, concise ways, (c) asking students questions relevant to the instructional objectives, (d) keeping students actively involved in relevant instructional activities, and (e) monitoring students' performance" (p. 3). What is remarkable here is not the content or phrasing of these tenets of teacher effectiveness, but rather the absence of any reference to information typically provided by school psychologists for classroom teachers. If the primary role for school psychologists is to serve as gatekeepers, deciding who is or is not eligible for psychological services, then discussion of teacher effectiveness as related to psychoeducational assessment is not relevant. As gatekeeper, the school psychologist is charged with decreasing the probability that a teacher's "suspicion of disability" does not result in referral of students simply because certain individual difference characteristics are bothersome to them (Ysseldyke et al., 1983).

Two points, however, argue against this view of the school psychologist's role. First, as Gerber and Semmel (1984) point out, school psychologists as gatekeepers may not serve a very useful or necessary function. Although teacher ratings are subjective and technically less valid than standardized measures, teachers are generally quite accurate in identifying those who need academic and behavioral programs beyond the scope of the regular classroom (Algozzine, Christenson, & Ysseldyke, 1981). For school psychologists to remain viable in the school marketplace, the role of the school psychologist must be seen as relevant to the needs of instruction, and the gatekeeper function may not long suffice.

Second, with the push to make school psychology a doctoral-level discipline, emphasis on the school psychologist as scientist/practitioner has reemerged (Fuchs & Fuchs, 1986; Pryzwansky, 1987). This view serves to expand the contributions of school psychologists to include the collection and interpretation of data that paint a rich and detailed picture of the status of a given child's academic development. A school psychologist functioning under this mandate should be prepared to help regular classroom teachers formulate and evaluate alternative instructional strategies for children referred for testing.

In a recent review of ability grouping and student achievement in elementary schools, Slavin (1987) asserts that available empirical evidence does not argue for the placement of children into self-contained classes, but instead supports the view that ability grouping is maximally effective when done for only one or two subjects. While Gamoran (1987) and Hiebert (1987) are critical of Slavin's conclusions on the grounds that he did not control for context of instruction or conceptual adequacy in evaluating effect sizes based on a "best-evidence synthesis" technique, the real impact of Slavin's comments are felt in his commentary on what makes ability grouping effective. When heterogeneity in a specific skill is greatly reduced, when group assignments are frequently reassessed, and when teachers vary the level and pace of instruction according to students' needs, then ability grouping and classroom instruction are maximally effective. For the classroom teacher to achieve these not so modest goals, we would argue that school psychologists need to be prepared to offer instructional support in the form of program evaluation techniques and data collection and interpretation skills. This type of preparation places school psychologists in a position to help (1) identify effective teaching practices, (2) provide instructional leadership, and (3) identify appropriate instructional materials. In essence, school psychologists can contribute to the development of what Hiebert (1987) and Rothrock (1961) view as the key to effective instruction: well-qualified teachers.

Given the position that school psychologists should function as problem solvers in their roles as scientist/practitioners, the primary purpose of testing should be to determine (1) where a given child is relative to the attainment of some fluent cognitive skill, (2) how individual difference variables affect skill development in a given academic area, and (3) what educational goals and objectives are crucial to promote steady academic progress at a given point in time. If the central goal for testing is to guide and monitor instruction, then determining those variables that have an impact on teacher effectiveness (e.g., equating time allocated with time engaged) and how those variables can be positively affected (e.g., addressing precise behavioral objectives at the correct level of difficulty) becomes important for the school psychologist who wants to make substantive contributions to the instructional needs of children (Deno, 1986; Howell, 1986; Lentz & Shapiro, 1986; Sewell, 1987).

As scientist/practitioner, the school psychologist needs a strong theoretical base. As a professional colleague of the school psychologist, the teacher needs to be conversant with the principles and concepts that form the theoretical base. But what is that theoretical base to be? The strict behaviorist approach to psychology is generally recognized as inadequate. Standardized tests used in our schools appear to be the products of atheoretical psychometric methodology. The diagnostic-prescriptive model that has been the cornerstone of special-education services over the past 30 years has received only tenuous theoretical support linking auditory or visual perceptual skills to reading acquisition, and almost no empirical support for diagnostic-prescriptive teaching based on contrasting auditory with visual methods of reading instruction (Kavale & Forness, 1987a, 1987b). There has been a call for a paradigm shift (Kuhn, 1970) that would provide a new theoretical base (Forness & Kavale, 1987). Fortunately, one has already taken place in psychology. The experimental study of learning has shifted from a behavioristic to a cognitive perspective.

Before one can examine how current work in cognitive psychology might provide a partial answer to the teacher's dilemma, one must first be familiar with the basic premises and constructs of the cognitive approach. Therefore, we have divided our treatment of information processing and cognitive assessment into two companion chapters. In this initial chapter, we will: (1) examine the origins of the current information-processing perspective in cognitive psychology, (2) provide a brief overview of some of the major constructs in cognitive psychology, and (3) outline a cognitive-instructional approach that guides educational applications. In Chapter 6, we will focus on a cognitive, information-processing analysis of academic assessment by presenting: (1) examples of how cognitive principles and techniques can be applied to the interpretation of students' performance on standardized ability tests, and (2) an alternative approach to assessment that is more in tune with cognitive tenets.

COGNITIVE PSYCHOLOGY:
THE INFORMATION-PROCESSING APPROACH

The experimental study of learning is now over 100 years old, yet our understanding of how people learn lags behind our understanding of other scientific areas such as cell biology, physics, and chemistry. Until recently, the psychology of learning has had little impact on classroom instruction beyond programmed texts and token economies. Two relatively recent developments promise to change that situation. First, cognitive psychology has once again emerged as the dominant approach to the description of human behavior. During its heyday, strict behaviorist orthodoxy had effectively maintained that the study of internal, unobservable, cognitive processes was inherently unscientific; but the emergence of new disciplines and developments have lent scientific credibility to the cognitive approach. Human factors research, information theory, and computer science provided the terminology, concepts, and models needed to breathe new life into the cognitive approach. With these new influences, however, cognitive psychology was not merely revived, it was transformed. Cognitive psychology has become information-processing psychology. Second, work in cognitive psychology has turned increasingly to the study of complex intellectual accomplishments such as the acquisition and use of knowledge in academic domains and the nature and development of academic skills such as reading and math. From an instructional perspective, the new cognitive psychology has relevance to assessment, teaching, and other classroom functions.

Origins of the Information-Processing Approach

Although current information-processing psychology is often represented as the result of a radical paradigm shift away from behaviorism, it does retain continuity in some respects with previous work in experimental psychology. Specifically, the new cognitive psychology draws heavily on the traditions of neobehaviorism, verbal learning, and human engineering (see Lachman, Lachman, & Butterfield, 1979). From neobehaviorism, information-processing psychology has taken the identification and statement of universal laws as its goal, empiricism as its method of proof, laboratory experiments as its mode of operation, and task analysis as a way of describing complex performance. Verbal learning's contribution to information-processing psychology has included a rich experimental data base, a focus on memory as a key research area, and many laboratory procedures and measurement techniques. Finally, from human engineering has come the view that humans are information processors and decision makers, and that there are limits to how much information humans can handle.

Information-processing psychology is often said to have begun with Broadbent's (1958) analysis of selective attention, although others such as Bruner, Goodnow, and Austin (1956), Miller (1956), Newell, Shaw, and Simon (1958), and Miller, Gallanter, and Pribram (1960) made important early contributions. One of the earliest applications of the information-processing approach was the development of information-processing or multistore models of human memory (Atkinson & Shiffrin, 1968; Broadbent, 1958; Waugh & Norman, 1965), which we will now sketch briefly.

These models identified the path by which information is input, or stored, and output, or retrieved. Information received at the receptors is initially held momentarily in sensory registers or sensory information store. The sensory information store serves as an input buffer that helps to maintain information from the receptors long enough for it to be perceived and analyzed.

Information that is attended to, or selected for further processing, is entered in short-term or working memory. Whereas the sensory registers are believed capable of handling all information received at the receptors, working memory can accommodate only a limited amount of information. A limited-capacity working memory is central to information-processing views of memory, whether that limitation is specified in terms of storage space or of processing power. Early descriptions of short-term memory specified a limited number of storage spaces, sufficient to hold only about seven "chunks" of information (Miller, 1956), which might be anything from digits or letters to words or even larger units, as long as they were meaningful, unitary packets of information. As is explicit in the term "short-term memory," this component of the memory system typically retains information only for a short time, say, less than half a minute. Recent characterizations have stressed the role of working memory as the central processor where information is manipulated, and have described the capacity limits of the system in terms of processing or attentional capacity.

For information to have any lasting impact or utility for the human information-tion processor, it must make it into long-term memory. Once in long-term memory, information can be stored for a very long time. In fact, current models often posit that long-term memory, is, within the lifetime of the individual, essentially permanent. Also, unlike working memory, long-term memory is viewed as having functionally unlimited capacity. It is clear that we cannot think about everything that we know at once, and the portion that we are currently thinking about is said to reside in working memory. Everything else that we know resides in long-term memory. To use this information, we must call it up to working memory, a process called "retrieval" or "activation."

Information is output by the effectors, which are guided by a response generator. Except for highly practiced responses, response output requires and competes for working memory or attentional capacity. Thus, for example, as students take notes in a lecture, their recording of the teacher's just-spoken words competes with their ability to listen to the teacher's next words. For students who are still learning to write, this interference would be so great that we would not expect them to take notes from a lecture.

Another important early landmark in the cognitive renaissance was the publication of Neisser's (1967) *Cognitive Psychology*, a highly readable synthesis of diverse and often conflicting areas of research, with many powerful insights into the workings of human cognition. Reflecting his own work and interests, Neisser (1967) devoted approximately 90% of the book to the analyses of perceptual processes. Neisser viewed perception (and also remembering) as a constructive act, emphasizing the role of elaboration and interpretation in imposing meaning on sensory inputs. For Neisser, "Visual cognition, then, deals with the processes by which a perceived, remembered, and thought-about world is brought into being from as unpromising a beginning as retinal patterns" (p. 4). He proposed analysis-by-synthesis as the means by which the perceiver actively constructs an internal cognitive representation of that which is being perceived. Neisser's emphasis on the constructive nature of human cognition served both to foreshadow the demonstrations of constructive memory processes by Bransford and others (e.g., Bransford & Johnson, 1972; see Bransford, 1979, for a review) and to revive earlier cognitive views of perception and memory, most notably those of Gestalt psychologists and of Bartlett (1932).

Neisser proposed that perception generally proceeds from preattentive processes to analysis-by-synthesis. Preattentive processes are both spatially and operationally parallel (i.e., capable of doing many operations independently and at the same time) and provide a general impression but little detail. "Analysis-by-synthesis" refers to the interpretation of perceptual inputs through the construction of an internal model. Analysis-by-synthesis requires focal attention, entails sequential and spatially serial processing, and is essential for the construction of a rich and detailed internal representation. Commenting on preattentive processes and analysis-by-synthesis, Neisser observed that "In terms of information processing, the whole is *prior* to its parts" (p. 91, emphasis in original). Thought and memory were said to involve the same sequencing of processes.

Much has happened since the publication of *Cognitive Psychology*. Information-processing psychologists have, for the most part, continued to concentrate on the "software" of the human information processor while neglecting the "hardware," as Neisser did, but the descriptions of the "software" have become increasingly sophisticated and elaborate. Cognitive processes remain a major topic of inquiry, but the descriptions of cognitive structures, strategies, and executive functions have become increasingly prominent. Perception, though still an active area of inquiry, must now share at least equal billing with the study of problem solving, comprehension, and memory. Although the continued availability of beginning college students as subjects has ensured continued study of their cognition, the cognitive development of children and adolescents and the development of expertise have come under increasing scrutiny. Cognitive psychologists have availed themselves of an increasingly rich data base, examining reaction times, speed–accuracy tradeoff curves, confusions (i.e., errors of commission), and verbal reports, as well as simple measures of accuracy of performance.

In order to provide a brief overview of these developments, recent theory and research will be partitioned, somewhat arbitrarily, into descriptions of cognitive structures, processes, strategies, and executive functions. Although no completely explicit, rigorous, and comprehensive cognitive theories currently exist (perhaps Anderson's 1983 ACT* model comes closest), it seems likely that any such theory would have to provide an account of structure, process, strategy, and executive function. Similarly, instructional application of the cognitive information-processing approach may be guided by analyses of the structures, processes, strategies, and executive functions involved in academic tasks. After reviewing these areas, we will briefly examine the cognitive instructional approach that embodies many of the educational implications emanating from information-processing research.

Cognitive Structures

By "cognitive structures" we mean models of the internal representation of information in memory, that is, the structures of knowledge. The need for the representation of large volumes of information in accessible and usable formats in artificial intelligence systems, advances in the study of semantics in linguistics, and the emergence of semantic memory as a major area of inquiry in cognitive psychology have spurred the development of increasingly sophisticated descriptions of cognitive structure. These structures not only code information already acquired, but also guide perception and the acquisition of new knowledge. Learning is described as the creation, alteration, and augmentation of knowledge structures.

Early models of semantic memory proposed network structures for the representation of knowledge. EPAM, the Elementary Perceiver and Memorizer (Feigenbaum, 1963; Simon & Feigenbaum, 1964) and SAL, the Stimulus and Association Learner (Hintzman, 1968) employed discrimination nets to recognize (i.e., discriminate between) stimuli and produce appropriate (i.e., associated) responses. The discrimination nets were networks of sequential, branching tests leading to a terminal node that constituted the internal representation of the stimulus and provided access to the associated response(s). Although these models suffered from a number of serious difficulties (see, for example, Anderson & Bower, 1973, pp. 74–77), they did introduce useful representational constructs that were employed in later structural models.

The model that served most directly as a prototype for network theories of semantic memory, however, is Quillian's (1968, 1969) Teachable Language Comprehender. The goal of the Teachable Language Comprehender, as with other language analysis programs (e.g., Schank, 1972; Winograd, 1971), was to develop a usable internal representation of the meaning of linguistic input. The linguistic analysis employed by these models was derived, for the most part, semantically rather than syntactically, and embodied the realization that comprehension of language requires much more than linguistic information. General or "world" knowledge, and in some cases the capacity to acquire it, was built into the programs and used extensively. Quillian's model was designed to store, and retrieve upon probing, linguistic information. The Teachable Language Comprehender, like other network models (e.g., Anderson, 1976; Anderson & Bower, 1973; Kintsch, 1972, 1974; Rumelhart, Lindsay, & Norman, 1972) represented the structure of knowledge as a set of propositions, or, equivalently, as a network of nodes and links. The nodes represented concepts, and the links represented the relationships between concepts.

An alternative approach to the structure of knowledge has been developed under the rubric of schema theory. Although related use of the term "schema" can be traced to Kant (1963–1787), Wulf (1922, translated 1938), Bartlett (1932), and Piaget (1926), the recent popularity of schema theories has been sparked by the work of Minsky (1975) and others (e.g., Norman & Rumelhart, 1975; Schank & Abelson, 1977; Winograd, 1975) in artificial intelligence. Minsky was interested in how people quickly construct an organized representation (i.e., perception) of an object as complex as a room. He became convinced that this nearly immediate organization must be based on preexisting knowledge structures that can be quickly mobilized and used to guide the processing of visual information. These structures, called "frames" by Minsky and "scripts," "plans," and "schemata" by others, have been promulgated as the type of knowledge structures required for machine perception and language comprehension. Schema theory has also attracted much attention in cognitive and educational psychology (e.g., Anderson, 1977, 1978; Anderson & Pearson, 1984; Bower, Black, & Turner, 1979; Rumelhart, 1980; Rumelhart & Ortony, 1977; Schallert, 1982).

Schemata are prototypical representations of objects and events that specify the component parameters and their interrelations. For example, the schema for an elementary classroom might include parameters such as *students, chairs, teacher,* and *desk,* and relationships such as *students belong in chairs, desk belongs to teacher, desk is at front of classroom.* A schema provides a ready-made structure into which information can be assimilated, much as slots or placeholders accept information that specifies relevant parameters. This process is termed "instantiation." Thus, upon entering a classroom, we can quickly encode information about the nature and location of students, chairs, teacher's desk, and the like. Schemata can exist at various levels of abstraction. They can: (1) self-embed, (2) code specific experiences as instantiated schemata, (3) guide processing during storage and retrieval, and (4) support inferencing through the use of default values for unspecified parameters.

Recently, it has become popular to distinguish between two basic types of knowledge, declarative and procedural (Anderson, 1982, 1983). This division reflects differing form and function. *Declarative knowledge* is represented in propositional networks, and it corresponds to our factual knowledge or knowledge *that.* When we recall *that* February has 28 days, or *that* George Washington was the first president, or *that* plants give off oxygen, we are drawing on our declarative knowledge structures. *Procedural knowledge* is represented in production systems and corresponds to our knowledge of *how* to do things, that is, our knowledge *how.* When we demonstrate that we know *how* to tie our shoes, or *how* to type a letter, or *how* to do long division, our performance is guided by procedural knowledge structures.

Production systems are composed of ordered sets of productions or condition–action pairs (Newell & Simon, 1972), that follow the logic of *if–then.* Certain conditions must be met *if* the production is to be applied. Once it has been determined that the conditions have been met, *then* certain actions are taken. In doing long division, for example, one checks to see *if* the divisor will go into the first digit: *if* it will, *then* division can proceed; if not, we must group the first two digits of the dividend together and once again test to see if the divisor can be accommodated. The sequencing of productions in a production system results from the fact that the actions of earlier productions help to produce the conditions required for the application of the later productions. In reviewing the distinction between declarative and procedural knowledge, one of Anderson's (1982, 1983) major contributions has been the specification of a theory of the development of procedural knowledge. We will examine this model and its implications for assessment and instruction later in this chapter.

Although there has been a great deal of concentration on cognitive structures, any structural model that predicts or stimulates human performance must specify processes that act on the postulated structures. In addition, a fair amount of theory and research has focused on cognitive processes. In the next section, we turn our attention to developments in the description of cognitive processes.

Cognitive Processes

In information-processing models, the function of cognitive processes is the manipulation of information. Basic processes include information storage, retrieval, recoding, reduction, and elaboration. As in the case of cognitive structures, current conceptions of cognitive processes strongly reflect the influences of the computer analogy and the analysis of general information systems. Postulated human cognitive processes are viewed as functionally equivalent to the data input, manipulation, and output functions of computers and other information systems. While early cognitive models focused on perceptual processes, subsequent work has provided detailed procedural models of comprehension (e.g., Kintsch & van Dijk, 1978), recall (e.g., Collins & Loftus, 1975), and problem solving (e.g., Simon, 1978).

Although the details of cognitive processes such as "spreading activation" (Collins & Loftus, 1975) and "processing cycles" (Kintsch & van Dijk, 1978) may differ, there are common issues to which many of the models can be related. For example, models of perception and comprehension can be classified as "bottom-up" or data-driven (e.g., Gough, 1972; La Berge & Samuels, 1974), "top-down" or conceptually driven (e.g., Norman & Bobrow, 1975), or interactive (e.g., Neisser, 1976; Rumelhart, 1975; Stanovich, 1980). Whether processing proceeds in a parallel or sequential fashion would appear to be another such common issue, but the issue has become increasingly cloudy. Some theorists assume that all human information processing occurs "essentially serially, one-process-at-a-time, not in parallel fashion" (Simon & Newell, 1971, p. 149), but others are not so certain.

Whereas Neisser (1967) originally posited parallel preattentive processes followed by sequential attentional processes, subsequent work has stressed the effect of extended practice in transforming attention-demanding sequential processing to processing requiring so little time or attention that it can run off simultaneously with other processing (e.g., Hirst, Spelke, Reaves, Caharack, & Neisser, 1980; La Berge & Samuels, 1974; Neisser, 1976; Schneider & Shiffrin, 1977; Shiffrin & Schnieder, 1977). This transformation has been described as the development of processing "automaticity" (e.g., La Berge & Samuels, 1974; Schneider & Shiffrin, 1977; Shiffrin & Schneider, 1977) but the use of this construct has been challenged on the grounds that it entails unjustifiably rigid attention capacity constraints (Hirst et al., 1980) and that it merely relabels (rather than explains) one set of research findings while glossing over contradictory results (Ryan, 1983). Further, it appears that automatic processes are both simultaneous and sequential. For example, in Schneider & Shiffrin's (1977) model, ability to run off in parallel (i.e., simultaneously) with other automatic or controlled (i.e., attentional) processes is one of the defining characteristics of automatic processes, and "An automatic process can be defined within this system as a *sequence* of nodes that nearly always become active in response to a particular input configuration . . . where the *sequence* is activated without the necessity of control or attention of the subject (Shiffrin & Schneider, 1977, pp. 155–156, emphasis added). The situation is further complicated by the fact that both automatic and controlled processes are required for many "real" cognitive acts. "Even more important, controlled processing is often used to initiate automatic processing. Particularly in complex processing situations (such as reading), an ongoing mixture of controlled and automatic processing is utilized" (Shiffrin & Schneider, 1977, p. 161). Finally, Anderson (1976) has asserted that "it is never possible to decide whether a process is serial or parallel" (p. 6) and provides a formal mathematical proof for the claim, along the lines that for any result that appears to implicate serial (or parallel) processing, an equivalent parallel (or serial) model can be found.

Recently, parallel memory search, a feature of spreading activation models (e.g., Anderson & Bower, 1973; Collins & Loftus, 1975; Collins & Quillian, 1969), has been elaborated and updated into current parallel distributed processing or neural net models (McClelland, Rumelhart, & the PDP Research Group, 1987; Rumelhart, McClelland, & The PDP Research Group, 1987). Before we discuss this work, it is important to remember that the network metaphor serves as a conceptual tool. As neurologists might be quick to point out, the anatomical basis of memory may be far different from these models, although there may be functional parallels between the human brain and current notions of parallel distributed processing or neural net models of memory.

"Spreading activation" is a term used to describe a hypothesized mechanism of memory retrieval. Activation spreads across ideas in the memory network, causing us to recall some information. In addition, activation primes other related ideas, making them more readily accessible for recall and use. In network models, concepts (declarative knowledge) are represented in memory as nodes, and conceptual relationships (procedural knowledge) are linked to nodes via associative pathways. All ideas are ultimately associated with one another in a propositional network. Although all knowledge may be interconnected, this connectedness is hidden from awareness by limitations of the information-processing system. If all pathways are interconnected, then, the pathways that bridge any two ideas may be long and complex. Thus, to get from one idea to another, many intervening ideas may have to be traversed. At any given time, almost all of the propositions in the network are inactive. In fact, because working memory is of such limited capacity, only a small portion of the propositions that are activated at any given time enter working memory (i.e., become fully activated or available to awareness).

Balota and Lorch (1987) presented four key properties of the spreading activation process that have empirical as well as theoretical support. First, the spread of activation is automatic, not subject to strategic control (Balota, 1983; Neely, 1977). Second, length of the associative pathway between a node and a source of activation determines the strength of association (i.e., the amount of activation that reaches a concept node from an activation source) (Lorch, 1982). Presumably, then, many associated propositions will not be activated when part of the memory network is activated because the associative strength for certain pathways does not exceed minimum threshold levels governing whether or not propositions become part of current working memory. Third, the amount of activation that spreads from a given node along a given pathway is a mathematical function of the associative strength of the activated pathway relative to the sum of the strengths of all the pathways that stem from the given node (Reder & Anderson, 1980). Finally, there is the multiple-step assumption of spreading activation. This property essentially accounts for the interrelatedness of all concepts within the propositional network and helps to explain a variety of memory retrieval phenomena. Activation may spread in multiple steps to concepts far across the memory network, thus accounting for category verification response latency (Collins & Quillian, 1969), mediated priming effects in pronunciation but not in lexical decision (Balota & Lorch, 1987), and episodic sentence recognition (Anderson, 1976).

In practical terms, what all this means is that students will have much more information potentially available to them in long-term memory than they can use or keep active in working memory at any one time. Further, two points regarding assessment and performance are underscored by this work. First, standardized instructions and static problem-solving environments characteristic of standardized tests may not provide the right primes to activate information that is crucial to the task at hand. Therefore, strict, quantitative interpretation of standardized ability test scores may lead to erroneous conclusions about cognitive capacity, when student difficulties are better understood in terms of cognitive competence (Bortner & Birch, 1970). Second, how children are prompted is likely to determine what and how much information gets primed for further processing. Thus, in instructional settings, it is important for teachers to adjust the level of prompting provided students to match their requirements for information organization and retrieval. Work in the area of process or dynamic assessment of ability is consistent with the notion of a reciprocal relationship between instruction and assessment (Brown & Ferrara, 1985; Brown & French, 1979; Delclos, Burns, & Kuewicz, 1987).

Cognitive Strategies

By "cognitive strategies" we mean planful, goal-oriented behavior (Flavell, 1970) that is employed in the performance of some cognitive task or in pursuit of some cognitive objective. That is, cognitive strategies are the cognitive means we select to accomplish our cognitive ends. With the advent of the information-processing approach, the nature, utility, and development of cognitive strategies has received a great deal of attention, particularly in areas such as problem solving and memory.

The work of Herbert Simon, Allen Newell, and their colleagues (e.g., Newell & Shaw, 1957; Newell & Simon, 1972; Simon, 1978, 1980; Simon & Newell, 1971) has had a tremendous impact on the study of problem solving in cognitive psychology and artificial intelligence. Their basic approach has been to develop detailed descriptions of problem-solving strategies (and structures, processes, and executive functions) based on "think aloud" protocols collected from individual human problem solvers and attempts to simulate human problem solving on the computer. The basic function of problem-solving strategies is *reduction*: reduction of the complexity of the problem representation and reduction of the disparity between the present and solution state in the problem space. Scan and search strategies bring in new information as needed. Heuristics constrain the search of possible solutions to some subset manageable under the serial-processing constraint, which they view as central to human problem solvers. Problem reduction procedures and means–ends analyses work to close the problem space by systematically identifying and fulfilling subgoals and by identifying and eliminating obstacles to solution.

In the study of memory, attention has been focused on strategies employed in information storage and retrieval. Memory strategies can be as simple as rehearsal (i.e., rote memorization) or as complex as the use of mnemonics such as the peg word or loci methods. Retrieval strategies include "dumping" or recalling the last item or two first in immediate free recall, and running through the alphabet in attempting to generate a forgotten name. The advantages of simple rehearsal and of mnemonics and other elaborative strategies such as imagery is that they increase the probability of retrieval through the construction of a distinctive, durable representation of the information encoded that is elaborately interconnected with preexisting knowledge structures. As a demonstration of the power of mnemonics as a retrieval strategy, try to recall the number of days in November—without resorting to the familiar rhyme. Although there is an extensive body of research establishing the utility of memorial strategies, there is also ample evidence that young children and less proficient learners often fail to employ even a simple rehearsal strategy in the service of memory. Brown (e.g., 1975) and others have argued that children must learn the requirements of strategies for memory tasks through exposure to the deliberate learning most often found in schools.

Cognitive Executive Functions

One effect of the advent of the information-processing approach, and of the computer as a model of the human information processor in particular, was that it provided scientific respectability for concepts that would have been attacked as rampant mentalism in earlier cognitive accounts. Before computer programming came of age, it was difficult to imagine how we could plan, orchestrate, monitor, and modify our own cognitive processes without little homunculi there to do it for us. Now we can rest assured that such executive functions can be accomplished perfectly mechanistically. Miller, Gallanter, and Pribram's (1960) *Plans and the Structure of Behavior* and their TOTE (Test–Operate–Test–Exit) unit represented an early attempt to show how an information-processing system might be given sufficient purposefulness and sophistication to regulate its own activities. The role of executive functions has received increasing emphasis in artificial intelligence (e.g., Hayes-Roth & Hayes-Roth, 1979) and in the description of the human information processor.

In cognitive psychology, and to an even greater extent in developmental psychology, executive functions have been elaborated under the rubric of metacognition, owing to the pioneering and extensive research and writing of John Flavell and Ann Brown (e.g., Brown, 1975, 1978, 1980; Flavell, 1970, 1976, 1979; Flavell & Wellman, 1977). Their research, and that of many others who have followed their lead, suggests that differences in the adequacy of planning, orchestration, monitoring, and modification of cognitive processes and strategies accounts for many of the observed differences between older and younger children, more and less "able" learners and problem solvers, and experts and novices.

Information Processing in Learning and Development: The Instructional Approach

The instructional approach was outlined by Belmont and Butterfield (1977) and further articulated by Butterfield and Belmont (1977); Brown and Campione (1978); Borkowski and Cavanaugh (1979); Brown, Campione, and Day (1981); Ryan (1981); and Brown, Bransford, Ferrara, and Campione (1983). The instructional approach was originally intended as a set of methodological principles to guide research on cognitive development. The basic idea was that the provision of instruction on the use of a cognitive strategy would provide the best evidence about a young learner's ability to use the strategy (Belmont & Butterfield, 1977). Although the implications of the instructional approach for developmental research are important, its implications for academic instruction are perhaps of greater value. Performance on school tasks can be enhanced in two ways: Either the task to be performed can be modified to accomodate the needs and skill level of the learner, or the learner can be modified to meet the prerequisite skill requirements of the task. Students experiencing academic difficulties evidence the same general pattern that has emerged from developmental and instructional research, that poor performance often results when the learner fails to bring to the problem-solving environment specific knowledge, strategies, or skills required for acceptable performance.

The instructional approach is, transparently enough, a set of guidelines useful for providing instruction on how to perform a task. As outlined by Belmont and Butterfield (1977), the development and delivery of this instruction was to be regulated by three principles: (1) direct measurement, (2) task analysis, and (3) standards of evaluation.

Direct measurement refers to the need to minimize the "logical distance" between the aspects of behavior observed and the inferred underlying cognitive processes and strategies. Although cognitive operations cannot be observed directly, it is important to use the best evidence available. The principle of direct measurement mandates that the best evidence is that which has the shortest inferential path to the student's cognitive processes and strategies. In this regard, the wealth of data collected and analyzed in information-processing research proves most helpful. Patterns of errors may reveal underlying "bugs" in students' knowledge of mathematical procedures (Brown & Burton, 1978). Response latencies may provide evidence regarding the nature and sequence of cognitive operations (Sternberg, 1985). Simply asking students to *think aloud* as they work on problems, or to provide retrospective self-reports of how they solved a problem just completed, can furnish useful evidence about task-specific cognitive processes and strategies (Ericsson & Simon, 1980, 1984).

Effective instruction, however, requires more than just an understanding of what students know and do when working on academic tasks. It also requires that we have a clear understanding of what they must know and do in order to be successful. The principle of task analysis represents this requirement. In her textbook examining school learning from an information-processing perspective, Gagne (1985) discussed two approaches to cognitive task analysis. We will refer to these approaches as prerequisite skills analysis and procedural analysis.

Prerequisite skills analysis (e.g., Gagne & Paradise, 1961) represents a hierarchy of knowledge and skills that must be acquired before you can perform a certain task. At the top of the hierarchy is the most advanced skill, the one that is the focus of the analysis. As you move down through the hierarchy, you find successively simpler skills. The idea is that to perform at any given level in the hierarchy, you must have acquired all the required skills at the lower levels. Thus, the emphasis is on the mastery of successively more complex and sophisticated skills, culminating in the ability to perform a given academic task. The prerequisite or required skills for a given task are those that appear at lower levels of the hierarchy and are linked to it.

Prerequisite skills analysis proceeds by repeatedly addressing the question, "What would the student need to know how to do to be able to perform this task independently?" For example, in order to add fractions, students must be able to identify a common denominator, multiply the numerator and denominator for each fraction by the same number, and add the fractions. Each of these skills, however, is complex and assumes mastery of simpler skills. Therefore, the question is repeated for each of the prerequisite skills identified, and the process is repeated until you reach a level of basic skill for which further reduction is unnecessary.

Procedural analysis specifies what a student must do while actually performing a task. This specification is often given in the form of underlying component processes. For example, Sternberg's (e.g., 1977) seminal work on the componential analysis of analogical reasoning specified that in order to solve an analogy problem (A:B::C:?), a student must *encode* the terms of the problem, *infer* the relationship between the A and B terms, *map* the relationship between the A and C terms, and *apply* the relationships identified through inferring and mapping to generate (or recognize) an appropriate answer. Procedural analysis can also be couched in more general, functional terms. For example, Flower and Hayes's (e.g., 1981) analysis of the task of writing includes the major functions of *planning* what is to be written (i.e., establishing a goal for writing, generating and organizing one's thoughts); *translating* one's thoughts into words, sentences, and text; and *reviewing* (i.e., evaluating and revising) what has been written.

Procedural task analysis often specifies the order in which the processes or operations occur during task performance. This specification can take a variety of forms. The familiar flowchart representations of cognitive processes were borrowed from computer programming and reflect the influence of the computer model in the information-processing approach. Procedural networks (e.g., Brown & Burton, 1978) are another example of computer modeling of human cognitive processes. As discussed earlier, Anderson (1982, 1983) represents cognitive procedures as production systems or procedural knowledge structures that follow conditional, if–then, rules.

Standards of evaluation address the need to be able to determine whether instruction has been successful. The information-processing approach suggests that there should be more to the evaluation of academic skill than normative comparison or percentage correct. Normative comparisons reveal nothing about *how* a student accomplishes an academic task. Instead, they reflect only how well performance stacks up against that of age- or grade-appropriate peers. An exclusive focus on response correctness can be misleading in at least two ways. First, incorrect or incomplete cognitive procedures can produce correct responses beyond those accounted for by guessing. Second, the elimination of errors is not sufficient to characterize the development of skill.

If an academic skill is to be of use to a student, its use must be fluent and require minimal effort. Students are unlikely to employ or benefit from academic skills that can be applied only haltingly and with excruciating effort.

Thus, the level of proficiency in an academic skill should be evaluated as directly as possible. Anderson's (1982, 1983) theory of development of procedural knowledge is suggestive in this regard.

Anderson (1982) has proposed a theory of the development of cognitive skill in which he recognized three general stages of knowledge representation in the acquisition of cognitive skill. In the first, or declarative stage, declarative knowledge (i.e., verbal rules or facts) guides cognitive procedures. Individuals, noting that certain new facts or pieces of information are important to learning a skill, engage in self-monitoring activities that serve to keep unlearned or unfamiliar information active in short-term memory. This information is then organized for use in interpretive procedures that form the rudiments of developing skilled behaviors.

In the second stage, knowledge compilation, knowledge is transformed from an understandable verbal form to a precise, efficient symbolic code. Whereas a declarative-knowledge description of a procedure must be interpreted before it can be put to use, information in the knowledge compilation stage is stripped of interpretation, directly guiding cognitive operations. Like a computer program written in machine language, the code is in the form of commands that elicit certain operations every time specific criteria (i.e., memory states) are encountered. The individual benefits in that cognitive operations are carried out with increased speed. As a skill becomes more automatic, however, conscious control over the skill is lessened, making the skill more difficult to describe or modify. For example, it is often difficult for an "expert" to find the right words to describe the sequence of automatic actions that will best illustrate how to hit a baseball, drive a car with manual transmission, or fill out a specialized form, because the fluent act is not easily reduced to components that were a part of the rudimentary, verbalized skill. In part, this is due to the development of two companion processes during the knowledge compilation stage: proceduralization and composition. For proceduralized, composed skills, performance is characterized by automaticity (e.g., La Berge & Samuels, 1974; Schneider & Shiffrin, 1977) that speeds up processsing and frees up cognitive or attentional resources. *Proceduralization* is the replacement of declarative-knowledge descriptions of a skill with procedural-knowledge structures that are represented as systems of condition–action pairs called "productions." This aspect of knowledge compilation is referred to as an automation process. In contrast, *composition* is the replacement of many small productions with a single comprehensive production. Composition thus is an abbreviation process. In general, the compilation stage is characterized by practice and reduction in the use of verbal mediators to guide performance. As noted by Fitts (1964), this is a "smoothing out" stage.

In the final stage, application of the skill is tuned or strengthened to the appropriate situations through the processes of generalization and discrimination. That is, procedural knowledge is tuned to the environment so that individuals do what they are supposed to do when the appropriate conditions are met. Where the procedure has been too broadly applied, discrimination acts to reduce the range of application through specification of additional necessary conditions. Where the procedure has been too narrowly applied, generalization increases the range of application by eliminating unnecessary conditions.

Admittedly, this brief synopsis oversimplifies Anderson's theory. Nonetheless, it serves to point out that evaluators must go beyond attempts to determine the relative presence or absence of some skilled behavior. We must seek to assess the skill in terms of its progress toward automatic, fine-tuned performance. The appropriate instructional support will differ depending on the student's stage of skill acquisition (Glaser, Lesgold, & Lajoie, 1987). In assessing skill development, it is essential to attend to the speed with which the task and/or its component processes are performed, as well as the accuracy of performance.

CONCLUSION

Our examination of information processing and cognitive assessment began with a consideration of the teacher's dilemma in evaluating and interpreting student performance, illustrated by an examination of Jonathan's story. We suggested that current cognitive psychology, the information-processing approach, may prove valuable in understanding what students have and have not learned, and in planning effective instruction. Much of this chapter has been devoted to providing background information regarding the cognitive, information-processing perspective, including its origins, major constraints, and instructional applications (i.e., the cognitive-instructional approach). In the following, companion chapter, we will examine, in some detail, the implications of this perspective for assessment in the schools.

REFERENCES

Algozzine, B., Christenson, S., & Ysseldyke, J. E. (1981). *Probabilities associated with the referral to placement process.* Minneapolis: Institute for Research on Learning Disabilities, University of Minnesota.

Anderson, J. R. (1976). *Language, memory and thought.* Hillsdale, NJ: Lawrence Erlbaum.

Anderson, J. R. (1982). Acquisition of cognitive skill. *Psychological Review, 89,* 369–406.

Anderson, J. R. (1983). *The architecture of cognition.* Cambridge, MA: Harvard University Press.

Anderson, J. R., & Bower, G. H. (1973). *Human associative memory.* Washington, DC: Winston.

Anderson, R. C. (1977). The notion of schemata and the educational enterprise. In R. C. Anderson, R. J. Spiro, & W. E. Montague (Eds.), *Schooling and the acquisition of knowledge* (pp. 415–431). Hillsdale, NJ: Lawrence Erlbaum.

Anderson, R. C. (1978). Schema-directed processes in language comprehension. In A. Lesgold, J. Pelligreno, S. Fokkema, & R. Glaser (Eds.), *Cognitive Psychology and Instruction*. New York: Plenum Press.

Anderson, R. C., & Pearson, P. D. (1984). A schema-theoretic view of basic processes in reading comprehension. In P. D. Pearson (Ed.), *Handbook of reading research* (pp. 255–291). New York: Longman.

Atkinson, R., & Shiffrin, R. (1968). Human memory: A proposed system and its control processes. In K. Spence & J. Spence (Eds.), *The psychology of learning and motivation: Advances in theory and research* (Vol. 2). New York: Academic Press.

Balota, D. A. (1983). Automatic semantic activation and episodic memory encoding. *Journal of Verbal Learning and Verbal Behavior, 22*, 88–104.

Balota, D. A., & Lorch, R. F., Jr. (1987). Depth of automatic spreading activation: Mediated priming effects in pronounciation but not lexical decision. *Journal of Experimental Psychology: Learning, Memory, and Cognition, 12*, 336–345.

Bartlett, F. C. (1932). *Remembering*. Cambridge: Cambridge University Press.

Belmont, J. M., & Butterfield, E. C. (1977). The instructional approach to developmental cognitive research. In R. V. Kail Jr. & J. W. Hagen (Eds.), *Perspectives on the development of memory and cognition* (pp. 437–481). Hillsdale, NJ: Lawrence Erlbaum.

Borkowski, J. G., & Cavanaugh, J. C. (1979). Maintenance and generalization of skills and strategies by the retarded. In N. R. Ellis (Ed.), *Handbook of mental deficiency: Psychological theory and research* (2nd ed.) (pp. 569–618). Hillsdale, NJ: Lawrence Erlbaum.

Bortner, M., & Birch, H. G. (1970). Cognitive capacity and cognitive competence. *American Journal of Mental Deficiency, 74*, 735–744.

Bower, G. H., Black, J. B., & Turner, T. J. (1979). Scripts in memory for text. *Cognitive psychology, 11*, 177–220.

Bransford, J. D. (1979). *Human cognition: Learning, understanding and remembering*. Belmont, CA: Wadsworth.

Bransford, J. D., & Johnson, M. K. (1972). Contextual prerequisites for understanding: Some investigations of comprehension and recall. *Journal of Verbal Learning and Verbal Behavior, 11*, 717–726.

Broadbent, D. E. (1958). *Perception and communication*. London: Pergamon Press.

Brown, A. L. (1975). The development of memory: Knowing, knowing about knowing, and knowing how to know. In H. W. Reese (Ed.), *Advances in child development and behavior* (Vol. 10, pp. 103–110). New York: Academic Press.

Brown, A. L. (1978). Knowing when, where, and how to remember: A problem of metacognition. In R. Glaser (Ed.), *Advances in instructional psychology* (pp. 77–165). Hillsdale, NJ: Lawrence Erlbaum.

Brown, A. L. (1980). Metacognitive development and reading. In R. J. Spiro, B. C. Bruce, & W. F. Brewer (Eds.), *Theoretical issues in reading comprehension: Perspectives from cognitive psychology, linguistics, artificial intelligence, and education* (pp. 453–482). Hillsdale, NJ: Lawrence Erlbaum.

Brown, A. L., Bransford, J. D., Ferrara, R. A., & Campione, J. C. (1983). Learning, remembering, and understanding. In J. H. Flavell & E. M. Markman (Eds.), *Handbook of child psychology: Vol. 3. Cognitive development* (pp. 77–166). New York: Wiley.

Brown, A. L., & Campione, J. C. (1978). Permissible inference from the outcome of training studies in cognitive development research. *Quarterly Newsletter of the Institute for Comparative Human Development, 2,* 46–53.

Brown, A. L., Campione, J., & Day, J. D. (1981). Learning to learn: On training students to learn from texts. *Educational Researcher, 10,* 2, 14–21.

Brown, A. L., & Ferrara, R. A. (1985). Diagnosing zones of proximal development. In J. V. Wertsch (Ed.), *Culture, communication, and cognition: Vygotskian perspectives* (pp. 275–304). Cambridge: Cambrige University Press.

Brown, A. L., & French, L. A. (1979). The zone of potential development: Implications for intelligence testing in the year 2000. *Intelligence, 3,* 255–277.

Brown, J. S., & Burton, R. R. (1978). Diagnostic models for procedural bugs in basic mathematical skills. *Cognitive Science, 2,* 155–192.

Bruner, J. S., Goodnow, J., & Austin, G. A. (1956). *A study of thinking.* New York: Wiley.

Butterfield, E. C., & Belmont, J. (1977). Assessing an improving the executive cognitive functions of mentally retarded people. In I. Bialer & M. Sternlicht (Eds.), *Psychological issues in mental retardation.* New York: Psychological Dimensions.

Collins, A. M., & Loftus, E. F. (1975). A spreading-activation theory of semantic processing. *Psychological Review, 82,* 407–428.

Collins, A., & Quillian, M. (1969). Retrieval time from semantic memory. *Journal of Verbal Learning and Verbal Behavior, 8,* 240–248.

Delclos, V. R., Burns, M. S., & Kulewicz, S. J. (1987). Effects of dynamic assessment on teachers' expectations of handicapped children. *American Educational Research Journal, 24,* 325–336.

Deno, S. L. (1986). Formative evaluation of individual student programs: A new role for school psychologists. *School Psychology Review, 15,* 358–374.

Ericsson, K. A., & Simon, H. A. (1980). Verbal reports as data. *Psychological Review, 87,* 215–251.

Ericsson, K. A., & Simon, H. A. (1984). *Protocol analysis: Verbal reports as data.* Cambridge, MA: MIT Press.

Feigenbaum, E. A. (1963). Simulation of verbal learning behavior. In E. A. Feigenbaum & J. Feldman (Eds.), *Computers and thought.* New York: McGraw-Hill.

Fitts, P. M. (1964). Perceptual–motor skill learning. In A. W. Melton (Ed.), *Categories of human learning.* New York: Academic Press.

Flavell, J. H. (1970). Concept development. In P. H. Mussen (Ed.), *Carmichael's manual of child psychology* (3rd ed.) (Vol. 1, p. 983–1060). New York: Wiley.

Flavell, J. H. (1976). Metacognitive aspects of problem solving. In L. B. Resnick (Ed.), *The nature of intelligence* (pp. 231–236). Hillsdale, NJ: Lawrence Erlbaum.

Flavell, J. H. (1979). Metacognition and cognitive monitoring. *American Psychologist, 34,* 906–911.

Flavell, J. H., & Wellman, H. M. (1977). Metamemory. In R. V. Kail, Jr., & J. W. Hagen (Eds.), *Perspectives on development of memory and cognition* (pp. 3–33). Hillsdale, NJ: Lawrence Erlbaum.

Flower, L., & Hayes, J. R. (1981). A cognitive process theory of writing. *College Composition and Communication, 32,* 365–387.

Forness, S. R., & Kavale, K. A. (1987). Holistic inquiry and the scientific challenge in special education: A reply to Iano. *Remedial and Special Education, 8,* 47–51.

Fuchs, L. S., & Fuchs, D. (1986). Linking assessment to instructional interventions: An overview. *School Psychology Review, 15,* 318–323.

Gagne, E. D. (1985). *The cognitive psychology of school learning.* Boston, MA: Little, Brown.

Gagne, R. M., & Paradise, N. E. (1961). Abilities and learning sets in knowledge acquisition. *Psychological Monographs: General and Applied, 75,* (Whole No. 518).

Gamoran, A. (1987). Organization, instruction, and the effects of ability grouping: Comment on Slavin's "best-evidence synthesis." *Review of Educational Research, 57,* 341–346.

Gerber, M. M., & Semmel, M. I. (1984). Teacher as imperfect test: Reconceptualizing the referral process. *Educational Psychologist, 19,* 137–148.

Glaser, R., Lesgold, A., & Lajoie, S. (1987). Toward a cognitive theory for the measurement of achievement. In R. R. Ronning, J. A. Glover, J. C. Conoley, & J. C. Witt (Eds.), *The influence of cognitive psychology on testing* (pp. 41–85). Hillsdale, NJ: Lawrence Erlbaum.

Goetz, E. T., & Hall, R. J. (1984). Evaluation of the Kaufman Assessment Battery for Children from an information-processing perspective. *Journal of Special Education, 18,* 281–296.

Goetz, E. T., Hall, R. J., & Fetsco, T. G. (in press). Implications of cognitive psychology for assessment of academic skill. In C. R. Reynolds & R. W. Kamphaus (Eds.), *Handbook of psychological and educational assessment* (Vol. 1). New York: Guilford Press.

Gough, P. B. (1972). One second of reading. In J. F. Kavanaugh & I. G. Mattingly (Eds.), *Language by ear and by eye.* Cambridge, MA: MIT Press.

Hayes-Roth, B., & Hayes-Roth, F. (1979). A cognitive model of planning. *Cognitive Science, 3,* 275–310.

Hiebert, E. H. (1987). The context of instruction and student learning: An examination of Slavin's assumptions. *Review of Educational Research, 57,* 337–340.

Hintzman, D. L. (1968). Explorations with a discrimination net model for paired-associate learning. *Journal of Mathematical Psychology, 5,* 123–162.

Hirst, W., Spelke, E. S., Reaves, C. C., Caharack, G., & Neisser, U. (1980). Dividing attention without alternation or automaticity. *Journal of Experimental Psychology: General, 109,* 98–117.

Howell, K. W. (1986). Direct assessment of academic performance. *School Psychology Review, 15,* 324–335.

Kant, E. (1963). *Critique of pure reason* (N. Kemp Smith, Trans.). London: MacMillan. (Original work published 1787.)

Kavale, K. A., & Forness, S. R. (1987a). The far side of heterogeneity: A critical analysis of empirical subtyping research in learning disabilities. *Journal of Learning Disabilities, 20,* 374–382.

Kavale, K. A., & Forness, S. R. (1987b). Substance over style: Assessing the efficacy of modality testing and teaching. *Exceptional Children, 54,* 228–239.

Kintsch, W. (1972). Notes on the structure of semantic memory. In E. Tulving & W. Donaldson (Eds.), *Organization of memory* (pp. 247–309). NY: Academic Press.

Kintsch, W. (1974). *The representation of meaning in memory.* Hillsdale, NJ: Lawrence Erlbaum.

Kintsch, W., & van Dijk, T. A. (1978). Toward a model of text comprehension and production. *Psychological Review, 85,* 363–394.

Kuhn, T. S. (1970). *The structure of scientific revolutions* (2nd ed.). Chicago: University of Chicago Press.

La Berge, D., & Samuels, S. J. (1974). Toward a theory of automatic information processing in reading. *Cognitive Psychology, 6,* 293–323.

Lachman, R., Lachman, J. L., & Butterfield, E. C. (1979). *Cognitive psychology and information processing: An introduction.* Hillsdale, NJ: Lawrence Erlbaum.

Lentz, F. E., Jr., & Shapiro, E. S. (1986). Functional assessment of the academic environment. *School Psychology Review, 15,* 346–357.

Lorch, R. F. (1982). Priming and search processes in semantic memory: A test of three models of spreading activation. *Journal of Verbal Learning and Verbal Behavior, 21,* 468–492.

Mastropieri, M. A., & Scruggs, T. E. (1987). *Effective instruction for special education.* Boston, MA: Little, Brown.

McClelland, J. L., Rumelhart, D. E., & The PDP Research Group. (1987). *Parallel distributed processing: Explorations in the microstructure of cognition: Vol. 2. Psychological and biological models.* Cambridge, MA: MIT Press.

Miller, G. A. (1956). The magical number seven, plus or minus two: Some limits on our capacity for processing information. *Psychological Review, 63,* 81–97.

Miller, G. A., Gallanter, E., & Pribram, K. (1960). *Plans and the structure of behavior.* New York: Holt.

Minsky, M. (1975). A framework for representing knowledge. In P. Evinston (Ed.), *The psychology of computer vision* (pp. 211–280). New York: Winston.

Neely, J. H. (1977). Semantic priming and retrieval from lexical memory: Roles of inhibitionless spreading activation and limited capacity attention. *Journal of Experimental Psychology, 106,* 226–254.

Neisser, U. (1967). *Cognitive psychology.* New York: Appleton-Century Crofts.

Neisser, U. (1976). *Cognition and reality: Principles and implications of cognitive psychology.* San Francisco: Freeman.

Newell, A., & Shaw, J. C. (1957). Programming the Logic Theory Machine. *Proceedings of the 1957 Western Joint Computer Conference (February 26–28),* pp. 230–240.

Newell, A., Shaw, J. C., & Simon, H. A. (1958). Elements of a theory of human problem solving. *Psychological Review, 65,* 151–166.

Newell, A., & Simon, H. (1972). *Human problem solving.* Englewood Cliffs, NJ: Prentice-Hall.

Norman, D. A., & Bobrow, D. G. (1975). On data limited and resource limited processes. *Cognitive Psychology, 7,* 44–64.

Norman, D. A., & Rumelhart, D. E. (1975). *Explorations in cognition.* San Francisco: Freeman.

Piaget, J. (1926). *The language and thought of the child.* New York: Harcourt Brace.

Pryzwansky, W. B. (1987). The school psychologist as scientist and practitioner. *The School Psychologist: Division of School Psychology Newsletter, 41* (June), 1–2.

Quillian, M. R. (1968). Semantic memory. In M. Minsky (Ed.). *Semantic information processing* (pp. 227–270). Cambridge, MA: MIT Press.

Quillian, M. R. (1969). The teachable language comprehender. *Communications for Computing Machinery, 12,* 459–476.

Reder, L. M., & Anderson, J. R. (1980). A partial resolution of the paradox of interference: The role of integrating knowledge. *Cognitive Psychology, 12,* 447–472.

Rothrock, D. G. (1961). Heterogeneous, homogeneous, or individualized approach to reading? *Elementary English, 38,* 233–235.

Rumelhart, D. E. (1975). Notes on a schema for stories. In D. G. Bobrow & A. M. Collins (Eds.), *Representation and understanding: Studies in cognitive science* (pp. 211–236). New York: Academic Press.

Rumelhart, D. E. (1980). Schemata: The building blocks of cognition. In R. J. Spiro, B. C. Bruce, & W. F. Brewer (Eds.), *Theoretical issues in reading comprehension* (pp. 33–58). Hillsdale, NJ: Lawrence Erlbaum.

Rumelhart, D. E., Lindsay, P., & Norman, D. A. (1972). A process model for long-term memory. In E. Tulving & W. Donaldson, *Organization of memory* (pp. 198–245). New York: Academic Press.

Rumelhart, D. E., McClelland, J. L., & The PDP Research Group. (1987). *Parallel distributed processing: Explorations in the microstructure of cognition: Vol. 1. Foundations.* Cambridge, MA: MIT Press.

Rumelhart, D. E., & Ortony, A. (1977). The representation of knowledge in memory. In R. C. Anderson, R. J. Spiro, & W. E. Montague (Eds.), *Schooling and the acquisition of knowledge* (pp. 99–135). Hillsdale, NJ: Lawrence Erlbaum.

Ryan, E. B. (1981). Identifying and remediating failures in reading comprehension: Toward an instructional approach for poor comprehenders. In G. E. MacKinnon & T. G. Waller (Eds.), *Reading research: Advances in theory and practice* (pp. 224–262). New York: Academic Press.

Ryan, E. B. (1983). Reassessing the automaticity–control distinction: Item recognition as a paradigm case. *Psychological Review, 90,* 171–178.

Schallert, D. L. (1982). The significance of knowledge: A synthesis of research related to schema theory. In W. Otto & S. White (Eds.), *Reading expository material* (pp. 13–48). New York: Academic Press.

Schank, R. C. (1972). Conceptual dependency: A theory of natural language understanding. *Cognitive Psychology, 3,* 552–631.

Schank, R. C., & Abelson, R. (1977). *Plans, scripts, goals, and understanding.* Hillsdale, NJ: Lawrence Erlbaum.

Schneider, W., & Shiffrin, R. M. (1977). Controlled and automatic human information processing: I. Detection, search, and attention. *Psychological Review, 84,* 1–66.

Sewell, T. (1987). Perspectives. *The School Psychologist: Division of School Psychology Newsletter, 41,* (June), 1, 3–5, 10.

Shiffrin, R. M., & Schneider, W. (1977). Controlled and automatic information processing: II. Perceptual learning, automatic attending, and a general theory. *Psychological Review, 84,* 127–159.

Simon, H. A. (1978). Information-processing theory of human problem-solving. In W. K. Estes (Ed.), *Handbook of learning and cognitive processes* (pp. 271–295). Hillsdale, NJ: Lawrence Erlbaum.

Simon, H. A. (1979). *Models of thought.* New Haven, CT: Yale University Press.

Simon, H. A. (1980). The behavioral and social sciences. *Science, 209,* 72–78.

Simon, H. A., & Feigenbaum, E. A. (1964). An information processing theory of some effects of similarity, familiarity, and meaningfulness in verbal learning. *Journal of Verbal Learning and Verbal Behavior, 3,* 385–396.

Simon, H. A., & Newell, A. (1971). Human problem solving: The state of the theory in 1970. *American Psychologist, 26,* 145–159.

Slavin, R. E. (1987). Ability grouping and student achievement in elementary schools: A best-evidence synthesis. *Review of Educational Research, 57,* 293–336.

Stanovich, K. E. (1980). Toward an interactive–compensatory model of individual differences in the development of reading fluency. *Reading Research Quarterly, 166,* 32–71.

Sternberg, R. J. (1977). *Intelligence, information-processing, and analogical reasoning: The componential analysis of human abilities.* Hillsdale, NJ: Lawrence Erlbaum.

Sternberg, R. J. (1985). *Beyond IQ: A triarchic theory of human intelligence.* Cambridge: Cambridge University Press.

Waugh, N. C., & Norman, D. A. (1965). Primary memory. *Psychological Review, 72,* 89–104.

Winograd, T. (1971). *Procedures as a representation for data in a computer program for understanding natural language.* Project MAC Report No. TR-84. Cambridge, MA: MIT Press.

Winograd, T. (1975). Frame representations and the declarative–procedural controversy. In D. G. Bobrow & A. M. Collins (Eds.), *Representation and understanding: Studies in cognitive science* (pp. 185–210). New York: Academic Press.

Wulf, F. (1922). Ueber die Veranerang von Vorstellungen (Gedachtnis und Gestalt), *Psychologische Forschung, 1,* 333 373. Translated and condensed by W. D. Ellis (1938) in *A sourcebook of Gestalt psychology.* London: Routledge & Kegan Paul.

Ysseldyke, J. E., Thurlow, M. L., Graden, J. L., Wesson, C., Deno, S. L., & Algozzine, B. (1983). Generalizations from five years of research on assessment and decision making. *Exceptional Education Quarterly, 4,* 75-93.

6

INFORMATION PROCESSING AND COGNITIVE ASSESSMENT II: ASSESSMENT IN THE SCHOOLS

ROBERT J. HALL
ERNEST T. GOETZ
Texas A&M University
THOMAS G. FETSCO
Dickinson State University

In the preceding chapter by Goetz, Hall, and Fetsco, we stated the need for more informative and instructionally relevant ways of assessing the performance of students like Jonathan. We argued that the cognitive, information-processing approach to this problem was promising, and attempted to present a brief primer on work in the area.

In this chapter, we would like to examine how information-processing concepts can be applied in school settings. First, we will present an information-processing analysis of how students perform on standardized ability tests. As we will see, this analysis contrasts markedly with the way such tests are often viewed. Second, we will examine how information-processing principles might be applied to more direct assessment of students' academic skills and difficulties.

STANDARDIZED ABILITY TESTS

The development of the study of individual differences (psychometrics) and of standardized tests is inextricably tied to the assessment of academic ability or intelligence. From Galton, Cattell, Spearman, and Binet (see Boring, 1950; Haney, 1984, for reviews) to the present, the development, administration, and interpretation of intelligence tests has attracted a great deal of attention and controversy. In schools, intelligence tests and other standardized ability tests are used to differentiate between types and degrees of severity of learning problems, to improve accuracy of referrals, to provide information that is useful for planning instruction, and to evaluate effectiveness of instructional programs (Goetz, Hall, & Fetsco, in press). In view of the impact of ability tests on students' academic experiences, and of all the controversy surrounding the use of such tests, it seems worthwhile to consider such instruments from an information-processing perspective.

In examining how an information-processing analysis might contribute to our understanding of how students perform across tasks and environments, we will focus on the Kaufman Assessment Battery for Children (Kaufman & Kaufman, 1983). We would like to state at the outset, however, that the approach described, and many of the conclusions reached, would apply equally well to other tests such as the Wechsler Intelligence Scales for Children or Adults, Revised (WISC-R, WAIS-R); the Stanford-Binet, Revised; or the Woodcock-Johnson Tests of Cognitive Ability. The primary motive for focusing on the Kaufman Assessment Battery for Children (K-ABC) is that it is a recently published test that was heralded as a synthesis of two diverse traditions in scientific psychology, a theoretically based test that represented a major departure from previous tests.

It is a duly noted and often decried historical fact that testing and the study of individual differences have evolved independently of experimental psychology and the study of learning and cognitive processes (e.g., Carroll, 1976; Cronbach, 1957; Resnick, 1976). Thus, psychometrics has developed primarily as an atheoretical methodology (e.g., Anastasi, 1967; Willson, 1987). Development of the K-ABC was intended to rectify this situation. The K-ABC purportedly is based on a "convergence" of theory and research in cognitive psychology and neuropsychology supporting the assertion that human cognitive processing can be classified as essentially simultaneous or sequential in nature (Kaufman & Kaufman, 1983, p. 25):

> Diverse avenues of research within cognitive psychology, neuropsychology, and related disciplines have come up with an intriguing variety of labels for the dichotomy between two basic types of information processing: sequential versus parallel or serial versus multiple (Neisser, 1967), successive versus simultaneous (Das, Kirby, & Jarman, 1975; Luria, 1966), analytic versus gestalt/holistic (Levy, 1972), propositional versus appositional (Bogen, 1969), verbal versus imagery or sequential versus synchronous (Pavio, 1975, 1976), controlled versus automatic (Schneider & Shiffrin, 1977; Shiffrin & Schneider, 1977), time-ordered versus time-independent (Gordon & Bogen, 1974), and other dichotomous labels associated with individuals such as Freud, Pavlov, Maslow, and James (Bogen, 1969).

This processing dichotomy is the foundation for interpreting results from assessment and for planning educational programs using the K-ABC and its companion instrument, the Kaufman Sequential or Simultaneous (K-SOS).

As noted previously (Goetz & Hall, 1984), however, our reading of the information-processing literature reveals no trace of convergence on a simultaneous–sequential processing dichotomy like that underlying the K-ABC.

Neisser (1967) talked of parallel preattentive processing followed by sequential attentive processing. Schneider and Shiffrin (1977) talked about controlled processes being replaced by automatic processes through extended practice under favorable (i. e., consistent) conditions. Further, Schneider and Shiffrin (also Shiffrin & Schneider, 1977) clearly and repeatedly state that they view both automatic and controlled processes as sequential. Simon and Newell (1971) claimed that all human information processing is sequential, and Anderson (1976) argued that the simultaneous–sequential controversy is empirically unresolvable. None of these theorists have considered simultaneous or sequential processing as preferred modes of processing characteristic of and varying between individuals, as in the K-ABC.

Although Neisser's (1967) distinction between parallel and sequential processes and Schneider and Shiffrin's (1977) characterization of automatic versus controlled processing reflect quite different models, neither of which appears closely aligned with the simultaneous–sequential dichotomy underlying the K-ABC, there is one area of convergence between Neisser and Schneider and Shiffrin. Both the studies reviewed by Neisser and the studies conducted and reported by Schneider and Shiffrin focused on response time as crucial in determining the nature of underlying processing. If response time increased with stimulus complexity or information load, processing was said to be sequential or controlled. If response time was independent of stimulus complexity, processing was characterized as parallel or automatic. Recently, we have embarked on a program of research to examine the Spatial Memory and Matrix Analogies subtests of the K-ABC from an information-processing perspective (Hall & Goetz, 1987; Hall, Goetz, Eckert, Stowe, and Kangiser 1987; Willson, Goetz, Hall, & Applegate, 1986). We would like to review this research briefly, beginning with Spatial Memory.

Spatial Memory

Our primary interest in conducting this line of research was to address two major issues of importance to school psychologists: (1) is performance on the Spatial Memory task of the K-ABC best viewed as an index of simultaneous processing ability? and (2) does a simple measure of correctness of response, like that collected in the standard administration of the K-ABC, represent an adequate data set for educational and psychological interpretation of performance? The latter question reflects an issue that should be of general concern to school psychologists and teachers as they interpret any standardized test. The former question is specific to the K-ABC and is important because differential diagnoses based on the sequential/simultaneous dichotomy are purported to have potential for specifying certain types of instruction. For example, simultaneous processors might be more likely to benefit from meaning emphasis or language experience approaches to teaching reading, while sequential processors might be more appropriately placed in code emphasis or phonetically based reading programs.

On the Spatial Memory subtest of the K-ABC, children are presented briefly with a page displaying several pictures of familiar objects in an array. The array is then replaced by a grid and children are asked to point to the locations where the pictures had been. Children's performance on this task is interpreted as a measure of proficiency at "simultaneous processing," one of the two components of general intelligence proposed by Kaufman and Kaufman (1983).

Spatial Memory was classified as a simultaneous processing task on the basis of factor analyses of the K-ABC subtests. Performance on these subtests was measured by the number of items correctly completed, ignoring other data that are important from the information-processing perspective, such as response time, error patterns, and self-reports. As we have previously noted (Goetz & Hall, 1984), the ordering of items on the K-ABC, based on increasing item difficulty (i.e., fewer correct answers), is more consistent with the assumption of sequential than of simultaneous processing. Relative difficulty of items on the Spatial Memory test increases as the number of objects whose locations must be remembered increases.

In our research, response times were recorded to provide a more sensitive test of the simultaneous versus sequential hypotheses. If Kaufman and Kaufman's (1983) notion of simultaneous processing is based on Neisser's parallel processing and Schneider and Shiffrin's automatic processing, and if Spatial Memory is a simultaneous-processing task, then response times should be independent of stimulus complexity once the time physically required to point to more grid locations is controlled. Converging evidence was sought from an examination of touch patterns and self-report data.

Although the K-ABC is normed for children 2½ to 12½ years old, our initial research has examined the performance of adult subjects. Adult subjects were chosen because (1) young children are less aware and/or less able to report how they perform a task and (2) analysis of adult performance will provide a developmental contrast for subsequent studies with children. Since the initial study with adults, we have tested first-, fourth-, and sixth-grade students.

In this research, we have used the original Spatial Memory task materials of the K-ABC. The materials for this task consist of sets of stimulus and response cards. On each stimulus card, several (2 to 7) familiar objects (e.g., apples, birds) are arrayed in various locations. The response cards present a grid of rectangles configured in either a 3×3 or a 3×4 array. A second set of stimulus cards was constructed for a motor task designed to control for the time required to point to various grid locations. These cards presented two to seven black boxes within grids identical to the test grids (3×3 or 3×4) of the Spatial Memory task. A microcomputer was used to regulate presentation time for the stimulus plates, to collect response times, and to record the sequence of pointing responses. In addition, a video recorder was used to provide a backup record of response sequence and posttask interview.

Procedures for the Spatial Memory task were kept as close to the standard administration procedures of the K-ABC as possible. Deviations from K-ABC administration procedures were introduced only where it was necessary to obtain information to evaluate the validity of the simultaneous-processing claim.

Each subject viewed and responded to all 21 stimuli in the K-ABC Spatial Memory task. For each item, an experimenter pushed a button starting an internal clock in the computer as he or she exposed the stimulus card. When the 5-second exposure period had expired, the computer emitted a beep, at which point the experimenter exposed the response card, simultaneously pressing a button to start a second clock. Subjects were instructed to rest their hand on a button during the presentation of the stimulus card. After the response card had been presented, subjects removed their hand from the button, pointed to the squares that corresponded to the location of the objects, and returned their hand to the button. When the subject initially touched the stimulus card, the experimenter pressed a button, registering the time to first touch. For each trial, the computer recorded three times: (1) release time (from exposure until the subject removed his or her hand from the button), (2) first-touch time (from exposure until the subject initially touched the response card), and (3) total time (from exposure until the subject returned his or her hand to the button). As the subject pointed to the response card, a second experimenter recorded the sequence of grid locations to which the subject pointed using a designated section of the computer keyboard in which each key corresponded to one of the grid cells.

Immediately after completing the Spatial Memory task, subjects were interviewed concerning their performance on the task. Initially they were asked a general question about how they remembered the locations: "Is there anything you did to help you remember where you saw the objects?" Then, for each item beginning with the final item, they were asked how they remembered where they had seen the objects.

Finally, subjects were given a perceptual-motor task designed to control for individual differences in motor speed and the extra time physically required to point to more locations. In this task, each item comprised a single card. In a 3×3 or 3×4 matrix identical in size to the response cards of the K-ABC Spatial Memory task, varying numbers of black boxes were presented. After viewing a card for 5 seconds, subjects were to remove their hand from the button on an auditory cue from the computer, point to each grid cell that contained a black box, and return their hand to the button. Release, first touch, and total times and response sequence were once again recorded.

For each subject, data from 21 spatial memory plates was collected. For the initial sample of 28 college students, this represented a total of 588 possible items for which correctness of response could be judged. Five hundred seventy-five (98%) of the possible items were available for analysis. The remaining 13 items were lost through computer malfunction or experimenter error. Evaluating the 575 responses according to the standard dichotomous scoring method suggested for the K-ABC resulted in 519 (90%) correct responses across all subjects. This represents a clear ceiling effect, reflecting the fact that this was a task for children administered to adults. Analyzed differently, however, the adult data are not uninformative relative to the question of whether or not a simple correct–incorrect judgment masks information that might be useful for interpreting performance on this task.

For each of the 21 plates, it is possible to perform more detailed analyses of correctness. Subjects were asked to recall and to touch between 2 and 7 locations on a blank grid. By preserving the touch sequence, we can generate scores reflecting approximations to correct performance across all items. Judging correctness in this fashion, subjects touched correctly 2,475 out of 2,546 (97%) possible locations. The difference between a dichotomous and a more detailed analysis of responding was even more dramatic when considering performance for only the last seven plates. The last seven plates (15–21) represent the most informationally complex arrays and contain 48% of the total possible correct touches. In addition, these last seven plates contained 97% (83 of 86) of all errors of omission and 94% (51 of 54) of all errors of commission. When scored dichotomously, 72% (138 of 191) of the responses to those plates were correct. Using the more detailed analysis, however, it was found that subjects pointed to 93% (1,143 of 1,226) of the total possible correct locations. From the detailed analysis, it was also noted that when subjects made errors, they tended to maintain or approximate the correct number of touches. That is, for the 53 plates on which errors occurred, subjects pointed to the correct number of locations 26 (49%) times. Subjects pointed to the correct number of locations ± 1 49 (92%) times.

Three measures of response time were collected for both the spatial memory and the motor tasks. For the memory task, release time and time to first touch were not strongly related to stimulus complexity ($R^2 < .02$). Total response time, however, was sensitive to stimulus complexity. The simple correlation between total time and grid size was .37 and between total time and number of locations to be recalled was .69. When between-subject variance was removed (see Anderson, Mason, & Shirey, 1984), it was found that grid size accounted for 19% of the within-subject variance for total time, and that number of correct locations contributed an additional 46%. Thus, the two indices of stimulus complexity accounted for 65% of the within-subject variance for total time on the memory task. When the motor task was used to control for time required to point to more locations, response time still increased with stimulus complexity.

Interview or introspective data have been characterized as useful for discovering psychological processes but unreliable for describing and verifying the specific characteristics of those processes (Nisbett & Wilson, 1977). Thus, verbal reports are often viewed as sources of interesting but suspect information that needs to be verified against objective performance measures. Ericsson and Simon (1980, 1984), taking a contrary position, argue that verbal reports are data and suggest that reliable and informative verbal report data are a function of: (1) how close in time subjects are interviewed following completion of a task and (2) whether or not the requested information requires subjects to infer rather than remember specific mental processing sequences.

In the present research, we attempted to follow the general guidelines offered by Ericsson & Simon (1980, 1984) for use of verbal report data. Inclusion of this data source is consistent with Ericsson's (1987) contention that verbal report data are important to understanding what psychometric tests really measure. Subjects were interviewed directly following completion of the spatial memory task, starting with the most complex and most recently seen plate (#21) and working backwards through less informationally complex plates to the beginning. Subjects were asked to recall if there was anything in or about the array that helped them to remember the locations of objects. Most informative were the data on the correspondence between touch pattern responses and verbal reports of how information was organized for retrieval for the last six plates. There was agreement between 141 of the 152 (93%) coded responses for plates 16 through 21. These six plates represented the most complex informational arrays of objects presented at the closest point in time to the interview. On the basis of the high percentage of agreement between performance and verbal report of performance, a further analysis of the interview data was warranted.

Subject responses were classified into one of the six strategic categories: rows, columns, corners, diagonals, shapes, or other. When subjects could not remember how they organized information for a specific plate, strategy use was classified as "don't know." In cases where subjects reported the use of more than one strategy, all responses were coded.

Use of a row or column strategy meant that subjects tried to chunk information by row or by column to help them remember the location of items in an array. For example, subjects using a row strategy might report that there were three objects in the first, second, and fourth positions of the first row, two objects in the middle of the second row, and two objects in the first and last positions of the third row. The use of a row or column strategy was predominant when there were 6 or 7 objects to be recalled on the 3 × 4 grid or 5 objects to be recalled on the 3 × 3 grid. It would appear that these sequential processing strategies are more likely to be used when subjects recognize that increasing stimulus complexity requires systematic organization of information if spatial locations are to be recalled accurately.

Corner and diagonal strategies tended to be used as secondary information organizers. For instance, a subject might chunk information according to a general row or column strategy, and then note that items in the first or last rows were in corners or that items in two rows were juxtaposed diagonally. For only two plates, numbers 5 and 4, were corner or diagonal strategies cited as the primary organizational aid. In plate 5 the four locations to be recalled were the four corners, and in plate 4 the two locations to be recalled formed a diagonal from the center to the lower right corner.

Shape or form was the only major strategy mentioned as an aid to recall. In general, shape strategies were used as secondary organizational sources for plates with high stimulus complexity (6 or 7 locations to be recalled) and primary sources of recall for plates of moderate stimulus complexity (3, 4, or 5 locations to be recalled). One or two objects do not represent enough locations to form recognizable shapes. Six or seven locations, on the other hand, represent enough data points that simple shapes such as boxes are not readily apparent unless the locations happen to be in straight lines such as the five data points included in the "X" in plate 20.

Finally, only about 17% of the responses were coded as "other" or "don't know." Responses such as "straight line" with no accompanying locator information (e.g., "in the middle") or "that one was just easy" were classified as "other" or "don't know," respectively. These responses typically occurred in situations of low stimulus complexity and generally reflected the fact that little or no effort was required by the adult subjects to recall locations in these arrays.

In summary, examination of the interview data is consistent with the interpretation that: (1) subjects report the use of a variety of reasonable strategies for remembering locations, (2) many of these strategies are inherently sequential (e.g., row and column strategies), and (3) strategy reports can often be directly verified against response sequences.

What we see from the analysis of adult data is that performance on a spatial memory task cannot be adequately characterized by simple measures of response correctness nor can it be described accurately as the result of simultaneous processing. A detailed analysis of performance revealed that even where subjects made mistakes, their performance was reasonably accurate with respect to the number and location of objects they had seen. If a dichotomous summary of the data were sufficient to account for all relevant response variance in performance, one would not expect to find widely discrepant response summaries upon detailed analysis of performance. Said more directly, simple and detailed performance protocols should be congruent if reliable interpretation of subject data is to be discerned. Analysis of adult data suggests an interpretation that children would be less likely to be characterized as deficient in their ability to recall spatial locations following a detailed as opposed to a dichotomous analysis of correct responses.

Analysis of response times and subjects' verbal reports failed to provide evidence for the contention that Spatial Memory is a simultaneous-processing task. Performance on the Spatial Memory subtest of the K-ABC is said to be most correctly defined in terms of a child's ability "to mentally integrate input simultaneously" (Kamphaus, Kaufman, & Reynolds, 1985, p. 178). This would mean that at the time of recall, no systematic search of short-term memory is necessary to ensure accuracy. Since information encoded simultaneously would exist in working memory as a chunk or unit, no manipulation of the information would be necessary for accurate retrieval to occur if time limits for memory traces in short-term store were not exceeded. In an integrated unit, even items in an informationally complex array should be equally available for recall. For subjects participating in this research, response times increased with item complexity in a manner that can be neither accounted for in terms of motor responses nor easily reconciled with the simultaneous-processing assumption. Under the assumption of simultaneity, controlling for motor speed in total response time should have resulted in constant decision times across information loads. This was clearly not the case in our data. As information load increased, the difference between motor and memory task times and the variance associated with those times also increased. We would interpret this to mean that subjects needed more time to respond to complex arrays because retrieval was guided by systematic search. Consistent with this interpretation were subjects' verbal reports citing the use of a variety of organizational strategies to aid recall.

In a task such as Spatial Memory, the question of whether processing is parallel or sequential might reasonably be asked with regard to input, output, and central processing (see Das, Kirby, & Jarman, 1975; Luria, 1973; and Neisser, 1967, for discussion of these topics). Although our research has focused only on direct assessment of output or retrieval processing, other memory research (e.g., mnemonics, encoding specificity) and interview data from this study support the notion that processing during input is consistent with and provides a retrieval plan for output. Presumably, by planning interventions based on presenting information sequentially or simultaneously, the K-ABC gives indication that the simultaneous versus sequential distinction applies to processing at input. We view this as problematic for the K-ABC, however, as the locus of the distinction has not been made clear. As would be expected, each of the sequential-processing tasks requires sequential recall of sequentially presented stimuli. What creates confusion is that many of the simultaneous tasks also involve sequencing. For example, Photo Series requires the proper sequencing of pictures depicting some event, and Magic Window requires identification of objects presented "sequentially" as they move past a window that reveals only a portion of the picture at any one time. To establish more clearly the nature of sequential and simultaneous processing on the K-ABC, we would argue that research investigating response time during input is needed.

Our intent in this portion of the chapter has been (1) to describe how an information-processing analysis can be overlaid on a standardized administration of a cognitive ability subtest and (2) to illustrate how detailed, information-processing analyses of performance can converge to provide more precise descriptions and clearer understandings of performance on psychometric tests. In the next section, we will turn our attention to the Matrix Analogies subtest.

Matrix Analogies

A second subtest of the K-ABC that we have examined is Matrix Analogies. In Matrix Analogies, the child must complete geometric analogy problems. Analogies generally are represented by the form A:B::C:D, read "A is to

B as C is to D." In the Matrix Analogies subtest, the A, B, and C terms are squares marked by varying geometric patterns. These patterns are arrayed in an incomplete 2 × 2 matrix:

A   B

C   ?

The child's task is to complete the analogy by selecting the appropriate pattern from seven response alternatives, orienting it properly, and placing it in the empty cell of the matrix.

Matrix Analogies, like Spatial Memory, is classified as a simultaneous-processing task on the basis of factor analyses. This classification is interesting in view of the fact that information-processing analyses of analogy problem-solving processes are decidedly sequential in nature. Sternberg's componential analysis of analogical reasoning (e.g., Sternberg, 1977; Sternberg & Rifkin, 1979) has yielded considerable support for a sequence of component processes in which the problem solver (1) *encodes* information about the terms of the analogy, (2) *infers* a relationship between the A and B terms, (3) *maps* a relationship between A and C, and (4) *applies* these relationships to determine the missing term and complete the analogy. Further support for Sternberg's analysis comes from the work of Alexander and her colleagues, who have had considerable success in improving children's performance on analogy problems through training based on Sternberg's model (Alexander, White, Haensly, & Crimmins-Jeanes, 1987; White & Alexander, 1986).

As we noted in our earlier critique of the K-ABC (Goetz & Hall, 1984), Matrix Analogies bears a striking resemblance to the geometric analogy problems studied by Mulholland, Pellegrino, and Glaser (1980). Mulholland and colleagues constructed a set of 460 true–false analogy problems by systematically varying the number of elements (e.g., circles, rectangles, or crosses) in the A term and the number of transformations (e.g., "rotate 45° to the right," "reflect on the *x* axis") required to specify the relationship between A and B. The number of elements and A–B transformations and their interactions had dramatic effects on response time, accounting for a total of more than 95% of the variance in the means of various types of true problems. Since Neisser (1967) and Schneider and Shiffrin (1977) argued that increases in response time with increasing item complexity indicated that the underlying processing was sequential or controlled in nature, Mulholland and co-workers' result would appear to contradict the assumption that Matrix Analogies is a simultaneous-processing task. Further, Mulholland *et al.* found that response correctness was strongly affected by the number of A–B transformations. They developed a model with three processing stages, each with recursive sequential processing, to describe their findings. There is perhaps no term less apt than "simultaneous processing" to describe this model.

Recently, we applied an item analysis to the K-ABC Matrix Analogies test (Willson *et al.*, 1986) based on the work of Mulholland *et al.* (1980). Through inspection of the K-ABC items, we determined the number of elements in the A term and the number of A–B and A–C transformations with reasonable interrater reliability. We then analyzed the original K-ABC norming data to determine the effect of these item parameters. Our analyses were constrained by the two limitations inherent in the data set. First, only binary correct–incorrect response data was available. Second, only 16 items were available for analysis. The subtest is made up of only 20 items, the first 4 of which present simple pictures rather than geometric forms. For younger children, only 8 of these items are administered. Further, whereas Mulholland *et al.* constructed their items to vary item parameters systematically, the K-ABC Matrix Analogy items were selected on the basis of psychometric properties, and thus do provide systematic variation of item parameters. In view of these limitations, it is noteworthy that our analyses revealed that the number of elements and the number of transformations in the items had a small but significant effect on children's performance. Therefore, even the original norming data of the K-ABC appear to suggest that the Matrix Analogies test is better interpreted in terms of a sequential, information-processing model, like those developed by Sternberg and Mulholland *et al.*, than as a reflection of simultaneous processing as assumed for the K-ABC.

In summary, investigations of Spatial Memory and Matrix Analogies suggest that an information-processing analysis of student's performance may diverge sharply from the standard psychometric interpretation or from the one presented in the test manual. The present results appear to contradict the assumption underlying the K-ABC and K-SOS, that performance on memory and other cognitive tasks can be reduced to simplistic explanations characterized by the simultaneous–sequential processing dichotomy. It appears that the simultaneous–sequential approach to differential diagnosis may prove no more successful than other diagnostic-prescriptive approaches that have characterized special education in the past (Forness & Kavale, 1987). The information-processing analysis illustrated in our studies of the K-ABC might easily be applied to tasks on other standardized tests such as the Concept Formation, Analysis/Synthesis, or Analogies subtests from the Woodcock-Johnson Tests of Cognitive Ability, or to Block Design from the WISC-R. In the next section, we will examine an alternative approach to assessment that is more in keeping with the implications of information-processing theory and research than are currently available standardized tests.

ALTERNATIVE APPROACHES TO ASSESSMENT

Dissatisfaction with the standard psychometric approach to testing and advances in cognitive psychology have led to the development of an alternative information-processing approach to assessment (Goetz, Hall, & Fetsco, in press; Ronning, Conoley, & Glover, 1987; Sternberg, 1984). Consistent with the principles of direct measurement from the instructional approach described earlier, information-processing analysis of students' performance will be most informative when applied directly to the tasks on which a student is experiencing difficulties. Further, given the nature of the limitations of working memory capacity and the vagaries of retrieval or activation of information from long-term memory, conclusions about students' knowledge base and cognitive skills are likely to prove most accurate when derived through a dynamic instructional interaction between teacher (or other educational professional, such as a school psychologist) and student. In this section we would like to describe briefly dynamic or process assessment techniques that appear directly to address these concerns.

Dynamic and Process Assessment

Several authors have concluded that the best method to deal with the inadequacies of standardized tests is to supplement or replace them with direct measures of learning (Budoff & Corman, 1976; Feuerstein, Rand, & Hoffman, 1979; Howell, 1986; Swanson, 1984; Vygotsky, 1978). These learning-based assessment procedures have been labeled "dynamic assessment procedures" by some (Brown & Ferrara, 1985; Carlson & Wiedl, 1980) and "process assessment procedures" by others (Haywood, Fuller, Shifman, & Chatelanet, 1975; Kratochwill, 1977; Meyers, Pfeffer, & Erlbaum, 1985). Traditionally included as dynamic or process assessment models are the works of Budoff and his associates at Cambridge (Budoff & Corman, 1976), Vygotsky's work with the zone of proximal development (Vygotsky, 1978), Haywood's work with the learning efficiency of children with cultural–familial retardation (Gordon & Haywood, 1969; Haywood & Switzky, 1974), and Feuerstein's work with mediated learning (Feuerstein, Rand, & Hoffman, 1979; Feuerstein, Rand, Hoffman, & Miller, 1980). Other recently developed process assessment models are Meyers, Pfeffer, & Erlbaum's (1985) process assessment model, Swanson's (1984) multidimensional assessment model, and the direct assessment or curriculum-based assessment model (Fuchs & Fuchs, 1986; Howell, 1986). In a recent examination of the implications of cognitive psychology for assessment of academic skill (Goetz et al., in press), we described some of the differences between the various approaches to dynamic and process assessment and summarized some of the major conclusions derived from the work. In this chapter, we would like to discuss briefly the seminal work in this area, Vygotsky's (1978) zone of proximal development (ZPD).

Assessment in the Zone of Proximal Development

Vygotsky's development of ZPD procedures was motivated in part by his concern with the use of standardized ability and achievement tests to assess learning efficiency (Griffin & Cole, 1984). Vygotsky believed that ability tests often underpredicted children's ability to profit from instruction (Campione, Brown, Ferrara, & Bryant, 1984). Although these tests were adequate for providing a primary orientation, they were relatively ineffective in differentiating between children at the same assessed ability level who had different learning efficiencies (Luria, 1961).

In response to this concern, Vygotsky and his associates suggested that assessment not only should look at what the child has learned previously, but also should assess children's learning efficiency directly (Brown & French, 1979). They believed that assessing what a child can learn to do with assistance and contrasting this with what a child can do alone provides a more sensitive measure of learning efficiency. This is basically the idea behind the ZPD as a philosophy of assessment.

In general, a ZPD assessment procedure consists of three steps. First, a measure is taken of what the child can accomplish independently in a given domain. Next, the child is provided assistance by a more competent learner. This assistance is usually provided in a series of gradually more explicit hints or cues. Finally, a measure of the child's ability to profit from this assistance is collected. The child's ability to profit from assistance is assumed to be a measure of that child's learning efficiency in that domain.

In designing ZPD procedures, there are two critical decisions to be made. First, it must be decided how to provide the assistance. Second, the method or methods of assessing the child's ability to profit from this assistance must be identified.

Regarding the first of those decisions, Vygotsky (1978) allowed that there were a variety of methods for providing assistance that could be useful for assessing learning efficiency. "Different experimenters might employ different modes of demonstration: Some might run through an entire demonstration and ask the child to repeat it, others might initiate the solution and ask the child to finish it, or offer leading questions" (p. 86). Current researchers, however, have preferred to use the method of graduated hints or prompts for supplying assistance (Brown & Ferrara, 1985; Bryant, Brown, & Campione, 1983; Burns, 1984; Campione et al., 1984; Wozniak, 1980).

In the method of graduated hints, a sequence of increasingly explicit hints is developed. When a child fails an item, the hints are given one at a time in sequence until the child can solve the item. As the hints are the major component of this type of ZPD procedure, they must be developed in a thoughtful manner. First, it is important that the hints be meaningful to the child. Rogoff and Gardner (1984) noted that adults and children may define critical elements of a problem in different ways. The hints must be developed in such a fashion that they create a common interpretation of the problem for the adult and the child. It is important that the child see the logic behind the hints.

Second, the hints not only should lead to the successful solution of a given problem type, but also should help the child develop the skills necessary to solve similar problems in the future. From a Vygotskian perspective, effective assistance is that which can be internalized by children and applied later on their own (Berk, 1985; Cazden, 1980; Luria, 1961).

According to Brown and Ferrara (1985), the most effective method for developing meaningful sequences of hints is to perform a comprehensive task analysis. The steps of the task analysis become the sequence of hints provided for children. These hints or steps are the same steps children would use in solving any problem of this type. This advice appears particularly useful when a problem lends itself readily to task analysis. For example, the inductive-reasoning tasks used by Brown and Ferrara can be task-analyzed rather easily. It is our contention that understanding of the student's underlying cognitive processes, such as the spreading activation retrieval mechanism, would further guide successful prompting.

After the method of providing assistance has been identified, the second major decision in designing a ZPD assessment procedure concerns how learning efficiency is to be measured. Day (1983) was able to identify seven different measures of learning efficiency in the literature that made use of ZPD procedures. These seven measures were:

1. How much improvement does a child demonstrate after receiving assistance?
2. How explicit must training be to produce improvement in performance?
3. How well does the child maintain learned skills?
4. How much additional help is necessary to get a child to maintain learning?
5. How well does a child transfer learning?
6. How easily does a child transfer learning with assistance?
7. How quickly does a child transfer learning across different types of problems?

In general, however, these seven measures can be organized into two different approaches for assessing learning processes with the ZPD. The first approach focuses on how much improvement children demonstrate after assistance or training. The second approach focuses on how much assistance children require from an adult to demonstrate a given level of improvement. In terms of Day's (1983) seven measures of learning efficiency just listed, the first approach is reflected in measures 1, 3, and 5, the second in measures 2, 4, 6, and 7. Fetsco (1987) has discussed advantages and limitations of these approaches.

Vygotsky believed that because of the reciprocal nature of the teaching–learning process, the dynamic interactive approach to assessment embodied in ZPD procedures is essential to effective instruction. For Vygotsky (1978, p. 89), "the only good learning is that which is in advance of development." Thus, ZPD assessment can help teachers and school psychologists determine the instructional zone of skill development in which effective instruction can produce "good learning." Following Vygotsky, teachers and school psychologists might view every instructional activity as a dynamic interaction between teacher and student, providing opportunities for both assessment and instruction of students' cognitive skills.

CONCLUSION

Our examination of information processing and cognitive assessment has come a long way (and many pages) since we recounted the tale of Jonathan's story in the preceding chapter. What have we learned along the way? We have argued that the cognitive psychology of information processing can provide a theoretical basis for scientist/practitioner school psychologists and professional-educator teachers. Information-processing task analysis of school tasks and cognitive assessment of students can help provide a better data base on which to anchor instruction and special services. By considering students' cognitive structures, processes, strategies, and executive functions, we get a glimmer of the cognitive complexity that underlies even seemingly trivial academic exercises.

We argued that the instructional approach from cognitive-development research has implications for classroom instruction and assessment, calling for direct measurement of students' cognitive processes, standards of evaluation for performance and instruction, and task analysis for understanding the regularities in relationships between strategies and task demands. We showed that an information-processing analysis of students' performance on standardized tests may reveal a very different picture from that presented by the test manual and norms. Dynamic and process assessment were seen to put assessment directly into an instructional context, giving a fuller, more accurate view of what a student can do.

If, as we have argued, the application of the information-processing approach holds great promise for improving the effectiveness of school psychologists and teachers alike, how realistic is it to expect that that promise might be kept? A partial answer to this question can be found in our analysis of Jonathan's literary effort. As we hope you noticed, we practiced some of what we preached. Detailed error analysis and use of verbal report data combined to help us approach direct assessment of his cognitive processing during writing. Evidence regarding his cognitive structure for stories was found in the structure of the story he produced. A second chance at the task, the revision with additional prompting from his father, provided dynamic or process assessment of Jonathan's ZPD for story writing. With a little prompt from his dad, Jonathan was able to retrieve just the right word. His shift of attention and processing effort toward punctuation and other niceties, which were ignored in the original draft as he concentrated on plot and character development, provided not only a more accurate assessment of his ability in these areas, but also evidence of metacognitive sophistication guiding the allocation of limited information-processing capacity. Thus, it seems the youngster's executive was functioning.

As an answer to a question about the feasibility of implementing the information-processing approach to assessment in the schools, however, a reference to our analysis of Jonathan's story is not altogether satisfying. As we acknowledged at the outset, the one-of-him-to-three-of-us odds we enjoyed reversed the many-to-one or many-to-few odds faced by most teachers and school psychologists. How are they to reap the benefits we ascribed to the information-processing approach? One answer is suggested by the cognitive literature itself: through the acquisition of skills in information-processing analyses, the development of expertise in cognitive assessment. Through the development of fine-tuned, automated analytical procedures and the accumulation of a richly detailed and organized knowledge base, the skilled, expert educational professional can very quickly assess what a student is doing on an academic task and what must be done to be successful. Simon and others have pointed to such development to explain how chess masters can move from one opponent to the next while conducting multiple games. Is it unreasonable to expect that school psychologists and teachers might move from one student to the next with such effectiveness and dispatch? Perhaps not, but cognitive research suggests that getting to that point is by no means easy. Simon has estimated that experts have some 50,000 or more complex chunks or knowledge structures for chess tucked away in long-term memory in a manner that permits ready access. He has repeatedly stated that truly notable expertise takes some ten years to acquire, regardless of the domain. There is little reason to hope that becoming a bona fide expert school psychologist or teacher will require any less.

It is important to remember, however, that chess players of less than world class expertise can sometimes play a fair game of chess. Look at the story Jonathan produced the first time out. Simply by being aware of the information-processing perspective and attempting to implement it in your work, you can improve the quality of services provided to your students, even while beginning the long and arduous pursuit of expert skill.

REFERENCES

Alexander, P. A., White, C. S., Haensly, P. A., & Crimmins-Jeanes, M. (1987). Training in analogical reasoning. *American Educational Research Journal, 24,* 387–404.

Anastasi, A. (1967). Psychology, psychologists, and psychological testing. *American Psychologist, 22,* 297–306.

Anderson, J. R. (1976). *Language, memory and thought.* Hillsdale, NJ: Lawrence Erlbaum.

Anderson, R. C., Mason, J., & Shirey, L. (1984). The reading group: An experimental investigation of a labyrinth. *Reading Research Quarterly, 20,* 6–38.

Berk, L. E. (1985). Why children talk to themselves. *Young Children, 40,* 46–52.

Bogen, J. E. (1969). The other side of the brain (Parts I, II, and III). *Bulletin of the Los Angeles Neurological Society*, *34*, 73–105, 135–162, 191–203.

Boring, E. G. (1950). *A history of experimental psychology* (2nd ed.). New York: Appleton-Century-Crofts.

Brown, A. L., & Ferrara, R. A. (1985). Diagnosing zones of proximal development. In J. V. Wertsch (Ed.), *Culture, communication, and cognition: Vygotskian perspectives* (pp. 275–304). Cambridge: Cambridge University Press.

Brown, A. L., & French, L. A. (1979). The zone of potential development: Implications for intelligence testing in the year 2000. *Intelligence*, *3*, 255–277.

Bryant, N., Brown, A. L., & Campione, J. C. (1983). *Preschool children's learning and transfer of matrices problems: A study of proximal development*. Unpublished manuscript, University of Illinois.

Budoff, M., & Corman, L. (1976). Effectiveness of a learning potential procedure in improving problem-solving skills of retarded and nonretarded children. *American Journal of Mental Deficiency*, *81*, 260–264.

Burns, M. S. (1984). Comparison of "graduated prompt" and "mediational" dynamic assessment with young children (doctoral dissertation, Vanderbilt University, 1983). *Dissertation Abstracts International*, *45*, 3216A.

Campione, J. C., Brown, A. L., Ferrara, R. A., & Bryant, N. R. (1984). The zone of proximal development: Implications for individual differences and learning. In B. Rogoff & J. V. Wertsch (Eds.), *Children's learning in the "zone of proximal development"* (pp. 77–91). San Francisco: Jossey-Bass.

Carlson, J. S., & Wiedl, K. H. (1980). *Dynamic assessment: An approach toward reducing test bias*. Paper presented at the annual meeting of the Western Psychological Association. (ERIC Document Reproduction Service No. ED 191 884).

Carroll, J. B. (1976). Psychometric tests as cognitive tasks: A new "structure of intellect." In L. B. Resnick (Ed.), *The nature of intelligence* (pp. 25–56). Hillsdale, NJ: Lawrence Erlbaum.

Cazden, C. B. (1980). Toward a social educational psychology with Soviet help. *Contemporary Educational Psychology*, *5*, 196–201.

Cronbach, L. J. (1957). The two disciplines of scientific psychology. *American Psychologist*, *12*, 671–684.

Das, J. P., Kirby, J. R., & Jarman, R. F. (1975). Simultaneous and successive syntheses: An alternative model for cognitive abilities. *Psychological Bulletin*, *82*, 87–103.

Day, J. D. (1983). The zone of proximal development. In M. Pressley & J. R. Levin (Eds.), *Cognitive strategy research psychological foundations* (pp. 155–175). New York: Springer-Verlag.

Ericsson, K. A. (1987). Theoretical implications from protocol analysis on testing and measurement. In R. R. Ronning, J. A. Glover, J. C. Conoley, & J. C. Witt (Eds.), *The influence of cognitive psychology on testing* (pp. 191–226). Hillsdale, NJ: Lawrence Erlbaum.

Ericsson, K. A., & Simon, H. A. (1980). Verbal reports as data. *Psychological Review*, *87*, 215–251.

Ericsson, K. A., & Simon, H. A. (1984). *Protocol analysis: Verbal reports as data*. Cambridge, MA: MIT Press.

Fetsco, T. G. (1987). *Assessing the zone of proximal development for spelling*. Unpublished doctoral dissertation, Texas A&M University.

Feuerstein, R., Rand, Y., & Hoffman, M. B. (1979). *The dynamic assessment of retarded performers: The learning potential assessment device, theory, instruments, and techniques.* Baltimore, MD: University Park Press.

Feuerstein, R., Rand, Y., Hoffman, M. B., & Miller, R. (1980). *Instrumental enrichment.* Baltimore, MD: University Park Press.

Forness, S. R., & Kavale, K. A. (1987). Holistic inquiry and the scientific challenge in special education: A reply to Iano. *Remedial and Special Education, 8,* 47–51.

Fuchs, L. S., & Fuchs, D. (1986). Linking assessment to instructional interventions: An overview. *School Psychology Review, 15,* 318–323.

Goetz, E. T., & Hall, R. J. (1984). Evaluation of the Kaufman Assessment Battery for Children from an information-processing perspective. *Journal of Special Education, 18,* 281–296.

Goetz, E. T., Hall, R. J., & Fetsco, T. G. (in press). Implications of cognitive psychology for assessment of academic skill. In C. R. Reynolds & R. W. Kamphaus (Eds.), *Handbook of psychological and educational assessment* (Vol. 1). New York: Guilford Press.

Gordon, H. W., & Bogen, J. E. (1974). Hemispheric lateralization of singing after intracarotid sodium amylocarbitone. *Journal of Neurology, Neurosurgery, and Psychiatry, 37,* 727–738.

Gordon, J. E., & Haywood, H. C. (1969). Input deficit in cultural–familial retardation: Effects of stimulus enrichment. *American Journal of Mental Deficiency, 73,* 604–610.

Griffin, P., & Cole, M. (1984). Current activity for the future: The zoped. In B. Rogoff & J. Wertsch (Eds.), *Children's learning in the zone of proximal development* (pp. 45–63). San Francisco: Jossey-Bass

Hall, R. J., & Goetz, E. T. (1987). *Encoding and retrieval processes in spatial memory performance of adults and children.* Paper presented at the meeting of the American Educational Research Association, Washington, DC.

Hall, R. J., Goetz, E. T., Eckert, S. P., Stowe, M. L., & Kangiser, S. M. (1987). Encoding and retrieval processes in the spatial memory performance of adults. In R. D. Zellner, J. J. Denton, M. J. Burger, & R. J. Kansky (Eds.), *Technology in education: Implications and applications* (pp. 110–121). Instructional Research Laboratory, College of Education, Texas A&M University, College Station.

Haney, W. (1984). Testing reasoning and reasoning about testing. *Review of Educational Research, 54,* 597–654.

Haywood, H. C., Fuller, J. W., Jr., Shifman, M. A., & Chatelanet, G. (1975). Behavioral assessment in mental retardation. In P. McReynolds (Ed.), *Advances in psychological assessment* (Vol. 3, pp. 96–136). San Francisco: Jossey-Bass.

Haywood, H. C., & Switzky, H. N. (1974). Children's verbal abstracting: Effects of enriched input, age, and IQ. *American Journal of Mental Deficiency, 78,* 556–565.

Howell, K. W. (1986). Direct assessment of academic performance. *School Psychology Review, 15,* 324–335.

Kamphaus, R. W., Kaufman, A. S., & Reynolds, C. R. (1985). Applications of the Kaufman Assessment Battery for Children to the study of individual differences. In C. R. Reynolds & V. L. Willson (Eds.), *Methodological and statistical advances in the study of individual differences* (pp. 95–118). Syracuse, NY: Syracuse University Press.

Kaufman, A. S., & Kaufman, N. L. (1983). *Kaufman Assessment Battery for Children: Interpretive manual.* Circle Pines, MN: American Guidance Service.

Kratochwill, T. (1977). The movement of psychological extras into ability assessment. *Journal of Special Education, 11,* 299–311.

Levy, J. (1972). Lateral specialization of the human brain: Behavioral manifestations and possible evolutionary basis. In J. A. Kiger (Ed.), *Biology of behavior.* Corvallis: Oregon State University Press.

Luria, A. R. (1961). Study of the abnormal child. *American Journal of Orthopsychiatry, 31,* 1–16.

Luria, A. R. (1966). *Higher cortical functions in man.* New York: Basic Books.

Luria, A. R. (1973). *The working brain: An introduction to neuropsychology.* London: Penguin Books.

Meyers, J., Pfeffer, J., & Erlbaum, E. (1985). Process assessment: A model for broadening assessment. *Journal of Special Education, 19,* 73–89.

Mulholland, T. A., Pellegrino, J. W., & Glaser, R. (1980). Components of geometric analogy solution. *Cognitive Psychology, 12,* 252–284.

Neisser, U. (1967). *Cognitive psychology.* New York: Appleton-Century-Crofts.

Nisbett, R. E., & Wilson, T. D. (1977). Telling more than we know: Verbal reports on mental processes. *Psychological Review, 84,* 231–259.

Pavio, A. (1975). Perceptual comparisons through the mind's eye. *Memory and Cognition, 3,* 635–647.

Pavio, A. (1976). Concerning dual-coding and simultaneous–successive processing. *Canadian Psychological Review, 17,* 69–71.

Resnick, L. B. (1976). Introduction: Changing conceptions of intelligence. In L. B. Resnick (Ed.), *The nature of intelligence* (pp. 1–10). Hillsdale, NJ: Lawrence Erlbaum.

Rogoff, B., & Gardner, W. (1984). Adult guidance of cognitive development. In B. Rogoff & J. Lave (Eds.), *Everyday cognition: Its development in social context* (pp. 95–116). Cambridge, MA: Harvard University Press.

Ronning, R. R., Conoley, J. C., & Glover, J. G. (1987). Introduction: The implications of cognitive psychology for testing. In R. R. Ronning, J. A. Glover, J. C. Conoley, & J. C. Witt (Eds.), *The influence of cognitive psychology on testing* (pp. 1–8). Hillsdale, NJ: Lawrence Erlbaum.

Schneider, W., & Shiffrin, R. M. (1977). Controlled and automatic human information processing: I. Detection, search, and attention. *Psychological Review, 84,* 1–66.

Shiffrin, R. M., & Schneider, W. (1977). Controlled and automatic information processing: II. Perceptual learning, automatic attending, and a general theory. *Psychological Review, 84,* 127–159.

Simon, H. A., & Newell, A. (1971). Human problem solving: The state of the theory in 1970. *American Psychologist, 26,* 145–159.

Sternberg, R. J. (1977). *Intelligence, information processing, and analogical reasoning: The componential analysis of human abilities.* Hillsdale, NJ: Lawrence Erlbaum.

Sternberg, R. J. (1984). What should intelligence tests test? Implications of a triarchic theory of intelligence for intelligence testing. *Educational Researcher, 13,* 5–15.

Sternberg, R. J., & Rifkin, B. (1979). The development of analogical reasoning processes. *Journal of Experimental Child Psychology, 27,* 195–232.

Swanson, H. L. (1984). Process assessment of intelligence in learning disabled and mentally retarded children: A multidirectional model. *Educational Psychologist, 19,* 149–162.

Vygotsky, L. S. (1978). *Mind in society: The development of higher psychological processes.* Cambridge, MA: Harvard University Press.

White, C. S., & Alexander, P. A. (1986). Effects of training on four-year-old's ability to solve geometric analogy problems. *Cognition and Instruction, 3,* 261–268.

Willson, V. L. (1987). *Cognitive psychology and test development: Out with the old.* Invited address, Division 5, annual meeting of the American Psychological Association, New York, August.

Willson, V. L., Goetz, E. T., Hall, R. J., & Applegate, B. (1986). *Effects of varying elements and transformations of matrix analogies on children ages 5–12.* Paper presented at the annual conference of the American Educational Research Association, San Francisco, May.

Wozniak, R. H. (1980). Theory, practice, and the "zone of proximal development" in Soviet psychoeducational research. *Contemporary Educational Psychology, 5,* 175–183.

7
A COGNITIVE-BEHAVIORAL MODEL FOR ASSESSING CHILDREN'S SOCIAL COMPETENCE

JAN N. HUGHES
Texas A & M University

THE ROLE OF PEER RELATIONS IN DEVELOPMENT

Psychologists' and educators' interest in children's social development is not of recent origin. Rather, the study of children's social development is one of the oldest and most respected disciplines within psychology, with important empirical investigations and theoretical developments occurring in the 1930s and 1940s (Jersild & Fite, 1939; Koch, 1933; Piaget, 1932). Much of this early research had a decidedly social-cognitive orientation. During the 30-year reign of behaviorism in American psychology, however, research investigations on children's social cognition and peer relationships waned. The late 1960s heralded the cognitive revolution in psychology, followed by a resurgence of research on children's social development (Damon, 1977; Schantz, 1975). Today, research on children's social cognition represents one of the most dynamic research fields in psychology.

Several factors contribute to the current interest among both psychologists and educators in children's social competence and social development. First, because social interactions are so important in everyday life, the possibility of improving the quality of these interactions and reducing loneliness and interpersonal conflict is appealing to psychologists and educators. Second, the view of personal competence as multifaceted, comprising intellectual, physical, and social competence (Greenspan, 1981), has challenged the practice of relying on a single index of competence (i.e., intellectual competence) in the evaluation of educational interventions such as Head Start (Putallaz & Gottman, 1982).

A third reason for the increase in research activity on peer relations is the accumulation of a large body of research documenting that childhood peer relationship problems are predictive of a variety of negative outcomes in adolescence and adulthood. Most of this longitudinal and retrospective research has focused on the long-term consequences of peer rejection (versus peer withdrawal or isolation). This research has documented that peer rejection predicts juvenile delinquency (Roff, Sells, & Golden, 1972), dropping out of school (Ullmann, 1957), bad-conduct discharges from the military service (Roff, 1961), and a variety of serious mental health problems in adulthood (Cowen, Pederson, Barbigian, Izzo, & Trost, 1973; Kohn, 1977; Strain, Cooke, & Apollini, 1976). In the most frequently cited longitudinal study, Emory Cowen and his colleagues (1973) found that the number of negative sociometric nominations received in the third grade was a better predictor of adult psychiatric disturbance than a battery that included school records, intelligence performance, and self-report data. Studies on the correlates of peer acceptance have documented that low peer acceptance is associated with poor academic achievement and school failure in the elementary school years (Green, Forehand, Beck, & Vosk, 1980; Laughlin, 1954; Muma, 1965).

Fourth, psychologists and educators recognize the importance of peer interaction in the socialization process. It is through interacting with peers that children develop important social skills. Thus, clinical concern for the neglected, socially withdrawn child is based on the view that children who interact infrequently with peers miss important opportunities to develop social skills, including social-cognitive and moral reasoning skills. Concern for these children is also based on the finding that socially isolated children tend to be depressed and lonely (Strauss, Forehand, Frame, & Smith, 1984) and to perform less well in school (Green et al., 1980).

A final reason for the resurgence of interest in children's social behavior is the demonstrated beneficial effect of social skills remediation interventions. Attempts to improve unpopular children's peer relationships through social skills training have resulted in treatment gains on measures of peer acceptance and teacher ratings of adjustment as well as on measures of the specific skills targeted in the intervention (for reviews, see Gresham, 1985; Hughes, 1986; Hughes & Sullivan, 1988; Urbain & Savage, Chapter 17, this volume).

DEFINITIONS OF SOCIAL COMPETENCE AND SOCIAL SKILLS

Recently, investigators have adopted McFall's (1982) distinction between the terms "social competence" and "social skills" (Gresham & Elliott, 1984; Putallaz & Gottman, 1983). According to McFall, "social competence" is an evaluative term referring to the overall effectiveness of social behaviors as judged by significant others. Perceptions of social competence are obtained via peer ratings of likability and teacher ratings of overall competence in peer relations. Evidence of the validity of peer sociometric ratings and teacher ratings as indices of social competence is supported by evidence linking them to socially important outcomes, such as academic achievement, special class placement, and psychological adjustment.

The term "social skills" refers to "those behaviors which, within a given situation, predict important social outcomes such as (a) peer acceptance or popularity, (b) significant others' judgments of behavior, or (c) other social behaviors known to correlate consistently with peer acceptance or significant others' judgments" (Gresham & Elliott, 1984, pp. 292–293). This empirical approach to defining social skills requires a documented relationship between specific skill measures and socially valid outcomes (i.e., sociometric measures or teacher ratings). Whereas McFall's (1982) and Gresham & Elliott's (1984) definitions of social skills focus on observed social behaviors, Ladd & Mize's (1983) definition of social skills distinguishes between social skills and social competence while also recognizing the importance of social-cognitive skills: "Social skills refer to children's ability to organize cognitions and behaviors into an integrated course of action directed toward culturally acceptable social or interpersonal goals" (p. 127).

The distinction between social competence and social skills is consistent with the recommendation that outcome assessment in behavior therapy includes measures at both the impact and specifying assessment levels (Kendall & Morrison, 1984). Measures at the specifying level identify exactly what did or did not change as a result of treatment. Behavior observations and task performance measures (e.g., measures of problem-solving skills or role-taking ability) are examples of specifying assessment measures. Measures at the impact level assess the impact of treatment on the perceptions of significant others in the child's environment (e.g., parents, teachers, peers) as well as on other socially consequential outcomes, such as academic achievement. Measures at both levels are necessary to establish the functional relatedness between specific skills targeted in an intervention and a socially valid outcome (such as peer acceptance). If a social skills intervention results in a change in target skills with no accompanying change in judgments made by significant others, the treatment may have changed socially inconsequential behaviors. Conversely, if treatment results in improved peer acceptance or teacher evaluative ratings with no evidence of improvement on measures of target skills, one does not know how to account for the improvement.

SCOPE OF CHAPTER

Much has been written on the assessment of children's social competence (Asher & Hymel, 1981; Dodge, 1985, 1986; Hops & Greenwood, 1988; Hughes, in press; Hymel, 1983). The purpose of this chapter is not to provide a comprehensive review of the various approaches and measures used in the assessment of social skills and social competence; rather, it is to recommend a model of social competence that can serve as a guide to assessing social skills. Toward this end, the remainder of this chapter is organized according to three objectives.

First, the three most prevalent school-based approaches to the assessment of children's peer relations are reviewed. These three approaches are (1) peer sociometrics, (2) teacher behavior ratings, and (3) behavior observations. This review concludes with a discussion of the limitations of the sociometric/behavioral assessment methodology.

Second, an information-processing model of social competence is presented. Selected research on social information processing is reviewed in order to illustrate the base of empirical support for the model.

Third, implications of the information-processing model for school-based assessment efforts are suggested. Specifically, a three-stage assessment methodology is recommended that includes measures at both the impact and specifying levels, takes into account the situational determinants of social behaviors, and links assessment data to interventions. This section concludes with a case study that illustrates the recommended assessment methodology.

SOCIOMETRIC AND BEHAVIORAL ASSESSMENT OF SOCIAL COMPETENCE AND SOCIAL SKILLS

Sociometric Assessment

The term "sociometric assessment" refers to a range of specific procedures, all of which have in common the involvement of a child's peers in the evaluation of social competence. These various sociometric procedures can be grouped for discussion purposes into two types: peer nominations and peer ratings (for an extended discussion of sociometric assessment, see Hughes, in press; Hops & Greenwood, 1988).

Peer Nominations

In the peer nomination procedure, each child in a classroom (or other socially defined group) is asked to select a restricted number of classmates (usually three) with respect to a given criterion (e.g., "like the most," "like the least," "best friend"). A child's score is the number of nominations received. The number of positive nominations received is an index of a child's popularity, and the number of negative nominations received (e.g., "like the least") is an index of a child's rejection. Researchers, parents, and educators have been reluctant to use negative nominations because their use might increase the saliency of the rejected child's status. However, the combined use of both positive and negative nominations is supported by data suggesting that positive and negative nominations measure different dimensions of social competence. For example, positive and negative nomination scores are only moderately negatively correlated (Gottman, 1977; Landau, Milich, & Whitten, 1984) or not at all (Hartup, Glazer, & Charlesworth, 1967). Furthermore, the combined use of positive and negative nominations permits a distinction to be made between two types of unpopular children, neglected and rejected children. Whereas both types of children receive few positive nominations, the rejected child also receives many negative nominations

Recently, Coie, Dodge, and Coppotelli (1982) proposed a classification system based on both positive and negative choice nominations. In this system, two new scores, social preference and social impact scores, are derived from the standardized raw score nominations for "like most" and "like least." The derived social preference and social impact scores are used to identify children for five distinct social status groups, (popular, average, controversial, neglected, and rejected). Although this classification system has only recently been proposed, a substantial amount of data has accumulated documenting its high reliability and concurrent and predictive validity (Coie *et al.*, 1982; Dodge, 1983; Dodge, Coie, & Brakke, 1982; Dodge, Murphy, & Buchsbaum, 1984; Dodge, Schlundt, Schocken, & Delugach, 1983). Specifically, neglected and rejected groups of children demonstrate different social behaviors (Coie & Kupersmidt, 1983; Dodge, 1983; Putallaz, 1983), are perceived differently by peers, (Coie & Dodge, 1983) and differ on measures of social cognition (Dodge, Murphy, & Buchsbaum, 1984).

A variation of the peer nomination procedure is the peer behavioral description method. The best known example of this procedure is the Class Play (Bower, 1969; Lambert & Bower, 1961). Children "cast" their classmates into a variety of positive and negative roles, such as bully or leader. Short behavioral descriptions accompany each role. For example, the leader role is described as "someone who is the leader when children do something in class or on the playground—someone everyone listens to." A revised version of the Class Play (Masten, Morison, & Pellegrini, 1985) consists of 15 positive and 15 negative roles and yields three factors: sociability-leadership, aggressive-disruptive, and sensitive-isolated. Evidence of the reliability and validity of the behavioral description method is good (Hughes, in press).

Peer Rating

The second type of sociometric procedure is the roster-and-rating method. In this procedure, each child in a classroom is asked to rate his or her degree of liking for every other same-sex child. A 5- or 7-point Likert-type rating scale is used, where a rating of 1 means "I don't like to play with this person at all" and a rating of 5 means "I like to play with this person a lot." Ratings minimize ethical concerns involved in asking children to list the names of persons they do not like. Evidence of the reliability and validity of peer ratings is good (see Hughes, in press). They are especially appropriate with preschool children because of their higher reliability with this group, compared to peer nominations (Hymel, 1983). A disadvantage of the rating method is that it does not permit the classification of children into sociometrically derived groups. Both the rejected and the neglected child may receive the same mean rating; yet they may experience very different amounts of rejection. Asher and Dodge (1986) have suggested a way to overcome this limitation of the rating method. They suggest combining a positive peer nomination question with a rating scale to distinguish between neglected and rejected children. According to their classification system, a liking rating of 1 a 5-point rating scale is treated as a rejection nomination for purposes of computing social preference scores. These social preference scores are plugged into Coie's (Coie et al., 1982) classification formulae. The agreement between Asher and Dodge's alternative method and the Coie et al. method is good, especially in classifying the rejected child (91% agreement).

In summary, sociometric procedures represent a reliable and valid method of identifying children with peer relations problems, and can reliably disciminate between two types of unpopular children, neglected and rejected children. Whereas both types of children experience peer relations problems, they have different patterns of social-cognitive and behavioral deficits. For example, rejected children engage in high levels of negative behavior, whereas neglected children engage in low levels of peer interaction. Rejected children, but not neglected children, tend to systematically distort social cues in the direction of overperceiving hostility (Dodge et al., 1984; Dodge & Frame, 1982).

Even though such differences exist between sociometric status groups, it is not recommended that these status groups be the basis for selecting target skills and treatment procedures. These classifications are too global to serve as the basis for target skill selection. Two children who share rejected status may differ in the specific skill deficits that result in others' negative reactions to them. In other words, there are many ways in which a child can be socially incompetent. Although sociometric procedures do a good job of classifying children according to the general nature of their peer relationships, they do not permit a specification of those social-cognitive and behavioral deficits that lead to others' judgments of incompetence. Similarly, in the case of popular children, sociometric procedures do not permit a specification of those social-cognitive and behavioral skills that lead to judgments of competence.

Behavior Ratings

Parent and teacher behavior rating scales and checklists are probably used more frequently in schools than any other measure of children's social competence. Their prevalence in school-based assessment is based on the fact that rating scales are economical, are easy to administer and score, and demonstrate good test–retest and interrater reliabilities (for reviews, see Asher & Hymel, 1981; Hughes, in press). Teacher ratings of social behaviors predict direct behavior observations (Algozzine, 1977; Balou, 1966; Quay, 1979; Schachar, Sandberg, & Rutter, 1986), diagnostic classifications (Behar & Stringfield, 1974; Stumme, Gresham, & Scott, 1982; Waksman, 1985), and peer sociometric measures (Green et al., 1980; Van Hasselt, Hersen, & Bellack, 1981).

Teacher rating scales differ on several dimensions, including the specificity of the items, the comprehensiveness of coverage, and item format. The most frequently used teacher rating scales include the Child Behavior Checklist—Teacher Report Form (Achenbach & Edelbrock, 1986), the Revised Behavior Problem Checklist (Quay & Peterson, 1983, 1984), and the Walker Problem Identification Checklist (Walker, 1976). These checklists obtain teachers' global perceptions, are comprehensive in scope, and ask teachers to rate problem behaviors rather than skilled behaviors. They are norm-referenced and yield factor scores in addition to a total score. The individual items are not directly useful as they refer to classes of behavior rather than to specific behaviors. For example, items on the Behavior Problem Checklist include "lacks self-confidence," "sulks and pouts," and "generally fearful." These measures are valid for purposes of assisting in diagnostic classification and for evaluating the impact of intervention programs. Like sociometric methods, however, teacher rating scales do not permit a specification of the nature of a social competence problem or, in the case of popular children, of the nature of their social skills.

Teacher rating scales that obtain teachers' perceptions of specific behaviors include the Teacher Rating of Social Skills (TROSS) (Clark, Gresham, & Elliott, 1985) and the Matson Evaluation of Social Skills for Youth (MESSY) (Matson, Rotatori, & Helsel, 1983). The purpose of these behaviorally specific scales is to specify the nature of a child's behavioral strengths and weaknesses. Therefore, evidence that the scale items predict behavior observations of specific behaviors as well as socially consequential outcomes is crucial to establishing the scale's potential usefulness. To date, this evidence has not been forthcoming for scales that attempt to measure a wide range of specific social behaviors.

Behavior Observations

Direct observation of behavior is the hallmark of behavior assessment (Bellack, 1979), and a number of excellent sources on conducting behavior observations exist (Barton & Ascione, 1984; Ciminero, Calhoun, & Adams, 1977). The advantages and limitations of direct observation are discussed in Asher & Hymel (1981) and Hughes (in press) and will only be summarized here.

Advantages of behavior observations include the low inference required for interpretation, their nonreactive nature, and their sensitivity to treatment effects. Of particular relevance to this chapter is the fact that direct observation permits the specification of both target behavior and important contextual variables (i.e., antecedents and consequences). The resulting data are, therefore, useful in selecting treatment targets and in determining what changes are needed in the child's environment to effect a desired change in child behavior. Relatedly, observational data can be used to estimate the functional relationship between specific social behaviors and socially consequential outcomes.

That is, those social behaviors that lead to peer or teacher global evaluations can be ascertained. Finally, behavior observation systems that code sequential social interactions permit a more refined analysis of interactional differences. For example, knowing that a shy child responds to peers' initiations at the same frequency as other children but does not initiate peer interaction has clear treatment implications. For example, peer priming (Strain, 1977, 1985) and instructions in joining in would be likely to increase her rate of social interaction.

Despite the advantages offered by behavior observations, they also have important limitations. Foremost, beyond the early childhood years, opportunities for adults to observe unobtrusively those behaviors critical to peer acceptance and friendship formation are seriously limited (Asher & Hymel, 1981). Whereas easily observed behaviors, such as rate of interaction and sharing, are related to peer acceptance in preschool populations, verbal behaviors and more subtle social skills become crucial to peer acceptance at older ages (Eisenberg & Harris, 1984). Accurate observation of these skills requires sophisticated observational systems and videotaping capabilities, limiting their usefulness in schools.

A limitation shared by both behavior observations and rating scales is that neither method can distinguish between topographically similar behaviors that have very different underlying causes. That is, they answer the question of "what" but not the question of "why." For example, two boys may each be rated as aggressive. Furthermore, both boys are observed to start fights, hit, and threaten others. One boy's aggressive behavior is the result of a systematic distortion of social cues relevant to inferring others' intentions. As a result of this systematic bias, he misperceives others as acting with hostile intent toward him, and he responds with counteraggression. The second boy believes aggression is an effective means to get his own way. He uses aggression selectively in peer interactions to obtain desired goals. It is likely these two boys would respond best to different interventions. The first boy might benefit from training in perspective taking and in attending to more of the available social cues (e.g., facial cues, body posture, past experiences with person). The second boy might benefit from a contingency management program and discussions focusing on the nonimmediate consequences of aggression.

In general, past assessment efforts have focused on measuring discrete facets of social competence. The specific facets selected for assessment have depended on the assessor's conceptualization of social competence. Thus, some investigators assess behavioral assertion skills, whereas others assess perspective-taking or social problem-solving skills. Although groups of socially competent and socially incompetent children may differ on these skill measures, it is unlikely that a given unpopular child is deficient in all of these skills. The long list of cognitive and behavioral skill differences between socially competent and incompetent children attests to the futility of this correlational approach as a method of selecting skills to be taught to an individual child experiencing a lack of peer acceptance. Furthermore, the correlational approach to the assessment/intervention process encourages a simplistic view of social competence defined in terms of discrete skills rather than as a complex, sequential process. Hughes and Hall (1987) argue that whereas the known-group approach identifies facets of social competence, it does not suggest methods for integrating these facets into a unified conceptual framework that can guide assessment and intervention efforts.

INFORMATION-PROCESSING MODEL
OF SOCIAL COMPETENCE

Hughes and Hall (1987) and Dodge and his colleagues (Dodge, 1986; Dodge & Murphy, 1984) have recommended that socially competent performance be viewed as the result of the successful application of specific social-cognitive and behavioral skills in the context of some social situation or some problem. According to this view, performance judged by others as competent results from the successful application of skills at each of three stages of social information processing. Borrowing from Greenspan's (1981) model of personal competence, Hughes and Hall labeled these stages Reading, Generating, and Applying. Borrowing from McFall (1982), Dodge and Murphy referred to these stages as Decoding, Decision Making, and Enactment. Later, Dodge (1986) divided the Decoding and Decision Making stages into two stages each, resulting in five total stages. Despite the different terminology, both models recognize that social competence is a social problem-solving process involving social-cognitive and behavioral skills. Although both models recognize the importance of identifying the situational determinants of social performance, the models differ in their relative emphasis on situational assessment. Hughes and Hall emphasize the assessment of generalizable skills, whereas Dodge and Murphy emphasize the assessment of skills in particular types of situations (a skill $\times$ context approach).

Recent research demonstrating the low cross-situational consistency and high within-situational consistency in aggressive children's responses to different types of social problem situations (Dodge, McClaskey, & Feldman, 1985a; Lochman & Lampion, 1986) suggests the usefulness of Dodge's two-dimensional, skill $\times$ content approach to assessing children's social competence. This approach is consistent with the view that a child might have difficulty applying social problem solving to group entry situations, but not to situations involving peer provocations.

Next, an information-processing model of socially competent performance is presented. Selected studies documenting differences between socially competent and socially incompetent children at each stage of the model are briefly reviewed to illustrate the type of research that undergirds the model. Implications of the information-processing model for school-based assessments of social competence and social skills are discussed in the final section.

Problems in Reading Social Situations

Socially competent performance requires the successful execution of skills at each of three sequential steps. First, the child must read (or encode) the social situation. Social situations are inherently ambiguous, and accurate interpretations of the situation require the child to attend to and interpret a variety of social cues. Consider the child who is bumped in the lunch line. In order to infer the other child's intentions, the bumped child must attend to the protagonist's facial expression (e.g., a surprised look would signal accidental intent), the velocity of the bump (a high velocity might signal aggressive intent), relevant situational cues (the lunch room is crowded and lots of jostling is occurring), and past history with the protagonist (the protagonist often acts aggressively). One's knowledge of social mores (for example, people usually say "sorry" when they accidentally bump into someone; young children bump into each other as a way of initiating social interaction) and ability to represent these social mores cognitively are also required at this step of social information processing. Problems in reading social cues could result from faulty role-taking ability, poor social comprehension, poor social inference skills, or poor representational skills. Reading includes both surface understanding of the event (the "what" of a social situation) and a deeper, more causal understanding (the "why" of a social situation). Kenneth Dodge and his colleagues (Dodge, 1980; Dodge & Frame, 1982; Dodge, Murphy, & Buchsbaum, 1984; Dodge & Newman, 1981; Dodge & Tomlin, 1983; Milich & Dodge, 1984; Steinberg & Dodge, 1983) have conducted a series of theoretically important and methodologically sound investigations on aggressive children's deficiencies and distortions related to social inference processes. This body of research has demonstrated that aggressive boys, relative to nonaggressive boys, overattribute hostile intent to peers in situations in which a peer's intention for a frustrating outcome is ambiguous. These biased attributions are the result of the aggressive boy's social information-processing errors. Specifically, aggressive boys selectively attend to and recall social cues consistent with hostile, versus nonhostile, intentionality (Dodge & Frame, 1982; Dodge & Newman, 1981). Additionally, aggressive boys do not utilize all available social cues and collect fewer pieces of information prior to making an attribution of a peer's intent in a situation resulting in a negative outcome (Dodge & Newman, 1981; Dodge & Tomlin, 1983; Milich & Dodge, 1984). Furthermore, when aggressive boys do attend to all the social cues and delay their decision as to a peer's intention, they do not overattribute hostility (Dodge & Newman, 1981). The picture that emerges of the aggressive boy's processing of social cues is one of interdependent errors and distortions in accurately reading, or encoding, social cues. The importance of these reading errors to the boy's aggressive behavior is demonstrated by research documenting that biased attributions are a direct antecedent of aggressive responding (Dodge, Murphy, & Buchsbaum, 1984; Dodge & Frame, 1982). In the Dodge *et al.* (1984) study, children classified according to sociometric status were shown videotapes of situations in which a peer caused a negative outcome or provocation. The peer was depicted as acting with one of five intentions: prosocial, hostile, merely present, accidental, or ambiguous. Socially deviant children (neglected and rejected) were less accurate than normal children (average and popular) in identifying peers' intentions, particularly in prosocial and accidental situations. Furthermore, when socially deviant children erred in identifying the peer's intention, they tended to misattribute hostile intent. Most important to the social information-processing model of social competence is the finding that deviant children's responses to the provocation varied directly as a function of the type of intention they identified and not as a direct function of the intention actually portrayed. This last finding underscores the fact that children respond to a perceived environment, not to a real one. Socially deviant children (especially aggressive children) perceive a more hostile environment.

Problems in Generating Solutions

The second stage in the model is anchored to the key word "generating." Given some perceived social situation, the child must decide how to respond to it. Problems at this stage in social information processing may occur as a result of deficiencies in the child's knowledge of effective responses to social situations, in ability to generate several alternative solutions, in sequential-planning skills (i.e., means–end thinking), or in consequential-thinking skills. Much of the research conducted by Spivack and co-workers (Spivack, Platt, & Shure, 1976; Spivack & Shure, 1974) on social problem solving has focused on skills essential to generating effective problem solutions (e.g., alternative thinking, means–end thinking, and consequential thinking). To follow the example of the child bumped in the lunch line, assume the child is unsure of the peer's intention. The children may generate only aggressive solutions ("hit") or ineffective solutions ("tell the teacher," "do nothing"). Additionally, problems may occur because the child lacks the ability to anticipate the consequences of specific solutions (e.g., "If I hit her, she will probably hit me back, and we'll both have to miss recess"). Part of evaluating the consequences of a solution is evaluating one's own competence for carrying out the solution. A poorly executed solution is unlikely to be effective. Finally, the child may experience problems at the generating stage because she has inadequate inhibitory control over responding. That is, she may respond impulsively to the problem with the first available response without stopping to think of its consequences or to consider alternative solutions and their consequences.

Illustrative Research

A great many research investigations have documented differences between socially deviant and normal children in the component skills required at this second stage of social information processing (Spivack et al., 1976; Richard & Dodge, 1982). Aggressive/rejected children generate fewer solutions to hypothetical social dilemmas (Asarnow & Callan, 1985; Richard & Dodge, 1982), and their solutions are less effective and more aggressive than those of nonaggressive children (Asarnow & Callan, 1985; Deluty, 1981; Lochman & Lampion, 1986; Richard & Dodge, 1982). In the Richard and Dodge study, groups of popular, aggressive, and isolate boys at two grade levels (second/third grades and fourth/fifth grades) were presented with six hypothetical problem situations and asked to generate alternative solutions to the problem. Three situations concerned a conflict with a peer, and three concerned a situation in which the child wanted to initiate a friendship with an unfamiliar peer. Popular children generated more solutions than either the aggressive or isolate groups, which did not differ. Although initial solutions generated by all groups were equally effective, subsequent solutions varied as a function of subject status. Popular children continued to generate effective solutions, whereas aggressive and isolate children's subsequent solutions were ineffective and aggressive. The premise that deviant boys are deficient in the specific skill of generating effective solutions and not in evaluating solutions was supported by the finding that groups did not differ in their ratings of effectiveness of solutions presented to them by the experimenter.

Asarnow and Callan (1985) investigated five social-cognitive skills in fourth- to sixth-grade boys with positive and negative (rejected) peer status. Four of these five processes involve skills relevant to the generating stage: (1) ability to generate a number of alternative solutions to social problems; (2) ability to generate nonaggressive, positive solutions to problems; (3) ability to evaluate possible solutions, and (4) ability to plan adaptively. After being presented with four social vignettes representing both aggressive and friendship situations, children were asked to generate solutions to the problem. Next, children were asked to evaluate solutions to the vignette problems. After children's responses to the situations and evaluations of responses to the four vignettes were obtained, the same situations were presented again, and the child was asked to describe what he would "feel and think" in each situation. Finally, the child was presented with six possible self-statements the "child in the story might be thinking and feeling" and asked to rate each one in terms of how likely the story child would be to feel and think that way. Compared to popular boys, rejected boys generated fewer solutions to the hypothetical problems, generated less mature, prosocial, and assertive solutions, generated more aggressive solutions, evaluated aggressive strategies more positively and prosocial strategies more negatively, and showed less adaptive and more maladaptive planning. Thus, Asarnow and Callan not only replicated the finding that rejected children generate fewer and more negative solutions, they also documented differences in rejected and popular children's characteristic planning, or means–end thinking. Specifically, rejected children were less likely to give a response indicating consequential thinking (e.g., "If I hit him, I'd get in trouble), anticipation of obstacles to a solution, reference to social rules, or goal setting.

Aggressive children's social problem-solving deficiencies do not occur equally in all types of situations. Researchers have found that aggressive/rejected children are especially likely to experience problems in situations involving peer provocation (Dodge *et al.*, 1985; Lochman & Lampion, 1986). For example, Dodge *et al.* (1985a) found that aggressive/rejected children's role play responses to different social situations were overall less competent than the responses of nonaggressive, adaptive children. However, the deficiencies of aggressive/rejected children were most evident in situations involving provocation by peers and in response to meeting social expectations. In addition to marked group differences in responding to problematic situations, low consistency of responding across situations was found among aggressive children. The researchers concluded that although general social problem-solving deficiencies characterize aggressive/rejected children, individual aggressive children will have particular problems with some situations and not with others.

Problems in Applying Solutions

Socially competent behavior requires not only the accurate interpretation of social cues and the generation and selection of effective solutions but also the competent execution of the chosen solution. "This component is characterized by the fluency with which skilled behaviors are summoned and executed in accordance with some strategic plan and by the ability to monitor efficiently one's own performance" (Hughes & Hall, 1987, p. 252). The girl bumped in the lunch line who infers (whether accurately or not) hostile intent may lack a strategic behavioral repertoire for responding to the provocation. She may decide that telling the peer to quit is the most effective solution, but her execution of this response in flawed. For example, she may whine, look at her feet, and speak softly.

Illustrative Research

Although a great deal of observational data document that socially deviant children behave less competently than socially normal children in a variety of situations (e.g., Dodge *et al.*, 1983; Putallaz, 1983; Rubin & Daniels-Beirness, 1983), this research does not permit an analysis of the specific social information processing deficits that result in incompetent performance. In order to assess a child's ability to enact a social solution, reading and generating processes must be held constant. Role play assessments offer a potentially useful method for assessing enactment skills. Most role play assessment measures present a hypothetical social situation to which the child responds. This procedure confounds reading, generating, and application skills. Dodge (1986) offered a procedure that holds events at the reading and generating stages constant. In this procedure, the child is presented with a videotaped hypothetical situation. After the child is asked questions pertinent to assessing social information processing stages, the child is asked to enact a particular solution provided by the assessor. Dodge rated children's behavioral execution of solutions to two types of situations, peer group entry and responding to peer provocation. Aggressive children's enactments were rated as less competent than those of nonaggressive peers. However, judgments of the effectiveness of children's role play enactments were not significantly related to judgments of the effectiveness of their behavior in actual provocations. In general, role play tests have not been successful in predicting naturalistic behaviors.

Summary

Research evidence supports differences between socially competent and socially incompetent children at each stage of the proposed model of social information processing. Although this evidence suggests these stages are important to successful social performance, correlational evidence of this sort does not demonstrate the clinical utility of the proposed model. The clinical utility of the model depends on the model's usefulness in deriving testable hypotheses as to the reasons for a particular child's social competence difficulties. Next, the use of the model in deriving such hypotheses is described.

IMPLICATIONS OF MODEL FOR ASSESSMENT

It is suggested that the three stages in the proposed information-processing model serve as decision points in assessing children's social behaviors. In this view, the assessment of social behavior involves obtaining information relevant to answering a series of questions yoked to each information processing stage. Figure 7-1 depicts a schematic of this decision-making process, starting from the social situation and moving through componential choice points to behavioral subtypes (Hughes & Hall, 1987, p. 252). Although the choice points are represented as dichotomous decisions, the underlying processes are assumed to be continuous. Nevertheless, these choice points are represented as dichotomous for purposes of delineating the possible errors and combinations of errors that may result in performance that is judged incompetent. The resulting subtypes should also have treatment implications. For example, a child with deficiencies at only one stage would be expected to require a more focused and briefer intervention that a child with deficiencies at each stage.

Importantly, the decision-making process is conducted in reference to a social problem. A "social problem" is defined as a class of social situations (e.g., responding to provocation, offering assistance/support) rather than as a specific social situation (e.g., telling a peer to stop drumming his pencil, complimenting a peer). Thus, an assessment of problematic social situations precedes the assessment of social information-processing skills. These skills are then assessed in the contexts in which the child's performance is judged unsuccessful.

Situational Assessment

Once the psychologist has determined that a child has difficulty in peer relations, as indicated by teacher ratings or sociometric assessments, it is important to identify those situations in which the child's performance is

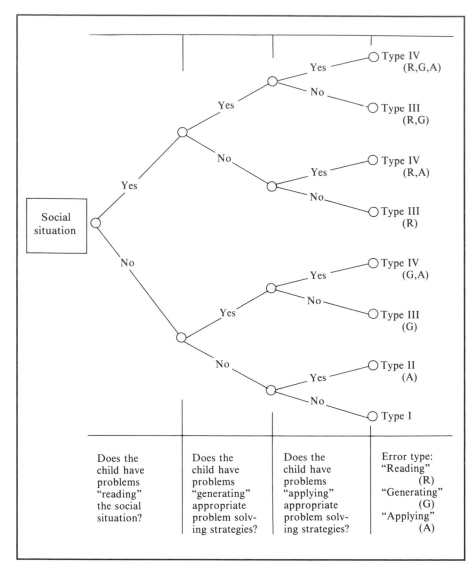

FIGURE 7-1. Schematic of the major components linking assessment to treatment/ intervention.

Source: From "Proposed Model for the Assessment of Children's Social Competence" by J. N. Hughes and R. J. Hall, 1987, *Professional School Psychology*, Vol. 2, pp. 254–255. Copyright © 1987 by Lawrence Erlbaum. Reprinted by permission.

judged incompetent. Several teacher-completed behavior rating scales supply information regarding the types of situations that are problematic for a child. The Social Behavior Assessment (SBA) (Stephens, 1981) is an example of a behaviorally and situationally specific rating scale. A total of 136 items are grouped into 4 broad categories and 34 subcategories on the basis of a logical, nonempirical analysis of item content. Though referred to as skill categories, these categories actually refer to types of situations (e.g., coping with conflict, helping others). A limitation of the SBA is that the situations and skills were not empirically derived. That is, they were not selected for inclusion based on evidence of the relationship of these situations and skills to indices of social competence.

Recently Dodge *et al.* (1985a) developed a teacher rating scale intended to identify the kinds of situations that are most likely to cause problems for a child. The authors used the behavior-analytic approach of Goldfried and d'Zurilla (1969) to develop the 44-item Taxonomy of Problematic Social Situations for Children (TOPS). Factor analysis of the taxonomy yielded six types of situations: peer group entry, response to peer provocation, response to failure, response to success, social expectations, and teacher expectations. Unlike other teacher rating scales, the TOPS asks teachers to rate how problematic given situations are for a child rather than to rate a child's skills. Teachers are instructed to rate social situations in terms of "how likely this child is to respond in an inappropriate manner (by hitting peers, aggressing verbally, crying, disrupting the group, withdrawing, appealing to the teacher for help, or behaving in some other immature, unacceptable, and unsuccessful way)." Three example items from the TOPS follow:

1. When this child is working on a class project that requires sharing or cooperation
2. When a peer performs better than this child in a game
3. When the teacher asks the child to work on a class assignment that will take a long time and will be difficult (Dodge, McClaskey, & Feldman, 1985b)

The TOPS has demonstrated high internal consistency and test–retest reliability and discriminates between socially rejected and adaptive children (Dodge *et al.*, 1985a).

Role play assessments can also be useful in identifying problematic situations. The Behavioral Test of Interpersonal Competence for Children (BTICC) (Hughes & Boodoo, 1987; Hughes & Hall, 1985) presents children with 24 videotaped social problem situations (18 in the revised BTICC). These situations require either positive assertive responses (e.g., expressing positive feelings, helping others, giving compliments) or negative assertive responses (e.g., refusing an unreasonable request, accepting blame, responding to teasing). The BTICC has demonstrated good interrater reliability and adequate test–retest reliability, and it discriminates between socially adjusted and maladjusted children. An advantage of the BTICC in individual child assessment is that it permits the assessor to observe a child's responses to a range of social problem situations not likely to be observed during a lengthy naturalistic observation. Evidence of comparability of a child's response in the role plays and *in situ*, however, has not yet been established. At best, role play assessments measure the child's optimal rather than customary performance in different situations.

Specifying Component Processes

Because social behavior is a result of a series of sequential steps, errors at one step are expected to affect the next step. For example, if a child misattributes hostile intent to a peer's accidental provocation, the child is likely to generate aggressive, as opposed to prosocial, responses to the provocation. Similarly, one cannot tell from observing a child's ineffective attempt to enter a play group whether the child lacks knowledge of effective entry strategies or has difficulty translating social knowledge to action. Thus, the sequential aspect of social information processing poses a challenge to the assessor. Dodge (1986) states that one assumption of the information-processing model is that the processes described at each step are separable and can be measured independently. Dodge (1986) presents an assessment procedure for holding each preceding step constant in assessing component processes. In this procedure, a child's stepwise processing of social cues is assessed via videotaped presentations of social interactions. Dodge has developed videotapes depicting two types of situations: peer group entry and responding to peer provocations. The child is asked to pretend he or she is in the situation presented on the tape. The tape is stopped at preinteraction, and the assessor asks questions relevant to each of the five steps in the Dodge (1986) social information processing model. Each step, in turn, yields between one and four processing variables. This procedure results in an accuracy score for each processing variable. Low to moderate correlations were found between scores on the information-processing steps and both sociometric status and actual behavior in entry and provocation situations. As the model predicts, greater predictive efficiency was obtained from multiple correlations using all of the information-processing variables.

The Dodge videotape assessment procedure is a laboratory procedure that is not easily transported to school-based assessments. Nevertheless, the basic procedure of presenting a child with hypothetical social dilemmas and asking questions posed by the decision-making scheme depicted in Figure 7-1 can be implemented in a school or clinic setting. Hughes & Hall (1987) describe a semistructured interview, the purpose of which is to collect data relevant to the decision-making model. The recommended interview format is structured around the social contexts that are thought to be problematic for the child (e.g., joining in, making friends, conflict resolution). First, the psychologist describes a particular social situation. It may be helpful to use pictures to represent the social situation. For example, a shy girl who has difficulty joining in with peers may be told a story about a girl who is watching her classmates jumping rope. The girl is depicted standing alone at some distance from the girls and is described as liking to jump rope. The psychologist then asks a series of questions about the story intended to obtain information on the child's sequential information processing. Table 7-1 presents a sample interview format. The specific questions and ordering of questions will depend on the child's answers. For example, if the girl says that the child in the story wants to watch the girls play, the psychologist would, at a later point, suggest a specific goal (the girl wants to play with them) and ask "What might the girl do if she wanted to play with them?" If the girl responded, "Tell the teacher," the psychologist would, at a later point, ask the child, "What might happen next if she asked them to play?" To assess application skills, the psychologist would instruct the child to role play the response "asking the girls to play."

The interview results in tentative hypotheses about specific cognitive and behavioral skill variables. Following the interview, the psychologist might administer selected measures of social-cognitive and behavioral skills to provide additional detail and documentation regarding these variables. Table 7-2 presents specific questions relevant to each decision-making juncture and assessment procedures that may provide data relevant to answering each question. For example, a child who generates few effective solutions to peer provocations might be administered the Problem Solving Measure for Conflict (PSMC) (Lochman & Lampion, 1986). A child who seems to have poor

TABLE 7-1. Sample Interview Format in RGA Model

R e a d	I. What is the story about?
	A. What does the child want?
	B. Why does the child want that?
	II. What are the other children thinking?
	III. What could the child do to get what he or she wants?
G e n e r a t e	A. What might happen next if the child did that?
	B. What else could the child do?
	1. What might happen if the child did that?
	2. What would be the best thing to do?
	3. What would be the best thing to do if the child wanted to play with other children?
A p p l y	IV. Is that what you would do?
	A. How good are you at doing that?
	B. Show me how you would do that?

Source: From "Proposed Model for the Assessment of Children's Social Competence" by J. N. Hughes and R. J. Hall, 1987, *Professional School Psychology*, Vol. 2, pp. 255–256. Copyright © 1987 by Lawrence Erlbaum. Reprinted by permission.

TABLE 7-2. Sample Questions, Procedures, and References for the RGA Model

Questions	Assessment Procedure	Reviews
Phase 1: Does the child have problems "reading" the social situation?		
1. Does the child accurately label others' intentions?	*Intention–Cue Discrimination Task (Dodge et al., 1984)	
2. Does the child accurately label others' emotions?	*Affective Perspective Taking Task (Marsh et al., 1980)	
3. Does the child sense social problems?	PEPSI (Feldhusen et al., 1972)	Butler & Meichenbaum, 1981
4. What goals does the child construct in social situations?	*Goals Interview (Renshaw, 1981)	
5. Does the child see the problem from multiple and differing social perspectives?	Chandler Role Taking Task (Chandler, 1971)	Enright & Lapsley, 1980; Kendall et al., 1981
	Interpersonal Understanding Interview (Selman et al., 1979)	Selman, 1980
6. Does the child seek information that would be useful in clarifying the problem?	PEPSI (Feldhusen et al., 1972)	Butler & Meichenbaum, 1981
Phase 2. Does the child have problems "generating" appropriate problem-solving strategies?		
1. Does the child generate different solutions to problems?	PIPS (Shure & Spivack, 1974)	Spivack et al., 1976; Butler & Meichenbaum, 1981
	Problem Solving Measure (Allen et al., 1976)	Butler & Meichenbaum, 1981
2. Does the child make step-by-step plans for achieving given problem resolutions?	MEPS (Platt & Spivack, 1975) and Children's MEPS (Shure & Spivack, 1972; Spivack et al., 1985)	Kendall & Braswell, 1985
3. Does the child anticipate consequences of different solutions to problems?	What Happens Next? Game (Spivack & Shure, 1974); The Awareness of Consequences Test (Shure & Spivack, 1978)	
4. Does the child use the evaluation of consequences in selecting a plan?		
Phase 3: Does the child have problems "applying" appropriate problem-solving strategies?		
1. Does the child "stop and think" before responding in social situations?	Teacher Self-control Rating Scale (Humphrey, 1972; direct observation; Conners's Parent and Teacher Rating Scales (Goyette et al., 1978)	Reynolds & Stark, 1986; Barton & Ascione, 1984; McMahon, 1984

(continued)

TABLE 7-2. (*continued*)

Questions	Assessment Procedure	Reviews
	Self-control Rating Scale (Kendall & Wilcox, 1979)	Reynolds & Stark, 1986
2. Does the child verify whether his or her solution was effective (self-monitoring)?	PEPSI (Feldhusen *et al.*, 1972); direct observation	Butler & Meichenbaum, 1981; Barton & Ascione, 1984
3. Does the child engage in the behavioral skills necessary to carry out the solution successfully?	Direct observation procedures; BAT-C (Bornstein *et al.*, 1977) Waksman Social Skills Rating Scale (1985)	Barton & Ascione, 1984; Michelson *et al.*, 1981

Source: From "Proposed Model for the Assessment of Children's Social Competence" by J. N. Hughes and R. J. Hall, 1987, *Professional School Psychology*, Vol. 2, pp. 254–255. Copyright © 1987 by Lawrence Erlbaum. Reprinted by permission.

Note: The assessment procedures and reviews of assessment procedures are for purposes of illustration and are not presented as an exhaustive listing.

*Procedures preceded by an asterisk have been developed for research uses and are not easily available.

perspective-taking ability might be administered Chandler's Bystander Cartoons (Chandler, 1971). The measures listed in Table 7-2 vary greatly in their evidence of reliability and validity. Furthermore, because most of these measures are not situationally specific, they may provide an indication of general skill level but may not predict performance in a specific type of situation.

The results of testing are integrated with results of the situational assessment and child interview to develop an individual model of the nature of the child's peer relationship difficulties. The clinical accuracy of the resulting model is best tested via documentation and evaluation of the child's progress before, during, and after the implementation of an intervention based on assessment results (Evans, 1985). Results of the interview and tests provide a preintervention baseline for the specific processes targeted in the intervention. The intervention can be evaluated by documenting changes in a child's impact on others (i.e., sociometric and teacher ratings) and changes in measures of component processes (i.e., interview and test data).

Next, the proposed assessment model is illustrated with a case study.

CASE STUDY IN ASSESSMENT OF SOCIAL COMPETENCE AND SOCIAL SKILLS

Background Information

Mark, age 9, was referred to the author by his parents on the recommendation of Mark's teachers. Mark's teachers and his parents were quite concerned about Mark's poor peer relations and oppositional behaviors. Mark, a boy of slight build with thick glasses, lives in a rural home with his parents and two brothers, ages 6 and 14. Because of the remoteness of the home, Mark's most frequent playmates were his two brothers. He rarely had friends over or visited friends, and when he did, Mark and his friend usually argued or played separately. Mark also frequently argued and fought with his younger brother.

Mark's problems were evident as early as age 4, when he entered preschool. He had difficulty separating from his mother, avoided playing with his peers, refused to comply with the teacher's directions, and "tested the limits." Throughout the elementary school years, Mark achieved adequately but was disliked or ignored by his classmates.

At the time of referral, Mark was completing fourth grade in a rural school. Because Mark was achieving adequately in school, he had not been referred by the school for consideration for special class placement.

Stage 1 Assessment: Impact Level Assessment

Both of Mark's teachers separately completed the Child Behavior Checklist–Teacher Report Form (Achenbach & Edelbrock, 1986). The results were quite consistent. Mark was rated as behaving much less appropriately than his classmates and as being much less happy. His school performance was rated as average. The teachers' written comments were especially revealing. One teacher wrote: "My major concern with Mark is his inability to interact with classmates. He seems to enjoy getting peers to argue or fight with him." The second teacher commented: "Other children dislike Mark intensely. Others can only stand to sit by him a short time. They all ask to be moved. He bothers them verbally and physically." Both teachers also commented on Mark's perfectionist tendencies and his frequent bids for approval.

Mark's scores on three of the behavior problem scales were in the clinically significant range. These scales are labeled Anxious, Unpopular, and Aggressive. The elevated anxiety scale reflects Mark's perfectionistic tendencies and low self-esteem (e.g., needs to be perfect, feels worthless, anxious to please, fears mistakes, worries).

A combination sociometric rating scale ("how much you like to play with") and nomination question ("like most") were administered to the 24 children in Mark's class. Using Asher and Dodge's procedure (1986), Mark was classified as rejected. He received seven ratings of "1" and no "like most" ratings.

Stage 2 Assessment: Situational Assessment

One of Mark's teachers completed the Taxonomy of Problem Situations (Dodge et al., 1985a). Mark experienced greatest difficulty in situations involving responding to provocation, meeting social expectations, and meeting teacher expectations.

On a videotape-administered role play test of social skills (Hughes & Hall, 1985), Mark performed ineffectively in situations involving peer provocation.

His most frequent responses to provocations were "telling the teacher" and "not listening to them." Importantly, Mark did not enact his responses, as requested, but told the examiner what he *would* do. He seemed unable to assume the "as if" attitude required to role play, possibly because of his high anxiety about giving the "correct" response.

Stage 3 Assessment: Componential Skills

In an interview format, Mark was presented with four hypothetical social dilemmas, two involving peer provocation and two involving meeting social expectations. A transcript of the interview for one of this provocations is provided below.

Interviewer: (*Presents first picture, which depicts the back of a boy in a lunch line. A second boy is walking toward the first boy with a food tray. The second boy is not looking where he is going.*) Pretend this is a picture of you standing in the lunch line at school. There are lots of kids in the cafeteria, and the line is crowded. This boy, Joe, is sorta a bully in your class. He has just got his tray and is trying to get through the line to a table. (*Interviewer presents second picture, depicting the food tray falling on the first boy. The second boy has a startled expression.*) Here Joe has bumped into you, spilling his food on you. What do you think happened?

Mark: I don't know.

Interviewer: Here you are with food on you. What do you think happened to cause that?

Mark: Joe spilled his food on me.

Interviewer: Why did Joe do that?

Mark: I don't know.

Interviewer: Did Joe spill his food on you by accident, or did he do it on purpose?

Mark: On purpose.

Interviewer: What makes you think he did it on purpose?

Mark: He's a bully.

Interviewer: What could you do if Joe spilled his food on you on purpose?

Mark: Tell the teacher.

Interviewer: What might happen next if you told the teacher?

Mark: She would punish him.

Interviewer: What else could you do?

Mark: I don't know. Nothing. Just do nothing.

Interviewer: What might happen if you did nothing?

Mark: I'd have to clean it up.

Interviewer: If Joe spilled his food on you by accident, what could you do?

Mark: Tell the teacher.

Interviewer: What might happen next?

Mark: She would punish him. I said that.
Interviewer: What else could you do?
Mark: I don't know. Ignore him. Do nothing.
Interviewer: What might happen next if you ignored him?
Mark: He would stop. I'd have to clean it up.
Interviewer: What would be the best thing to do if Joe spilled his tray on purpose?
Mark: Tell the teacher.
Interviewer: What would be the best thing to do if Joe spilled his tray by accident?
Mark: Tell the teacher.

Interviewer: One thing you could do if Joe spilled his food by accident is ask him to help you clean it up. Show me how you would do that. Pretend I'm Joe and ask me.
Mark: (*Eyes downcast, pulling at crotch of pants*) You'd better help me clean this up.

Mark's responses to the dilemmas suggested he had deficiencies at each of the three stages of social information processing. Thus, his subtype, according to the decision-making schematic in Figure 7-1, is Type IV. These deficiencies were most evident in provocation situations. He selectively attended to hostile cues (e.g., reputation as bully) and ignored cues inconsistent with hostile intent (crowded room, startled expression). He generated few solutions, and his solutions tended to be socially inappropriate and ineffective. Finally, his behavioral social skills were poor. His behavioral execution of solutions was marked by poor eye contact and nervous mannerisms.

To obtain additional information on Mark's skills, the Children's Means–End Problem Solving Test (MEPS) (Spivack, Shure, & Platt, 1985) and Children's Action Tendency Scale (CATS) (Deluty, 1979) were administered. On the MEPS, Mark generated an average number of solutions and demonstrated average step-by-step problem-solving ability. His responses to situations on the CATS requiring assertive responses tended to be either aggressive or submissive.

On the basis of the results of this assessment, a comprehensive intervention program was developed. This program involved weekly sessions over 5 months (May–September). Additionally, the parents participated in 6 sessions focusing on child management strategies. The first 8 child sessions addressed Mark's problems in cue utilization and cue detection. During these sessions, stories were presented and story characters' perceptions and intentions discussed. The same story was discussed from the perspective of different story characters, and social cues consistent with different attributions were highlighted. Mark kept a diary of disagreements and conflicts with others, and these incidents plus incidents reported by his parents were used to practice role taking and inferring attributions. The next 12 sessions focused on increasing Mark's social knowledge and behavioral skills. These sessions included a second boy who had also been referred for difficulties in peer relations. Social dilemmas were presented via role plays, the therapist modeled effective responses to those dilemmas, the two boys rehearsed the modeled solutions, and the therapist provided corrective feedback. Because of Mark's difficulty responding in uncertain situations and desire for detailed instructions, behavioral solutions were presented as specific steps, as in the Goldstein, Sprafkin, Gershaw, and Klein (1980) training program. Mark's role play responses were videotaped, and he evaluated his performance from the videotapes.

Because of the intervening summer vacation, data on Mark's school behavior could not be collected continuously during training. Mark's role play performance showed consistent improvement, as measured by increases in the proportion of effective solutions generated and decreases in nervous mannerisms. He demonstrated improved information-processing skills at each of the three stages, according to interview assessments completed in September. In October, Mark's fifth-grade teacher completed the Child Behavior Checklist and Taxonomy of Problem Situations, and the sociometric measures taken the preceding spring were readministered. Mark was rated as behaving as appropriately as his classmates and as being somewhat less happy than his classmates. His school performance continued to be average. Once again, the teacher's comments were helpful:

> Mark is well behaved in my class. A little girl came up to me at the football game Friday night and told me that Mark's behavior had improved a lot since last year. When other children notice an improvement, I think it means a great deal. I told Mark what the little girl said, and he was quite pleased.

> Mark is a good worker but worries too much about making mistakes. I wish he would just relax!

Mark showed improvement on all of the behavior problem scales and scored in the clinically significant range on only one scale, the anxious scale. Mark's sociometric classification was "average," and he received four ratings of "1" and two "like most" ratings.

On the Taxonomy of Problem Situations (Dodge et al., 1985a), Mark was no longer rated as having difficulty in peer provocation situations or in meeting social or teacher expectations.

In summary, Mark's behavior and peer acceptance improved. Unfortunately, this uncontrolled case study does not permit an experimental validation of the assessment model. It does, however, illustrate a systematic approach to the assessment of social competence that can be implemented in schools. It also illustrates a framework for selecting treatments on the basis of assessment data. The clinical utility of the hypotheses generated from the assessment model is supported by the efficacy of the treatment.

CONCLUSION

A model for assessing children's peer relations difficulties was presented. According to the proposed model, socially skilled performance is the result of proficient processing of information at each of three sequential stages, labeled Reading, Generating, and Applying. Proficient performance at each stage requires the application of specific information-processing skills. Assessment procedures must take into account the sequential nature of these skills by attempting the independent measurement of skills at each stage. An interview procedure was described and illustrated that facilitates the independent assessment of componential skills at each stage. Additionally, a decision-making schematic was presented to serve as a framework for classifying children with social competence problems according to error types. Finally, the recommended approach to assessing social competence problems and matching subtypes to treatments was illustrated with a case study.

Dodge (1986) has begun the experimental validation of the social information processing model. His preliminary investigations demonstrate that a combination of skill measures at each step predicts children's actual behavior in similar situations and judgments of social competence. Experimental validation of the clinical utility of the assessment model requires a finding that the subtypes generated by the model respond differentially to different treatments. Although matching subtypes to treatments is speculative at this point, the model's ability to specify subtypes and treatments means the model is testable. While awaiting further experimental validation of the model, psychologists can use the model as a framework for the systematic collection of data relevant to assessing and treating children's social competence problems.

REFERENCES

Achenbach, T. M., & Edelbrock, C. (1986). *Manual for the Teacher's Report Form and Teacher's Version of the Child Behavior Profile.* Burlington, VT: University Associates in Psychiatry.

Algozzine, B. (1977). The emotionally disturbed child: Disturbed or disturbing? *Journal of Abnormal Child Psychology, 5,* 205–211.

Asarnow, J. R., & Callan, G. A. (1985). Depression self-rating scale: Utility with child and psychiatric inpatients. *Journal of Consulting and Clinical Psychology, 53,* 491–499.

Asher, S. R., & Dodge, K. A. (1986). Identifying children who are rejected by their peers. *Developmental Psychology, 22,* 444–449.

Asher, S. R., & Hymel, S. (1981). Children's social competence in peer relations: Sociometric and behavioral assessment. In J. D. Wine & M. D. Smye (Eds.), *Social competence* (pp. 125–157). New York: Guilford Press.

Balou, B. (1966). The emotionally and socially handicapped. *Review of Educational Research, 36,* 120–133.

Barton, E. J., & Ascione, F. R. (1984). Direct observation. In T. H. Ollendick &

M. Hersen (Eds.), *Child behavioral assessment* (pp. 166–194). New York: Pergamon Press.

Behar, L. B., & Stringfield, S. (1974). A behavior rating scale for the preschool child. *Developmental Psychology, 10,* 601–610.

Bellack, S. A. (1979). A critical appraisal of strategies for assessing social skills. *Behavioral Assessment, 1,* 157–176.

Bornstein, M., Bellack, A. S., & Hersen, B. (1977). Social skills training for unassertive children: A multiple-baseline analysis. *Journal of Applied Behavior Analysis, 10,* 183–195.

Bower, E. M. (1969). *Early identification of emotionally handicapped children in school* (2nd ed.). Springfield, IL: Charles C. Thomas.

Butler, L., & Meichenbaum, D. (1981). The assessment of interpersonal problem-solving skills. In P. C. Kendall & S. D. Hollon (Eds.), *Assessment strategies for cognitive-behavioral interventions* (pp. 197–225). New York: Academic Press.

Chandler, M. J. (1971). *Egocentrism and childhood psychopathology: The development and application of measurement techniques.* Paper presented at the biennial meeting of the Society for Research in Child Development, Minneapolis, March.

Ciminero, A. R., Calhoun, K. S., & Adams, H. E. (Eds.). (1977). *Handbook of behavioral assessment.* New York: Wiley.

Clark, L., Gresham, F. M., & Elliott, S. N. (1985). Development and validation of a social skills assessment measure: The TROSS-C. *Journal of Psychoeducational Assessment, 4,* 347–356.

Coie, J. D., & Dodge, K. A. (1983). Continuities and changes in children's social status: A five-year longitudinal study. *Merrill-Palmer Quarterly, 29,* 261–282.

Coie, J. D., Dodge, K. A., & Coppotelli, H. (1982). Dimensions and types of status: A cross-age perspective. *Developmental Psychology, 18,* 557–570.

Coie, J. D., & Kupersmidt, J. B. (1983). A behavioral analysis of emerging social status in boys' groups. *Child Development, 54,* 1400–1416.

Cowen, E. L., Pederson, A., Barbigian, H., Izzo, L. D., & Trost, M. A. (1973). Long-term follow-up of early detected vulnerable children. *Journal of Consulting and Clinical Psychology, 41,* 438–446.

Damon, W. (1977). *The social world of the child.* San Francisco: Jossey-Bass.

Deluty, R. H. (1979). Children's action tendency scale: A self-report measure of aggressiveness, assertiveness, and submissiveness in children. *Journal of Consulting and Clinical Psychology, 47,* 1061–1071.

Deluty, R. H. (1981). Adaptiveness of aggressive, assertive, and submissive behavior for children. *Journal of Clinical Child Psychology, 10,* 149–155.

Dodge, K. A. (1980). Social cognition and children's aggressive behavior. *Child Development, 51,* 162–170.

Dodge, K. A. (1983). Behavioral antecedents of peer social status. *Child Development, 54,* 1386–1399.

Dodge, K. A. (1985). Facets of social interaction and the assessment of social competence in children. In B. H. Schneider, K. H. Rubin, & J. E. Ledingham (Eds.), *Children's peer relations: Issues in assessment and intervention* (pp. 3–22). New York: Springer-Verlag.

Dodge, K. A. (1986). A social information processing model of social competence in children. In M. Perlmutter (Ed.), *Cognitive perspective on children's social and behavioral development* (pp. 77–125). Hillsdale, NJ: Lawrence Erlbaum.

Dodge, K. A., Coie, J. D., & Brakke, N. P. (1982). Behavior patterns of socially rejected and neglected preadolescents: The roles of social approach and aggression. *Journal of Abnormal Child Psychology, 10*, 389–410.

Dodge, K. A., & Frame, C. L. (1982). Social cognitive biases and deficits in aggressive boys. *Child Development, 53*, 620–635.

Dodge, K. A., McClaskey, C. L., & Feldman, E. (1985a). Situational approach to the assessment of social competence in children. *Journal of Consulting and Clinical Psychology, 53*, 344–353.

Dodge, K. A., McClaskey, C. L., & Feldman, E. (1985b). *Taxonomy of problem situations*. (Available from K. A. Dodge, Department of Psychology, Indiana University, Bloomington, 47405.)

Dodge, K. A., Murphy, R. R., & Buchsbaum, K. C. (1984). The assessment of intention-cue detection skills in children: Implications for developmental psychology. *Child Development, 55*, 163–173.

Dodge, K. A., & Newman, J. P. (1981). Biased decision-making processes in aggressive boys. *Journal of Abnormal Psychology, 90*, 375–379.

Dodge, K. A., Schlundt, D. C., Schocken, I., & Delugach, J. D. (1983). Social competence and children's sociometric status: The role of peer group entry strategies. *Merrill-Palmer Quarterly, 29*, 309–336.

Dodge, K. A., & Tomlin, A. (1983). *The role of cue-utilization in attributional biases among aggressive children*. Unpublished paper, Indiana University.

Eisenberg, N. J., & Harris, J. O. (1984). Social competence: A developmental perspective. *School Psychology Review, 13*, 267–277.

Enright, R. P., & Lapsley, D. K. (1980). Social role-taking: A review of the constructs, measures, and measurement properties. *Review of Educational Research, 50*, 647–674.

Evans, I. M. (1985). Building systems models as a strategy for target behavior selection in clinical assessment. *Behavioral Assessment, 7*, 21–32.

Feldhusen, J., Houtz, J., & Ringenbach, S. (1972). The Purdue Elementary Problem-Solving Inventory. *Psychological Reports, 31*, 891–901.

Goldfried, M. R., & d'Zurilla, T. J. (1969). A behavioral-analytic model for assessing competence. In C. D. Spielberger (Ed.), *Current topics in clinical and community psychology* (Vol. 1, pp. 151–196). New York: Academic Press.

Goldstein, A. P., Sprafkin, R. P., Gershaw, N. J., & Klein, P. (1980). *Skill-streaming the adolescent*. Champaign, IL: Research Press.

Gottman, J. M. (1977). The effects of a modeling film on social isolation in preschool children: A methodological investigation. *Journal of Abnormal Child Psychology, 5*, 69–68.

Green, K. P., Forehand, R., Beck, S. J., & Vosk, B. (1980). An assessment of the relationship among measures of children's social competence and children's academic achievement. *Child Development, 51*, 1149–1156.

Greenspan, S. (1981). *The clinical interview of the child*. New York: McGraw-Hill.

Gresham, F. M. (1985). Utility of cognitive-behavioral procedures for social skills training with children: A critical review. *Journal of Abnormal Child Psychology, 13*, 411–423.

Gresham, F. M., & Elliott, S. N. (1984). Assessment of children's social skills: A review of methods and issues. *School Psychology Review, 13*, 292–301.

Hartup, W. W., Glazer, J. A., & Charlesworth, R. (1967). Peer reinforcement and sociometric status. *Child Development, 38*, 1017–1024.

Hops, H., & Greenwood, C. R. (1988). Social skill deficits. In E. J. Mash & L. G.

Terdal (Eds.), *Behavioral assessment of childhood disorders* (2nd ed.) (pp. 263–314). New York: Guilford Press.

Hughes, J. N. (in press). Assessment of children's social competence. In C. R. Reynolds & R. L. Kamphaus (Eds.), *Handbook of psychological and educational assessment of children*. New York: Guilford Press.

Hughes, J. N. (1986). Methods of skill selection in social skills training: A review. *Professional School Psychology, 1*, 235–248.

Hughes, J. N., & Boodoo, G. (1987). *Development and validation of a role play test of children's social competence*. Unpublished paper, Texas A&M University.

Hughes, J. N., & Hall, D. M. (1985). Performance of disturbed and nondisturbed boys on a role play test of social competence. *Behavioral Disorders, 11*, 24–29.

Hughes, J. N., & Hall, R. J. (1987). A proposed model for the assessment of children's social competence. *Professional School Psychology, 2*, 247–260.

Hughes, J. N., & Sullivan, K. (1988). Outcome-assessment in social skills training with children. *Journal of School Psychology, 26*, 167–183.

Hymel, S. (1983). Preschool children's peer relations: Issues in sociometric assessment. *Merrill-Palmer Quarterly, 29*, 237–260.

Jersild, A. T., & Fite, M. D. (1939). The influence of nursery school experience on children's social adjustment. *Child Development Monograph*, No. 21.

Kendall, P. C., & Braswell, L. (1985). *Cognitive-behavioral therapy for impulsive children*. New York: Guilford Press.

Kendall, P. C., & Morrison, P. (1984). Integrating cognitive and behavioral procedures for the treatment of socially isolated children. In A. W. Meyers & W. E. Craighead (Eds.), *Cognitive behavior therapy with children* (pp. 261–288). New York: Plenum Press.

Kendall, P. C., Pellegrini, J. S., & Urbain, E. S. (1981). Approaches to the assessment for cognitive-behavioral intervention with children. In P. C. Kendall & S. D. Hollon (Eds.), *Assessment strategies for cognitive-behavioral interventions* (pp. 227–285). New York: Academic Press.

Koch, H. L. (1933). Popularity in preschool children: Some related factors and a technique for its measurement. *Child Development, 4*, 164–175.

Kohn, M. (1977). The Kohn Social Competence Scale and Kohn Symptom Checklist for the preschool child: A follow-up report. *Journal of Abnormal Child Psychology, 5*, 249–263.

Ladd, G. W., & Mize, J. (1983). A cognitive–social learning model of social skill training. *Psychological Review, 90*, 127–157.

Lambert, N. M., & Bower, E. M. (1961). *A process for in-school screening of children with emotional handicaps*. Princeton, NJ: Educational Testing Service.

Landau, S., Milich, R., & Whitten, P. (1984). A comparison of teacher and peer assessment of social status. *Journal of Clinical Child Psychology, 13*, 44–49.

Laughlin, F. (1954). *The peer status of sixth- and seventh-grade children*. Bureau of Publication, Teachers College, Columbia University, New York.

Lochman, J. E., & Lampion, L. B. (1986). Situational social problem-solving skills and self-esteem of aggressive and nonaggressive boys. *Journal of Abnormal Child Psychology, 14*, 605–617.

Marsh, D. T., Serafica, F. C., & Barenboim, C. (1980). Effect of perspective-taking training on interpersonal problem solving. *Child Development, 51*, 140–145.

Masten, D. T., Morison, P., & Pellegrini, D. S. (1985). A revised class play method of peer assessment. *Developmental Psychology, 21*, 523–533.

Matson, J. L., Rotatori, A. F., & Helsel, W. J. (1983). Development of a rating scale to measure social skills in children: The Matson Evaluation of Social Skills with Youngsters (MESSY). *Behavior Research and Therapy*, *21*, 335–340.

McFall, R. M. (1982). A review and reformulation of the concept of social skills. *Behavioral Assessment*, *4*, 1–33.

McMahon, R. J. (1984). Behavioral checklists and rating scales. In T. H. Ollendick & M. Hersen (Eds.), *Child behavioral assessment* (pp. 80–105). New York: Pergamon Press.

Michelson, L., Foster, S., & Ritchey, W. (1981). Social skill assessment of children. In B. B. Lahey & A. E. Kazdin (Eds.), *Advances in clinical child psychology* (pp. 119–165). New York: Plenum Press.

Milich, R., & Dodge, K. A. (1984). Social information processing patterns in child psychiatric population. *Journal of Abnormal Child Psychology*, *12*, 471–490.

Muma, J. R. (1965). Peer evaluation and academic achievement performance. *Personnel Guidance Journal*, *44*, 405–409.

Piaget, J. (1932). *Moral judgment of the child*. New York: Harcourt, Brace.

Putallaz, M. (1983). Predicting children's sociometric status from their behavior. *Child Development*, *54*, 1417–1426.

Putallaz, M., & Gottman, J. (1983). Social relationship problems in children: An approach to intervention. In B. B. Lahey & A. E. Kazdin (Eds.), *Advances in clinical child psychology* (Vol. 6, pp. 1–44). New York: Plenum Press.

Quay, H. C. (1979). Classification. In H. C. Quay & J. S. Werry (Eds.), *Psychopathological disorders of childhood* (2nd ed.) (pp. 1–42). New York: Wiley.

Quay, H. C., & Peterson, D. R. (1983). *Interim manual for the Revised Behavior Problem Checklist*. University of Miami, Coral Gables, FL.

Quay, H. C., & Peterson, D. R. (1984). *Appendix I to the Interim Manual for the Revised Behavior Problem Checklist*. University of Miami, Coral Gables, FL.

Renshaw, P. D. (1981). *Social knowledge and sociometric status: Children's goals and strategies for peer interaction*. Unpublished doctoral dissertation, University of Illinois, Champaign, IL.

Reynolds, W. M., & Stark, K. D. (1986). Self-control in children: A multimethod examination of treatment outcome measures. *Journal of Abnormal Child Psychology*, *14*, 13–24.

Richard, B. A., & Dodge, K. A. (1982). Social maladjustment and problem solving in school-aged children. *Journal of Consulting and Clinical Psychology*, *50*, 226–233.

Roff, M. (1961). Childhood social interactions and young adult bad conduct. *Journal of Abnormal and Social Psychology*, *63*, 331–337.

Roff, M., Sells, S. B., & Golden, M. M. (1972). *Social adjustment and personality development in children*. Minneapolis: University of Minnesota Press.

Rubin, K. H., & Daniels-Beirness, T. (1983). Concurrent and predictive correlates of sociometric status in kindergarten and grade 1 children. *Merrill-Palmer Quarterly*, *29*, 337–351.

Schachar, R., Sandberg, S., & Rutter, M. (1986). Agreement between teachers' rating and observations of hyperactivity, inattentiveness and defiance. *Journal of Abnormal Child Psychology*, *14*(2), 331–345.

Schantz, C. U. (1975). The development of social cognition. In E. M. Hetherington (Ed.), *Review of child development research* (Vol. 5). Chicago: University of Chicago Press.

Selman, R. L. (1980). *The growth of interpersonal understanding.* New York: Academic Press.

Selman, R. L., Jaquette, D., & Bruss-Saunders, E. (1979). *Assessing interpersonal understanding: An interview and scoring manual.* Cambridge, MA: Harvard–Judge Baker Social Reasoning Project.

Shure, M. B., & Spivack, G. (1972). Means–end thinking, adjustment, and social class among elementary school-aged children. *Journal of Consulting and Clinical Psychology, 38,* 348–353.

Shure, M. B., & Spivack, G. (1974). *Problem-solving techniques in childrearing.* San Francisco: Jossey-Bass.

Spivack, G., Platt, J. J., & Shure, M. B. (1976). *The problem solving approach to adjustment.* San Francisco: Jossey-Bass.

Spivack, G., & Shure, M. B. (1974). *Social adjustment of young children: A cognitive approach to solving real-life problems.* San Francisco: Jossey-Bass.

Spivack, G., Shure, M. B., & Platt, J. J. (1985). *Means–Ends Problem-Solving stimuli and scoring procedures supplement.* Hahnemann University, Department of Mental Health Sciences, Philadelphia.

Steinberg, M. D., & Dodge, K. A. (1983). Attributional bias in aggressive adolescent boys and girls. *Journal of Social and Clinical Psychology, 1,* 312–321.

Stephens, T. M. (1981). *Technical information: social behavior assessment.* Columbus, OH: Cedars.

Strain, P. S. (1977). An experimental analysis of peer social initiations on the behavior of withdrawn preschool children: Some training and generalization effects. *Journal of Abnormal Child Psychology, 5,* 445–455.

Strain, P. S. (1985). Programmatic research on peers as intervention agents for socially isolate classmates. In B. H. Schneider, K. H. Rubin, & J. E. Ledingham (Eds.), *Children's peer relations: Issues in assessment and intervention* (pp. 193–205). New York: Springer-Verlag.

Strain, P. S., Cooke, T. P., & Apollini, T. (1976). *Teaching exceptional children.* New York: Academic Press.

Strauss, C., Forehand, R., Frame, C., & Smith, K. (1984). Characteristics of children with extreme scores on the Children's Depression Inventory. *Journal of Clinical Child Psychology, 13,* 227–231.

Stumme, V. S., Gresham, F. M., Scott, N. A. (1982). Validity of social behavioral assessment in discriminating emotionally disturbed from nonhandicapped students. *Journal of Behavioral Assessment, 4,* 327–341.

Ullmann, C. A. (1957). Teachers, peers, and tests as predictors of adjustment. *Journal of Educational Psychology, 48,* 257–267.

Van Hasselt, V. B., Hersen, M., & Bellack, A. S. (1981). The validity of role play tests for assessing social skills in children. *Behavior Therapy, 12,* 202–216.

Waksman, S. A. (1985). The development and psychometric properties of a rating scale for children's social skills. *Journal of Psychoeducational Assessment, 3,* 111–121.

Walker, H. M. (1976). *Walker Problem Behavior Identification Checklist manual.* Los Angeles: Western Psychological.

8
CONCEPTUAL AND METHODOLOGICAL ISSUES IN THE ASSESSMENT OF CHILDREN'S ATTRIBUTIONS

DOUGLAS J. PALMER
WILLIAM S. RHOLES
Texas A&M University

An important historical trend in psychology is the increased attention given to cognitive models of behavior control. Attribution theory (Abramson, Seligman, & Teasdale, 1978; Kelley, 1971) has made significant contributions to this development. This theoretical approach is largely defined by its attention to a single type of cognition, that is, cognitions related to perceptions of causality. Initially, attribution research focused on the cognitive operations involved in inferring causality, but over time it has become heavily involved in attempts to understand the cognitive processes that regulate behaviors. Consequently, attribution theory has become an important part of the cognitive-behavior modification (CBM) field. As such, it provides a theoretical framework for CBM techniques related to modifying children's causal perceptions in an attempt to alter problem behavior (cf. Dodge, 1980; Dweck, 1975).

Attribution theory has generated a substantial body of research related to both applied and theoretical issues, but relatively little attention has been devoted to assessment questions. In our view, this inattention may have a variety of negative consequences. With this in mind, the present chapter discusses issues relevant to the assessment of attributions, particularly assessment of children's attributions. (There is a limited discussion of the adult literature because in some cases relevant issues are not addressed in the childhood literature). The present chapter does not attempt to provide an exhaustive review of attributional studies. Studies have been selected that highlight important assessment questions. Moreover, the goal of the chapter is to address these questions from a largely pragmatic perspective. Although material related to theoretical concerns is included as background, the greater part of the chapter is devoted to "hands on" issues. Our goal is to address researchers and clinicians who may assess attributions in their work and to bring to their attention methodological issues that they may need to bear in mind when involved in assessing attributions.

We will first discuss the place of attributions in personality theory, and then will discuss concerns about the validity of verbal report data from an information-processing viewpoint. This will be followed by a description and critique of methodologies used to assess situationally specific attributions and attributional style. Finally, we will address a selected set of developmental considerations that may have an impact on the assessment of attributions in children.

PERSONALITY THEORY AND THE STUDY OF ATTRIBUTIONS

Self and other perception and motivational processes have been and continue to be an important area of study for personality researchers and theorists (Burnham, 1968; Ekehammar, 1974). Within the field of personality, research and theory have been guided primarily by four models: trait psychology, psychodynamics, situationism, and interactionism (see Endler & Magnusson, 1976, for an excellent review of these models). Although there continues to be substantial disagreement concerning the relative strengths and weaknesses of each of these models, there is a growing body of empirical support for an interactional model (Bandura, 1978; Bowers, 1973; Ekehammar, 1974; Endler & Magnusson, 1976; Mischel, 1973; Sameroff & Chandler, 1975). This section of the chapter will briefly describe the interactional model and discuss attribution theory within this context.

Interactional Model

Interactional psychology is concerned with the interplay of persons and situations in determining behavior (Ekehammar, 1974). According to Endler and Magnusson (1976), there are four essential features of modern interactionist models.

1. *Behavior is seen as a function of multidirectional interactions between individuals and the situations they encounter.* Advocates of this model propose that there is reciprocal interaction between environmental events and a person's behaviors. Not only do events affect behavior, but an individual's behaviors influence the environment as well. For example, teachers' selection of instructional tasks and procedures may influence pupils' behaviors. Pupils' subsequent classroom performance, however, may modify teachers' behaviors.

2. *Individuals are seen as intentional, active agents in these interactions.* That is, individuals interpret situations and assign meaning to them. They choose, to some extent, situations in which to participate. Individuals also select specific aspects of these situations as cues for their behavior.

3. *On the person side of the interaction, cognitive factors within the individual are the essential determinants of behavior.* Mischel (1973) arued that a

viable theory of personality must attend to person variables that are products of individuals' histories and that mediate their reactions to new situations. On the basis of his review in the areas of cognition and social learning, Mischel proposed a series of "cognitive" variables that mediate behavior. These variables include individuals' ability to generate thoughts and behaviors, and their self-perceptions, expectations, and personal rules for their behavior.

4. *From the situation side of the interaction, psychological meaning of the situation for the person is the important determining factor.* Interactional psychologists have adopted a distinction between the physical and the psychological environment (Ekehammar, 1974). The "physical" environment refers to the world outside the individual and can be described in terms of physical and social variables. In contrast, the "psychological" environment refers to individuals' perceptions and constructions of the physical environment and can be described with psychological variables. Endler and Magnusson (1976) suggest that these perceptions of the nature of environmental events are the basis of individuals' reactions. Examples of variables that may influence how individuals perceive their situation may be noted from Mischel's (1973) review. Specifically, he suggests that the manner in which individuals organize and categorize environmental events, perceive stimulus–outcome expectations, and value environmental stimuli will affect their behavior.

Attributions and the Interactional Model

Attributional cognitions may be characterized as a particular component of the person–situation interaction process. Interactionism and attribution theory have common roots in the work of Kurt Lewin (Ekehammar, 1974; Weiner, 1972). Interactionism in general, and attribution theory in particular, contend that human behavior is a function of the interaction between person and environment. For attribution theorists, the nature of the current environmental situation and individuals' personal histories form the psychological environment. The characteristics of this environmental context influence the development of individuals' attributional cognitions. These attributions mediate behaviors, which, in turn, affect the environment. As such, attributional cognitions are both a produce and an ingredient of person–environment interactions.

As a product of interactions, attributions are affected by a variety of personal and environmental antecedents (Weiner, 1972, 1979, 1985). A list of attributional antecedents most relevant to educational issues would include individuals' current performance, their history of performance on similar tasks, performance of others, characteristics of the instructional context and task, sex differences, and the use of behaviorally relevant medication (such as stimulant use for the control of attentional problems) (Palmer, 1983; Weiner, 1985).

As one of the "person" ingredients of the interaction, attributional perceptions influence behavior in two ways. First, as previously noted, attributions for specific events mediate subsequent thoughts and behaviors. These attributional consequences affect the nature of future interactions, which, in turn, may influence future attributional cognitions. Second, as a result of this complex interplay of personal and situational characteristics, attributions, and their consequences, individuals may over time develop a preferred set of attributional explanations. These preferential causal cognitions are referred to as "attributional styles." Children may, for example, view themselves in positive terms as bright, popular individuals. Despite their poor performance on a particular class assignment or the fact that some child may have snubbed their friendly overtures, they may continue to view themselves as bright and popular. These self-perceptions serve as one of the person characteristics that interact with situational factors and affect the formulation of situationally specific attributions. Attributional style may be viewed, in part, as an attributional mediator of the impact of environmental events on self-perceptions.

In sum, much of the recent theoretical and empirical work in personality psychology points toward a person–environment interactional model. Attribution theory is seen as one specific framework within this model. Situationally specific attributions and a somewhat enduring attributional style are both ingredients and products of this interactional process.

ATTRIBUTIONS AND VERBAL REPORT

Attribution theorists are concerned with the relationship between environmental events and the perceived reasons for these events (Weiner, 1972). These perceptions of causality are ascriptions made by observers or participants and, as such, are not directly observable. When we ask a child to explain why she did well on her spelling test, we are asking her to make public a private reflection of her thoughts and beliefs. Precisely because of the private nature of these cognitions, they are difficult to validate. The mere fact that she says she had a particular thought does not mean she did so, nor does failure to report indicate the absence of a thought. Moreover, even if individuals are motivated to report accurately, not all attributional processes may be available for conscious inspection. In this section, we will review briefly the arguments against the utility of verbal report data and make recommendations from recent work in cognitive psychology that may increase the reliability and validity of individuals' inferential reports. This information will be reflected on later sections of this chapter when we review various methodologies that have been used to collect attributional information from children and adults.

Criticisms of Verbal Report

In their attempt to understand mental functioning, early experimental psychologists relied on introspective reports. In the face of a variety of challenges, however, introspectionism soon was dropped as a method of scientific inquiry. Its demise was due, in part, to the impact of Freud's theories of the unconscious (Lieberman, 1979; Weiner, 1972). If the important determinants of behavior were unconscious, then introspective accounts of the conscious mind would be of limited utility. A second, rather potent attack came from the early behaviorists. Watson (1913) argued that understanding human behavior requires direct objective observation of behavior. From this perspective, reflections on one's own mental activities are of questionable value. Forty years later, Skinner (1953) accepted verbal reports of mental events as objects of scientific study but did not believe they could be used to study other behavior. He argued that introspective reports are inherently inaccurate in that they require individuals to match words to internal states that are in large part inaccessible. Skinner also objected to the use of mental events in explaining behavior because, in his view, they are not needed, to predict behavior. Furthermore, he was concerned that preoccupation with the mind would lead to the neglect of environmental factors. Although some forms of verbal report were not suspect—for example, performance on paired associate learning tasks—verbal reports generally came to be viewed as inadmissible evidence. Behaviorists expressed particular concern for the utility of retrospective inference-based verbal reports (Skinner, 1953; Watson, 1913).

Until the 1970s, few investigators examined the utility of verbal report information (e.g., Greenspoon, 1955). Recently, however, Nisbett and Wilson (1977) cited a number of experiments indicating that people often do not report accurately the effects of stimuli on higher order inferential processes. Nisbett and Wilson contend that individuals frequently are unaware of influences on their behavior. When asked, however, individuals will still generate reasons for their actions on the basis of implicit causal theories that they have formed. Nisbett and Wilson argue that these reports are unreliable and idiosyncratic, and as a consequence do little to further our understanding of behavior. Since assessment of attributions generally involves retrospective reporting of causal inferences, Nisbett and Wilson's conclusions are particularly challenging to researchers or practitioners who are concerned with youngsters' attributions.

In response to these various attacks on verbal report, Ericsson and Simon (1980, 1984) reflected on information-processing literature and proposed a model that specifies the conditions under which the previously noted criticisms of verbal report do and do not hold. They contend that the existence of invalid verbal reports should not force investigators to discard these data generally. Ericsson and Simon proposed a theory of verbalization that specifies when, where, and with what instructions informative verbal reports can be obtained. Although their review addresses a variety of content domains and methodologies, we will focus on their discussions and the features of their model that concern the reporting of higher order cognitive processes.

Ericsson and Simon's Model

Within the context of information-processing models (see Newell & Simon, 1972), Ericsson and Simon (1980, 1984) propose that information recently attended to is kept in a short-term memory store (STM) and is directly accessible for further processing, including the production of verbal reports. In contrast, information from a long-term memory store (LTM) must be retrieved and then transferred to STM before it can be reported. They hypothesize that, because of the limited capacity of STM, only the most recently attended-to information is directly accessible. However, a portion of the contents of STM is stored in LTM before being lost. This can later be retrieved from LTM. Verbal reporting is seen as bringing information from LTM and STM into attention and then converting it into verbalizable code. Ericsson and Simon contend that the crucial issue for verbal reporting is what information is attended to.

They propose that two forms of verbal report procedures can closely reflect cognitive processes. The first procedure is *concurrent* verbal reports—that is, talk-aloud or think-aloud procedures, where cognitive activities are verbalized as they occur. The second procedure is *retrospective* reporting. A durable memory trace of the cognitive activity is stored in LTM as individuals complete the task. After the task is completed, this trace can be accessed from STM or retrieved from LTM and verbalized. Since attributional assessments primarily involve retrospective reports, discussion of this procedure will be emphasized.

Retrospective reports on immediately preceding cognitive activity can be accessed without the experimenter having to provide cues as to what the individual is to retrieve. For example, when asked to report everything they can remember after they had just received feedback on their exams, students will still retain the necessary retrieval cues in STM. Although this reporting procedure may closely reflect cognitive processes, people may have difficulty separating recall of their cognitive activities in a specific instance from their recall of information from related episodes. Ericsson and Simon suggest that this problem may be eliminated by telling subjects to focus on the immediately preceding context or episode.

Another issue that is relevant to assessment of attributions concerns the use of directed probes or questions. In an attempt to assist individuals in retrieving the desired information from memory and to facilitate the completeness of their reports, investigators will frequently provide subjects with questions or verbal probes to aid their recall. Ericsson and Simon argue that people may generate thinking processes rather than reflect actual cognitive activities when the probes provide an inadequate set of alternatives. Their argument suggests that probes for youngsters' attributions should follow careful delineation of possible causal inferences gathered by open-ended procedures and in similar contexts. This recommendation has, in fact, been proposed by Elig and Frieze (1979).

Accuracy of verbal reports may depend, in large part, on the methodology used to gather them. Ericsson and Simon suggest that invalid reports like those discussed by Nisbett and Wilson (1977) may be due to inadequate procedures for eliciting verbal reports. For example, in many of the studies cited by Nisbett and Wilson, general probes such as "Why did you engage in certain behaviors during the experiment?" did not direct subjects to reflect on characteristics of the experiment. Subjects may have had relevant background information related to the probes and the experimental situation. Consequently, they may prefer to generate plausible responses on the basis of their experiences rather than attempt to retrieve information from their memory of the experimental situation. Many of the studies reviewed by Nisbett and Wilson also contained procedures that make the cognitive activities less accessible. For example, Ericsson and Simon note that there was limited incentive for subjects to recall their thoughts accurately. Further, in most of the studies reviewed by Nisbett and Wilson there was a substantial time lag between the end of the task and the probe. This lag may have affected the ability of subjects to recall their thoughts accurately.

Although individuals may, at times, be inaccurate in their verbal reports of higher cognitive processes, this inaccuracy appears to be the result of methodological concerns rather than some inherent inability of individuals to provide insight into their cognitive processes. Furthermore, when the experimental procedures facilitate veridical reporting, these reports provide valuable insight into important cognitive processes that mediate performance (Ericsson & Simon, 1980, 1984; Lieberman, 1979).

Implications for Assessment of Attributions

This brief review of issues and recommendations concerning the collection of verbal report data has implications for practitioners and researchers interested in obtaining attributional responses from children. Although investigation of children's attributional statements under a variety of experimental conditions may be a topic of interest unto itself, the outcomes from many of these studies may tell us little about their causal thoughts and beliefs when the events took place. As noted in later sections of this chapter, a number of studies have used methodologies that may have produced verbal reports of questionable utility. Reflecting primarily on Ericsson and Simon's (1980, 1984) reviews and their proposed model of verbalization, the following recommendations for eliciting attributions are presented.

1. Use "think-aloud" to examine children's causal thoughts at the time of the specific incident. This procedure will provide a more direct on-line assessment as specific information is heeded in STM. Unfortunately, in many real-world contexts such as classrooms, talking aloud may be disruptive. In addition, many youngsters may feel awkward or embarrassed about either the procedure or the content of what they are saying. Consequently, a retrospective method that allows for greater anonymity and less disruption may be preferable.

2. Use open-ended, more general probes such as, "Tell me everything you were thinking when you were not picked for the softball team." These retrospective probes should be administered immediately after the event of interest

has occurred and should refer directly to the event. These probes may be particularly useful when there is little available information on a particular populations' open-ended attributional responses for a specific event. For older children, open-ended probes may take a written format. This procedure allows for a greater sense of anonymity on the part of the respondents. Either an oral or a written general probe enables individuals to respond without the constraints of a fixed set of alternative responses that were established by the examiner.

3. If a substantial body of open-ended attributional information on a specific population for a specific set of events is available, researchers should be able to present a rather complete set of structured retrospective attributional probes. Using many of the same recommendations noted for the open-ended probes, structured probes need to refer directly to the specific event that has just occurred.

SITUATIONALLY SPECIFIC ATTRIBUTIONS

Since the early 1970s there has been substantial interest in the study of individuals' causal ascriptions in a variety of experimental conditions. Despite this interest, little systematic work has focused on *how* to gather valid attributional responses for specific events. Papers that have addressed methodological concerns in attributional research focus primarily on issues outside the context of attributional assessment (e.g., Covington & Omelich, 1984; Weiner, 1983). Elig and Frieze's (1979) study is one of the few methodological investigations that has addressed assessment of attributions. They examined convergent and discriminant validities of open-ended and structured approaches to assessment of adults' achievement attributions. Unfortunately, investigators assessing attributions in children have had little empirical or theoretical basis on which to examine the validity of their assessment approaches. As a result, there has been a proliferation of methodologies resulting in procedural confusion and conflicting sets of findings across studies. On the basis of our previous discussion of verbal report, we will critique a variety of procedures that have been used to assess attributions.

In our attempt to survey the current state of attributional assessment of children, we examined studies primarily from three major journals: *Child Development*, *Developmental Psychology*, and *Journal of Educational Psychology*. We focused on these publications because they contained a large number of studies with children. In addition, contributors to these journals are often the most active and respected researchers in their field. Consequently, a review of attribution studies in these journals should provide an overview of the procedures used to assess attributions in children. Because we were not interested in specific findings but, rather, in how children's attributions for particular events were assessed, the citations do not represent all possible attribution studies. Experiments are cited when they used some unique approach to attributional assessment. Finally, to provide an overview of current methodologies, we primarily reviewed studies that have been published within the last 15 years.

Review of Sampled Investigations

Methodologies of 38 studies were reviewed (see Table 8-1). A large majority of these articles assessed attributions for achievement events, with only 10 of the 38 studies examining children's attributions for social outcomes.

Attributions for Achievement Outcomes

For many of the studies, the achievement event of interest was an academic outcome. But a number of studies of achievement attributions did consider performance on a variety of cognitive nonacademic tasks and in sports. Approximately half of these achievement events were hypothetical in nature; that is, youngsters are asked to *imagine* that they or other children succeed or fail on a task. With these procedures, youngsters are required to generate attributional responses from long-term memory that may not reflect their thoughts if the achievement event had actually occurred (see Ericsson & Simon, 1984; Nisbett & Wilson, 1977). Studies using hypothetical situations can reveal children's logic in simulated situations. Findings from these studies, however, may not reveal the logic children may use in actual situations. Consequently, studies with hypothetical achievement events (e.g. Pearl, Bryan, & Donahue, 1980) may provide little insight into children's attributions for actual achievement outcomes. In fact, results from these studies may conflict with findings from investigations using actual achievement situations (e.g. Palmer, Drummond, Tollison, & Zinkgraff, 1982).

Six of the achievement attribution studies used open-ended probe procedures, as recommended by Elig and Frieze (1979) and Ericsson and Simon (1984). Of these six studies, Bar-Tal and Darom's (1979) and Diener and Dweck's (1978) investigation were the only studies that assessed open-ended attributional responses in an actual achievement situation. Bar-Tal and Darom's decision rule for inclusion of pupils' statements into the final list of attributions was that the ascriptions were mentioned at least twice in their pilot study. Although this procedure placed few constraints on the raw data, it is not a naive, intuitive, or systematic analysis that will produce a comprehensive listing of attributions. Judgments concerning the conceptual similarity of individuals' responses depend, in part, on the nature of the population who are doing the categorizing (Hartke, 1978). Categorization of children's attributional responses by psychologists (e.g., Bar-Tal & Darom, 1979) may differ greatly from the categories generated by children.

An alternative approach to analyzing free-response attributional responses is Latent Partition Analysis (Willson & Palmer, 1983). In the Willson and

Palmer study, college students received feedback on a class exam and were asked an open-ended attribution probe concerning their performance. Other college students from a different section of the same course were asked to categorize these attributional responses. Latent Partition Analysis of attributions assumes that individual categorizations are based on an individual probability matrix. It is also assumed that individuals' matrices can be averaged to obtain a group probility matrix. Each attributional category for each subject is formed into a vector representing the absence or presence of attribution statements. The vectors of all the attribution categories from the matrix to be examined (see Hartke, 1978; 1979; Wiley, 1967) This procedure allows for a naive and systematic approach to the analysis and categorization of open-ended attributional responses.

An additional issue concerning the gathering of free-response attributions from young children is whether the children have sufficient verbal fluency to communicate their attributional cognitions. When asked to tell what they were thinking, many children may respond, "Don't know." Ericsson and Simon (1984) suggest that this response may not be due to an inability to respond. Bretherton and Beeghly (1982) report that even 2- and 3-year-old children are able to communicate about their internal states, including concepts of ability and volition. Therefore, the issue may not be youngsters' capacity but, rather, their willingness to communicate. A potential solution to this problem could be the assessment of young children's concurrent verbalizations. Recording and categorizing these responses may provide valuable insight into children's attributions without being obtrusive. Of the studies reviewed, Diener and Dweck (1978) were the only investigators to use a talk-aloud procedure for achievement-related attributions. Although mastery-oriented pupils engaged in different verbalizations than helpless pupils, both groups of youngsters did verbalize attributions.

The most prevalent manner used by the studies we reviewed to collect attributional data from children involved the use of retrospective structured probes. Of the probe procedures used, Likert-type scales were the most popular, but multiple-choice and paired-comparison formats were also used with some frequency. The Likert scales ranged from 4- to 11-point scales and assessed degree of importance (influence) or amount of the factor. In addition, some of the scales used visual or manipulative cues, whereas others presented only a linear scale. With the exception of references to previous studies or to the Elig and Frieze (1979) research with adults, little rationale was given for the nature and structure of the assessment procedure. In fact, in reviewing a series of studies by the same authors, we found variation in methodology used with little accompanying explanation for the changes.

In regard to the attributions assessed, there was remarkable consistency in the specific attributions that were assessed by specific probes. In large part, this consistency appears to be due to the common reference to Weiner's (1972) early work. In addition, there have been a variety of studies with adults that support the use of effort, ability, and task characteristics as achievement

TABLE 8-1. Methodologies for Attributional Assessment

Experiment	Sample	Attributional Context	Type[a]	Attributional Event: Description	Attribution	Probe[b]
Ames, 1978	M & F; 5th grade	Self	Act	Solvable and insolvable puzzles	Ability Effort Luck Task difficulty	Likert 9 pt. with visual cue (amount)
Ames, 1984	M & F; 5th–6th grade; low/medium/high achievers	Self	Act	Solvable and insolvable puzzles	Ability Effort Self-instruction	Circle statement they are thinking
Ames & Ames, 1981	M & F; 5th–6th grade	Self	Act	Solvable and insolvable puzzles	Ability Effort Task difficulty Luck	PC
Ames & Felker, 1979	M & F; 1st–5th grade	Other	Hyp	Stories of child performing puzzle task	Ability Effort Task difficulty Luck	Likert 9 pt with visual cue (amount)
Amirkhan, 1982	M & F; medium/normal hyperactive; LD and nonhandicapped; 11–12.5 yr	Other	Hyp	Six stimulus vignettes of medicated/nonmedicated hyperactive and nonhandicapped boys who experienced failure or success on test	Ability Effort Difficulty of test Medication Nourishing breakfast Teacher intervention	OE/pilot Likert 7 pt (importance)

Study	Sample	Source	Type	Task	Attributions	Method
Bar-Tal & Darom, 1979	M & F; 5th–6th grade	Self	Act	Returned graded class test	Ability Interest Difficulty of material Effort during test Difficulty of test Preparation for test Teaching explanation of material Learning conditions at home	OE/pilot Likert 4 pt. (influence)
Bar-Tal, Raviv, Raviv, & Bar-Tal, 1982	6th grade; low/middle/upper SES	Self	Act	Returned graded class tests	Ability Interest Attributions Luck	Likert 7 pt. (influence)
Bird & Williams, 1980	M & F; 7–18 yr	Other	Hyp	Performance in sports	Ability Hard work Difficulty of sport Luck	Likert 7 pt. (importance)
Bugental, Whalen, & Henker, 1977	M; medicated/non-medicated hyperactive 7–12 yr	Self	Hyp	Interview concerning school success and failure	Effort Teacher bias Luck	Likert 4 pt. (importance) with visual cue
Callaghan & Manstead, 1983	M & F; average age = 16.7 yr	Self	Act	Outcome for certificate exam	Ability Preparation Effort Mood Help from teachers Help from home Difficulty of exam Luck	Likert 11 pt. (importance)
		Self	Act	Randomly assigned to easy/difficult anagrams for success/failure condition	Effort Ability Task difficulty Luck	Likert 11 pt. (amount)

(continued)

177

TABLE 8-1. (continued)

Experiment	Sample	Attributional Context	Attributional Event		
			Type[a]	Description	Attribution	Probe[b]
Diener & Dweck, 1978 Study 1:	M & F; 5th grade	Self	Act	Experimenter provided failure feedback on a two-choice discrimination task	Ability Effort Luck Experimenter not fair Task harder	OE; categorized by two raters
Study 2:	M & F; 5th grade (did not participate in Study 1)	Self	Act	(See Study 1)	Useful/ineffectual task strategy Self-instruction Loss of ability	No probe. Talk-aloud procedure was used
Dix & Grusec, 1983	M & F; 5–13 yr	Other	Hyp	A brief tape recorded story with pen & ink sketch of story about family member needing help	Internal trait (being nice) External causes for the reason they behaved (mother's influence)	PC
Dodge, 1980 Study 1:	M; aggressive/nonaggressive; 2, 4, & 6 yr	Other	Hyp	Stories of a peer spilling milk on/hitting a child	Intentionality	OE interview in which responses were called as intentional/accidental
Dollinger, Staley, & McGuire, 1981	M & F; 5th–6th grade	Other	Hyp	Story about 4 players having a playoff softball game	Situational factor (losing game) Internal factors (characteristics of player)	PC Likert 5 pt. (confidence) for each factor OE

Study	Subjects			Task		Measure
Dweck & Bush, 1976	M & F; 5th grade	Self	Act	Failure on 3 trials of digit-letter substitution problems	Ability / Effort / Experimenter not fair	MC
Erwin & Kuhn, 1979	M & F; 4th, 8th, & 12th grade	Other	Hyp	Seven stories with pictures concerning social events		OE: Response determined by reference to more than a simple cause
Etaugh & Brown, 1975	M & F; 5th–8th grade & college	Other	Hyp	Stories of success or failure in mechanics or athletics	Ability / Effort / Task difficulty / Luck	MC
Friend & Neale, 1972	M & F; 6th grade; middle/low SES; black/white	Self	Act	Randomly assigned feedback on reading comprehension task	Ability / Effort / Task difficulty / Luck	Likert / 9 pt. with manipulate cue (amount) / Rank order (importance)
Frieze & Snyder, 1980	M & F; 1st, 3rd, & 5th grade	Other	Hyp	Four stories with pictures concerning success or failure: Academic exam / Football / Catching frogs / An art project		OE: Response categorized by Elig & Frieze (1975) Coding scheme
Harris, 1977	M & F; 1st, 3rd, 6th, & 8th grade	Other	Hyp	Videotape scenes concerning damage of an item and a child. Scenes represent different levels of responsibility	Child's responsibility	Likert / 9 pt. with visual cue
Heller & Berndt, 1981	M & F; K, 3rd, 6th grade, & college	Other	Hyp	Stories concerning sharing behavior	Sharing / Helpful / Nice / Bad / Smart / Neutral	Likert / 5 pt. with visual cue (amount)

(continued)

TABLE 8-1. (*continued*)

Experiment	Sample	Attributional Context	Attributional Event		Attribution	Probe[b]
			Type[a]	Description		
Hiebert, Winograd, & Danner, 1984	M & F; 3rd & 6th grade	Self	Hyp	24 items concerning evaluation of reading & comprehension situations, half with success and half with failure outcomes	Ability Studying Task difficulty Luck Paying attention Assistance	Likert 5 pt. with visual cue (agree/disagree)
Karabenick & Heller, 1976	M & F; 1st, 3rd, 5th grade & college	Other	Hyp	Stories about pupils described as differing in effort or ability and performance on puzzle task	Effort Ability	PC
Keasey, 1977	K & 1st grade	Other	Hyp	Stories of children differing in intention and damage to items		OE: Concerning why children were naughty or not. Responses were coded as intentionality, chance, or consequence oriented.
Kun, 1977 Study 1:	M & F; 3rd & 5th grade	Other	Hyp	Stories of boys' performance on a set of 7 puzzles. Puzzles were shown to subjects.	Ability Effort	Ability—bipolar Likert 9 pt. scale with visual cue Effort—unipolar Likert 9 pt. scale with visual scale

Licht, Kistner, Ozkaragox, Shapiro, & Clausen, 1985	M & F; LD & non-LD; 3rd–5th grade	Self	Hyp	Items concerning failure performance on reading comprehension activities	Ability Effort External causes	FC
Marsh 1984	5th grade	Self	Hyp	24 brief scenarios representing academic success/failure	Ability Effort External causes	Likert 5 pt. (false/true)
Nicholls, 1979	1st, 3rd, 5th, & 7th grade	Self	Hyp	Items concerning success or failure on reading tasks	Ability Effort Task difficulty Luck	PC
Pearl, 1982	3rd–4th grade	Self	Hyp	Six hypothetical situations dealing with success/failure in reading, putting together a puzzle, and getting along with other children	Ability Effort Task difficulty Luck	PC
Pearl, Bryan, & Donahue, 1980 Exp. 2	1st–8th grade; under achievers normal achievers	Self	Hyp	Six situations described in Pearl (1982)	Effort Ability Task difficulty Luck	Likert 4 pt. (importance)
Rholes & Walters, 1982	M & F; 5–10 & 18–22 yr	Other	Hyp	18 short stories concerning achievement, affective responses, and decisions on choices	Stimulus (task or setting) Person (ability) Circumstance (luck)	Likert 4 pt. with visual cue (importance)
Ruble, Parsons, & Ross, 1976 Exp. 2	M & F; 4–5.8 & 7.5–9 yr	Self	Act	Randomly assigned performance feedback on Matching Familiar Figures Task	Ability Effort Task difficulty	Likert 9 pt. scale with visual cue (amount)
Schunk, 1984	M & F; 3rd grade	Self	Act	Performance on subtraction problems	Ability Effort Task difficulty Luck	Likert 10 pt. (importance)

(continued)

TABLE 8-1. *(continued)*

Experiment	Sample	Attributional Context	Type[a]	Attributional Event Description	Attribution	Probe[b]
Shultz & Butkowsky, 1977	M & F; Kindergarten	Other	Hyp	Stories or videotapes of child solving puzzles		OE: Response analyzed to determine use of causal schemes
Shultz, Butkowsky, Pearce, & Shanfield, 1975	M & F; K, 4th–8th grade	Other	Hyp	Stories about a variety of social events	Internal / External	Absence/presence
Smith, Gelfand, Hartmann, & Partlow, 1979	M & F; 2nd–3rd grade	Self	Act	Participation in a game in which donation opportunities were available to help an unknown other player		OE: Response categorized according to intrinsic/extrinsic motivation; Likert 7 pt.
Stipek & Hoffman, 1980	M & F; 1st & 3rd grade; top/middle/low achievers	Self	Act	Insolvable anagrams	Ability / Effort / Task difficulty / Luck	PC
Tollefson et al., 1982	M & F; 7th–9th grade; LD & non-LD	Self	Act	Performance on spelling task	Ability / Effort / Task difficulty / Luck	MC

[a]Act indicates actual event took place. Hyp indicates use of a hypothetical situation.

[b]PC indicates paired comparison. OE indicates open-ended procedure. MC indicates multiple-choice probe.

attributions (Weiner, 1985). Consequently, investigators do have a substantial data base from which to derive attributions, but it is unclear whether these attributions accurately reflect children's naturally occurring causal ascriptions for achievement.

Attributions for Social Outcomes

Only 1 of 10 studies that assessed attributions for social events used actual outcomes (Smith, Gelfand, Hartmann, & Partlow, 1979). In view of the concerns raised earlier about verbal reports of hypothetical events, one should have little confidence that the findings reported from these investigations do reflect actual cognitive processes that children use when encountering social events.

Four of the 10 studies did use open-ended procedures to gather attributional information. In some of these studies, however, (Dodge, 1980; Shultz & Butkowsky, 1977; Smith et al., 1979), a series of categorical constraints was placed on the verbal reports to determine use of causal schemes, intrinsic/extrinsic motives, and intention/accident attribution, respectively. As a result, the naive, intuitive organization of children's causal statements was not available.

For the remaining 6 studies, a variety of structured probe procedures were used. As with the achievement attributions, there was no theoretical or empirical rationale provided for the selection of particular probe procedures. Selection of the attributions for study reflected, to a large extent, the specific interests of the investigators and the nature of the experimental setting.

Summary

On the basis of our sample of recent attributional investigations with children, it appears that a variety of methodological features of these studies may affect the validity of their attributional responses. Despite the growing interest in children's attributions, particularly for achievement outcomes, few studies have gathered data on youngsters' attributions for actual social or academic outcomes. Although the use of hypothetical situations allows one to explore a variety of events of interest in a short time period, the utility of verbal reports from these investigations is questionable (Ericsson & Simon, 1984). A second concern involves the lack of systematic efforts to gather and organize free-response attributions. Much of the children's attribution literature has drawn on experimentation with adults that contains many of the same methodological concerns previously noted. Further, even if the conclusions from the adult literature are valid, there is a need to assess and categorize children's attributions without placing a series of methodological constraints on their open-ended verbal responses. There also needs to be greater study of the different structured probe procedures used with children. Although there is some, albeit limited, information in this area with adults (Elig & Frieze, 1979) and this information is referenced in the children's literature, there has not been any direct study of the effects of various probes on children's attributional responses.

Although children's attributions have been assessed in a number of studies, because of the variety of potential methodological problems inherent in these investigations, we may in fact know little about children's attributions for real-world achievement or social events. To further our knowledge of children's attributions for specific situational outcomes, we propose the following methodological recommendations:

1. If investigators are interested in children's attributional cognitions of actual achievement or social outcomes, then they must study real-world events. Not only may attribution findings be inherently flawed because of the use of hypothetical situations (see Ericsson & Simon, 1984), but investigators frequently overgeneralize their results. With some regularity, simulation procedures were used, but the rationale and discussions within the studies referred to practical concerns and applications. Although this may appear to be a rather pedestrian recommendation, we feel it should be noted that accurae assessment of children's attributions for meaningful achievement and social outcomes in their lives requires the use of experimental procedures that reflect these activities.

2. Investigations should monitor children's on-line verbalizations while they are engaged in activities. This procedure may be particularly helpful for assessing attributions with young children. The use of concurrent verbalization procedures provides a more complete corpus of attributional cognitions for children and may give an indication of the antecedents of specific attributional statements.

3. When concurrent verbalizations are not feasible, use general, open-ended probes immediately after the event has occurred.

4. It is also recommended that "unbiased" procedures such as Latent Partition Analysis be used to categorize free-response attributional statements.

5. On the basis of the results of concurrent verbalization and/or general open-ended probe procedures, a set of structured attributional probes may be derived. However, the effects of various probe formats on children's responses will have to be investigated prior to recommending a particular format.

ATTRIBUTIONAL STYLE

The term "attributional style" (AS) refers, on the one hand, to universal or near universal biases in the attributional process, such as the actor–observer difference and the self-serving bias (Jones & Nisbett, 1971; Nisbett & Ross, 1980). It also is used, however, to refer to personality-based differences in patterns of attribution. In this second sense, the one with which we will be concerned in this chapter, it is viewed as a mediator of individual differences in responses to environmental inputs. It has been used most often in recent years to explain differences in vulnerability to depression (Abramson, Seligman, &

Teasdale, 1978) and in reactions to achievement-related situations (Dweck & Elliott, 1983).

Prior to discussing AS measures, the following two points should be noted. First, researchers frequently confuse the concepts of "attribution" and "attributional style." As noted earlier, "attributions" refer to individuals' unique causal assumptions for a *specific* event. A variety of characteristics associated with a particular event can affect attributions (e.g., Frieze, 1976). In contrast, AS is a preferential set of causal beliefs that individuals may reflect on across a variety of situations. Therefore, using AS measures in an attempt to assess attributions for a specific situation would be inappropriate and may result in spurious conclusions. Second, because of the conceptual differences between AS and attributions, the issues raised concerning verbal report are only partially applicable to AS. That is, AS measurement is *not* concerned with the assessment of ongoing cognitive process in specific situations. Consequently, although many of the previously noted criticisms concerning assessment of situationally specific attribution may be indirectly related to AS assessment, they will not be a focal point of this discussion.

A number of AS measures have been developed and used for research purposes. The various measures, despite their common linkage to attribution processes, are not interchangeable. They were developed with different conceptual rationales and with different purposes and populations in mind. The most widely used instruments fall into two broad classes: locus-of-control (LOC) scales and attributional style scales proper. Widely used locus-of-control scales have been developed by Rotter (1966); Levenson (1973); Wallston, Wallston, Kaplan, and Maides (1976); Norwicki and Strickland (1973); Crandall, Katkovsky, and Crandall (1965); and Mischel, Zeiss, and Zeiss (1974). The last three of these are for use with children. Examples of attributional style scales are the *Attributional Style Questionnaire* (ASQ; Peterson, Semmel, von Baeyer, Abramson, Metalsky, & Seligman, 1982; Seligman, Abramson, Semmel, & von Baeyer, 1979); the *Attributional Style Assessment Test* (ASAT; Anderson, Horowitz, & French, 1983; Anderson, Jennings, & Arnoult, 1987); the *Multidimensional–Multiattributional Causality Scale* (MMCS; Lefcourt, von Baeyer, Ware, & Cox, 1979); the *Content Analysis of Verbatim Explanations* measure (CAVE; Peterson, Luborsky, & Seligman, 1983; Peterson & Seligman, 1984b); and the *Children's Attributional Style Questionnaire* (CASQ; Seligman *et al.*, 1984), also referred to as the KASTAN. Of these, only the CASQ is designed specifically for children; but the CAVE technique, which is used for coding verbal data, can be used with data obtained from children, and older children and adolescents may well be able to respond to the adult instruments. Finally, one additional AS scale also should be mentioned because of its wide use. It is an adaptation of Crandall's IAR (Crandall *et al.*, 1965) developed by Dweck and her colleagues (Dweck & Elliott, 1983) to measure the helpless/mastery attributional style. Like the CASQ, this measure is intended for use with children.

Contrasting Locus of Control and Attributional Style

Locus-of-control (LOC) scales were developed by proponents of the cognitive social learning school of personality (e.g., Mischel, 1973). Their purpose is to measure generalized expectations for personal control over events. The development of attributional style scales, on the other hand, was guided by attribution theory (Heider, 1958; Kelley, 1971). The purpose of these measures is to assess individual differences in perceptions of the causes both of one's own behavior and of the events (outcomes, reinforcements, etc.) of one's life. AS is thought to be an antecedent of expectations regarding future behavior or events, emotional responses to events, and self-concept and self-esteem (Abramson et al., 1978; Weiner, 1985).

Although causality (AS) and control (LOC) are related, there are important differences between LOC and AS measures. For example, both scales make reference to the concept of internality, but in different ways. With LOC scales, "internal" responses are associated with personal control; but on AS scales, responses indicating internal causality may or may not imply control. Some internal responses (e.g., attributing failure to lack of effort) imply personal control, whereas other internal responses (e.g., attributing failure to lack of ability) imply the opposite. LOC scales appear to have been developed without a clear distinction between causality and control in mind. As Ickes and Layden (1978) point out, some of their items refer to personal control without personal causality, some refer to personal causality without control, and some make reference to both personal causality and control. The development of attributional style measures has helped clarify the causality–control distinction.

Attributional Style Measures

The most widely known and used AS measure, and therefore the benchmark measure in this area, is the Attributional Style Questionnaire (ASQ; Seligman et al., 1979). Its format represents a compromise between the need to avoid imposing attributions on respondents and the need for uniformity and clarity of responses. Each item begins with a hypothetical event, such as "You have been looking for a job unsuccessfully for some time." Half of the events (six) are positive and half are negative. Three of the positive and three of the negative items concern achievement, and the others concern interpersonal events. Respondents first decide on the single most important cause of the hypothetical event, if they were the actor in the scenario (the job seeker in the example item). Thus, the ASQ involves processes that are not unlike those tapped by Thematic Apperception Tests (TATs), in that it calls for a creative response to an ambiguous (in this case, causally ambiguous) stimulus. After deciding on the cause, respondents rate it in terms of their own perceptions of its (1) internality–externality, (2) stability over time, and (3) globality (i.e., the breadth of its influence). At present, it is not known at what point individual differences manifest themselves in this two-part response process. It may be in the selection of the cause, or in decisions about internality, stability, and globality, or both. The ASQ is designed to reveal a hypothesized "depressive" attribution style, which consists of characteristic attributions of negative events to internal, stable, and global causes and (secondarily) attribution of positive events to external, unstable, and specific causes. This overall style supposedly maximizes both expectations for future negative events and self-derogatory responses to such events. Thus, it implies both an inability to avoid aversive events (lack of control) and some form of personal responsibility for their occurrence.

The Content Analysis of Verbatim Explanations (CAVE) technique is different from that of the ASQ. It is used to categorize written or oral statements that are not specifically attributional in nature. For example, it was used in one recent study to code attributional content in interviews that appeared in newspaper articles (Peterson & Seligman, 1984b) and in another to code subjects' unstructured discussions of stressful events they had experienced (Peterson, Bettes, & Seligman, 1982, cited in Peterson & Seligman, 1984b). In using the CAVE, judges first select from a written transcript those statements that describe a negative event for which a causal explanation is provided. The explanation is then rated by judges for degree of internality, stability, and globality of the causal entity. The following excerpt is drawn from a study by Peterson, Bettes, and Seligman (1982; cited in Peterson & Seligman, 1984b). The causal explanations identified by the raters are shown in italics. Both explanations in this material were judged to imply higher levels of internality and stability but lower levels of globality.

About four months ago, he called me on the telephone from _____, where he's been working. He told me that our relationship was over, that he didn't want to see me anymore. I felt devastated. I tried to argue, but what could I say? I'm still flipped out. I guess *I'm just no good at relationships. I've never been able to keep a man interested in me.* I talked to my roommate about it all night after he called me. She knows me real well, plus she went to high school with _____. She told me to forget about him and find someone else. She said I made a mistake and the best thing to do was move on. There was never a chance for a lasting thing. *But how could I misjudge things so badly? When I get stars in my eyes I get carried away* [emphasis in original].

The CAVE technique is not specifically designed to assess AS. The attributions contained in material like the foregoing example may be partly a function of an individual's style, but other factors may also influence the explanations given. At best, AS might be inferred from verbal materials if a consistent pattern of explanations emerges over a range of coded materials.

Like the CAVE measure, the Children's Attributional Style Questionnaire (CASQ) yields the same three dimensions as the original ASQ: internality, stability, and globality. The major differences between the ASQ and CASQ involve the question format. The CASQ lists a large number of hypothetical events that are relevant to young people, and for each event respondents choose one of two possible causes as the better explanation. The pairs of causes systematically vary in the degree of internality, stability, or globality that they imply. An example event is, "You get an "A" on a test." Possible explanations of the event are: (a) "I am smart" or (b) "I am good in the subject that the test was in." Both options are internal and stable, but they vary in globality. This format was chosen because the format of the ASQ was found to confuse children. Finally, like the ASQ, the CASQ is intended to reveal the presence of the "depressive" attributional style, as described before.

Anderson's Attributional Style Assessment Test (ASAT; Anderson *et al.*, 1983) and the Multidimensional–Multiattributional Causality Scale (MMCS; Lefcourt *et al.*, 1979) both differ from the measures developed by Seligman and colleagues in a number of ways. Events contained in the MMCS fall into the same categories as the ASQ—positive and negative achievement and interpersonal events—but the response format is different. Respondents are asked in the MMCS to agree or disagree with quasi-attitudinal statements— for example, "I feel that my good grades reflect directly on my ability" and "My enjoyment of a social occasion is almost entirely dependent on the personalities of the people who are there." The statements were selected to reflect ability, effort, circumstances, and luck as causal alternatives. Thus, the scale corresponds to the attributional dimensions contained in Weiner's earlier writings on attribution theory (e.g., Weiner *et al.*, 1971). The items and format of the MMCS may tap cognitive processes that are substantially different from those associated with the ASQ. The ASQ attempts to simulate naturalistic attribution processes: Respondents imagine a specific event and then generate hypothetical attributions. The MMCS, on the other hand, asks respondents to state previously established beliefs about a general class of events (e.g., getting good grades). Persons using AS measures should at least be aware of potential differences in outcomes that may result from this difference in format.

The ASAT includes to-be-explained events that fall into the same groups as those on the ASQ and MMCS: positive and negative achievement and inter-personal events. In terms of format, the ASAT presents an event followed by several options regarding causality. The options vary as a function of internality/externality and stability. An example item is: "You have just attended a party for new students and failed to make any new friends. Why did this happen?"

(a) I used the wrong strategy to meet people. [strategy]
(b) I am not good at meeting people at parties. [ability]
(c) I did not try hard to meet people. [effort]
(d) I do not have the personality traits necessary for meeting new people. [trait]
(e) I was not in the right mood for meeting people. [circumstances]
(f) Other circumstances (people, situations, etc.) produced this outcome. [circumstances]

The ASAT can be scored in a number of ways. Often, a single summary score called "controllability" is computed. It equals the total number of strategy choices plus the total number of effort choices minus the total number of ability and trait attributions. The degree to which the ASAT attempts to simulate naturalistic attribution processes appears to fall between the extremes defined by the ASQ and the MMCS.

Finally, Dweck's adaptation of the IAR differs from all other measures described here in a number of ways (see Diener & Dweck, 1978). It is short, only 10 items. It is confined to one type of event, negative outcomes in school-related achievement, and assesses only one attributional dimension, effort. A typical test item asks respondents to select one of the two causal alternatives. One option always deals with effort or lack of effort. This option is then paired with a potential circumstantial or ability cause. Scores on this measure indicate how often effort is perceived to be causal. A "mastery" attributional style emphasizes effort, and a "helpless" style deemphasizes effort as a cause of poor performance.

To summarize, a number of AS instruments have been developed. Two are designed for children, but the majority are intended for use with adult popula-tions. The content of the attributional events shows substantial consistency. Most instruments include items pertaining to both positive and negative events, and most can be scored to assess achievement and interpersonal events separately. The AS measures are also similar to one another in terms of the attributional dimensions assessed. They all include, in one form or another, an internal–external dimension, and most include a stability dimension as well. The ASQ, CASQ, and CAVE measures add a globality dimension to these two. Finally, in terms of format, the measures vary considerably in their attempts to simulate naturally occurring attributions, with the ASQ and re-lated measures most clearly attempting to do this.

Measurement Questions

It is difficult to write about the measurement of attributional style without dealing with the substantive questions that have been studied by AS theorists, because measurement issues have rarely been a focal point of studies in AS literature. The measurement questions that have been addressed typically have arisen as secondary to research on substantive behavioral questions. For this reason, we will deal with measurement issues as they have appeared in research on topics such as the relationship of AS to depression and achievement behavior.

There are perhaps more recent studies of the relationship of AS to depres-sion than any other topic. Most of these studies deal with depression among adults, and most measure AS with the Attribution Style Questionnaire (ASQ). Although this research is somewhat controversial, AS appears to be moder-ately correlated with the severity of depressive symptomology when AS and depressive symptoms are measured concurrently (Benfield, Palmer, Pfefferbaum, & Stowe, 1988; Riskind, Rholes, Brannon, & Burdick, 1987). More important, AS predicts future levels of depression over 2- to 3-month intervals independent of current levels of depression (Peterson & Seligman, 1984a), especially for some subpopulations (Riskind et al., 1987). Finally, preexisting AS moderates reactions to potentially depressogenic experiences. For example, persons with a "depressive" attributional style as described above respond to academic failure experiences more adversely (Metalsky, Hulberstadt, & Abramson, 1987). Although this constitutes substantial evidence in favor of AS as a determinant of depression, it is nevertheless the case that the magnitude of the AS–depression relationship is relatively small (cf. Cutrona, 1983). This may be an accurate reflection of the importance of AS, or it may reflect problems in the measurement of AS with currently available instruments.

There are two major concerns regarding AS measures. The first involves internal and cross-situational consistency of attributions. The idea of an attributional style implies a congruent pattern of attributions in terms of both test item responses and real-world attributions, but there are serious questions about the degree of consistency. The second concern involves the content validity of AS measures. Are AS measures actually indicative of real-world attributions? Related to this is the question of whether the relationship of AS responses to phenomena such as depression is actually mediated by real-world attributional activities. Attribution-based theories of depression and achievement argue that AS is correlated with behavior because it is an index of the attributions that an individual actually makes. Although substantial evidence exists linking AS test responses to depression and achievement behavior, it is at least possible that the relationship does not emerge because AS indexes attributional activity.

Beginning with consistency, serious concerns have been raised about the internal consistency and cross-situational consistency of the depressive attributional style as measured by the most widely used measure, the ASQ. The internal consistency of the six subscales of the ASQ (internality, stability, and globality subscales for positive and negative events) is modest at best. A study by Peterson, Semmel, von Baeyer, Abramson, Metalsky, & Seligman (1982) reported alpha coefficients ranging from .44 to .69, with a mean of .54. (See Table 8-2 for information about the internal consistency of other measures.) A much larger study by Cutrona, Russell, and Jones (1984) with 1,133 respondents reported alpha coefficients of .33 (internality), .59 (stability), and .62 (globality) for the negative events subscales. (The positive events scales were not discussed in the article.) In part, these coefficients may be a result of the relatively small number of items per subscale. A revised ASQ with 24 items per subscale has proved to have much greater consistency (Peterson & Seligman, 1984a); its reported alpha coefficients are .66 (internality), .85 (stability), and .88 (globality). Unfortunately, most of the research done to date has used the original, shorter instrument.

Cross-situational consistency is central to the concept of an attributional style. The essential issue is what are the "equivalence classes" for attributions.

TABLE 8-2. Internal Consistency Information on Selected Measures of Attributional Style

Study	Instrument	Sample	Subscale and Internal Consistency Estimate
Lefcourt et al., 1979	MMCS	Undergraduates (N = 241)	Achievement (internality/externality) = .61 Affiliation (internality/externality) = .61 Total scale = .77
Anderson et al., 1987	ASAT	Undergraduates (N = 420)	Interpersonal failure = .60 Noninterpersonal failure = .53 Interpersonal success = .56 Noninterpersonal success = .58
Peterson et al., 1982	ASQ	Undergraduates (N = 130)	Positive events, internality = .50 Positive events, stability = .58 Positive events, globality = .44 Negative events, internality = .46 Negative events, stability = .59 Negative events, globality = .69 Positive events, composite = .75 Negative events, composite = .72
Seligman et al., 1984	CASQ	Elementary school children 3rd–6th grade (N = 96)	Positive events, internality = .38 Positive events, stability = .55 Positive events, globality = .48 Negative events, internality – .50 Negative events, stability = .28 Negative events, globality = .35 Positive events, composite = .70 Negative events, composite = .52
Peterson & Seligman, 1984[a]	ASQ expanded version	—	Negative events, internality = .66 Negative events, stability = .85 Negative events, globality = .88 Positive events not included in this measure

Do people who attribute events internally, for example, do so equally for all types of events? One question in this regard is whether positive and negative events elicit similar attributional tendencies. Studies of the ASQ indicate that, in fact, there is little relationship between attributional style for positive and negative events (Peterson, Semmel, et al., 1982). Analyses involving the ASAT (Anderson, Jennings, & Arnoult, 1987) also show little systematic relationship between attributional style for positive and negative events.

The most extensive psychometric study of consistency was carried out by Cutrona et al. (1984). Using a confirmatory factor-analytic strategy, Cutrona and her colleagues examined the consistency of response to the three subscales (internality, stability, and globality) associated with the negative items on the ASQ. Several factor models were tested. The authors began with a simple hypothesized model in which each subscale—internality, stability, and globality—constituted a separate but intercorrelated factor. Individual items were not hypothesized to separate into different factors in this model. When the analysis showed that this model was not an adequate representation of the relationships among the test items, it was discarded and others were tested. The model that proved most adequate hypothesized that both cross-situational consistency (i.e., consistency across items) and situational specificity (i.e., specificity to question items) underlie responses to the ASQ. Specifically, factors corresponding to the three attributional dimensions were postulated, with allowance for their intercorrelation, but six additional factors, corresponding to each of the six negative items on the ASQ, were also hypothesized. With minor modifications, this model was found to provide a good fit to the data.

Implications of the Cutrona et al. study are at best only moderately encouraging. Consistent with the theoretical position of Seligman and colleagues, the three dimensions of attribution were found to be significantly interrelated. Individuals tend to make either internal, stable, global attributions or external, unstable, and specific ones. On the other hand, the amount of variance account for by "cross-situational" factors in the model was small to moderate, suggesting that there is not substantial consistency across content areas in the attributions elicited by the ASQ. Thus, the psychometric evidence does not encourage one to conceptualize attributional style as measured by the ASQ to be a broad, cross-situationally consistent construct. This, of course, applies only to the original, smaller version of the ASQ. It is possible that modifications of this measure or other AS measures may yield greater cross-situational consistency. In fact, Anderson's ASAT promises to demonstrate somewhat greater consistency across content domains (Anderson, Jennings, & Arnoult, 1987), but it has not received the extensive examination given to the ASQ, and more research is needed before firm conclusions can be drawn.

The work of Cutrona et al. (1984) suggests that future attempts to measure AS must give careful attention to attributional content domains. AS measures may need to be confined to relatively narrow domains. It may be necessary, in other words, to move away from the notion of a very general attributional style. An objection to this, however, is that the concept of a style loses its utility if content domains are very narrow. We, however, suggest that style remains a useful construct even with narrowly defined categories of behavior if the behaviors in question (1) occur consistently over time in the experience of the relevant population and (2) play an ecologically important role in the lives of a substantial number of the target population. Dweck's research (e.g., Dweck & Elliott, 1983) is an example of work that has attended to a narrowly defined content area for AS—that is, attributions for negative academic outcomes. Despite this narrow focus, however, her research has made a substantial applied and theoretical contribution because of the persuasiveness and ecological importance of children's academic experiences.

There have been only a few behavioral studies of cross-situational consistency. One of the most intriguing (Dweck & Bush, 1976) also suggests narrow equivalence classes. In this study, the generality of sex differences in attributions for task-related failures was examined. Fifth-grade children worked in a school-like task and were given failure feedback by one of four evaluators, either peer or an adult of either the same or the opposite sex. Previous research on sex-linked attributional style had shown that girls are more likely than boys to respond to failure with attributions to their own lack of ability (cf. Deaux, 1976; Lefcourt et al., 1979) Dweck and Bush (1976) examined the consistency of this sex difference across different evaluators. The study found that the previously mentioned sex difference was clearly apparent with only one of the evaluators, the female adult. Boys, in fact, were more likely to make low-ability attributions and to manifest helpless behavior with peer, rather than adult, evaluators. This indicates that sex differences in attributional style may best be regarded as situation × sex interactions, or that the sex-linked attributional style is not highly consistent across situations, at least among children in the present age range. This is consistent with Mischel's (1973) observation that seemingly minor variations in situations can substantially undermine cross-situational consistency. Although the equivalence class reported in Dweck's study is indeed narrow, pertaining to failure in a school-related task as defined by an adult female evaluator, it seems nevertheless to be an important sex-linked personality difference because adult females frequently serve as evaluators in elementary school settings and because of the ecological importance of reactions to failure in school.

In one of the few other behavioral studies of cross-situational consistency, Lefcourt et al. (1979) also found that AS is relatively domain specific. AS measured by achievement items on the MMCS predicted achievement behavior but not interpersonal behavior. AS as measured by interpersonal items had the opposite effect; it predicted interpersonal but not achievement behaviors. In summary, the small literature available concerning cross-situational consistency suggests that AS is consistent only within a rather narrowly defined class of situations.

The second question regarding the ASQ is its construct validity. Specifically, how does AS relate to naturalistic attributional activities? Cutrona et al. (1984) and Peterson and Seligman (1984a) both address this question and give different answers. Cutrona and colleagues asked mothers of newborns to describe stressful events and negative mood states that they had experienced and to rate the perceived causes of the events in terms of internality, stability, and globality. Although several of the correlations between ASQ and actual attributions were significant, the relationships were weak. The mean correlation reported in the study was .18, and only a few correlations were greater than .20. This suggests that the ASQ is only very modestly related to attributional activity and, consequently, that the relationship between ASQ and depression many not in fact be mediated by real-world attributional processes.

Other studies, however, are more encouraging. Peterson, Bettes, and Seligman (1982, cited in Peterson & Seligman, 1984a) asked college students to write an essay describing their most stressful experiences of the past year. Causal explanations were not solicited but were spontaneously included in the descriptions by every subject. Using the CAVE method, the experimenters coded these explanations for internality, stability, and globality. The correlations between the ASQ dimensions and the corresponding dimensions in the descriptions ranged from .41 to .19, with a mean correlation of .28 ($p < .05$). In a study of depressed persons in therapy, Catellon, Ollove, and Seligman (1982, cited in Peterson & Seligman, 1984a) examined the relationship between the ASQ and patient's explanations of why they sought therapy and the origins of their symptoms. The correlation between the composite ASQ score and composite explanation score was .38 ($p < .02$).

These studies present a mixed picture. Cutrona and co-workers (1984) suggest little construct validity. The two studies of Seligman and his colleagues are slightly more optimistic. There are, however, important differences among the studies that may account for the different results. The assumption underlying AS research is that attributions are determined by two major factors—first, by situational aspects of the attributor's current experience, and second, by attributional style. In general, one can suggest that the impact of AS will increase as the number and importance of situational factors decrease (see Mischel, 1973, for a related discussion). One class of attributions that may be relatively unaffected by situational factors includes what may be called "life history" attributions. These are attributions that seek to explain broad themes in experience. When an attributor seeks to explain a single, specific experience, a number of situational factors may be salient and therefore may influence the attribution made. When an attributor seeks to explain cross-situational themes in behavior, however, specific situational factors may not as readily provide an explanation. In this case, the influence of attributional style may be more potent. This may help reconcile the different findings reviewed above. The studies that found a stronger AS–attribution relationship, especially the Castellon et al. (1982) study, seem to deal with explanations of events that might minimize the relevance of situational factors in attributions.

Finally in regard to validity, Diener and Dweck (1978) introduce one further important question. The ongoing cognition of children with helpless and mastery attributional styles was assessed in this study using a thought list methodology. Children listed their thoughts while working on very difficult problem-solving tasks. Previous research had shown that, under these conditions, children with the helpless style were more likely to manifest behavior characteristic of the learned-helplessness syndrome (Abramson et al., 1978). The thoughts reported by the two groups while working on the task were substantially different, and one of the differences concerned attributions. The helpless group, as anticipated, made more low-ability attributions than the mastery group. This is consistent with the idea that the assessment instrument used in the study in fact measured attributional style. However, there were also a number of nonattributional differences in the thoughts reported by the two groups. For example, the mastery group reported more thoughts having to do with problem-solving strategies, and the helpless group reported more thoughts about task-irrelevant matters. Similarly, the mastery group reported more thoughts involving positive emotions, while the helpless group reported more thoughts involving negative affect. It was not clear from this study how the various cognitions were related to one another. For example, were the affective differences derivative of the attributional differences, or vice versa? Moreover, it was not clear which cognitive differences were responsible for the proclivity for helpless behavior on the part of the helpless AS groups. The mastery group's greater focus on task strategies, for instance, rather than the attributional differences, may have been crucial in connection with the behavioral differences. The point made by this study is that even if AS scales do in fact measure real-world attributional activities, they may also tap into a variety of other cognitive differences among individuals, and this possibility makes it difficult to determine which cognitions mediate the behavioral correlates of attributional style scores.

To summarize the preceding material, little attention has been given to validity issues in the attributional style literature. Existing studies raise questions about the degree to which AS measures actually index attributional activity (Cutrona, 1983) and whether, when they can be shown to measure attributions as in Diener and Dweck (1978), they measure attributions discriminatively. These questions are of substantial importance to the AS literature as a whole. As was mentioned, AS has been shown to be correlated with a range of behavior, including achievement and affect-related behavior. However, concern about the validity of AS measures makes it difficult to determine how AS–behavior relationships arise. The AS literature implies that the relationships are mediated by real-world attributional activities; but, as we have seen, that implication is not at present well established.

Developmental Considerations

In studying children's attributions, it is important to be aware of potential developmental differences. Much research has been conducted on children's use of inferential principles in attribution, and this work is reviewed elsewhere (Ruble & Rholes, 1981). Less research has been devoted to children's understanding of causal constructs such as ability or luck. One construct that seems particularly relevant to the theme of this chapter concerns children's understanding of the cross-situational stability of the dispositional concept. Among adults and older children, dispositions (personality traits, abilities, etc.) are viewed as cross-situationally stable entities. A person whose behavior reveals him or her to be kind, for example, is expected to demonstrate behaviors in a range of situations that also are consistent with dispositional kindness. Like older children and adults, younger children (4 to 6 years old) can label many behaviors with relevant and appropriate dispositional labels when asked to do so. Nevertheless, a number of studies suggest that the significance of dispositional labels differs for younger children. Specifically, younger children may not understand that dispositions are stable, abiding elements of the self or of other persons.

Evidence for this conclusion comes from three sources. First a number of recent studies have examined younger and older children's use of dispositions as a basis for predicting an actor's future behavior. In these studies, children typically are presented with an action or sequence of actions that are intended to reveal a trait or an ability of the actor. Next, children are asked to predict how an actor would behave in a new situation that is relevant to the disposition revealed in the original behavior. For example, a child might observe an actor behaving altruistically and then be asked to predict whether the actor would exhibit a different form of altruism in a new situation. A number of studies have found that children between the ages of 4 and 6 years, in contrast to older children and adults, do not expect substantial consistency across situations (MacLennon & Jackson, 1985; Rholes & Ruble, 1984; Rotenberg, 1980, 1982). That is to say, they do not form strong expectations that behaviors in the new situations will be congruent with previous behaviors. Persons who act altruistically or selfishly are not necessarily viewed as locked into a pattern of behavior. These findings suggest that dispositional attributions made by younger children do not carry the same meaning as those made by adults and older children.

In contrast to those mentioned previously, some studies have found that younger children, at least under some circumstances, do expect cross-situationally consistent patterns of behavior (Heller & Berndt, 1981; Ruble, Newman, Rholes, & Altschuler, 1987). Thus, the findings regarding younger children in this area are mixed. Taken as a whole, however, they suggest that older children hold a more firmly established belief in disposition-based consistency across situations, but that younger children can, under some still not completely specified conditions, use an actor's prior behavior as a basis for forming expectations for behavior in new situations.

In a related series of studies, Nicholls and his colleagues have examined children's understanding of one particular disposition, intellectual ability, in great detail (Nicholls & Miller, 1984). The methods of this research are different from those used in the studies mentioned before. Children in these studies observed videotaped episodes in which actors obtained varying degrees of success with varying degrees of effort. These episodes served as the basis for interviews designed to reveal children's understanding of ability. The general conclusion of Nicholls's work is that younger children only gradually come to view ability and effort as separate constructs. Early conceptions of ability confuse ability with effort and view ability as an unstable causal factor that is under voluntary control. This finding is consistent with the idea stated previously that younger children do not regard dispositions as fixed, abiding determinants of behavior, at least not to the same extent that older children do.

Finally, a number of studies in the person perception literature also suggest important age differences in connection with dispositional constructs (Shantz, 1983). In these studies, children typically are asked to describe persons whom they know well. The descriptions are then coded for evidence of dispositional reasoning. These studies find a very consistent age-related increase in children's use of dispositional constructs in their descriptions. Instead of psychological dispositions, younger children tend to rely primarily on objective, superficial qualities of the other, such as physical appearance, possessions, group memberships, and the like, in their descriptions. In reviewing these studies, Shantz (1983) was led to conclude that up to 7 to 8 years of age, children view others from the perspective of "a demographer and behaviorist, defining persons in terms of their environmental circumstances and observable behavior" (p. 506). Taken together, children's limited use of dispositions in naturalistic description, their tentative use of them in the formation of expectations, and their conceptualization of intellectual ability as an unstable construct suggest an important shift in younger children's attributional thinking which takes place in the early elementary school years.

These findings make it important for researchers to take age into account when assessing children's attributions. The most obvious implication of this research is that younger children's sense of their own dispositions will be more fluid and unstable than that of older children. Younger children can and do at times label themselves and others in dispositional terms, usually when they are prompted to do so. A younger child who says he or she is "not smart," however, may not view this as a permanent condition that will place limits on his or her behavior across a range of intellectual activities. Consequently, the emotional and behavioral consequences of dispositional labels may be quite different for younger children, and in fact a number of studies suggest that this is the case (e.g., Grusec & Redler, 1980; Miller, 1985; Rholes, Blackwell, Jordan, & Walters, 1980; Rholes, Jones, & Wade, 1987; Weiner, Graham, Stern, & Lawson, 1982).

A second implication of this developmental research concerns the accuracy of younger children's self-perceptions. Even among older children, there is a need to view oneself as having desirable traits and abilities that leads to overly optimistic self-assessments. For example, Kagan, Hans, Markowitz, Lopez, & Sigal (1982) found in a study of third- and fourth-graders that approximately 75% of the members of an elementary school classroom rated themselves as above average on five desirable traits: attractiveness, reading ability, dominance, popularity, and athletic ability. This optimism, however, seems to be even more pronounced among younger children (Nicholls, 1978; Stipek, 1984). Several studies, for example, have found that children's perceptions of their academic ability become more closely associated with the assessments of an objective evaluator (usually a teacher) as children grow older. Younger children disagree with objective evaluations primarily by viewing themselves in excessively positive terms. From an assessment point of view, these findings suggest that younger children may fail to assess their experience accurately when making self-relevant attributions, and that these self-perceptions may stem in part from the younger child's conception of dispositions as unstable.

Viewing qualities of self or other persons as unstable may obscure the importance of paying close attention to patterns of behavior across situations. Without the constraint of the idea of stable disposition, thinking about the self or about other persons may be based on either wish fulfillment (Stipek, 1984) or the belief that one's abilities are based on one's efforts, goals, and desires (Nicholls & Miller, 1984).

CONCLUSION

One of the prerequisites for the development of effective CBM programs with children is adequate assessment of the children themselves (Harris, 1985). A cognitive characteristic of children that has received significant attention in the CBM literature involves youngsters' thoughts and beliefs about the causes of events in their environment (Pearl, 1985). Modifying children's attributions has been an important component of many CBM programs (e.g., Andrews & Debus, 1978; Fowler & Peterson, 1981; Thomas & Pashley, 1982). Although there has been substantial interest in children's attributions and attributional retraining, there are significant problems in the current status of attributional assessment of children. It appears that theory has developed and interventions have been tested using flawed assessment procedures.

A series of methodological concerns associated with the assessment of children's attributions has been identified in this chapter. For example, limited attention has been given to children's attributions for real-world events. Preference for simulation procedures over actual achievement or social events is understandable given the difficulty of gathering information on children's cognitions in real-life settings. Unfortunately, however, the results from these simulated procedures may have limited validity for real-world applications that are essential to CBM work. Second, individuals who have conducted attribution research with children have drawn heavily on the theory, content, and methodology of attributional studies with adults. As a result, there is an inadequate data base on children's naturally occurring attributional cognitions. Investigators may have distorted children's attributional reports by constraining youngsters' responses to a set of causal ascriptions and a methodology derived from work with adults. Third, little attention has been given to the psychometric qualities of AS measures in general. It is important to note that the major measure of adult AS in current use, the ASQ, has relatively poor psychometric qualities. To date, there is little psychometric information available on children's measures of AS. Fourth, there are serious questions about the cross-situational stability of AS and the relationship of AS to individuals' actual attributions in specific situations.

Establishing a coherent body of information on children's attributions will require, in part, the use of sound methodologies. With more systematic attention given to how attributions are to be assessed, we will have a better basis on which to develop theory and practice involving attributional constructs.

REFERENCES

Abramson, L. Y., Seligman, M. E. P., & Teasdale, J. D. (1978). Learned helplessness in humans: Critique and reformulation. *Journal of Abnormal Psychology, 87,* 49–74.

Ames, C. (1978). Children's achievement attributions and self-concept and competitive reward structure. *Journal of Educational Psychology, 70*(3), 345–355.

Ames, C. (1984) Achievement attributions and self-instructions under competitive and individualistic goal structures. *Journal of Educational Psychology, 76*(3), 478–487.

Ames, C., & Ames, R. (1981). Competitive versus individualistic goal structures: The salience of past performance information for causal attributions and affect. *Journal of Educational Psychology, 76*(3), 411–418.

Ames, C. & Felker, D. W. (1979). An examination of children's attributions and achievement-related evaluations in competitive, cooperative, and individualistic reward structures. *Journal of Educational Psychology, 71*(4), 413–420.

Amirkhan, J. (1982). Expectancies and attributions for hyperactive and medicated hyperactive students. *Journal of Abnormal Child Psychology, 10*(2), 265–276.

Anderson, C. A., Horowitz, L. M., & French, R. (1983). Attributional style of lonely and depressed people. *Journal of Personality and Social Psychology, 45,* 127–136.

Anderson, C. A., Jennings, D. L., & Arnoult, L. H. (1987). *The validity and utility of the attributional style construct at a moderate level of specificity.* Manuscript submitted for publication.

Andrews, G. R., & Debus, R. L. (1978). Persistence and the causal perception of failure: Modifying cognitive attributions. *Journal of Educational Psychology, 70,* 154–166.

Bandura, A. (1978). The self system in reciprocal determinism. *American Psychologist, 33*(4), 344–358.

Bar-Tal, D., & Darom, E. (1979). Pupils' attributions of success and failure. *Child Development, 50,* 264–267.

Bar-Tal, D., Raviv, A., Raviv, A., & Bar-Tal, Y. (1982). Consistency of pupil's attributions regarding success and failure. *Journal of Educational Psychology, 74*(1), 104–110.

Benfield, C. Y., Palmer, D. J., Pfefferbaum, B., & Stowe, M. L. (1988). A comparison of depressed and non-depressed disturbed children of measures of attributional style, hopelessness, life stress, and temperament. *Journal of Abnormal Child Psychology, 16*(4), 397–410.

Bird, A. M., & Williams, J. M. (1980). A developmental-attributional analysis of sex role stereotypes for sport performance. *Developmental Psychology, 16*(4), 319–322.

Bowers, K. S. (1973). Situationism in psychology: An analysis and a critique. *Psychological Review, 80*(5), 307–336.

Bretherton, I., & Beeghly, M. (1982). Talking about internal states: The acquisition of an explicit theory of mind. *Developmental Psychology, 18*(6), 906–921.

Bugental, D. B., Whalen, C. K., & Henker, B. (1977). Causal attributions of hyperactive children and motivational assumptions of two behavior-change approaches: Evidence for an interactionist position. *Child Development, 48,* 874–884.

Burnham, J. C. (1968). Historical background for the study of Personality. In E. F. Borgatla & W. Lambert (Eds.), *Handbook of personality theory and research* (pp. 3–81). Chicago: Rand McNally.

Callaghan, C., & Manstead, A. S. R. (1983). Causal attributions for task performance: The effects of performance outcome and sex of subject. *British Journal of Educational Psychology, 53,* 14–23.

Castellon, C., Ollove, M., & Seligman, M. E. P. (1982). Unpublished data, University of Pennsylvania.

Covington, M. V., & Omelich, C. L. (1984). An empirical examination of Weiner's critique of attribution research. *Journal of Educational Psychology, 76*(6), 1214–1225.

Crandall, V., Katkovsky, W., & Crandall, V. (1965). Children's beliefs in their own control of reinforcements in intellectual-academic achievement situations. *Child Development, 36,* 91–109.

Cutrona, C. E. (1983). Causal attributions and perinatal depression. *Journal of Abnormal Psychology, 92,* 161–172.

Cutrona, C. E., Russell, D., & Jones, R. D. (1984). Cross-situational consistency in causal attributions: Does attributional style exist? *Journal of Personality and Social Psychology, 47,* 1043–1058.

Deaux, K. (1976). Sex: A perspective on the attribution process. In J. Harvey, W. Ickes, & R. Kidd (Eds.), *New directions in attribution research* (Vol. 1, pp. 335–352). Hillsdale, NJ: Lawrence Erlbaum.

Diener, C. I., & Dweck, C. S. (1978). An analysis of learned helplessness: Continuous changes in performance, strategy, and achievement cognitions following failure. *Journal of Personality and Social Psychology, 36*(5), 451–462.

Dix, T., & Grusec, J. E. (1983). Parental influence techniques: An attributional analysis. *Child Development, 54,* 645–652.

Dodge, K. A. (1980). Social cognition and children's aggressive behavior. *Child Development, 51,* 162–170.

Dollinger, S. J., Staley, A., & McGuire, B. (1981). The child as psychologist: Attributions and evaluations of defensive strategies. *Child Development, 52,* 1084–1086.

Dweck, C. S. (1975). The role of expectations and attributions in the alleviation of learned helplessness. *Journal of Personality and Social Psychology, 31,* 674–685.

Dweck, C. S., & Bush, E. S. (1976). Sex differences in learned helplessness: I. Differential debilitation with peer and adult evaluators. *Developmental Psychology, 12*(2), 147–156.

Dweck, C. S., & Elliott, E. S. (1983). Achievement motivation. In E. M. Hetherington (Ed.), *Handbook of child psychology: Vol. 4. Socialization, personality, and social development* (4th ed.) (pp. 643–691). New York: Wiley.

Ekehammar, B. (1974). Interactionism in personality from a historical perspective. *Psychological Bulletin, 81*(12), 1026–1048.

Elig, T. W., & Frieze, I. H. (1975). A multi-dimensional scheme for coding and interpreting perceived causality for success and failure events: The CSPS. *JSAS Catalog of Selected Documents in Psychology, 5,* 313.

Elig, T. W., & Frieze, I. H. (1979). Measuring causal attributions for success and failure. *Journal of Personality and Social Psychology, 37*(4), 621–634.

Endler, N. S., & Magnusson, D. (1976). Toward an interactional psychology of personality. *Psychological Bulletin, 83*(5), 956–974.

Ericsson, K. A., & Simon, H. A. (1980). Verbal reports as data. *Psychological Review, 87*(3), 215–251.

Ericsson, K. A., & Simon, H. A. (1984). *Protocol analysis* (pp. 1–62). Cambridge, MA: MIT Press.

Erwin, J., & Kuhn, D. (1979). Development of children's understanding of the multiple determination underlying human behavior. *Developmental Psychology, 15*(3), 352–353.

Etaugh, C., & Brown, B. (1975). Perceiving the causes of success and failure of male and female performers. *Developmental Psychology, 11*(1), 103.

Fowler, J. W., & Peterson, P. I. (1981). Increasing reading persistence and altering attributional style of learned helpless children. *Journal of Educational Psychology, 73*, 251–260.

Friend, R. M., & Neale, J. M. (1972). Children's perceptions of success and failure: An attributional analysis of the effects of race and social class. *Developmental Psychology, 7*(2), 124–128.

Frieze, I. H. (1976). Causal attributions and information seeking to explain success and failure. *Journal of Research in Personality, 10*, 293–305.

Frieze, I. H., & Snyder, H. N. (1980). Children's beliefs about the causes of success and failure in school settings. *Journal of Educational Psychology, 72*(2), 186–196.

Greenspoon, J. (1955). The reinforcing effect of two spoken sounds on the frequency of two responses. *Journal of American Psychology, 50*, 409–416.

Grusec, J. E., & Redler, E. (1980). Attribution, reinforcement, and altruism: A developmental analysis. *Developmental Psychology, 16*, 525–534.

Harris, B. (1977). Developmental differences in the attribution of responsibility. *Developmental Psychology, 13*(3), 257–265.

Harris, K. R. (1985). Conceptual, methodological, and clinical issues in cognitive-behavioral assessment. *Journal of Abnormal Child Psychology, 13*(3), 373–390.

Hartke, A. R. (1978). The use of latent partition analysis to identify homogeneity of an item population. *Journal of Education Measurement, 15*, 43–47.

Hartke, A. R. (1979). The development of conceptually independent sub-scales in the measurement of attitudes. *Educational and Psychological Measurement, 39*, 585–592.

Heider, F. (1958). *The psychology of interpersonal relations.* New York: Wiley.

Heller, K. A., & Berndt, T. J. (1981). Developmental changes in the formation and organization of personality attributions. *Child Development, 52*, 683–691.

Hiebert, E. H., Winograd, P. N., & Danner, F. W. (1984). Children's attributions for failure and success in different aspects of reading. *Journal of Educational Psychology, 76*(6), 1139–1148.

Ickes, W., & Layden, M. A. (1978). Attributional styles. In J. Harvey, W. Ickes, & R. Kidd (Eds.), *New directions in attribution research* (Vol. 2, pp. 121–157). Hillsdale, NJ: Lawrence Erlbaum.

Jones, E. E., & Nisbett, R. E. (1971). The actor and the observer: Divergent perceptions of the causes of behavior. In E. E. Jones, D. E. Kanouse, H. H. Kelley, R. E. Nisbett, S. Valins, & B. Weiner (Eds.), *Attribution: Perceiving the causes of behavior* (pp. 79–94). Morristown, NJ: General Learning Press.

Kagan, J., Hans, S., Markowitz, A., Lopez, D., & Sigal, H. (1982). Validity of children's self-reports of psychological qualities. In B. A. Maher & W. B. Maher (Eds.), *Progress in experimental personality research* (pp. 124–162). New York: Academic Press.

Karabenick, J. D., & Heller, K. A. (1976). A developmental study of effort and ability attributions. *Developmental Psychology, 12*(6), 559–560.

Keasey, B. C. (1977). Young children's attribution of intentionality of themselves and others. *Child Development, 48*, 261–264.

Kelley, H. H. (1971). Attribution in social interaction. In E. E. Jones, D. E. Kanouse, H. H. Kelley, R. E. Nisbett, S. Valins, & B. Weiner (Eds.), *Attribution: Perceiving the causes of behavior* (pp. 1–26). Morristown, NJ: General Learning Press.

Kun, A. (1977). Development of the magnitude-covariation and compensation schemata in ability and effort attributions of performance. *Child Development, 48,* 462–873.

Lefcourt, H. M., von Baeyer, C. L., Ware, E. E., & Cox, D. J. (1979). The multidimensional-multiattributional causality scale: The development of a goal specific locus of control scale. *Canadian Journal of Behavioral Science, 11,* 286–304.

Levenson, H. (1973). Multidimensional locus of control in psychiatric patients. *Journal of Consulting and Clinical Psychology, 41,* 397–404.

Licht, B. G., Kistner, J. A., Ozkaragox, T., Shapiro, S., & Clausen, L. (1985). Causal attributions of learning disabled children: Individual differences and their implications for persistence. *Journal of Educational Psychology, 77*(2), 208–216.

Lieberman, D. A. (1979). Behaviorism and the mind. *American Psychologist, 34*(4), 319–333.

MacLennon, R. N., & Jackson, D. N. (1985). Accuracy and consistency in the development of social perception. *Developmental Psychology, 21,* 30–36.

Marsh, H. W. (1984). Relations among dimensions of self-attribution, dimensions of self-concept, and academic achievement. *Journal of Educational Psychology, 76*(6), 1291–1308.

Metalsky, C. I., Hulberstadt, L. J., & Abramson, L. Y. (1987). Vulnerability to depressive mood reactions: Towards a more powerful test of the diathesis–stress and causal mediation components of the reformulated theory of depression. *Journal of Personality and Social Psychology, 52,* 386–393.

Miller, A. T. (1985). A developmental study of the cognitive basis of performance improvement after failure. *Journal of Personality and Social Psychology, 49,* 529–538.

Mischel, W. (1973). Toward a cognitive social learning reconceptualization of personality. *Psychological Review, 80*(4), 252–283.

Mischel, W., Zeiss, R., & Zeiss, A. (1974). Internal and external control and persistence: Validation and implications of the Stanford Preschool Internal–External Scale. *Journal of Personality and Social Psychology, 29,* 265–278.

Newell, A., & Simon, H. A. (1972). *Human problem solving.* Englewood Cliffs, NJ: Prentice-Hall.

Nicholls, J. G. (1978). The development of the concepts of effort and ability, perceptions of academic attainment, and the understanding that difficult tasks require more ability. *Child Development, 49,* 800–814.

Nicholls, J. G. (1979). Development of perception of own attainment and causal attributions for success and failure in reading. *Journal of Educational Psychology, 71*(1), 94–99.

Nicholls, J. G., & Miller, A. T. (1984). Development and its discontents: The differentiation of the concept of ability. In J. G. Nicholls (Ed.), *The development of achievement motivation* (pp. 138–159). Greenwich, CT: JAI Press.

Nisbett, R. E., & Ross, L. (1980). *Human inference: Strategies and shortcomings of human inference.* Englewood Cliffs, NJ: Prentice-Hall.

Nisbett, R. E., & Wilson, T. D. (1977). Telling more than we can know: Verbal reports on mental processes. *Psychological Review, 84*(3), 231–259.

Norwicki, S., & Strickland, B. (1973). A locus of control scale for children. *Journal of Consulting and Clinical Psychology, 40,* 148–154.

Palmer, D. J. (1983). An attributional perspective on labeling. *Exceptional Children, 49*(5), 423–429.

Palmer, D. J., Drummond, F., Tollison, P., & Zinkgraff, S. (1982). An attributional investigation of performance outcomes for learning-disabled and normal-achieving pupils. *Journal of Special Education, 16*(2), 207–219.

Pearl, R. (1982). LD children's attributions of success and failure: A replication with a labeled LD sample. *Learning Disability Quarterly, 5,* 173–176.

Pearl, R. (1985). Cognitive-behavioral interventions for increasing motivation. *Journal of Abnormal Child Psychology, 13*(3), 443–454.

Pearl, R., Bryan, T., & Donahue, M. (1980). Learning disabled children's attributions for success and failure. *Learning Disability Quarterly, 3*(1), 3–9.

Peterson, C. M., Bettes, B. A., & Seligman, M. E. P. (1982). *Spontaneous attributions and depressive symptoms.* Unpublished manuscript, Virginia Polytechnic Institute and State University, Blacksburg.

Peterson, C. M., Luborsky, L., & Seligman, M. E. P. (1983). Attributions and depressive mood shifts: A case study using the symptom-context method. *Journal of Abnormal Psychology, 92,* 96–103.

Peterson, C. M., & Seligman, M. E. P. (1984a). Causal explanations as a risk factor in depression: Theory and evidence. *Psychological Review, 91,* 347–374.

Peterson, C. M., & Seligman, M. E. P. (1984b). *Content analysis of verbatim explanations: The CAVE technique for assessing explanatory style.* Unpublished manuscript, Virginia Polytechnic Institute and State University, Blacksburg.

Peterson, C. M., Semmel, A., von Baeyer, C., Abramson, L. Y., Metalsky, G. I., & Seligman, M. E. P. (1982). The attributional style questionnaire. *Cognitive Therapy and Research, 6,* 287–300.

Rholes, W. S., Blackwell, J., Jordan, C., & Walters, C. (1980). A developmental study of learned helplessness. *Developmental Psychology, 16,* 616–624.

Rholes, W. S., Jones, M., & Wade, C. (1987). Children's understanding of personal dispositions and its relationship to behavior. *Journal of Experimental Child Psychology, 45,* 1–17.

Rholes, W. S., & Ruble, D. N. (1984). Children's understanding of dispositional characteristics of others. *Child Development, 55,* 550–560.

Rholes, W. S., & Walters, J. (1982). Schematic patterns of causal evidence. *Child Development, 53,* 1046–1057.

Riskind, J. H., Rholes, W. S., Brannon, A. M., & Burdick, C. A. (1987). Attributions and expectations: A confluence of vulnerabilities in mild depression in a college student population. *Journal of Personality and Social Psychology, 53,* 349–354.

Rotenberg, K. J. (1980). Children's use of intentionality in judgments of character and disposition. *Child Development, 51,* 282–284.

Rotenberg, K. J. (1982). Development of character constancy of self and other. *Child Development, 53,* 505–515.

Rotter, J. B. (1966). Generalized expectancies for internal vs. external control of reinforcement. *Psychological Monographs, 80,* 1–28.

Ruble, D. N., Newman, L. S., Rholes, W. S., & Altshuler, J. (1987). Children's naive psychology: The use of behavioral and situational information for the prediction of behavior. *Cognitive Development, 3,* 89–112.

Ruble, D. N., Parsons, J. E., & Ross, J. (1976). Self-evaluative responses of children in an achievement setting. *Child Development*, *47*, 990–997.

Ruble, D. N., & Rholes, W. S. (1981). The development of children's perceptions and attributions about their social world. In J. Harvey, W. Ickes, & R. Kidd (Eds.), *New directions in attribution research* (Vol. 3, pp. 4–40). Hillsdale, NJ: Lawrence Erlbaum.

Sameroff, A., & Chandler, M. (1975). Reproductive risk and the continuum of caretaking casualty. In F. D. Horowitz (Ed.), *Review of child development research* (Vol. 4, pp. 197–244). Chicago: University of Chicago Press.

Schunk, D. H. (1984). Sequential attributional feedback and children's achievement behaviors. *Journal of Educational Psychology*, *76*(6), 1159–1169.

Seligman, M. E. P., Abramson, L. Y., Semmel, A., & von Baeyer, C. (1979). Depressive attributional style. *Journal of Abnormal Psychology*, *88*, 242–247.

Seligman, M. E. P., Peterson, C., Kaslow, N. J., Tannenbaum, R. L., Alloy, L. B., & Abramson, L. Y. (1984). Attributional style and depressive symptoms among children. *Journal of Abnormal Psychology*, *93*, 235–238.

Shantz, C. (1983). Social cognition. In J. H. Flavell & E. Markman (Eds.), *Carmichael's manual of child psychology: Vol. 3. Cognitive development* (4th ed.) (pp. 495–555). New York: Wiley.

Shultz, T. R., & Butkowsky, I. (1977). Young children's use of the scheme for multiple sufficient causes in the attribution of real and hypothetical behavior. *Child Development*, *48*, 464–469.

Shultz, T. R., Butkowsky, I., Pearce, J. W., & Shanfield, H. (1975). Development of schemes for the attribution of multiple psychological causes. *Developmental Psychology*, *11*(4), 502–510.

Skinner, B. F. (1953). *Science and human behavior*. New York: Macmillan.

Smith, C. L., Gelfand, D. M., Hartmann, D. P., & Partlow, M. E. Y. (1979). Help giving. *Child Development*, *50*, 203–210.

Stipek, D. J. (1984). Young children's performance expectations: Logical analysis or wishful thinking? In J. Nicholls (Ed.), *Advances in motivation and achievement* (pp. 33–56). Greenwich, CT: JAI Press.

Stipek, D. J., & Hoffman, J. M. (1980). Children's achievement-related expectancies as a function of academic performance histories and sex. *Journal of Educational Psychology*, *72*(6), 861–865.

Thomas, A., & Pashley, B. (1982). Effects of classroom training on LD students' task persistence and attributions. *Learning Disability Quarterly*, *5*, 133–144.

Tollefson, N., Tracy, D. B., Johnsen, E. P., Buenning, M., Farmer, A. W., & Barke, C. R. (1982). Attribution patterns of learning disabled adolescents. *Learning Disability Quarterly*, *15*, 14–20.

Wallston, B. S., Wallston, K. A., Kaplan, G. D., & Maides, S. (1976). Development and validation of the health locus of control scale. *Journal of Consulting and Clinical Psychology*, *44*, 580–585.

Watson, J. B. (1913). Psychology as the behaviorist views it. *Psychological Review*, *20*, 158–177.

Weiner, B. (1972). *Theories of motivation: From mechanism to cognition*. Chicago: Markham.

Weiner, B. (1979). A theory of motivation for some classroom experiences. *Journal of Educational Psychology*, *71*(1), 3–25.

Weiner, B. (1983). Some methodological pitfalls in attributional research. *Journal of Educational Psychology, 75*(4), 530–543.

Weiner, B. (1985). An attributional theory of achievement motivation and emotion. *Psychological Review, 92*(4), 548–573.

Weiner, B., Frieze, I., Kukla, A., Reed, L., Rest, S., & Rosenbaum, R. M. (1971). Perceiving the causes of success and failure. In E. E. Jones, D. E. Kanouse, H. H. Kelley, R. E. Nisbett, S. Valins, & B. Weiner (Eds.), *Attribution: Perceiving the causes of behavior* (pp. 95–120). Morristown, NJ: General Learning Press.

Weiner, B., Graham, S., Stern, P., & Lawson, M. (1982). Using affective cues to infer causal thoughts. *Developmental Psychology, 18*, 278–286.

Wiley, D. E. (1967). Latent partition analysis. *Psychometrika, 32*, 183–193.

Willson, V. L., & Palmer, D. J. (1983). Latent partition analysis of attributions for actual achievement. *American Educational Research Journal, 20*(4), 581–589.

PART THREE
Teaching and Direct Intervention Practices

9
ON COGNITIVE TRAINING: A THOUGHT OR TWO

BERNICE Y. L. WONG
Simon Fraser University

The contents of the chapters by Alexander and Hare (Chapter 10), Graham and Harris (Chapter 11), Keller and Lloyd (Chapter 12), and Zentall (Chapter 13) suggest an obvious scheme for my commentary. It is to group the first three chapters together since they concern academic areas, and to treat Zentall's chapter separately because it concerns the clinical area of hyperactivity. I shall begin with two general comments, followed by more specific comments on the individual chapters by Alexander and Hare, Graham and Harris, and Keller and Lloyd, respectively. Then I shall conclude the section on these three chapters with comments applicable to all of them. Finally, I will turn my focus to Zentall's chapter.

ACADEMIC INSTRUCTION

The chapters on academic instruction center on cognitive training. "Cognitive training" is a broad term. It covers intervention research that targets cognitive processes purported to mediate successful learning and problem solving. Typically, researchers conduct a cognitive task analysis of the component processes in a task, and then set forth to design a training procedure that would either elicit or enhance subjects' use of those component processes. The cognitive task analysis is guided by theoretical models—for example, a theory of reading processes.

Cognitive training is very much a product of the current cognitive zeitgeist in psychology and education. The scope of cognitive training varies. There are cognitive-training programs with substantially more breadth and, therefore, more ambitious in scope—for example, DeBono's CoRT program, Feuerstein's Instrumental Enrichment Program, and the Venezuelan Project (Schwebel & Maher, 1986). In contrast, the chapters on cognitive training here have a more modest and focused scope. They bear respectively on a single academic area: reading, writing, arithmetic.

Theoretical Status

One general problem with research in cognitive training is the status of the theoretical frame (Wong, 1988). Regarding the chapters here, the research reported appears to embrace either adequate process models (in reading and in writing) or loosely framed cognitive principles (as in the Learning Strategies Curriculum at Kansas University). A common theme in all three chapters (on reading, writing, and arithmetic) is the topic of cognitive-behavior modification and the self-instructional approach associated with it. Cognitive-behavior modification (CBM) is basically a framework for therapy (Meichenbaum, 1977, pp. 215–227). It is also a very flexible therapeutic framework because it accommodates diverse conceptualizations of client problems. Put differently, it can be used by therapists with diverse training perspectives who may interpret the same client's problem in very different ways. But in and of itself it is not a theory in the scientific sense (see Swanson, 1988). However, one can use it legitimately as a training approach, having hitched it to a particular theory— for example, a process theory in reading or writing.

In general, cognitive-training research (cognitive strategy intervention research) in learning disabilities suffers from the lack of coherent theoretical frameworks. The most widely adopted Cognitive Strategies Curriculum is a case in point. Although it is most ingeniously designed, it lacks an explicit and tight conceptual frame, which may detract from the eventual accumulation of empirical validation of the curriculum.

Similarly, much intervention research in learning disabilities has ensued from the notion of the "inactive learner." (My own earlier work is a culprit here, and I sorely regret having led or contributed to the use of that notion as a framework for research.) The inactive learner notion is a description of one aspect of learning-disabled students' general task approach. It is conceptually too loose to serve as a research-engendering framework. We should realize this and not perpetuate intervention research that uses such loose conceptions of theoretical frames.

The obvious conclusion to this general issue of the theoretical status of cognitive training is for researchers in learning disabilities to generate theory-based interventions. It is myopic to focus merely on the use of effective training procedures. These procedures must ensue from sound theoretical conceptualizations that provide the rationale and foci for training, as well as providing explanations for the efficacy of the given training.

Generalization

A second general issue in cognitive training is generalization. What is generalization of learned strategies, and why is it so important in cognitive training? Generalization of learned strategies occurs when trainees demonstrate spontaneous use of those strategies in new settings and new tasks, the successful completion/execution of which requires the use of those previously learned strategies. Such unprompted generalization of previously learned strategies is important because the whole point of learning new strategies that promote academic learning is for learners not only to build up their strategic repertoires, but also to use their learned strategies adaptively in future learning and problem solving. If they cannot generalize learned strategies, however, they will not become adaptive learners and problem solvers because what they learn cannot be extended flexibly beyond the original context of learning. To use Ann Brown's words, the learned strategies are "wielded" to the training context. They remain isolated and fragmented strategies and are therefore of limited use. There will be no savings in time or effort or increase in metacognition about learning for the students when strategy generalization does not occur.

Generalization is still a problem for researchers who attempt to apply cognitive-behavior modification (CBM) to academic domains. Although CBM originated as a treatment approach for clinical problems in psychology, its use was soon extended to academic domains involving mildly handicapped students (Hallahan, 1980). At that time, however, Meichenbaum (1980) shrewdly observed that the application of CBM to deal with academic problems of mildly handicapped students was promising, but that until generalization is obtained, it remains "A Promise Yet Unfulfilled." Meichenbaum's earlier caveat still obtains. Generalization of strategies induced through CBM has yet to be unequivocally and consistently demonstrated. The interesting finding is that trainees could recall nicely the CBM strategy despite absence of strategy transfer (see Graham & Harris, Chapter 11, this volume; Wong, Wong, Perry, & Sawatsky, 1986). How can we explain this apparent paradox?

Let me first trace the various ways researchers have attempted to analyze trainees' problem of lack of generalization and then propose a fresh way of analyzing the problem. Strategy trainers have tried to eliminate the problem of generalization by emphasizing the use of multiple training settings, multiple trainers, and different tasks (the University of Kansas; Meichenbaum & Asarnow, 1979). Faithful implementation of this procedure does not appear to ensure foolproof or consistent generalization. Then researchers concentrated on using informed plus self-control training (Brown & Palincsar, 1982). In this approach, intervention researchers emphasize explicit explanation of the rationale and significance of strategy training, as well as practice in using the strategy and in evaluating (monitoring) use of strategy. Basically, Brown and Palincsar (1982) were advocating a metacognitive perspective to strategy training. Again, adding the component of self-control training to CBM strategy training does not guarantee trainees' strategy generalization (Graham & Harris, Chapter 11, this volume). The most current perspective in explaining trainees' problems in strategy generalization is a motivational one (Wong, 1986). Trainees are considered to lack the motivation to generalize learned strategies. The proposed causes are diverse. They include attributional problems (Borkowski, Johnston, & Reid, 1987); trainees' lack of appreciation of the value of the learned strategies (Wittrock, 1988); trainees' failure to share and hence lack of commitment to trainers' instructional goals (Wong *et al.*, 1986); and the fact that trainees' own cost–benefit analysis does not encourage generalization of learned strategy (e.g., use of the strategy is too time-consuming or appears to involve too much effort). Any of these motivational problems is indeed a plausible cause for the trainees' lack of strategy transfer. More important, recent intervention research has shown increasing attention to them. Thus, we will be able to see how effective incorporation of these motivational variables has been in solving the problem of strategy generalization.

I suspect, however, that we may need to attend to yet another aspect of cognitive training before we can effectively solve trainees' problem in strategy generalization. I propose that we attend to teaching subjects how to identify and define their learning problems. Hitherto, we have concentrated totally on teaching students strategies that promote efficient learning, but we have not made them into *strategic* learners. Strategic learners consciously select task-appropriate strategies from among their strategy repertoires. Such flexible and adaptive use of learned strategies must involve strategy generalization. One reason we have not yet produced strategic learners may be that we have neglected to teach them to understand the nature of their own learning obstacles as these are encountered in their learning. Problem identification, definition or crystallization is an important skill for learning (Bransford, Sherwood, Vye, & Rieser, 1986; Getzels & Csikszentmihalyi, 1975). I think we need to teach students to understand clearly the nature of the learning problems they encounter in the course of their own learning, so that they can select the most appropriate strategy from among those they have learned from us, to deal with their individual learning problems. Currently, cognitive intervention researchers do try to impart "conditional knowledge" (Simon, 1980) regarding when and where a cognitive strategy would be usefully applied. Such knowledge, however, may be too global and conceived entirely from the viewpoint of the researcher. For students to apply learned strategies flexibly and appropriately—that is, to generalize learned strategies—they first need to learn to define for themselves exactly what is impeding their own learning. Otherwise, the given "conditional knowledge" may amount to a bunch of rote-memorized rules, which may contribute minimally to learners' strategy generalization.

Let me elaborate. Often we teach our subjects a strategy or several strategies. For example, we teach a group of subjects debugging strategies such as look-backs (Garner, 1981), and we carefully explain to them when and where to use the strategies. In short, we attend to Simon's (1980) pointer on providing "conditional knowledge," but we forget to teach them *concurrently* in analyzing their comprehension problems. If we do teach them such analysis, we may increase students' strategy generalization. Imagine this training scenario: "Students, when you find you don't understand a particular sentence as you are reading this passage, ask yourselves: What is it that makes this sentence hard for me to understand? Is it a word (vocabulary) that's bugging me? Is it something to do with grammar (like a double negative in the sentence)? Is it because I don't know enough about the topic?" Essentially, I am proposing that we teach students to identify and define clearly for themselves the nature of their reading comprehension breakdowns and then show them respective debugging strategies that match the defined comprehension problem. For learning-disabled students who daily encounter such problems in their school tasks, it is particularly important to teach them to analyze the nature of their learning problems.

If we add the foregoing instructional component to our current conceptualized intervention perspectives of metacognition and motivation, we may move one step closer to making students strategic in the deployment of selective and generalized learning strategies. For with understanding of the nature of their learning problems as these arise in the course of independent learning, and solving them effectively, students develop metacognition not only about strategy use, but also about themselves as learners and about the learning process. This increased awareness in and about learning should surely loop back profitably onto students' strategy generalization.

The Individual Chapters

Let me now turn to the individual chapters. Alexander and Hare (Chapter 10) provide an excellent summary on reading processes. Particularly praiseworthy is their emphasis on affective aspects of reading comprehension. Within the context of reading processes, they expounded on various training approaches with illustrative studies. In the section on the CBM approach to enhancing reading comprehension, Alexander and Hare were unable to provide illustrative studies. This is understandable because to date there are few reading comprehension intervention studies that have used a CBM approach. An unpublished study by Bommarito and Meichenbaum, reported in Meichenbaum and Asarnow (1979) was the first such study. The subjects were seventh- and eighth-graders who were either reading about one year below grade or who had reading comprehension problems not due to decoding problems. Through modeling by the experimenters, they were taught to generate relevant self-instructions in reading a story. These self-instructions involved: "What is the story about? Learn the important details of the story (sequence of main events). How do the characters feel and why?" In sum, the subjects learned to "get the main idea. Watch sequences. And learn how the characters feel and why."

Recently, Graham (1986) used CBM to enhance reading test performance in fifth- and sixth-graders. Specifically, she modified Taffy Raphael's work on text-explicit, text-implicit, and script-implicit questions. To facilitate children's learning the prompts, Graham created simpler mnemonics of "here," "hidden" and "in my head" to parallel Raphael's prompts for the three comprehension question types. She then used the CBM approach to teach Raphael's strategy in question analysis to the subjects. She obtained positive results for both average and poor readers.

The chapter on writing by Steve Graham and Karen Harris contains an excellent exposition of writing processes. They show a thorough grasp of the issues in current writing theories. Instructive to readers is their careful and systematic intervention research in writing with learning-disabled students. Specifically, Graham and Harris anchored their intervention firmly in trainees' demonstrated deficits in writing processes. The design of their self-instruction intervention procedure drew from CBM, Ann Brown's self-control training, and the Kansas Cognitive Strategies Curriculum. Thus, Graham and Harris explicitly linked an effective instructional procedure to Flower and Hayes's theoretical model of writing. They wrapped up their chapter with some very thoughtful pointers about future research on writing with the learning-disabled.

Keller and Lloyd (Chapter 12) have brought a fresh and important perspective to arithmetic instruction with their emphasis that such instruction should incorporate information from research by cognitive psychologists and mathematics educators. Specifically, they highlight the role of knowledge needed for competent performance in mathematics. Citing Mayer, Larkin, and Kadane (1984), Keller and Lloyd specify that in solving algebraic story problems, students need at least four kinds of knowledge:

1. They need linguistic and factual knowledge in order to translate the words of the problem properly so that they can form internal representations of the algebraic story problem.
2. They must then combine the representations with their schematic knowledge to represent both the explicitly stated and the implied relationships in the problem.
3. They need strategic knowledge, which governs the plan to solve the missing components in the relationships.
4. They need algorithmic knowledge to implement the problem-solving plan.

Clearly, then, there is much more involved in solving computation and word problems than simply reading the problem and writing the answer.

Keller and Lloyd also provide a good literature review on children's development and use of addition strategies. Similarly, they give a very good review of cognitive interventions in mathematics education. Both of these reviews should provide good grounding for graduate students interested in those particular areas of research.

The most salubrious pointer from Keller and Lloyd's chapter concerns their call for teachers to heed the findings of how children develop and use addition strategies, and to incorporate the implications into their own teaching. Likewise, the research on the importance of knowledge should alert teachers not to focus exclusively on imparting procedural knowledge.

I will now comment generally on Chapters 10 by Alexander and Hare, 11 by Graham and Harris, and 12 by Keller and Lloyd. These chapters share the theme of cognitive training in academic domains.

Cognitive training as it was first introduced by Meichenbaum and Goodman (1971) contained very general executive self-instructions, which served primarily the function of orienting or focusing the child on the task at hand and enabling him or her to self-monitor his or her performance. There were no task-specific self-instructions that guided the individual's task performance. Cognitive training studies involving academic areas, however, have typically involved *both* general metacognitive and more task-specific self-instructions. This can readily be seen in studies in arithmetic instruction by Johnston, Whitman, and Johnston (1981), Leon and Pepe (1983), Whitman and Johnston (1983), and in writing by Harris and Graham (1985). Thus, task-specific self-instructions play an explicit role in cognitive training of academic skills.

Metacognitive Components

Metacognitive components play an important role in cognitive training of academic skills. They are purpose-setting; they bring about the individual's smooth execution of the steps in cognitive training; they help the individual to monitor/self-check his or her learning/performance and to evaluate the learning/performance outcome. The important functions of metacognition in cognitive training of reading comprehension skills (Bommarito's study cited by Meichenbaum & Asarnow, 1979) and of writing skills (Harris & Graham, 1985) are readily understandable. However, in arithmetic instruction where a cognitive-training approach was not used, the role of metacognition is equivocal. Specifically, Keller and Lloyd pointed out that research on children's development and use of addition strategies has not examined the role of metacognitive processes. As they explained, the researchers might not have considered metacognition in relation to the topic of solving basic addition facts. In short, it is a function of specific research interest. Alternatively, the components involved in addition strategies may be too automatized, in which case it would be difficult to tap the child's metacognition about them. Keller and Lloyd then concluded that perhaps metacognition may not be appropriate content for cognitive-behavioral interventions on some types of mathematics content. They then reviewed some successful arithmetic intervention studies that had not included metacognitive components.

Obviously, there are constraints to the use of metacognitive components in intervention studies, just as there are constraints to the use of cognitive training (Wong, 1985). But before one contends that a metacognitive component or components should or should not be included in cognitive training on arithmetic skills, one should consider the rationale for their inclusion. Metacognitive components are included in intervention studies solely because they are purported to promote maintenance and generalization of learned skills (Brown, 1978). In the studies that Keller and Lloyd reported to contain successful arithmetic interventions, excepting the study by Haupt, Van Kirk, and Terraciano (1975), none of them contained measures of skill maintenance or generalization, at least not reported by Keller and Lloyd. The study by Haupt *et al.* had one follow-up (maintenance) measure in which the data were not clean. My point is that a proper test of whether or not inclusion of metacognitive component(s) plays a significant role in children's arithmetic learning is through appropriate experimentation in which particular groups of children are randomly assigned to particular instructional conditions. These instructional conditions should comprise the following: one including meta-cognitive component(s), one excluding it (them). One can jazz things up by throwing into the design the between-group variable of learning-disabled versus normally achieving non-learning disabled! The dependent variables would involve immediate posttests, at least two maintenance tests, and transfer tests. This design can be replicated across different types of arithmetic concepts and computational skills and across different age groups. Through such experimental manipulations, we would attain a clearer understanding of the role of metacognition in mathematics instruction. Keller and Lloyd's suggestion that metacognition may not be appropriate content for cognitive interventions for some types of mathematics content was based on an improper comparison: They pit a bunch of studies devoid of any metacognitive components against those that included them and simply looked at acquisition outcomes. Such comparison is invalid and reflects simplistic extrapolation of data because the two sets of studies represented different research foci/questions. Nevertheless, research into metacognition in mathematics education is called for.

Verbalization

Another prominent component in cognitive training is verbalization. Typically, verbalization of self-instructions proceeds from overt to covert in the trainees. But the ubiquitous inclusion of verbalization may be questioned. For example, Lloyd (1980) reported in teaching arithmetic and reading skills success with "attack strategies" in which verbalization plays no role. On the other hand, Schunk and Cox (1986) reported that requiring learning-disabled children to verbalize as they solved division problems enabled those children to score higher. Clearly, we need to research the conditions in which trainees' verbalization of instructions or self-instructions critically affects acquisition of targeted skills. At present, it is difficult to predict when verbalization is important since task difficulty and type of subjects do not explain why attack strategies are just as effective as cognitive training. One way of researching this issue is to pit different treatments against each other (e.g., attack strategy versus cognitive training) in the *same* study (see Wong, 1985). The obvious problems for such a complex intervention lie in funding, in amassing sufficient subjects and keeping them until the end of intervention, and in executing the instructional treatment and follow-ups.

HYPERACTIVITY

There are two highlights in Chapter 13 by Zentall. The first is her application and extension of Berlyne's optimal stimulation theory to hyperactive children. Berlyne's original theory proposes that all organisms would work to maintain optimal levels of arousal through instrumental responses. The theory hypothesizes that when an imbalance of arousal occurs for an organism, for example, through environmental deprivation, activity mediates as a homeostatic regulator of that arousal. In other words, an organism will initiate stimulation-seeking behavior/activity when there is inadequate stimulation/arousal.

Zentall applies Berlyne's optimal stimulation theory to hyperactive children in this way. She proposes that hyperactive children have a greater need for stimulation, which is presumed to originate from an inadequate physiological arousal. Zentall further proposes that hyperactive children satiate this need for stimulation through instrumental activity and attention that is focused outward to environmental novelty. Thus verbal activity, attentional changes, attraction to environmental novelty, response variability, failure to inhibit responses (impulsivity), and provocative social responses (aggression) all function to increase or maintain adequate levels of stimulation for hyperactive children.

Zentall's achievement is that in one elegant and parsimonious theory, she relates the three primary characteristics of hyperactivity (ADD-H): excessive activity, impulsivity, and inability to sustain attention to tasks/activities. Her theory also serves as a viable framework for interpreting the vast and varied literature on treatment.

The second highlight of Zentall's chapter is the refreshing way in which she analyzes factors that underlie successful treatments of hyperactive children. Zentall displays an impressive knowledge of the treatment literature, but she does not bore the reader with a litany of empirical studies. Rather, she sifts the empirical evidence with a critical eye and a lucid mind for alternative possibilities of data interpretation. Consequently, she spellbinds the reader with detailed, reflective analyses of various treatment approaches to hyperactivity. The reader comes away with an enlightened view of the fascinating complexities in the treatment of hyperactivity.

REFERENCES

Borkowski, J. G., Johnston, M. B., & Reid, M. K. (1987). Metacognition, motivation, and controlled performance. In S. J. Ceci (Ed.), *Handbook of cognitive, social and neuro-psychological aspects of learning disabilities* (pp. 147–174). Hillsdale, NJ: Lawrence Erlbaum.

Bransford, J., Sherwood, R., Vye, N., & Rieser, J. (1986). Teaching thinking and problem-solving: Research foundations. *American Psychologist*, October, pp. 1078–1089.

Brown, A. (1978). Knowing when, where, and how to remember: A problem of metacognition. In R. Glaser (Ed.), *Advances in instructional psychology* (pp. 77–165). Hillsdale, NJ: Lawrence Erlbaum.

Brown, A. L., & Palincsar, A. S. (1982). Inducing strategic learning from texts by means of informed, self-control training. In B. Y. L. Wong (Ed.), *Metacognition and Learning Disabilities: Topics in Learning and Learning Disabilities, 2,* 1–17.

Garner, R. (1981). Monitoring of passage inconsistency among poor comprehenders: A preliminary test of the "piecemeal processing" explanation. *Journal of Educational Research, 74*, 159–162.

Getzels, J. W., & Csikszentmihalyi, M. (1975). From problem solving to problem finding. In I. A. Taylor & J. W. Getzels (Eds.), *Perspectives in creativity* (pp. 90–116). Chicago: Aldine.

Graham, L. (1986). *The comparative effectiveness of didactic teaching and self-instructional training of a question-answering strategy in enhancing reading comprehension.* Unpublished master's thesis, Simon Fraser University, Burnaby, British Columbia.

Hallahan, D. P. (Ed.). (1980). Teaching exceptional children to use cognitive strategies. *Exceptional Education Quarterly, 1.*

Harris, K., & Graham, S. (1985). Improving learning-disabled students' composition skills: Self-control strategy training. *Learning Disability Quarterly, 8*, 27–36.

Johnston, M. B., Whitman, T. L., & Johnston, M. (1981). Teaching addition and subtraction to mentally retarded children: A self-instructional program. *Applied Research in Mental Retardation, 1*, 141–160.

Leon, J. A., & Pepe, H. J. (1983). Self-instructional training: Cognitive-behavior modification for remediating arithmetic deficits. *Exceptional Children, 50*, 54–60.

Lloyd, J. (1980). Academic instruction and cognitive behavior modification: The need for attack strategy training. *Exceptional Education Quarterly, 1*, 53–63.

Mayer, R. E., Larkin, J. H., & Kadane, J. B. (1984). A cognitive analysis of mathematical problem-solving ability. In R. J. Sternberg (Ed.), *Advances in the psychology of human intelligence* (Vol. 2, pp. 231–273). Hillsdale, NJ: Lawrence Erlbaum.

Meichenbaum, D. (1977). *Cognitive behavior modification: An integrative approach.* New York: Plenum Press.

Meichenbaum, D. (1980). Cognitive behavior modification with exceptional children: A promise yet unfulfilled. *Exceptional Education Quarterly, 1*, 83–88.

Meichenbaum, D., & Asarnow, J. (1979). Cognitive behavior modification and metacognitive development: Implications for the classroom. In P. C. Kendall & S. D. Hollon (Eds.), *Cognitive-behavioral interventions: Theory, research, and procedures* (pp. 11–35). New York: Academic Press.

Meichenbaum, D., & Goodman, J. (1971). Training impulsive children to talk to themselves: A means of developing self-control. *Journal of Abnormal Psychology, 77*, 115–126.

Schunk, D. H., & Cox, P. D. (1986). Strategy training and attributional feedback with learning-disabled students. *Journal of Educational Psychology, 78*, 201–209.

Schwebel, M., & Maher, C. A. (Eds.). (1986). *Facilitating cognitive development: International perspectives, programs, and practices.* New York: Haworth Press.

Simon, H. A. (1980). Problem solving and education. In D. T. Tuma & R. Reif (Eds.), *Problem solving and education: Issues in teaching and research* (pp. 81–96). Hillsdale, NJ: Lawrence Erlbaum.

Swanson, H. L. (1988). Toward a metatheory of learning disabilities. In B. Y. L. Wong & L. Wiederholt (Eds.), Forum on Basic Research in Learning Disabilities, *21(4)*, 196–209.

Whitman, T., & Johnston, M. B. (1983). Teaching addition and subtraction with regrouping to educable mentally retarded children: A group self-instructional training program. *Behavior Therapy, 14*, 127–143.

Wittrock, M. C. (1988). A constructive review of research on learning strategies. In C. E. Weinstein, E. T. Goetz, & P. A. Palmer (Eds.), *Learning and study strategies: Issues in assessment, instruction, and evaluation* (pp. 287–297). New York: Academic Press.

Wong, B. Y. L. (1985). Problems and issues in cognitive behavior modification applications in academics. In K. R. Harris, B. Y. L. Wong, & B. Keogh (Eds.), Cognitive behavioral interventions: A critical review of the state of the art. *Journal of Abnormal Child Psychology, 13*, 425–442.

Wong, B. Y. L. (1986). Metacognition and special education: A review of a view. *Journal of Special Education, 20*, 9–29.

Wong, B. Y. L. (1988). Issues in cognitive programs in facilitating cognitive development. Book review on Schwebel & Maher (Eds.), Facilitating cognitive development: International perspectives, programs, and practices. *Contemporary Psychology, 33*(7), 617–619.

Wong, B. Y. L., Wong, R., Perry, N., & Sawatsky, D. (1986). The efficacy of a self-questioning summarization strategy for use by underachievers and learning-disabled adolescents in social studies. *Learning Disabilities Focus, 2*, 20–35.

10
COGNITIVE TRAINING: IMPLICATIONS FOR READING INSTRUCTION

PATRICIA A. ALEXANDER
Texas A&M University

VICTORIA C. HARE
University of Illinois, Chicago

For the vast majority of those who will read this chapter, the processing of print is generally a meaningful, fairly effortless, and often rewarding activity. For many others who are younger or less proficient, however, the act of reading can better be described as meaningless, difficult, and frustrating. It is hoped that through effective instruction, many who initially approach the reading task with less than optimal results will eventually gain the knowledge, skills, and attitudes necessary for success. In this chapter we will provide information that may help in moving less proficient readers closer to the goal of reading proficiency. We will begin by examining the nature of the reading process. We will describe the attributes of effective reading and consider how these attributes influence cognitive training in reading. Once the theoretical framework for reading instruction has been established, we will present an overview of certain exemplary instructional programs in reading with either a general or a specific focus. Finally, we will discuss the future of reading and the effects that such a future is apt to have on reading instruction.

THE NATURE OF READING

Simply stated, reading is the process of deriving meaning from print. At no other time in recorded history has the interest in reading been greater from either a theoretical or a practical standpoint (Anderson, Hiebert, Scott, & Wilkinson, 1985). Indeed, in the past 15 years there has been a concerted effort to understand the nature of the reading process and to translate that theoretical knowledge into more effective classroom instruction. The outcomes of reading as a cognitive task require the successful achievement of many linguistic skills, both simple and complex (Perfetti, 1983). As we will see, it is also dependent on the knowledge, attitudes, and motivations that readers bring to the task. Therefore, in general, we can say that reading is the interaction of two types of information, visual and nonvisual (Smith, 1979). Visual information includes the linguistic aspects of the process—that is, what we can see on the printed page. Nonvisual or metalinguistic information is that knowledge of the world or about language that helps us make sense of the print. These two types of information interact to make reading a constructive, active, strategic, and affective undertaking.

As we noted at the outset, for most of us reading has become an effortless, routinized activity. Except in those instances when we are called on to process text that is unfamiliar or highly complex, we take our reading abilities for granted. The analogy of driving a car illustrates this point. If you have been driving for some time, it is probably a simple task for you to get into a car, turn it on, and proceed safely to your destination. You would have little problem climbing behind the wheel of a friend's car even if you had never driven that model of car before. Such ease and automaticity have been achieved through hundreds or thousands of successful driving experiences and from the ability to relate prior experiences to the present undertaking. Most of us, however, will also remember that our initial attempts to drive were anything but easy or automatic. Just turning the key in the ignition without grinding the motor was quite an accomplishment, and it seemed likely that we would never be able to steer the car while using the gas or brake pedal at the same time.

Teaching someone to read effectively, like teaching someone to drive a car, requires not only a phenomenal amount of fortitude but also an understanding of how a novice might approach the task at hand. There is so much to know, to remember, and to coordinate. There are so many physical, cognitive, and emotional conditions that can either facilitate or inhibit successful reading (Rupley & Blair, 1983). The effective instructor is one who understands and can anticipate the novice's problems and concerns. Indeed, reading is a far more complex cognitive activity than driving a car. Success or failure of the reading process can be affected by innumerable conditions relating to either visual or nonvisual sources of information. To identify better some of the potential sources of reading success or failure, we will describe the salient attributes of reading. Specifically, we will consider reading as a *constructive, active, strategic,* and *affective* process.

Reading Is Constructive

To read effectively, we must combine our understanding of the linguistic elements of text, the "on the page" components, with our knowledge of the world, the "in the head" components of reading. No piece of print is complete in and of itself. It is up to the reader to interpret, to clarify, or to elaborate the printed message—that is, to *construct* the meaning of the text.

For years it was believed that, to read, the individual needed only to recognize and produce the sounds of the letters correctly; combine those sounds into words; and then link the words together into sentences, into paragraphs, and so on until the text had been appropriately deciphered. Any experience or knowledge the reader had relative to the piece of text was viewed as irrelevant. This bottom-up view of the reading process was fueled by early behaviorial models of instruction, in which the complex task of reading was broken down and sequenced into small, isolated, measurable skills. Instructional programs were carefully orchestrated to follow sequenced lists of skills; once these skills were successfully mastered, the individual was proclaimed a proficient reader. With the resurgence of cognitive psychology, however, it has been demonstrated that such instructional models of reading fail to account for variability in reading performance, in large measure because they consider language to be unambiguous and because they tend to ignore the role of the reader in the process.

This is not to say that the letters, sounds, words, or punctuation are unimportant. Without the printed language, after all, there can be no reading. Still, meaning does not arise from a one-directional process that moves from the page to the reader. Rather, it occurs, as we have said, from the interaction of the visual information with nonvisual information. To demonstrate, let's try a simple experiment. Read the following passage:

> Just as Mary grabbed her things out of the locker, the bell sounded. She was late again. As she ran down the hall, she hoped that miraculously no one would be aware of her absence. No such luck. She opened the door, and there stood Mr. Jenkins. All she could do now was wait for the ax to fall.

Now, if we assume that reading is merely the process of taking in and appropriately deciphering the words on the page, then all of us should arrive at the same interpretation of this passage. How would you paraphrase what you just read? Who was Mary? What things did she grab from the locker? Where was Mary going? Who was Mr. Jenkins? What did it mean when it said that she was waiting for the ax to fall? Perhaps you assumed that Mary was a student late for a class, that she grabbed her school books, that Mr. Jenkins was her teacher, and that she was expecting to be punished for being late. None of this essential information is explicitly stated in the passage. To have such an interpretation, you must know something about schools, about lockers, about class schedules, and about the consequences of being late. Without this preexisting knowledge, you would find your understanding of the passage flawed.

Perhaps you had an alternative, albeit equally appropriate, interpretation of this passage. Maybe you thought that Mary was a worker, not a student; that she was grabbing her gear, not her books, that Mr. Jenkins was a foreman, not a teacher; and that she was waiting to be fired, not just reprimanded. Without further information, both interpretations seem feasible. Perhaps you had yet another interpretation. Maybe you interpreted the sentence, "All she could do now was wait for the ax to fall," literally rather than figuratively. In order to do so, you needed to construct a more gothic framework for the passage. Such an interpretation of the passage seems much more likely if for example, you had just finished reading a Stephen King novel. Clearly, then, reading is a *constructive* process. However you interpreted this passage, your understanding was assembled through the interaction of what was on the page and what you know or have experienced.

What are the implications of this particular attribute for cognitive training? That is, what effect does knowing that reading is a constructive process have on reading instruction? Many school curricula still view reading from a strongly behavioristic viewpoint. Reading instruction follows closely the set of prescribed, simple ordered skills that make up scope and sequence charts. Missing from these curricula is adequate attention to the nonvisual components of reading, such as the reader's background knowledge or experiences. Teachers must be careful not to assume that the meaning of any passage is apparent to any student or that all students reading the same passage will come away with the same interpretation.

Further, teachers need to take care to prepare students conceptually or experientially for the reading of text. This is particularly true when we are dealing with students whose background experiences do not match well with the content of the passage. In such instances, teachers should give students a framework into which the content can be placed. For example, before reading a story about the game of cricket, the teacher may relate the game to a game that is a bit more familiar to them, baseball (Hayes & Tierney, 1980). Before reading, it would also be helpful to activate students' prior knowledge by calling to mind related experiences through questioning or dialogue. Using our cricket example, students could be encouraged to talk about their experiences playing or watching baseball (if, as is highly likely, they have never seen or played cricket). In this way, teachers can help students to use the knowledge that they have more effectively in understanding print.

Reading Is Active

What we have also learned from the research of Wittrock (1983), Ausubel (1963), and others is that reading demands the active involvement of the individual. You cannot read effectively if you approach the task in a passive manner. Even though the reading act sometimes seems almost effortless to us, we do exert what Bartlett (1932) called "effort after meaning." We regulate and maintain our attention to the task at hand. We think about what we are reading as we read it, generating images in our heads, formulating questions, confirming or altering predictions. We must work to understand print, and the more actively we engage in the process, the more we are apt to understand and remember. Certainly, we have all experienced the situation where we are reading along beside the pool or on a plane, only to realize that we cannot remember a word. While our eyes were on the page, our minds were definitely elsewhere. This simple example illustrates the fact that reading cannot take place effectively if the reader does not take an active role in the process.

Of course, our level of activity is often a consequence of what we are asked to read and why we are asked to read it. Many people enjoy reading on the airplane, by the pool, or in bed. Although this type of recreational reading still requires attentiveness, it is far less demanding than the reading you are asked to do in school in order to pass a test (Anderson, 1980). Similarly, if you are asked to read something that is familiar or written at an easier level, the task will require less of your time and attention. The purposes of these types of reading are vastly different, as should be the level of activity they engender in the reader.

Wittrock (1983), in his generative theory of comprehension, has suggested various ways that the student can become more actively involved in the reading process. In general, Wittrick suggests that the more the individual manipulates, elaborates, or transforms the information read, the more likely he or she is to have a deeper understanding of the content, and to recall that information. Too often, however, students approach many tasks, including reading tasks, with an apparently passive attitude. They assume that if they go through the motions of learning the information somehow will find its way into their heads. A look at undergraduate classrooms confirms this perception of passive learning. Students sit with pencils flying as the instructor lectures on a topic, or they diligently underline information in the text. These students appear to assume that if they just write down or underline what seems important, they will understand and remember it. In other words, their reaction to learning seems much more of a motor activity that a cognitive one.

The implications of the active nature of reading are significant. As we provide students with instruction in the reading process, we must structure our teaching to involve them more directly in learning and must help them see reading as an active rather than a passive process. Instead of making students only question-answerers, we should make them question-askers as well. Rather than having students read headings or titles, we should give them the opportunity to create their own. Instead of having students look at the pictures, tables, or charts in the text, we should give them the chance to generate their own. The payoff of this type of learner involvement should be an increase in students' understanding of print.

Reading Is Strategic

Related to the notion of active processing is the concept of reading as a strategic process. Research has consistently demonstrated that more effective readers not only are actively involved in the process, but also are more strategically competent than their less effective counterparts. By "strategic competence" we mean that these readers have a well-developed strategic repertoire which they can draw as the situation demands. In many ways, this view of strategic competence is closely aligned with the theory of metacognition. Further, these students are good at monitoring their performance and determining what strategies should be applied and when. Let's go back to the situation we described earlier, where we discovered that we could not recall the content of the book we were reading by the pool. For most of us, this situation could be easily corrected by acknowledging our lack of understanding and then rereading those less-than-memorable pages.

Other situations, however, are not so simple to monitor or to control. In many of the readings we do as part of schooling, we are asked to read and remember much more detailed and complex materials than are found in the pages of some best-seller. This special form of reading, known as studying (Anderson, 1980), requires learners to assess their understanding accurately and apply whatever strategy is most suitable to the demands of text and task. Some of these text-processing strategies are general strategies that can be applied to a wide variety of texts or reading tasks. *Look-backs*, or the reaccessing of text, *self-questioning*, and *paraphrasing* are examples of these general text-processing strategies. There are also other strategies that function better within certain subject domains (Chi, 1985). For example, experts in mathematics seem to develop their own ways of processing highly specialized texts, as do experts in physics or computer technology. Most of the research on the strategic processing of text, however, has focused on the differential use of and training in general learning strategies.

In classrooms, we must help students, particularly those who are more at risk, to develop the self-monitoring skills and strategic repertoires necessary to function effectively in the school environment. Later in this chapter we will be looking at several models of strategy training. We must help students to recognize when they do not sufficiently understand, and then teach them what strategies would assist them in comprehending. Further, we must become strategic models for our students, demonstrating as well as describing what strategic competency looks like.

Reading Is Affective

Intertwined with the cognitive and metacognitive aspects of reading are its affective components. To be successful at reading, learners must be motivated. They must possess the desire and the emotional stability to perform such a complex cognitive activity. To attend only to the cognitive or metacognitive components of reading, without regard to its affective elements, is analogous to treating only part of a disease: The likelihood of a cure is greatly diminished. Likewise, to focus on the learner's self-concept or motivation without providing the cognitive or metacognitive support necessary for success is not apt to produce long-term positive effects either.

We would agree that, for most problem readers, the processing of print is anything but a positive experience. Print represents failure and frustration.

Indeed, some readers have even reached a state of learned helplessness when it comes to processing print (Weiner, 1983). Under cognitive models of reading, consequently, there should be explicit attention paid to affect.

Several of the comprehensive training programs, such as those conducted by McCombs (1988) and Paris and his colleagues (Paris, Lipson, & Wixson, 1983), have incorporated affective dimensions. In addition, students are furnished with motivating materials to read, are encouraged to share their readings in whatever form is most comfortable, and are given the opportunity to write and share their own stories. Students are also given the chance to share their understandings with other students in reciprocal-teaching, peer-tutoring, or cooperative learning situations (Dansereau, 1988; Judy, Alexander, Kulikowich, & Willson, 1987; Palinscar & Brown, 1984). These student-to-student teaching sessions have been found to be rewarding and instructive not only for the students who receive instruction but for those who deliver that instruction as well (Judy *et al.*, 1987).

Of course, the impact of affective aspects of reading extends beyond the learners' attention or persistence to task. Just as text must be interpreted in light of our prior knowledge and experiences, so too is that text filtered through our feelings and emotions. The meaning we construct from text is, therefore, as much a reflection of our affective state as it is of our cognitive or metcognitive abilities.

Summary

As we investigate the implications of cognitive training for reading instruction, it is important to consider the nature of reading itself. As we have attempted to show, reading is a complex process. Through active involvement, the reader seeks to construct meaning from the text, a meaning that is consistent not only with the text but also with the reader's view of the world. When gaps exist between what the learner needs to understand and remember and what he or she can recall effectively, then the reader must engage in strategic behavior that will remedy the existing situation. Yet, effective remediation is predicated on the learner possessing and using general or content-specific strategies. Although these strategies can be obtained indirectly, they can also be taught explicitly as we will see later in this chapter.

Although we have discussed each of these attributes of reading separately, in reality these attributes are intricately intertwined in reading performance. The strategies that we choose to employ relate directly to how much we feel we know about a particular topic, how much we feel we need to know, and how willing we are to undertake the task at hand. In other words, reading performance is a consequence of the interactive nature of all these essential attributes as much as it is the result of any one of them. In the next section we will begin an examination of various academic training programs that have been shown to be successful in teaching cognitive skills.

EFFECTIVE COGNITIVE-TRAINING PROGRAMS IN READING

In this section we will take a closer look at training programs that have been shown in the research literature to be successful at bringing poorer or less proficient readers to higher levels of proficiency. We have been selective in our presentation, choosing those programs that we feel have greater applicability to special learners such as the learning-disabled and to special contexts such as the resource room, and to those programs that have been influenced by the cognitive-behavioral modification approach. We will first examine the general characteristics of such effective reading programs that may contribute to their success. Next, we will consider exemplary programs that focus training on general comprehension strategies, on specific reading comprehension strategies, on teacher explanations, and then on word comprehension processes.

Characteristics of Effective Academic Training Programs

Cognitive-Behavioral Modification Programs

Cognitive-behavioral modification (CBM) programs, described by Meichenbaum and Asarnow (1979), have been applied to reading tasks as well as to tasks to help alleviate impulsivity, hyperactivity, and other problems of self-control. Typically, academic programs begin with the type of cognitive-functional analyses of target task performance inherent in CBM. Automatized task performances of successful readers are decomposed into their component processes, which in turn are incorporated into a training program. Teachers enact task processes, and their students follow their examples, first overtly, then covertly. In this way, students gradually take control of their own learning. It is not surprising that cognitive-behavioral modification programs are also called self-instructional programs.

Several assumptions are inherent in this approach to learning. One is that modeling and overt rehearsal of deautomatized reading processes may help poor readers dismantle ineffective or inefficient strategies in favor of more efficient ones. Another is that deautomatized reading processes will eventually be reassembled or automatized through practice. The activity of overt rehearsal or thinking aloud is itself assumed to accelerate problem solving and to bolster self-control of learning because it demands active, strategic attention to tasks on the student's part. Whether poor readers necessarily should execute tasks in ways similar to good readers is another matter. Scardamalia and Bereiter (1983) caution that novices may be unable or unwilling to follow experts' rules, either because they lack the requisite knowledge to apply a rule or because they are unable to appreciate what a particular rule can do for them.

Nevertheless, CBM interventions have demonstrated success when a number of problem-solving skills are modeled for students, specifically self-interrogation to identify the problem, attention focusing and response guidance, self-reinforcement based on self-evaluation, and coping skills to deal with detected problems (Meichenbaum & Asarnow, 1979). Modeling appropriate problem-solving behaviors that include coping strategies for dealing with difficulties is of crucial importance in the program, although the modeled activity is not meant to be copied directly by the students. Rather, the modeling is meant to provide students with "windows" on teachers' thinking processes as they adjust problem-solving activity relative to different task demands. Over time, as teachers cede control of the problem-solving activity to students, the approach resembles an interactive Socratic dialogue. Teachers replace modeling with soliciting problem-solving behavior from students and supplying them with information about the nature of their responses relative to the tasks at hand.

Because generalizability or transfer of strategy use has always been difficult to achieve in cognitive-behavioral modification programs, Meichenbaum and Asarnow (1979) advocate eliciting strategy use across a variety of tasks, setting, and people. In this way, students are able to acquire conditional knowledge (i.e., knowledge of when and where strategy use is appropriate) as well as procedural knowledge (knowledge of how a strategy operates) in relation to particular strategies (Paris et al., 1983).

Related Instructional Models

You may have noticed that the principles of cognitive-behavioral modification sound somewhat familiar. Its tenets are found in other instructional approaches applied to reading problems, among them: self-control training (Brown, Campione, & Day, 1981); informed strategies for learning (Paris, Cross, & Lipson, 1984); reciprocal teaching (Palincsar & Brown, 1984); explicit comprehension training coupled with metacognitive awareness (Pearson & Gallagher, 1983); and recent versions of direct instruction (Duffy et al., 1986; White & Alexander, 1986). Some models, such as direct instruction, emphasize more teacher explanation than teacher modeling. Others, such as reciprocal teaching, stress more interaction early on between teachers and students. All these instructional approaches, however, share a common metacognitive theme, learners taking charge of their own learning by internalizing teachers' models.

Exemplary Training Programs in Reading

The majority of academic applications of cognitive-behavioral modification and similar programs have been in the area of reading comprehension, converging with an interest in applying schema-theoretic training studies that exemplify key principles of a CBM approach. The description of each intervention includes specifics of how teachers enabled students to take control of their learning.

General Reading Comprehension Strategies

Reading comprehension instructional research reflects both broad-based efforts to improve comprehension generally and efforts deliberately restricted to improve use of a particular comprehension strategy. Of the broad-based efforts, one ambitious program was developed by Paris and his colleagues (Paris, Cross, DeBritto, Jacobs, Oka, & Saarno, 1984; Paris, Cross, & Lipson, 1984). Called Informed Strategies for Learning (ISL), the program had a twofold purpose. One aim was to increase third- and fifth-graders' awareness of declarative, procedural, and conditional knowledge about reading strategies. A second aim was to model for students how to evaluate, plan, and regulate their reading comprehension. These aims were tackled in a three-phase, 4-month program that began with raising students' consciousness about reading goals, plans, and strategies; continued with teaching specific strategies for text comprehension; and ended with informing students about comprehension monitoring strategies. The 20 modules, listing both metaphors and strategies, are presented in Table 10-1.

Each module described one comprehension strategy over separate lessons, the last one being a "bridging" lesson intended to help students generalize the strategy to content area reading. Strategy training emphasized learner control from the start. Students not only received a good deal of information about declarative, procedural, and conditional aspects of strategies, but also practiced taking charge of strategy choice and use from the onset of the ISL program. Twice-weekly group lessons taught by one of the investigators utilized teacher–student dialogues around the topics of reading goals and strategies that could be used to reach these goals. Paris and colleagues contend that this forum enabled teacher and students to "make thinking public," to share and compare perspectives about making meaning, and to straighten out misconceptions or modify viewpoints. Group interactions were supported by the preplanned use of concrete metaphors to make students aware of the different strategies and to impress upon them the utility of each strategy for reading specific reading goals.

For instance, as shown in Table 10-1, comprehension strategies were compared to a bagful of tricks for reading. Metaphors were incorporated into group lessons and reinforced in bulletin board displays. Group discussions were further reinforced by the application of strategies in worksheet exercises and by immediate feedback via discussions about strategy choice and use. Further, the likelihood of generalization of strategies to other situations was increased by providing classroom teachers with descriptions of strategy modules that suggested how to integrate the strategy instruction with other teaching strategies and other content areas.

ISL students in the Paris, Cross, and Lipson (1984) research displayed greater declarative, procedural, and conditional knowledge of reading strategies than did non-ISL students. In addition, the researchers inferred that ISL students learned how to evaluate, plan, and regulate their reading more effec-

TABLE 10-1. Comprehension Skill Training Modules

I. *Awareness of Reading Goals, Plans, and Strategies*
   1. Goals and purposes of reading
     "Hunting for reading treasure"
   2. Evaluating the reading task
     "Be a reading detective"
   3. Comprehension strategies
     "A bag full of tricks for reading"
   4. Forming plans
     "Planning to build meaning"
   5. Review

II. *Components of Meaning in Text*
   6. Kinds of meaning and text content
     "Turn on the meaning"
   7. Ambiguity and multiple meanings
     "Hidden meaning"
   8. Temporal and causal sequences
     "Links in the chain of events"
   9. Clues to meaning
     "Tracking down the main idea"
  10. Review

III. *Constructive Comprehension Skills*
  11. Making inferences
     "Weaving ideas"
  12. Preview and review of goals and task
     "Surveying the land of reading"
  13. Integrating ideas and using context
     "Bridges to meaning"
  14. Critical reading
     "Judge your reading"
  15. Review

IV. *Strategies for Monitoring and Improving Comprehension*
  16. Comprehension monitoring
     "Signs for reading"
  17. Detecting comprehension failures
     "Road to reading disaster"
  18. Self-correction
     "Road repair"
  19. Text schemas and summaries
     "Round up your ideas"
  20. Review
     "Plan your reading trip"

tively, judging by their success on cloze and error detection tasks that required use of reading strategies. Echoing Meichenbaum and Asarnow (1979), Paris *et al.* believe the program fostered self-control learning on the part of students: "This kind of functional learning represents a fusion of cognitive skill and motivational will into self-controlled learning that occurs with persuasive teaching and repeated practice" (p. 1250).

Palincsar and Brown (1984), using a mode of instruction they termed "reciprocal teaching," worked with seventh-grade poor comprehenders to improve comprehension-fostering and comprehension-monitoring activities. Reciprocal teaching is predicated on the notion that teaching "in advance of competence" (pp. 122–123) provides a supportive social context wherein students are encouraged to try out challenging cognitive activities—activities they are not able to perform unaided. Students' responses provide on-line diagnostic information about their levels of competence and enable teachers to build cognitive scaffolding initially through responsive modeling and eventually by taking on the role of sympathetic critic. Palincsar and Brown (1984) refer to this process as "continuous trial and error on the part of the student, married to continuous adjustment on the part of the teacher to their current competence" (p. 169).

Like ISL, reciprocal teaching emphasized learner control from Day 1. In two studies of reciprocal teaching, students and their teachers spent about 20 days taking turns conducting dialogues around four activities believed simultaneously to foster comprehension and enable comprehension monitoring. Whereas one of the investigators initially took on the adult teacher role in the first study, in a subsequent study classroom teachers led and guided discussions on their own. Segments of expository texts were assigned to be read silently, after which whoever was assigned to be teacher or dialogue leader (either the adult teacher or a student) asked a "teacher" a test question about the segment, summarized the material, discussed and clarified any troublesome material, and predicted what material might be forthcoming.

Adult teachers modeled the four activities when it was their turn to teach. Students participated as teachers from the beginning, although initially adult teachers needed to provide paraphrases and questions for them to mimic. When students were bogged down, adult teachers also guided them by prompting, instructing, switching around the order of activities as necessary, and providing informative feedback. Students were regularly reminded of the applicability of the comprehension strategies to other reading situations.

Effects of reciprocal teaching were reliable and durable. Students who underwent teaching activities clearly improved in their abilities to perform the four activities independently. Their questions and summaries became paraphrases of texts rather than verbatim selections from texts. The content they described reflected more and more top-level ideas over low-level details. Their scores on daily and classroom comprehension assessments rose dramatically relative to control groups'. Benefits also accrued on transfer tasks, where students' ability to summarize, predict questions, and detect incongruous sentences improved. In Tables 10-2 and 10-3, sample dialogues showing distinct changes in students' performances are represented. The first series of exchanges (Table 10-2) is between Charles, a poor seventh-grade reader, and his teacher; the second series (Table 10-3) is between Sara, a good seventh-grade reader, and her teacher. In both cases, clear improvements in students' questioning can be noted.

TABLE 10-2. Segment of Reciprocal Teaching Dialogues with a Poor Reader

Day 1

(*C* = Charles; *T* = Teacher)

Text: The water moccasin, somewhat longer than the copperhead, is found in the southwestern states. It lives in swampy regions. It belongs, as do also the copperhead and the rattlesnakes, to a group of poisonous snakes called pit vipers. They have pits between their eyes and their nostrils which, because they are sensitive to heat, help the snakes tell when they are near a warm-blooded animal. Another name for the water moccasin is "cottonmouth." This name comes from the white lining of the snake's mouth.

C: What is found in the southeastern snakes, also the copperhead, rattleshakes, vipers—they have. I'm not doing this right.

T: All right. Do you want to know about the pit vipers?

C: Yeah.

T: What would be a good question about the pit vipers that starts with the word "why"?

C: (*No response*)

T: How about, "Why are the snakes called pit vipers?"

C: Why do they want to know that they are called pit vipers?

T: Try it again.

C: Why do they, pit vipers in a pit?

T: How about, "Why do they call the snakes pit vipers?"

C: Why do they call the snakes pit vipers?

T: There you go! Good for you.

Day 7

Text: Perhaps you are wondering where the lava and other volcanic products come from. Deep within our earth there are pockets of molten rock called *magma*. Forced upward in part by gas pressure, this molten rock continually tries to reach the surface. Eventually—by means of cracks in the crustal rocks or some similar zone of weakness—the magma may break out of the ground. It then flows from the vent as lava, or spews skyward as dense clouds of lava particles.

C: How does the pressure from below push the mass of hot rock against the opening? Is that it?

T: Not quite. Start your question with, "What happens when?"

C: What happens when the pressure from below pushes the mass of hot rock against the opening?

T: Good for you! Good job.

Day 15

Text: Scientists also come to the South Pole to study the strange lights that glow overhead during the Antarctic night. (It's a cold and lonely world for the few hardy people who "winter over" the polar night.) These "southern lights" are caused by the Earth acting like a magnet on electrical particles in the air. They are clues that may help us understand the Earth's core and the upper edges of its blanket of air.

C: Why do scientists come to the South Pole to study?

T: Excellent question! That is what this paragraph is all about.

Source: Reprinted by permission from "Reciprocal teaching of comprehension-fostering and comprehension-monitoring activities" by A. M. Palincsar and A. L. Brown, 1984, *Cognition and Instruction*, Vol. 1, pp. 138–139.

TABLE 10-3. Segment of Reciprocal Teaching Dialogues with a Good Reader

Day 1

(*S* = Sara; *T* = Teacher)

Text: How Can Snakes Be So Flexible?
The snake's skeleton and parts of its body are very flexible—something like a rubber hose with bones. A snake's backbone can have as many as 300 vertebrae, almost ten times as many as a human's. These vertebrae are connected by loose and rubbery tissues that allow easy movement. Because of this bendable, twistable spinal construction, a smake can turn its body in almost any direction at almost any point.

S: Snakes' backbones can have as many as 300 vertebrates—almost _____ times as many as humans.

T: Not a bad beginning, but I would consider that a question about a detail. Try to avoid "fill in the blank" questions. See if next time you can find a main idea question and begin your question with a question word—how, why, when . . .

Day 3

Text: There are snakes in nearly all parts of the world. Some snakes prefer warm, arid desert areas. Others prefer leafy forests, fields, and woodlands. Some stay in areas near water and are fine swimmers. Then there are several varieties that live all their lives in the sca.

S: Can snakes live their whole lives in seas?

T: See if you can ask a question using your own words.

Day 11

Text: The young caterpillar's first meal is its own eggshell. Then it eats a leaf and each day eats more and more food. After a few days, the caterpillar becomes too large for its skin. A new skin forms beneath the first one, the old skin comes open and, like a snake, the caterpillar wriggles its way out of the split skin. Then the caterpillar goes on eating leaves or other kinds of food. When the new skin becomes too tight for the growing body, it again splits and comes off. By then the caterpillar is covered by another skin. This eating and shedding goes on for several weeks. The old skin may be replaced by a new one four or five times. Each time the skin is shed, the size and color of the caterpillar change.

S: Why does the caterpillar's skin split?

T: Excellent question. That was the point of the entire paragraph.

Source: Reprinted by permission from "Reciprocal teaching of comprehension-fostering and comprehension-monitoring activities" by A. M. Palincsar and A. L. Brown, 1984, *Cognition and Instruction*, Vol. 1, pp. 140–141.

Miller (1985) compared the effects of three one-to-one sessions of either general or specific self-instruction training on average fourth-graders' reading comprehension monitoring performance, here operationalized as error detection. The two types of training differed in whether or not an explicit rationale for the training sequence was included along with the task-specific statements. It was thought that including information about the utility of the strategy might affect the durability of strategy use. The self-verbalization involved in the training was predicated to guide ongoing cognitive processing by actively involving the reader.

Specific Self-Instruction enabled students to take control of learning by internalizing five task-specific self-statements (worded in the first person) via a four-phase procedure. Initially, the experimenter modeled the instructions with a training passage. Next, both the experimenter and the student together read and used the instructions. Third, the student alone whispered and applied the instructions, and finally, the student used the instructions covertly. Self-statements required students to operationalize or define the problem, approach the problem, evaluate the problem, reinforce themselves, and check for task completion. As the student completed each self-statement, he or she placed a checkmark beside the relevant step on a separate sheet of paper. The General Self-Instruction included a general self-statement that described a rationale for each step along with each of the five specific self-statements.

Both groups who received self-instructions uncovered more embedded text inconsistencies than groups who had not received self-instructions, immediately after instruction as well as 3 weeks later. Because one of the control groups received the same task-specific instructional content without the self-verbalization structure (rewritten in the second person), Miller concluded that self-verbalization was crucial to the success of the intervention.

Specific Reading Comprehension Strategies

Of efforts with more modest aims—that is, to improve use of a single comprehension strategy—attention to shifting control of learning from teacher to student is also notable. The following main idea and summarization studies exemplify this work.

Day (1986) examined the effects of coupling general self-management procedures with specific strategy instruction on junior college students' summarization ability. Training conditions included self-management alone, summarization rules alone, rules plus self-management, and rules integrated with self-management. Of interest was whether less able students required more explicit pairing of general and specific strategy training than more able students.

All training conditions moved from greater to lesser teacher explication on each day, as students were asked to work more independently. On Day 1, the teacher highlighted the usefulness of the relevant training steps listed on a handout differently written for each training condition. In all training conditions except the self-management alone, she next explained and applied summarization rules to a text. Students then applied the summarization rules under the explicit direction of the teacher, after which all students were requested to summarize still another text on their own. On Day 2, students received written feedback about their summaries, and Day 1, procedures were again followed.

Results showed that self-management alone was insufficient to affect students' summarization ability. The most effective training was the rules integrated with self-management, followed by rules plus self-management and then rules alone. Interestingly, effects of linking self-management instructions to strategy instruction varied with the difficulty of the summarization rule, with greater effects for the more difficult selection and invention of topic sentence rules. Day speculated that self-regulatory instructions may be most beneficial in learning moderately difficult rules or in learning very difficult rules that have been partially mastered. With easier rules, self-regulatory instructions may either be unnecessary or redundant.

Hare and Borchardt (1984) implemented a similar summarization program that was based on Day's program. Self-management steps were combined with an adapted list of summarization rules and taught to high school juniors by means of either a deductive or an inductive mode of instruction. Although objectives remained constant for both modes of instruction from day to day, deductive instruction teachers began with extremely detailed explanations, whereas inductive instruction teachers aimed for the same objectives by extremely directed questioning.

Shifting responsibility for learning from teacher to student occurred from within and across days of instruction in the deductive instruction groups. On Day 1, the objective was to describe what a summary was and to make students aware of the summarization rules and management steps, and how they worked. Only passages to which rules could be readily applied, Day's specially written ones, were utilized. Teachers explained and modeled rules, and students practiced applying the rules, first in groups and then independently. On Day 2, the objective was to review the rules and steps and to apply them to a short, real-world high school passage. Teachers modeled appropriate rule application in a good summary and rule misapplication in a poor summary. Students thereafter practiced in groups and then independently on high school passages.

On Day 3, the objective was to model coordination of all rules in summarizing a high school passage similar in length to those students might encounter in school. Teachers thought aloud through the summarization of a typical text, capitalizing on a previously developed worksheet. Modeling revealed, for example, that texts often offer hints as to what might be included in a summary, or that poorly structured texts can really impede summarization progress. Students summarized a final passage on their own. Inductive instruction groups achieved the same objectives, but as dialoguing was the constant mode of interaction during 3 days of instruction, learners had more control over learning from Day 1.

Students in both groups improved considerably in summarization skill over a control group, with improvements maintaining over a 2-week period. Compared with Day's population, this younger population showed improvement on easy as well as difficult rules. Specific summarization training coupled with self-management instructions improved performance both on rules that were fairly unambiguous in their deployment and on rules that relied on learners' sensitivity to importance in text.

Taylor and Beach (1984) examined the effects of text structure instruction on students' reading and writing skills. Their hierarchical summary procedure was hypothesized to increase students' awareness of text structure as signaled by headings and subheadings to enable students to capitalize on text structure when recalling and writing about text.

Over a period of 7 weeks, teachers helped students take control of the summarization process. For the first 4 weeks, students summarized assigned texts, discussed their summaries with the teacher, and compared their summaries against templates developed by the investigators. Summaries were constructed by filling in a skeleton outline based on the assigned text's structure. Discussions about thesis statements, main ideas in support of thesis statements, and details in support of main ideas also ensued. By Week 5, students were on their own in constructing summaries. Control group students received conventional reading instruction that also began with teacher–student group discussion about questions and then gradually moved to independent student question-answering.

Results favored the hierarchical summary group for recall of relatively unfamiliar social studies material, but not of relatively familiar material. The investigators believed that the procedure helped students by providing a set of specific steps to follow in summarizing what was read. Both groups fared well on recall of familiar material, suggesting to Taylor and Beach that written responses generally may keep students on task.

Baumann (1984) devised an instructional program to foster sixth-grade students' main idea comprehension. He worked within the framework of a direct instruction paradigm that initially required the teacher to take responsibility for student learning but that transferred responsibility to the students themselves as each lesson progressed.

Over a series of eight lessons, students mastered increasingly difficult applications of knowledge about main ideas, from finding explicit main ideas and details in paragraphs, to inferring implicit main ideas and details in passages, to constructing main idea outlines of passages. The teacher followed a five-step procedure each day: introduction, exemplification, and direct instruction of the skill, followed by teacher-directed application and then independent practice of the skill. During the introduction and exemplification phases, students were made aware of the purpose and value of the instruction. During the direct instruction phase, teachers used various heuristics to model the skill to be learned (e.g., main idea on a tabletop and supporting details on the table legs). Such heuristics were intended to give students some structured means to figure out future main ideas and details, when they applied main idea skills during teacher-directed application and independent practice.

Students receiving strategic main idea instruction performed better than students receiving massed basal reader instruction or vocabulary development exercises, in terms of recognition and generation of explicit and implicit main ideas at both paragraph and passage levels. Baumann attributed these results to the instructional model that moved from full teacher responsibility to shared student–teacher responsibility to full student responsibility.

Teacher Explanations

Duffy et al. (1986) used an intervention model similar to cognitive-behavioral modification to train teachers to make more explicit verbal explanations during reading skill instruction. It was hypothesized that better explanations would make students more aware of what is to be learned, which in turn would effect greater achievement on standardized reading measures. Teachers were trained to recast basal reader skills as strategies that could be used by readers to eliminate reading problems.

Fifth-grade teachers were recipients of 10 hours of training on making explicit explanations during reading skill instruction. First, information about strategy instruction was provided and tied to teachers' background experiences and expected student responses. Second, strategy instruction was modeled and teachers were assisted in working out their instructional plans. Third, teachers were guided in analyzing and critiquing transcripts of their prior lessons. Last, teachers were given oral feedback following observations of their explaining behavior.

The content of the training emphasized how to recast basal skills as strategies for unlocking meaning; how to make explicit statements about the skill, when it would be used, and how to use it; and how to organize these statements effectively for students. Teachers were advised to organize their instruction according to the following structure: introduction, modeling, guided interaction, practice, and application. Teachers were shown how to reveal readers' mental processing by talking aloud about their own use of the skill in actual reading situations. Additionally, they were informed about how to attend to key features of the skill, how to focus student attention during instruction, how to review, how to provide practice, and how to assist students in applying the skill.

Although experimental teachers' students took more time to complete subsequent achievement tests, possibly indicating greater attention to reading strategies, statistically significant differences between treatment and control teachers' students were not apparent on these tests. More encouragingly, however, experimental teachers' verbal explanations had a definite impact on poor readers' awareness of lesson content, relative to control teachers' explanations. As a result, although more studies are needed, Duffy and colleagues emphasized that the nature of instructional talk has a strong relationship with what students understand and remember.

Word Comprehension Processes

Up to this point we have been discussing successful training programs involving both general and specific comprehension strategies applied to connected discourse or text, programs influenced by the cognitive-behavioral modification approach. We would like to turn our attention briefly to a program that has focused more on the understanding and strategic manipulation of words via the training of the component processes of analogical reasoning. As with the previously described programs, this analogy training has adopted some of the principles of cognitive-behavioral modification. Further, this program has many of the characteristics of the new direct instruction paradigm as employed in the Baumann (1984) study of main idea and the Duffy et al. (1986) research on teacher explanation.

In a series of training studies, Alexander and her colleagues have successfully improved the analogical reasoning performance of preschoolers (White &

Alexander, 1986), middle and high school students (Alexander, White, Haensly, & Crimmins-Jeanes, 1987), and students of gifted and nongifted ability levels (Alexander, White, *et al.*, 1987; Judy *et al.*, 1987). In addition, significant effects for training have resulted whether training was administered by the researchers (Alexander, White, *et al.*, 1987; White & Alexander, 1986) by the classroom teachers (Alexander, Wilson, White, Willson, Tallent, & Shutes, 1987) or by the children themselves (Judy *et al.*, 1987). Besides consistent direct effect for training, as demonstrated on tests composed of verbal and nonverbal analogy problems, the training program has also been found to transfer to the comprehension of texts containing embedded analogies (Judy *et al.*, 1987).

The core of the analogy training, applied to analogy problems of the form A:B::C:?, were performance components of analogical reasoning specified by Sternberg (1977). Specifically, those components trained were: encoding (the identification of important attributes of each term), inferring (the establishment of the relationship between the A:B terms), mapping (the development of a rule relating the A and C terms), and applying (the resolution of the best response the basis of prior relationships generated). The success of the analogy training program, according to Alexander and her colleagues, is attributable to several factors: (1) effective teacher modeling combined with explicit teacher explanation; (2) clear specification of the underlying component processes of analogical reasoning as a framework for problem solution; (3) ordered practice from simpler, more concrete problems to more difficult, and more abstract problems; and (4) immediate and positive feedback to students.

The first several sessions of the analogy training centered on simple analogy problems of the form A:B::C:?. Once the component processes were effectively applied by the students to such problems, the training moved to establishing a relationship between analogical reasoning and text comprehension. Students were shown how the same component processes applied in the solution of analogy problems were used by good readers when they make sense of print. For example, students were told how good readers not only sound out or decode words as they read, but encode them as well. That is, good readers put meanings as well as sounds to the words that they read. Students were given opportunities to apply the component processes in their basal reading lessons and were encouraged to look for instances in their other classes where the component processes could be employed.

In the same manner as the Baumann (1984) training, the analogy training program is organized around the idea that multiple training sessions should move systematically from more to less teacher control and direction. Also, each of the sessions was developed to include occasions of group participation and independent practice where students were encouraged to verbalize their reasoning throughout problem solution. Throughout the training, students were shown that effective processing was at least as important, if not more so, than correct answer.

Throughout this section we have been describing several successful training programs in reading that reflect many of the principles of cognitive-behavioral modification. We have also seen how the success of these various programs relates in many ways to their attention to the essential characteristics of the reading process. These effective programs have acknowledged the complexity of reading, have required active learner participation, and have been aimed at providing students with strategic behavior that would increase their reading proficiency. In other words, these effective reading training programs, which represent the state of the art in instructional research, are linked directly to the nature of the reading process.

In the final section of this chapter, we will move from a discussion of the state of the art to what we might term the state of the future. We will consider some of the influences on training in reading that have begun to emerge as powerful forces, forces that are likely to have a significant impact on reading instruction in the years to come.

FUTURE DIRECTIONS IN COGNITIVE TRAINING IN READING

For the moment, we would like to put aside our normal roles as reading researchers and take on a new role as reading prognosticators. Our crystal ball has been replaced by well-worn copies of research journals, however, and by a fine-tuned intuition built around years of observing, engaging in, and discussing reading instruction with teachers, administrators, and fellow researchers. Although there may be many new directions we could describe, we have narrowed our discussion in this chapter to the following: (1) the growing impact of computer technology, (2) the development of cognitive models of assessment in reading, (3) the resurgence of attention to the affective domain in reading instruction, and (4) the consideration of the relationship between background knowledge and strategic knowledge in reading performance.

The Growing Impact of Computer Technology

Computers are becoming more and more a part of our everyday existence. Advances in computer technology have altered the way we function in the workplace, in our homes, and, to a lesser extent, in schools. As a result of sophistication in both computer hardware and software, more information can be processed quickly and easily. Our computers are becoming more intelligent and more user-friendly.

As we noted, however, the potential impact of computer technology has not yet been fully realized in the classroom. No one can argue that computers and computer software are very common sights in our schools. But the abundance of computers in our classrooms is only the catalyst for significant changes in reading instruction. It is the use that we make of this computer technology that is capable of altering the face of reading diagnosis and instruction. Today, computers are generally employed in rather limited ways in reading instruction. Computers serve more as electric gradebooks, microchip managers, and video worksheets. Even with a room full of computers, it is basically business as usual during reading instruction.

Even when testing or instruction are provided via computer terminals, we find that the nature of the test or the instruction is altered little from that provided without computer assistance. For example, computers are most often used in the elementary classrooms for drill and practice exercises that are only one step above the unguided practice that has plagued reading instruction for decades (see Durkin, 1978–1979). We are all familiar with the cute feedback displays that are part of many computer instruction packages. "Nice try" or "Way to go" may be somewhat motivational to the learner, but represents a major underuse of computer capabilities.

The situation in assessment is similar. Although computers can be used to administer and score reading tests to individuals or groups, the content or format of the test is not adapted to match the capabilities of the computer into which it is programmed. For example, computer technology is already at the stage of development where test items of varying levels of difficulty can be stored in a test bank. As a student works through a randomly selected subset of these test questions, his or her response to one item could be used by the computer as data to determine the appropriate level of difficulty for the next item selected, and so on until adequate response data have been generated. From these stored data, the computer could use the accumulated response information to generate a diagnostic profile for a specific student.

Several researchers have begun to explore the potential of the computer as an assessment and instructional aid in reading (Garner, Gillingham, Guthrie, Sawyer, & King, 1987; Palmer, Stowe & Kueker, 1987). These researchers have employed computer technology to track students strategic behaviors during text processing. By means of the computer, such variables as the time spent on each text segment, which lines of text are reaccessed, and the type of strategic resources requested by the student have been calculated. Even such aspects as heart rate as a measure of reader anxiety or stimulation have been monitored by means of computer technology (Palmer et al., 1987). All such information then becomes valuable in planning cognitive training to match the reader's particular strengths and needs. Eventually, elaborate training programs can be programmed into the computer to be activated as a gap in learner strategic behavior becomes identified. Certainly, such advances would be a far cry from computer-generated messages like "Sorry, try again."

The Development of Cognitive Models of Assessment in Reading

All of us who have sought to devise effective cognitive-training programs in reading have come face to face with the realization that our instructional capabilities have not been matched by the development of assessment tools. Paris, Cross, and Lipson (1984), Alexander, White, et al. (1987) and others have complained that existing instrumentation may not be sensitive enough to register the subtle changes in cognitive processes that may result from cognitive training. Indeed, whereas training programs in reading fall squarely within the realm of cognitive psychology and information-processing theory, assessment remains strongly within the realm of the psychometric tradition. The result is a significant theoretical gap between instruction and assessment. This issue is extensively explored in the section of this book dealing with assessment practices.

For the most part, when we employ standardized measures to assess reading comprehension, we are limited to data only about the correctness or incorrectness of student responses. In the composition of such tests, the test constructors have made the judgment that such dichotomous data are the only information of importance. Even on multiple-choice tests, where the correct response is compared to several very different distractors, the score received by the learner considers all those distractors to be of the same degree of wrongness.

An illustration of this situation can be drawn from the work of Goodman and Burke (1980) on miscue analysis. The research of Goodman and Burke awakened the reading community to the realization that oral reading errors were a valuable source of processing information. In some instances, those errors reflected an understanding of the content of the text being read, while at other times the word produced had no apparent relationship to the printed word either in form or in meaning. By using errors, then, as sources of information, diagnosis of reading patterns could be more accurately made and suitable remediation planned.

Alexander and her colleagues (Alexander, Willson, White, & Fuqua, 1987, Judy et al., 1987; White & Alexander, 1986) have begun to cope with the gap between training and assessment by constructing their own measures that provide cognitive-processing data. For example, in their assessment of analogical reasoning in very young children, Alexander, Willson, et al. (1987) developed a gamelike task that measures not only children's proficiency at reasoning analogically but also the type of rule structure children follow when errors are made. This error analysis can then be applied in the provision of effective training for these less proficient reasoners (White & Alexander, 1986). In their work with older students, Judy et al. devised a multiple-choice test for a text containing embedded analogies as a transfer task. Each of the distractors on the test was taken either from the intended domain (the game of cricket), from the related domain (baseball), or from an unrelated domain. Students' incorrect responses were coded for domain, and response profiles were developed from these codings. One finding of this study was the fact that the errors made by students of higher ability tended to be within the intended domain, whereas those of lesser ability were more apt to respond to questions in terms of their knowledge of baseball. It should also be noted that in the studies just described, most errors did not appear to be random, but followed rather consistent patterns even for less proficient learners.

Until reading tests are generally constructed in such a way that error analysis can be undertaken more systematically, reading educators and researchers will remain hampered in their attempts to assess process as well as product. It is hoped that the influence of cognitive psychology will soon begin to have a greater impact on the construction of comprehension measures. In this way, we will be able to coordinate our efforts in cognitive training in reading with instruments devised to be sensitive to processing differences. The presence of a section on this very topic in this book is certainly cause for optimism that such a future is not too far away.

The Resurgence of Attention to the Affective Domain

Interest in affect is by no means new. At this outset of this chapter, in the discussion of the nature of the reading process, we observed that reading is an affective process. The feelings, emotions, attitudes, and beliefs of readers are as key to success as their cognitive and metacognitive strategies. It would seem, however, that the strong focus on cognitive and metacognitive components of the reading process in recent years has overshadowed the concern for affect. Although there are some exemplary training programs, such as Paris, Cross and Lipson's (1984) ISL program, that address the affective dimensions along with the cognitive and metacognitive, the majority of training studies we have described in this chapter have largely ignored or at least not explicitly addressed affective components of reading.

Yet, as Palmer and Goetz (1988) have observed, even the strategies we select or the effort we exert is linked strongly to our self-perceptions. If we attribute our success to external and stable factors, we will likely be unwilling to employ strategies that require effort and that may not demonstrate immediate effects. Further, issues of motivation remain of primary concern with certain problem reader population—for example, those who suffer from learned helplessness. Without the marriage of affective training with training in cognitive or metacognitive strategies, the hope for success for such disabled readers seems dim.

The work of Dweck and Bempechat (1983), Weiner (1983), and others has maintained the concern for the affective domain and has rekindled other researchers' attention to the affective elements of the reading process (e.g., Palmer & Goetz, 1988). We predict that this trend will continue (see McCombs, 1988) and that models of the reading process will be developed that attend to all aspects of the reader—cognitive, metacognitive, and affective.

Consideration of the Relationship between Background Knowledge and Strategic Knowledge

The resurgence of cognitive psychology has produced two indisputable findings with regard to reading proficiency. First, those who know more about a particular topic read and remember more than those with only limited knowledge in that topic area (e.g., Anderson, Reynolds, Schallert, & Goetz, 1977; Glaser, 1984). Second, students who monitor and regulate their cognitive processing during task performance do better than those who do not engage in such strategic processing (e.g., Flavell, 1981; Garner, 1987). Although these two findings have been consistently supported in the research, there is little understanding of how these two forms of knowledge interact during learning. Intuitively, it would appear that reading as it most often occurs in the classroom is an interplay between what students already know (background knowledge) and the techniques they employ to make print more understandable and memorable (strategic knowledge). The studies of experts and novices (e.g., Chi, 1985) have demonstrated the importance both knowledge types play in differentiating the highly proficient from those who are less proficient. This research must be expanded to include the learning that occurs in the reading classrooms.

For example, Alexander and her colleagues (Alexander, Pate, Kulikowich, Farrell, & Wright, 1988) have begun a multiyear project with the purpose of assessing the interactive role of these two knowledge types in school learning. The goal of this project is a model of learning that better addresses the relationship of background and strategic knowledge. The domain under investigation in this research is human biology. Vocabulary tests in the domain of human biology have been generated to test background knowledge, figural analogy tests are used to assess strategic knowledge, and analogy tests composed of human biology terms and passages presented with and without embedded analogies are employed as measures involving both background and strategic knowledge. Performance on these various tests will be analyzed before and after training, and will be compared to student performance on existing standard measures of aptitude and achievement to determine relative contributions of background and strategic knowledge to school learning. Information of this type seems crucial if researchers and practitioners are to deliver more effective training to students in the area of reading instruction.

Summary

In this last section, we have been looking into our crystal ball (or better, our reading journals) and projecting several important trends to emerge in reading research in the years to come. We have considered that advancements in computer technology, development of cognitive approaches to assessment, interest in affective dimensions, and an awareness of interaction between background and strategic knowledge will exert powerful influences on the nature of reading instruction. As evidenced by chapters in this book, we have already begun to move in these directions, and the result should be more effective techniques and models of reading instruction in the decade to come.

CONCLUSION

It has been our intent in this chapter to present an overview of cognitive training as applied to the area reading instruction. A theoretical framework for this discussion was provided through an examination of the nature of reading, with emphasis on characteristics of the reading process. Next, we presented several exemplary programs in reading, of both general and more specific types. As could be seen in these model programs, which were influenced in part by the cognitive-behavioral approach, particular attention was paid to the salient characteristics of the reading process. There was an effort to make readers more actively and strategically involved, and a concern that the crucial aspects of the training be clearly and explicitly conveyed by the teacher. Further, in several of the training programs there was consideration of affective factors of the reader as well as cognitive and metacognitive ones. Finally, in the last section of the chapter we looked ahead to trends that seem to be emerging in reading research, trends that are likely to influence reading instruction in the future.

As we have seen throughout this chapter, reading is a complex, cognitive-demanding process. It is also an essential tool for amassing knowledge in our information-laden society. By effectively translating reading research into instructional programs that can be successfully initiated in schools and with problem readers, we have a chance to make print meaningful and rewarding for all students.

REFERENCES

Alexander, P. A., Pate, P. E., Kulikowich, J. M., Farrell, D. M., & Wright, N. L. (1988). *Domain-specific and strategic knowledge: The effects of training on students of differing ages or levels of competence.* Manuscript submitted for publication.

Alexander, P. A. White, C. S., Haensly, P. A., & Crimmins-Jeanes, M. (1987). Training in analogical reasoning. *American Educational Research Journal, 24,* 387–404.

Alexander, P. A., Willson, V. L., White, C. S., & Fuqua, J. D. (1987). Analogical reasoning in young children. *Journal of Educational Psychology, 79,* 401–408.

Alexander, P. A., Wilson, A. F., White, C. S., Willson, V. L., Tallent, M. K., & Shutes, R. E. (1987). Effects of teacher training on children's analogical reasoning performance. *Teaching and Teacher Education, 3,* 275–285.

Anderson, R. C., Hiebert, E. H., Scott, J. A., & Wilkinson, I. A. G. (1985). *Becoming a nation of readers: The report of the commission on reading* (Contract No. 400-83-0057). Washington, DC: National Institute of Education.

Anderson, R. C., Reynolds, R. E., Schallert, D. L., & Goetz, E. T. (1977). Frameworks for comprehending discourse. *American Educational Research Journal, 14,* 367–381.

Anderson, T. H. (1980). Study strategies and adjunct aids. In R. J. Spiro, B. C. Bruce, & W. F. Brewer (Eds.), *Theoretical issues in reading comprehension* (pp. 483–502). Hillsdale, NJ: Lawrence Erlbaum.

Ausubel, D. P. (1963). *The psychology of meaningful verbal learning.* New York: Grune & Stratton.

Bartlett, F. C. (1932). *Remembering: A study in experimental and social psychology.* London: Cambridge University Press.

Baumann, J. F. (1984). The effectiveness of a direct instruction paradigm for teaching main idea comprehension. *Reading Research Quarterly, 20,* 93–115.

Brown, A. L., Campione, J. C., & Day, J. D. (1981). Learning to learn: On training students to learn from texts. *Educational Researcher, 10,* 14–21.

Chi, M. T. H. (1985). Interactive roles of knowledge and strategies in the development of organized sorting and recall. In J. W. Segal, S. F. Chipman, & R. Glaser (Eds.), *Thinking and learning skills: Relating instruction to basic research* (pp. 457–483). Hillsdale, NJ: Lawrence Erlbaum.

Dansereau, D. F. (1988). Cooperative learning strategies. In C. E. Weinstein, E. T. Goetz, & P. A. Alexander (Eds.), *Learning and study strategies: Issues in assessment, instruction, and evaluation* (pp. 103–120). San Diego: Academic Press.

Day, J. D. (1986). Teaching summarization skills: Influences of student ability and strategy difficulty. *Cognition and Instruction, 3,* 193–210.

Duffy, G. G., Roehler, L. R., Meloth, M. S., Vavrus, L. G., Book, C., Putnam, J., & Wesselman, R. (1986). The relationship between explicit verbal explanations during reading skill instruction and student awareness and achievement: A study of reading teacher effects. *Reading Research Quarterly, 21,* 237–252.

Durkin, D. (1978–1979). What classroom observations reveal about reading comprehension instruction. *Reading Research Quarterly, 14,* 481–533.

Dweck, C. S., & Bempechat, J. (1983). Children's theories of intelligence: Consequences for learning. In S. G. Paris, G. M. Olson, & H. W. Stevenson (Eds.), *Learning and motivation in the classroom* (pp. 239–256). Hillsdale, NJ: Lawrence Erlbaum.

Flavell, J. H. (1981). Cognitive thinking. In W. P. Dickson (Ed.), *Children's communication skills* (pp. 35–60). New York: Academic Press.

Garner, R. (1987). *Metacognition and reading comprehension.* Norwood, NJ: Ablex.

Garner, R., Gillingham, M. G., Guthrie, J. T., Sawyer, R., & King, S. (1987). *Use of knowledge base and strategic resources in answering questions about text.* Manuscript submitted for publication.

Glaser, R. (1984). Education and thinking: The role of knowledge. *American Psychologist, 39,* 93–104.

Goodman, Y. M., & Burke, C. (1980). *Reading strategies: Focus on comprehension.* New York: Holt, Rinehart & Winston.

Hare, V. C., & Borchardt, K. M. (1984). Direct instruction of summarization skills. *Reading Research Quarterly, 20,* 62–78.

Hayes, D. A., & Tierney, R. J. (1980). *Increasing background knowledge through analogy: Its effects on comprehension and learning* (Technical Report No. 228). Champaign, IL: University of Illinois, Center for the Study of Reading.

Judy, J. E., Alexander, P. A., Kulikowich, J. M., & Willson, V. L. (1987). Effects of two instructional approaches and peer tutoring on gifted and nongifted sixth-grade students' analogy performance. *Reading Research Quarterly, 23,* 236–256.

McCombs, B. L. (1988). Motivational skills training: Combining metacognitive, cognitive, and affective learning strategies. In C. E. Weinstein, E. T. Goetz, & P. A. Alexander (Eds.), *Learning and study strategies: Issues in assessment, instruction, and evaluation* (pp. 141–169). San Diego: Academic Press.

Meichenbaum, D., & Asarnow, J. (1979). Cognitive-behavioral modification and metacognitive development: Implications for the classroom. In P. C. Kendall & S. D. Hollon (Eds.), *Cognitive-behavioral interventions: Theory, research, and procedures* (pp. 11–35). New York: Academic Press.

Miller, G. (1985). The effects of general and specific self-instruction training on children's comprehension monitoring performances during reading. *Reading Research Quarterly, 20,* 616–628.

Palincsar, A. M., & Brown, A. L. (1984). Reciprocal teaching of comprehension-fostering and comprehension-monitoring activities. *Cognition and Instruction, 1,* 117–175.

Palmer, D. J., & Goetz, E. T. (1988). Selection and use of study strategies: The role of the studier's beliefs about self and strategies. In C. D. Weinstein, E. T. Goetz, & P. A. Alexander (Eds.), *Learning and study strategies: Issues in assessment, instruction, and evaluation* (pp. 41–61). San Diego: Academic Press.

Palmer, D. J., Stowe, M. L., & Kueker, H. J. (1987). *A computer assisted investigation of good and poor readers' use of multiple semantic standards for evaluating comprehension.* Manuscript submitted for publication.

Paris, S. G., Cross, D. R., DeBritto, A. M., Jacobs, J., Oka, E., & Saarno, D. (1984). *Improving children's metacognition and reading comprehension with classroom instructions.* Research colloquium presented at the annual meeting of the American Educational Research Association, New Orleans, Louisiana, April.

Paris, S. G., Cross, D. R., & Lipson, M. Y. (1984). Informed strategies for learning: A program to improve children's reading awareness and comprehension. *Journal of Educational Psychology, 76,* 1239–1252.

Paris, S. G., Lipson, M. Y., & Wixson, K. K. (1983). Becoming a strategic reader. *Contemporary Educational Psychology, 8,* 293–316.

Pearson, P. D., & Gallagher, M. C. (1983). The instruction of reading comprehension. *Contemporary Educational Psychology, 8,* 317–344.

Perfetti, C. A. (1983). Individual differences in verbal processes. In R. F. Dillon & R. R. Schmeck (Eds.), *Individual differences in cognition* (Vol. 1, pp. 65–104). New York: Academic Press.

Rupley, W. H., & Blair, T. R. (1983). *Reading diagnosis and remediation: Classroom and clinic* (2nd ed.). Boston: Houghton Mifflin.

Scardamalia, M., & Bereiter, C. (1983). Child as coinvestigator: Helping children gain insight into their own mental processes. In S. G. Paris, G. M. Olson, & H. W. Stevenson (Eds.), *Learning and motivation in the classroom* (pp. 61–82). Hillsdale, NJ: Lawrence Erlbaum.

Smith, F. (1979). Conflicting approaches to reading research. In L. B. Resnick & P. A. Weaver (Eds.), *Theory and practice of early reading* (Vol 2, pp. 31–42). Hillsdale, NJ: Lawrence Erlbaum.

Sternberg, R. J. (1977). *Intelligence, information processing, and analogical reasoning: The componential analysis of human abilities.* Hillsdale, NJ: Lawrence Erlbaum.

Taylor, B. M., & Beach, R. W. (1984). The effects of text structure instruction on middle-school students' comprehension and production of expository text. *Reading Research Quarterly, 19,* 134–146.

Weiner, B. (1983). Some thoughts about feelings. In S. G. Paris, G. M. Olson, & H. W. Stevenson (Eds.), *Learning and motivation in the classroom* (pp. 165–178). Hillsdale, NJ: Lawrence Erlbaum.

White, C. S., & Alexander, P. A. (1986). Effects of training on four-year-olds' ability to solve geometric analogy problems. *Cognition and Instruction, 3,* 261–268.

Wittrock, M. C. (1983). *Generative reading comprehension.* Invited address presented at the annual meeting of the American Educational Research Association, Montreal, April.

11
COGNITIVE TRAINING: IMPLICATIONS FOR WRITTEN LANGUAGE

STEVE GRAHAM
KAREN R. HARRIS
University of Maryland

This present chapter examines the use of cognitive-behavioral approaches in the teaching of writing. Particular attention is directed at examining the use of these procedures with students who receive school psychology and/or special-education services. Although investigators have only recently begun to examine the effects of cognitive-behavioral approaches in improving writing performance, the available evidence demonstrates that these procedures hold great promise as a means for helping inefficient learners develop the skills and abilities necessary to carry out more sophisticated composing processes (Graham & Harris, 1987a, 1988a). Students with writing difficulties have been taught to make successful use of strategies and self-management routines designed to increase active task involvement during writing, to activate a search of appropriate memory stores for writing content, to establish intentional control over sentence and paragraph production, to facilitate advanced planning, and to boost the quantity and quality of text revisions.

Although we will advance the proposition that the writing of handicapped students and other inefficient learners can be improved by teaching them to make independent use of appropriate strategies and self-management routines, this should not be interpreted to imply that cognitive-behavioral approaches should supplant traditional writing pedagogy or other remedial methods that have proved to be effective. Instead, these approaches should be incorporated as an integral part of an instructional regime designed to facilitate the development of a variety of writing skills, ranging from the automatization of the lower level skills of getting language onto paper, to using writing as a tool for exploring and extending thought (see Graham, 1982, and Graham & Harris, 1988a, 1988b, for recommendations on developing a writing program for exceptional students). Within this framework, cognitive-behavioral techniques may be particularly useful in helping students develop more mature and complex composing behaviors as well as security in the cognitive processes and subprocesses central to effective writing.

Cognitive-behavioral approaches that have been used to improve writing performance are elaborated in later sections of this chapter, including a review of the application of self-regulation and strategy training in the treatment of writing difficulties. First, we offer an overview on the nature of the composing process. The cognitive processes and subprocesses crucial to effective writing are highlighted, providing a general framework to which the specific strategies and routines presented next can be anchored.

THE NATURE OF THE COMPOSING PROCESS

During the last decade, researchers and theorists have developed reasonably coherent descriptions of the mental processes that writers employ when composing (Humes, 1983), resulting in the construction of several general models of the composing process (e.g., Beaugrande, 1984; Hayes & Flower, 1986). The most influential model developed to date, provided by Hayes and Flower (Flower & Hayes, 1980; Hayes & Flower, 1980), is an explicit account of the mental operations used by mature writers. According to this model, writing is a goal-directed activity, writing goals are hierarchically organized, and writers accomplish their goals by employing three major cognitive processes—planning, sentence generation, and revision. Each of these cognitive processes and their relationships are presented in more detail below.

Planning

Of the three cognitive processes identified in the Hayes and Flower model, planning has been the most thoroughly investigated (Humes, 1983). Planning involves setting goals and determining the content of a paper (Flower & Hayes, 1981). During planning, writers draw on a set of mental operations or subprocesses that include generating, organizing, and goal-setting (Hayes & Flower, 1980). *Generating* involves accessing information to write about, either from the writer's own background or from external sources. *Organizing* entails culling and arranging information, providing structure to the written product. *Goal-setting* includes generating criteria for judging text and developing en route tactics for completing a paper.

When planning a composition, writers must deal with two principal problems (Flower & Hayes, 1980). First, they must generate an organized set of concepts for a paper by selecting, culling, and arranging ideas from a potentially large body of information. Second, the information gathered must be made to fit the constraints of formal prose and the characteristics and needs of the reader. In order to deal effectively with these two constraints, mature writers often develop a number of specialized goals or plans to guide their actions (Flower & Hayes, 1981; Humes, 1983). Two types of goals that writers typically draw on are *content* goals, which direct what to say (e.g., "I'll describe where the story takes place"), and *process* goals, which govern what the writer does (e.g., "Write an opening sentence"). A goal can also be directed at governing both what the writer does and what he or she says (e.g., "I want to close with a statement about the moral of this story").

The plans that writers use have at least three sources (Hayes & Flower, 1986). One obvious source is the writer's knowledge of the topic under consideration. A fan writing a description of a basketball game, for instance, would know what to observe, and such knowledge can provide organizing concepts that aid in selecting and structuring relevant information. A second source involves the use of textual conventions, genre patterns, or other discourse schema. A well-known writing format offers a prefabricated plan for directing the writing process and can be used to produce sentences, paragraphs, or even whole text. A final source for planning entails the writer's development of new or novel plans when known writing formats are inadequate to deal with the immediate writing problem. This may necessitate the activation and orchestration of a repertoire of strategies that support planning and problem solving—searching for constraints, testing hypotheses, and so forth (Voss, Greene, Post, & Penner, 1983).

Sentence Generation

Sentence generation involves translating the writing plan into acceptable written English (Hayes & Flower, 1980, 1986). This includes putting nonverbal ideas into written form, expanding briefly sketched ideas or notes, and carrying out specific goals or plans (e.g., "Write an introduction"). Translation places considerable demands on writers' processing capabilities. When transforming ideas into written language, the writer is faced with a variety of problems related to discourse coherence and structure (Humes, 1983). These include, but are not limited to, factors such as handwriting, spelling, punctuation, capitalization, word choice, textual connections, syntax, clarity, and the possible reaction of the reader. Fortunately, the mental load imposed by translation "becomes lighter as an increasing number of writing skills become automatic rather than consciously driven" (Bridwell, 1981, p. 96). The automatization of skills such as handwriting, spelling, or language usage, however, takes years of practice (Graham & Miller, 1979, 1980; Humes, 1983).

In translating ideas into text, writers generally produce sentences in parts (Kaufer, Hayes, & Flower, 1986). Furthermore, sentence parts are commonly assembled in a left to right fashion. In other words, each new sentence part is added to the right of the preceding sentence or is generated to replace it.

Revision

Revision involves the writer's attempt to improve the text. It is a highly complex process that entails a range of behaviors from simple editing for violations of written conventions to reformulating whole texts (Humes, 1983).

A revision may be initiated for a variety of different reasons (Hayes & Flower, 1986). Writers may perceive a mismatch between what they intended to say and what is actually written; this recognition leads them to attempt to change their textual material. Revisions can also be triggered because a writer, through the act of composing, has discovered something better to say. In addition, revisions can be applied to plans or goals for producing text. Finally, when writers revise other people's text, revisions may be triggered by the difficulties encountered in comprehending the author's intentions and/or text material.

Hayes and his colleagues (Flower, Hayes, Carey, Schriver, & Stratman, 1986) have identified two strategies that writers use frequently to revise text. The most common strategy involves revising without diagnosis; the writer detects a problem in text and rewrites, rather than revises, the problematic section without formally diagnosing the problem. This approach (labeled the "rewrite" strategy) may be particularly useful when (1) it is not necessary to save the original text, (2) so many problems are evident that diagnosis requires too much effort, or (3) the author has such a clear grasp of the purpose of the text that rewriting an alternative is easy.

The most commonly used alternative to the "rewrite" strategy is to diagnose textual problems and to fix them. This approach (labeled the "revise" strategy) may be preferable when (1) as much as possible of the original text needs to be saved, (2) textual problems are infrequent and diagnosis is easy, or (3) the author has such a poor grasp of the purpose of the text that writing an alternative is not easy.

The Relationships among Cognitive Processes in Writing

The cognitive processes and subprocesses identified in the Hayes and Flower (1980) model are overlapping and recursive. Planning, for example, may occur before, during, or after words are written on paper. Similarly, revising can be initiated at any point during the composing process—an idea might be reformulated before the act of translation begins, a sentence might be erased and rewritten as the author is in the act of putting words on paper, or a first draft may be reread and modified. Thus, mature writing is not a simple linear process in which planning precedes writing and writing precedes revision.

As writers engage in the process of composing, they bring into play various cognitive moves and strategies for completing the writing task; activate different levels of processing, ranging from the unconscious and automatic to the highly intentional and conscious; and deploy processing capacity to a variety of functions enabling the act of composing to proceed (Bereiter, 1980). Effective writing requires much more than mastering the dialectical properties of written English and the mechanics of handwriting, capitalization, punctuation, and spelling. Writers must be able to monitor and regulate the composing process successfully. Cognitive activities such as planning, sentence generation, and revising must be managed and orchestrated so that the writer can switch attention between these functions and a host of mechanical and substantive concerns (Scardamalia & Bereiter, 1986). This requires deploying attention to a number of ongoing and competing tasks without serious lapses or interferences (Bereiter & Scardamalia, 1982). Bereiter (1980) indicated that writers are able to execute this exceedingly complex process by putting into operation several different schemas. There is an executive schema for managing the overall writing process, a genre schema that activates and directs knowledge and strategies for certain kinds of writing (e.g., an essay rather than a story), a content-processing schema that retrieves material from memory and organizes it so that it is compatible with the writer's knowledge of the genre under consideration, and a language-processing schema that transfers ideas into explicit language. The operation of these schemas is interrelated; for example, "difficulty in finding the right word starts a chain of adjustments at successively higher levels until finally the intention of the whole composition is altered" (Bereiter, 1980, pp. 79).

COMPOSING BEHAVIOR OF INEXPERIENCED AND POOR WRITERS

As can be seen from the previous section, writing is a complex task. Not surprisingly, then, learning to write effectively is a process that develops gradually through the refinement and elaboration of various skills and mechanisms. As children move from speaking to writing, a radical conversion takes place. They must cultivate the ability to generate language in the absence of a conversational partner, learn to activate certain memories without having their memories triggered by what someone else says, produce text in units larger than what is included in a conversational turn, and develop the capability to examine what is produced from the perspective of both the writer and the reader (Bereiter & Scardamalia, 1982). As a result, learning to write requires more than adding special knowledge and skills to already existing oral language abilities; it involves the development of a production system capable of functioning autonomously (Scardamalia & Bereiter, 1986).

In a recent review of literature examining differences between mature writers and children, Scardamalia and Bereiter (1986) identified five areas of competence that are especially problematic for developing writers. As school-age children learn to compose, they must develop the ability to (1) generate writing content or gain access to the knowledge they have, (2) create an organizing structure or frame for their compositions, (3) quickly and efficiently execute the mechanical aspects of writing, (4) formulate goals and higher-level plans for their compositions, and (5) revise text and reformulate goals. Although the written language problems of students who receive school psychology and/or special-education services have not been investigated extensively (Graham & MacArthur, 1987), evidence gathered to date provides some support for the contention that these students have greater difficulty developing competence in these areas than do normally achieving students. This supposition will be illustrated by examining relevant literature on the writing characteristics of students labeled "learning-disabled" (LD). LD students were targeted for illustration because much of the writing research with handicapped students has been conducted with this population (Graham & MacArthur, 1987), learning disabilities represent the largest category of exceptionality (Algozzine & Korinek, 1985), and almost all of the cognitive-behavioral writing research has been aimed at this group of students.

Generating Content

For mature writers, the greater part of their effort in writing is directed at content generation (Hayes & Flower, 1980; Scardamalia & Bereiter, 1986). Good writers generate more ideas than they will eventually use in their compositions and employ metamemorial search strategies that allow them to retrieve ideas from memory associatively (Bereiter & Scardamalia, 1982).

Learning-disabled students, in contrast to normally achieving children, have a great deal of difficulty finding enough to say; their compositions are much shorter (cf. Deno, Marston, & Mirkin, 1982; Nodine, Barenbaum, & Newcomer, 1985; Poteet, 1979). Although the content generation problems of LD students may be due in part to a lack of knowledge about the topics on which they are asked to write (Scardamalia & Bereiter, 1986), it also appears that they have difficulty expressing the knowledge they do have. For example, Graham (1989) found that simply encouraging LD students to write more doubled to tripled their output. Additional evidence that LD students possess far more knowledge than is reflected in their *written* compositions was reported by MacArthur and Graham (1987). They found that LD students' dictated compositions were approximately three to four times as long as their stories composed via handwriting or the word processor.

Englert and her colleagues (Englert & Raphael, 1988; Englert, Raphael, & Anderson, 1986; Thomas, Englert, & Gregg, 1987) proposed that LD students have difficulty with content generation because they are less successful than normally achieving students in employing strategies for self-directed memory search. In a study by Thomas and co-workers (1987), LD students had difficulty in sustaining their thinking about topics, as evidenced by their failure to produce multiple statements about familiar subjects. Englert and Raphael (1988) indicated that these findings can be interpreted to indicate that LD students have distinct problems in retrieving ideas and using relevant schemas to maintain their thinking and writing in generative ways.

Once an idea is produced, however, LD students appear to be reluctant to discard it. MacArthur and Graham (1987) reported that only a small amount of LD students' revisions involved deletions. For instance, when LD students were composing on the word processor, only about one in every 60 revisions involved the deletion of textual material.

Framing Text

Framing text involves the active process of developing an ongoing structure for a composition (Scardamalia & Bereiter, 1986). Good writers frequently use their knowledge of genre patterns or other discourse schema to regulate what will go where in a particular piece of writing. Knowledge of genre patterns or other discourse schema is also important in formulating goals, making strategic decisions, and developing high-level representations of text (Scardamalia & Paris, 1985).

Examinations of LD students' compositions reveal considerable difficulty generating text that conforms to the common text structures found in different types of discourse (see Englert & Thomas, 1988; Graham & Harris, in press a; Graham & Harris, in press b; Nodine et al., 1986; Thomas et al., 1987). Graham and Harris (in press b), for example, found that essays written by LD students often contained reasons and elaborations of those reasons, but that a stated premise and concluding statements were frequently missing. Similarly, Graham and Harris (in press a) reported that LD students' creative stories almost always included a main character, a locale, and some action, but that common story grammar elements such as a starter event, response, or ending were often missing from their stories. Although LD students appear to have at least some understanding concerning text structure, as evidenced by their ability to develop compositions that contain at least some of the content that is common to the type of writing task they are assigned, their knowledge is incomplete and/or they are unable to gain conscious access to the structural knowledge they do possess (Graham & Harris, 1988a). Regardless, LD students' ability to use genre patterns or other discourse schema as an organizing structure for framing text is limited.

Mechanics

When writing, students must attend to a variety of mechanical demands, including penmanship/typing, spelling, punctuation, and capitalization. The need to attend consciously to the lower level skills of getting language onto paper may interfere with higher order cognitive processes such as planning and content generation (Scardamalia & Bereiter, 1986). For instance, young writers' handwriting/typing is seldom fast enough to keep up with their thoughts; consequently, potential textual material may be lost during the time it takes to translate it into print.

Mastery of mechanics among normally achieving students in the upper elementary grades appears to be sufficiently developed that interference and cognitive overload are not a serious problem (Scardamalia, Bereiter, & Goelman, 1982). For most LD students, however, this does not appear to be the case. MacArthur and Graham (1987) reported that when the mechanical requirements of composing are removed via dictation, LD students in the fifth and sixth grades wrote longer and better stories. Moreover, in the students' written compositions at least one in every ten words was misspelled and, on average, every third sentence contained a capitalization and punctuation error. These findings are consistent with the results from other research studies documenting significant differences between LD and normally achieving students on mechanical skills (cf. Deno *et al.*, 1982; Moran, 1981).

The importance of mastering the mechanics of writing can be further highlighted by examining the performance of LD students as they learn to use the word processor. In a study by MacArthur and Graham (1987), LD students who had considerable experience using word processors, but relatively little formal typing instruction, were asked to compose stories under three methods of text production: handwriting, word processing, and dictation. Handwritten stories were produced twice as fast as stories composed on the word processor. Similar results were obtained on copying tasks administered before students composed; handwriting speed was twice as fast as typing speed. More important, however, students who were more adept at typing, and/or composed more quickly when using the word processor, concurrently developed compositions that were longer, more complete structurally, and superior in overall quality. Similar results were not found for either handwriting or dictation.

Planning Text

Skilled writers plan by working through their compositions at an abstract level prior to going through them concretely (Scardamalia & Bereiter, 1986). They actively construct high-level goals that direct the writing process, and these are translated into a network of subgoals. Planning may occur at any point throughout the composing process, in advance of or during the course of writing. Thus, high-level goals and subgoals may undergo change (reconstruction, elimination, reordering, and so forth), resulting in a composition that differs considerably from what the writer was initially attempting.

Very little is known about how LD students plan their compositions. MacArthur and Graham (1987) reported that even though the fifth- and sixth-grade students in their study were prompted to plan their stories in advance, the average amount of time between the end of the examiner's instructions and the physical start of writing, typing, or dictation was less than one minute. Similar results have been obtained with normal students (Graves, 1983; Scardamalia & Bereiter, 1986).

If LD students do not plan their compositions in advance, then it must be assumed that they plan during the course of writing. Such an assumption, however, reveals little about the nature and extent of their plans. A recent model developed by Bereiter and Scardamalia (1985), termed "knowledge telling," may shed some light on these matters. They propose (Scardamalia & Bereiter, 1986) that school-age as well as many college students approach writing by using a greatly reduced version of the "generating" subprocess in the Hayes and Flower (1980) model. This involves converting writing tasks into simply telling whatever one knows—that is, writing-as-remembering or writing-by-pattern. Text is generated in a linear and associative fashion; ideas are produced as they come to mind, with each preceding word or sentence stimulating the development of the succeeding text. Little attention is directed at whole-text organization, the needs of the reader, or the constraints imposed by the topic.

Englert and her colleagues (Englert & Raphael, 1988; Thomas *et al.*, 1987) suggested that LD students exhibit the "knowledge-telling" strategy to an even greater extent than normally achieving school-age children. Their proposal is supported by the results of a study that examined the errors that LD and normally achieving students committed while composing different types of text (Thomas *et al.*, 1987). The findings from this study were consistent with several of the characteristics that exemplify the knowledge-telling strategy (see Bereiter & Scardamalia, 1983, and Brown, Day, & Jones, 1983, for a discussion of these characteristics). For instance, they found that LD students were more likely than normally achieving students to include redundant and irrelevant information in their writing. A large number of redundancies and irrelevancies reflects a lack of interconnectedness in writing and suggests that one sentence may be as deletable as the next, two key features of the knowledge-telling strategy. Furthermore, it appears that many of the LD students in their study converted the assigned writing tasks into a question-answering task, telling whatever they could think of and then terminating their response or answering in short choppy phrases. Although there is currently not enough evidence to determine whether the knowledge-telling strategy provides a cogent description of how LD students plan and execute their compositions, the model is not inconsistent with the available information.

Revisions

Attempts to revise a composition can occur as the text is being created or after an initial draft is developed. Words, phrases, sentences, text structure, goals, and so forth can be added, deleted, rearranged, or substituted. Most revisions, even by college-age students, involve minor changes in text (e.g., spelling, word usage, punctuation), with little change in content or meaning (Scardamalia & Bereiter, 1986).

Only one study has taken a close look at the revising behavior of LD students (MacArthur & Graham, 1987). Fifth- and sixth-grade LD students wrote and revised two stories: one on the word processor and one with paper and pencil. Both the initial writing and subsequent revision session were videotaped. Revisions made during the process of composing the first draft (in process) were identified, as well as changes made in preparing the second draft (between-draft revisions). Revisions involving typing or handwriting errors were excluded from the analysis.

Although LD students made approximately the same number of revisions (20 per 100 words) when preparing and revising their handwritten and word-processed stories, the two methods of text production yielded different patterns of revising. When composing on the word processor, LD students tended to make most of their revisions as they generated the initial draft of their story. When asked to revise this draft, they generally made a few minor surface adjustments (e.g., spelling) and in some instances added new textual material. In contrast, these same students made relatively few changes while they were in the process of generating the first draft of their handwritten stories. Most of their revisions occurred during the composing session; the majority of these changes involved minor surface-level adjustments or word substitutions.

It is also important to note that revisions made during handwriting and word processing did not differ in terms of the type of unit of text that was revised or in the proportion of revisions that changed textual meaning. It was much more common, however, for students to delete material when revising handwritten stories. Although students rarely used this capability when using the word processor (even though they had developed this skill), they did take advantage of the text-editing operations for inserting new material. All the stories composed on the word processor became longer when students were directed to revise their initial drafts. Only half of the handwritten stories became longer following revision, and a few actually were shorter.

The most frequent type of revision involved surface-level changes (57%), followed by changes in words (20%), T-units (13%), and phrases (13%). It is not surprising, therefore, that the type of changes LD students made had little impact on the quality of their compositions. Most of the revisions involved surface-level changes and word substitutions, and it appears that these changes were relatively ineffective: The first and second drafts of handwritten/typed stories did not differ in terms of spelling, capitalization, punctuation, or grammatical errors. More important, only a small percentage of the total number of revisions in either handwriting (10%) or word processing (28%) effected a meaningful change in what was written.

The MacArthur and Graham (1987) study also demonstrated the difficulty LD students have in overcoming the saliency of what is already written. Their first choice when revising text was to add new sentences, phrases, or words. The next most common strategy involved small word and phrase substitutions, followed by the deletion of textual materials. In no instances did LD students restructure or rearrange textual material. Thus, when revising text, LD students seem to employ what Bereiter and Scardamalia (1982) referred to as a "least effort" strategy: Change what is easiest to change. Left to their own devices, LD students will elaborate, substitute, and/or delete from what they have already produced; but they do not restructure or rearrange their language once it has assumed written form.

Summary and Implications

The research presented in this section suggests that LD students have difficulty generating, planning, framing, producing, and revising text. Five factors have been identified, one or more of which may account for the difficulties LD students have with these mental operations. First, LD students simply may not know enough about the subjects on which they are asked to write and/or may be unable to retrieve effectively what they do know. Second, they may have failed to develop adequate knowledge of the characteristics of different types of writing genres (e.g., purpose, conventions, types of content, and so forth) and/or may be unable to gain conscious access to the knowledge they do possess. Third, LD students' difficulties in producing text (handwriting, spelling, etc.) may interfere with the execution of other processes such as planning or revising. Fourth, the cognitive moves or task-specific strategies that LD students employ when engaging in a cognitive process such as generating or planning may be ineffective. Fifth, their difficulties may be a result of problems in executive control. Effective writing requires more than the development of effective task-specific strategies for planning, drafting, and revising; it is also dependent on executive procedures for bringing these strategies into use at the right time and in proper relation to other processing demands (Scardamalia & Bereiter, 1986). According to Englert and her colleagues (Englert & Raphael, 1988; Englert et al., 1986), LD students lack metacognitive control in terms of strategy awareness, implementation, and regulation.

If LD students' writing can be used as a benchmark for other exceptional students' writing, then many children who are provided special education or school psychology services can benefit from the application of cognitive-behavioral principles to the teaching of composing. Cognitive-behavioral modification (CBM) involves "the selective, empirically based combination of affective, behavioral, and/or cognitive principles and procedures" (Harris, 1985, p. 386). Two assumptions underlying the models and strategies subsumed under this approach are important here. First, instruction aimed at changing a person's cognitions is an effective component of behavior change, because cognitive events mediate behavior. Second, individuals are active participants in their own learning. Writing involves a variety of complex mental processes (many of which appear to be problematic for exceptional students) and necessitates active involvement on the part of the author (the behavior of exceptional students has often been characterized by a lack of active task engagement; see Harris, 1982). Thus, cognitive-behavioral procedures provide a mechanism for promoting active task involvement on the part of poor writers and for advancing the development of mental processes central to effective writing. Students can be taught the independent use of appropriate strategies for gaining access to writing content and their knowledge of different types of discourse. They can learn routines designed to provide intentional control over text production procedures such as sentence and paragraph generation. They can be instructed in the use of cognitive moves or strategies for planning, framing, and revising compositions. They can learn to develop procedures for regulating mental operations and their own behavior during writing.

Before discussing specific cognitive-behavioral procedures that have been used to modify exceptional students' writing performance, it should be noted that these procedures may not be appropriate for all individuals. There is a great deal of variability in the writing performance of exceptional children. In our own work with students labeled learning-disabled, we have occasionally encountered children who write as well as their normally achieving counterparts. In contrast, we have also seen children who are unable to produce even one coherent sentence. For the former, cognitive-behavioral procedures may not be necessary; for the latter, further development may be required before strategies or procedures for planning, drafting, or revising text are taught (see Moran, 1988, for suggestions on teaching students with severe writing difficulties.)

SELF-REGULATION TRAINING

Even though professional writers have developed a considerable repertoire of skills, knowledge, and experience, many still find the process of regulating the composing act and their own writing behavior a formidable task (Wallace & Pear, 1977). As a result, many well-known writers have developed various strategies to assist them in maximizing their performance. Some authors have self-regulated their literary output by monitoring and recording their daily production, establishing writing goals, and/or rewarding or punishing themselves depending on their performance (Wallace & Pear, 1977). Charles Darwin, for example, controlled the quantity of work that he produced by implementing a rather simple management strategy (Stone, 1978). Before writing each day, he would decide how many points he wished to make (represented by flint pebbles) and kick one pebble away each time a point was proved and footnoted.

Self-regulation has been described as a general cognitive strategy in which an individual determines a criterion and then observes his or her performance, compares the two, and appropriately self-reinforces or self-punishes (Craighead, Wilcoxon-Craighead, & Meyers, 1978). Self-regulation training can be used to help students become more independent during their writing, thus reducing demands on teacher time. The use of self-regulation skills may also increase task engagement, thereby indirectly reducing disruptive behavior during writing. In addition, some evidence suggests that self-regulation procedures promote maintenance and generalization effects (Harris, 1982, 1985; Harris & Graham, 1985).

Self-regulation procedures include the following:

1. *Self-instruction*: Self-instruction has been used effectively to prompt, direct, and maintain behavior (Harris, 1982, 1986a).
2. *Self-determined criteria*: Though not especially effective alone, when used in conjunction with other self-regulation procedures, self-determined criteria can lead to increased maintenance effects (O'Leary & Dubey, 1979), although guidance in initially determining criteria may be necessary.

3. *Self-assessment*: Self-assessment procedures such as self-monitoring, self-recording, or self-evaluation used alone have produced equivocal results (cf. Hallahan, Kneedler, & Lloyd, 1983; O'Leary & Dubey, 1979). Combining self-assessment with other self-regulation procedures, however, may facilitate maintenance and generalization.
4. *Self-reinforcement*: Based on a comparison to a criterion, self-reinforcement can significantly augment the impact of self-assessment and self-determined criteria (O'Leary & Dubey, 1979).

Although these same procedures represent the basic building blocks that have been used in designing self-regulation training programs in the area of writing, researchers have commonly used a combination of these procedures, making it difficult to determine the effects of individual self-regulation procedures.

Most of the self-regulation research conducted to date has concentrated on increasing the output and/or task involvement of exceptional students as they compose. In a study by Seabaugh and Schumaker (1981), learning-disabled and non-learning-disabled students who had histories of noncompliance were introduced to a self-regulation package designed to increase the number of lessons completed each day. The pacakge included the four self-regulation skills. One skill, *behavioral contracting*, required students to target an academic area (writing, reading, or math) to be improved; to identify reasons that this area was in need of improvment; to analyze the task demands and sequence of behaviors surrounding the target area (i.e., conduct a task analysis); and to specify the procedures for recording, evaluating, and reinforcing behavior. Once the student became familiar with the written behavioral contract, a goal sheet was introduced, which served as an addendum to the contract. This provided an annotated contract that was less formal and allowed students to establish new goals and change or revise their old goals. A second skill, *self-recording*, involved providing a rationale for the use of self-recording, modeling of self-recording procedures, and practice in graphing baseline data on lesson completion. *Self-evaluation* also involved establishing a rationale for the use of self-evaluation, as well as the modeling and practice of self-evaluative statements regarding students' accomplishments. Students were prompted to evaluate their performance from one week to the next and to examine their success in terms of the sequence of events outlined during the task analysis for the behavioral contract. Finally, *self-reinforcement* was introduced by encouraging the student to visualize the events surrounding the successful completion of a lesson in order to identify possible reinforcing variables. Students were prompted to verbalize and record the rewards they would administer to themselves and encouraged to withhold delivery until lessons were completed each day.

The self-regulation package was delivered via a series of teacher–student conferences: three conferences to introduce the components of the treatment sequence, followed by a series of conferences that provided review, corrective feedback, amendments to the original contract, and the completion of new goal sheets. Following training, both the learning-disabled and non-learning-disabled students increased the number of lessons completed. Furthermore, several students were observed to change goals from one academic area to another or to self-initiate a change in their goals independent of the student–teacher conferences. Thus, the training package developed by Seabaugh and Schumaker (1981) appears to provide an effective means for increasing written productivity.

In another study, Rumsey and Ballard (1985) investigated the use of self-regulation procedures not only as a means for increasing written output, but also as a way of increasing task involvement and decreasing disruptive behaviors. Seven students with a past history of behavior difficulties and a low level of written productivity were instructed to use several self-management strategies during their classroom story writing sessions. These included: (1) counting the number of words written during each session and recording them on a bar graph, (2) recording whether they were working or not working when a tone sounded at variable intervals, and (3) self-evaluating their effort during the lesson. Following introduction of the experimental procedures, the mean number of words written and the on-task behavior of the target children increased dramatically, while off-task disruptive behaviors decreased. As expected, subsequent removal of the experimental procedures resulted in a slight decrease in on-task behavior and a large decrease in number of words written; disruptive behaviors returned to original baseline levels. Reintroduction of experimental procedures, however, did not return the behaviors of interest to the same level as when treatment was first introduced; there were slight increases in both on-task behavior and number of words written, while disruptive behaviors showed only a small drop. A further factor limiting the strength and generality of the findings was that individual students demonstrated a great deal of variability in their performance. In addition, the inclusion of two different monitoring systems as well as self-evaluation makes it difficult to determine the effects of individual self-regulation components (see Harris, 1986b, for a comparison of self-monitoring of attention to self-monitoring of productivity on a written language task).

Five of the seven students in the Rumsey and Ballard (1985) study, who demonstrated a great deal of variability during the second introduction of the experimental procedures, received correspondence training. Correspondence training involved the examiner presenting a list of four desired behaviors ("I will work on my story"; "I will try to write a really good story"; "I will not talk to others"; "I will ignore people who try to interrupt me"), followed by prompts designed to solicit a student's response that they would exhibit the identified behaviors during story time. Following introduction of correspondence training, on-task behavior and number of words written increased dramatically, and disruptive behaviors were significantly decreased.

In a study involving regular third-grade children, Ballard and Glynn (1975) found that having students self-assess and self-record the number of sentences, different action words, and different describing words they wrote did not affect their performance on these variables. With the addition of contingent self-determined and self-administered reinforcement, however, the rates of responding for each of these measures increased substantially. Moreover, an increase in on-task behavior and story quality was correlated with the addition of self-reinforcement to self-assessment and recording. Consequently, self-regulation procedures can be used not only to foster task involvement and boost how much is written, but also to direct what is written.

In our research with learning-disabled students, we have used self-regulation procedures in conjunction with strategy training. In a study by Harris and Graham (1985), for example, students were taught a strategy for increasing vocabulary diversity in their compositions. In addition, they set specific goals on the amount and type of vocabulary items that they would include in their stories; and, after each writing period, they graphed their performance, evaluated their success in reaching their goals, and established a new goal for their next story. In a second study (Graham & Harris, in press a), students were taught a strategy for generating content related to the elements commonly found in short stories. Half of the students in this study used the same self-regulation procedures (goal setting, graphing, and evaluation of success) employed in the previous study, but the other half did not. Although strategy training produced significant improvements in creative writing, training was not enhanced by the inclusion of the self-regulation training. However, students reported that they enjoyed using these procedures and were able to monitor and evaluate their performance accurately. This study did not determine what effect the self-regulation procedures alone would have had on students' written products.

In summary, the available evidence suggests that self-regulation training can be used to increase task engagement, raise productivity, and shape what children write; exceptional students have also reported that they enjoy using these procedures. Although these findings are encouraging, it must be pointed out that the application of self-regulation training to the writing problems of exceptional children has been narrow in focus. As Scardamalia and Bereiter (1985) have indicated, self-regulation can contribute to both immediate performance and further cognitive and metacognitive development. In terms of the former, self-regulation mechanisms may be thought of as building blocks that can be combined with other mental operations into a program for accomplishing a task. With the latter, the introduction of self-regulatory mechanisms such as planning or evaluation "may constitute change-inducing agents that will have the effect of altering the rules by which the system operates" (Scardamalia & Bereiter, 1985, p. 566), resulting in the acquisition of new rules and leading to a change in strategic behavior. Most of the research reviewed in this section has concentrated on the use of self-regulation training as a way of improving immediate performance. More attention needs to be directed at developing mature cognitive strategies by promoting self-regulatory functions that will enable students to acquire rules as a result of their own activity.

STRATEGY TRAINING

A recent emphasis in writing instruction for both normally achieving and exceptional students is strategy instruction (Graham & Harris, 1987a; Scardamalia & Bereiter, 1986). This approach is based primarily on the belief that writing is a cognitive process and students should be provided with explicit instruction in cognitive strategies. For exceptional students, this viewpoint has been operationalized by teaching them writing strategies for planning, generating, revising, and so forth. In this section, both strategy-training procedures developed at the University of Kansas Institute for Research in Learning Disabilities (Learning Strategies Curriculum) and Self-Instructional Strategy Training, which we have developed, will be reviewed.

Learning Strategies Curriculum

Based on their extensive research demonstrating that learning-disabled adolescents in secondary schools are severely deficient in basic academic skills and in the skills needed to cope with the broad variety of demands encountered in secondary settings (Schumaker, Deshler, Alley, & Warner, 1983), the Research Institute at the University of Kansas has developed a curriculum for secondary students with reading and other academic problems based on the learning strategies approach. "Learning strategies" refer to "techniques, principles, or rules that will facilitate the acquisition, manipulation, integration, storage, and retrieval of information across situations and settings" (Alley & Deshler, 1979, p. 13). Thus, the curriculum emphasizes teaching students how to learn rather than specific content. As a result, "the overall intent of learning strategies instruction, therefore, is to teach students skills that will allow them not only to meet immediate requirements successfully but also to generalize these skills to other situations over time" (Schumaker *et al.* 1983, p. 49).

At present the curriculum consists of a series of task-specific strategies designed to enable students to: (1) gain information from written material; (2) organize, store, and retrieve information; and (3) complete assignments, take tests, and *express themselves in writing* (Schumaker, Nolan, & Deshler, 1985). For the purposes of this chapter, we will concentrate on the strategies for promoting written expression. Before examining each strategy individually, however, the principles for teaching these strategies will be outlined.

Instructional Methodology

The teaching methodology for the learning strategies curriculum consists of two basic components, acquisition and maintenance/generalization (Schumaker *et al.*, 1983). The purpose of the instructional procedures incorporated under the acquisition step is to provide students with the knowledge, motivation, and practice needed to apply the strategy to materials or situations that would normally be encountered in their regular secondary classrooms. The maintenance and generalization component is designed to allow students to transfer the strategy learned in the special-education setting to both academic and nonacademic contexts over time. Both components have undergone extensive experimental analysis and can be modified for use with small groups (see Schumaker *et al.*, 1985; Schumaker & Sheldon, 1985).

The acquisition component consists of seven basic steps:

1. *Pretest and commitment to learn*: Student's current functioning on the task of interest is determined, and this information is shared with the student; the student is asked to sign a written agreement to develop a new skill to remedy the weaknesses.
2. *Describe*: The new skill or strategy is described, and the student and teacher discuss why and when the strategy is used.
3. *Model*: The teacher demonstrates the strategy while thinking aloud.
4. *Verbal rehearsal*: The student memorizes the steps in the strategy;
5. *Controlled practice*: Students practice using the strategy with ability-level material; reinforcement and corrective feedback are provided.
6. *Grade-appropriate practice*: Student practice using the strategy with materials and situations drawn from the regular classroom; reinforcement and corrective feedback are provided.
7. *Posttest and commitment to generalize*: A posttest is administered, and students are informed of their progress; the student is asked to agree to generalize the use of the strategy to other settings.

The generalization component consists of three phases. First, students are made aware of situations and circumstances in which the target strategy can be used and how the strategy can be adjusted to meet unique situations. Second, students are given specific assignments that require that they practice and use the strategy in a variety of situations. Third, students are periodically monitored to ensure that they use the strategy appropriately.

Written Expression Strategies

To date, four written expression strategies have been developed. Two of the strategies, Sentence Writing and Paragraph Writing, teach students to use a series of steps independently for generating different types of sentences and paragraphs, respectively. A third strategy, Error Monitoring, is a self-directed executive procedure for detecting and correcting errors of capitalization, punctuation, spelling, and overall appearance. The fourth strategy, Theme Writing, includes a routine for organizing and writing a five-paragraph theme. The strategies are taught in the order presented, with the first three being taught in the late junior high grades and the last in the early high school grades (Schumaker *et al.*, 1985)

With the Sentence Writing strategy, students are taught to apply a series of steps and formulas for writing four basic types of sentences: simple, compound, complex, and compound-complex (Schumaker & Sheldon, 1985). There are 14 different formulas, each corresponding to a different sentence structure. The student first *picks* a formula and then *explores* words to fit the formula. Once the student decides on a set of appropriate words, these are *noted* or written down and the sentence is checked to ensure that a *subject* and verb are present. The mnemonic PENS (Picks, Explores, Noted, Subject) is used to help students remember the strategy.

Prior to introducing the formulas for each of the basic sentence types, students are taught to name and identify various parts of speech. For instance, when learning the formulas for compound sentences, students are also required to master: (1) the definitions for independent clause, coordinating conjunction, and compound sentence; (2) the names of different coordinating conjunctions, and (3) the use of commas and semicolons.

Evidence to support the use of the Sentence Writing strategy is meager. In an unpublished study by Schmidt, Deshler, Schumaker, and Alley (reported in Schumaker *et al.*, 1983), it was found that for four of seven LD students, 100% of their sentences in a paragraph generated in their regular classroom were complete, and at least 50% were compound and/or complex after they received instruction in the Sentence Writing strategy, which included the acquisition and maintenance/generalization steps described in the previous section. The other three students were able to reach the same level of mastery as their cohorts after the inclusion of additional procedures for promoting generalization.

Several factors limit the value and utility of the Sentence Writing strategy. First, it is not clear that LD students have difficulty generating basic sentence types or that, it they do have difficulties, these are severe enough to warrant the use of this strategy. For instance, Blair and Crump (1984) found that half or more than half of eighth- and tenth-grade LD students' sentences were compound, complex and compound/complex when they were writing in the argumentative mode. Furthermore, LD and normally achieving students cannot be distinguished in terms of written syntactic fluency (Deno *et al.*, 1982; Morris & Crump, 1982; Nodine *et al.*, 1985), and it is not clear that LD students use different words while composing (cf. Morris & Crump, 1982) or make more syntactical miscues (Hemereck, 1979; Poteet, 1979). Second, the Sentence Writing strategy does not appear to be very cost-effective. It takes approximately 30 minutes a day, for 9 to 10 weeks, to teach (Schumaker & Sheldon, 1985). As a result, a less complicated and better established practice, such as sentence combining (Hillocks, 1984) may represent a more parsimonious approach for helping exceptional students gain more intentional control over sentence generation. Third, the evidence currently available suggests that much of the preskill training (naming and identifying various parts of speech) incorporated into this strategy is not a necessary prerequisite for learning to write sentences (Hillocks, 1984). Finally, the Sentence Writing strategy is so complicated and requires the memorization of such a large host of formulas and terms that it may be expecially susceptible to misuse or modification by students.

For the Paragraph Writing strategy, students are taught a procedure for writing four types of paragraphs. These include paragraphs that list or describe, show sequence, compare and/or contrast, or demonstrate cause and effect. In order to help students remember the strategy, the mnemonic SLOW CaPS is used. Each letter except for the small "a" in CaPS is designed to remind the student to carry out a specific action: (S)—show the type of paragraph in the first sentence; (L)—list the type of details you plan to write about; (O)—order the details; (W)—write the details in complete sentences; and cap off the paragraph with a (C) concluding, (P) passing, or (S) summary sentence. Evidence on the effectiveness of the strategy has been promising; both Moran, Schumaker, and Veter (1981) and Schmidt et al. as reported in Schumaker et al. (1983) have reported that LD students' paragraph writing skills improve following training.

The Error Monitoring strategy includes six steps that students use to direct the composing process, from generation of an initial draft to editing for mechanical errors (Schumaker *et al.*, 1985). The mnemonic WRITER is used to help students remember the six steps. First, in developing their initial draft, students *write* on every other line using the Sentence Writing strategy (PENS). Second, the rough draft is *read* for meaning, and inappropriate sentences (e.g., those that are not related to the topic or are unclear) are deleted and changed. Third, students *interrogate* themselves using the COPS strategy: (C)– Have I capitalized the first word and proper nouns; (O)—Have I made any handwriting, margin, messy, or spacing errors; (P)—Have I used end punctuation, commas, and semicolons correctly; and (S)—Do the words look like they're spelled right, can I sound them out, or should I use the dictionary? Fourth, if students are unsure about an error, they are directed to *take* their paper to someone else (teacher, parent, friend, etc.) for help. Fifth, students *execute* a final copy of their paper, incorporating corrections made on the rough draft and writing as neatly as possible on every line. Sixth, the composition is *reread* and final corrections are made.

Schumaker, Deshler, Alley, Warner, Clark, and Nolan (1982) have shown that LD students trained in using the COPS portion of the Error Monitoring strategy improved in their ability to detect and correct mechanical errors in others' writing. Additionally, they found that these same students were able to detect and correct mechanical errors in their own writing following instruction in a modified version of the overall strategy (Step 2—read for meaning and delete or change inappropriate sentences—was not included). It is not clear whether this strategy has an impact on *what* students write. Although correct form and appearance is an important part of writing for others (Graham, 1982), it is secondary to the content of the message.

The last strategy, Theme Writing, involves a series of five steps for writing an integrated composition. The mnemonic TOWER is used to help students remember the strategy. First, students *think* of content: write a title, major areas to be discussed, and details for each area. Second, the major topics and details under each topic are hierarchically *ordered*. Third, a rough draft is *written*. Fourth, students check for *errors* using the COPS portion of the Error Monitoring strategy. Fifth, the rough draft is rewritten or *revised*.

We were unable to obtain any evidence on the effectiveness of the Theme Writing Strategy. Nonetheless, one advantage of this strategy is that it emphasizes the importance of planning as a preliminary facet of writing and of editing in terms of form and appearance. Moreover, by dividing the composition process into a series of relatively discrete stages, it may make the writing task more manageable for poor writers and reduce cognitive strain (Graham, 1982; Graham & Harris, 1988a). On the other hand, revising for meaning is not emphasized and the strategy is not reflective of the typically complex intermixing of planning, writing, and revising demonstrated by more mature writers.

Summary

The writing strategies developed by the Research Institute at the University of Kansas represent an ambitious effort to help poor writers develop intentional control over the processes of generating and editing written discourse. The training materials are well designed, and the strategies are hierarchically organized and interrelated. Additional research, however, needs to be undertaken to validate the effectiveness of these strategies, particularly the Error Monitoring and Theme Writing strategies. Moreover, there is some question of the utility and cost-effectiveness of the Sentence Writing strategy.

Self-Instructional Strategy Training

We have also developed a series of writing strategies that have been field-tested with students classified as learning-disabled. The strategies have been designed for poor writers in the upper elementary grades and are taught via a set of training procedures labeled "self-instructional strategy training." A detailed examination of the training procedures (which can be used to teach a variety of academic skills) is provided, followed by a presentation of the various strategies.

Instructional Methodology

Our training regime and approach to strategy instruction (Graham & Harris, 1987a; Graham, Harris, & Sawyer, 1987; Harris & Graham, 1988) has been heavily influenced by three important developments. These include cognitive-behavior modification training (Meichenbaum, 1977), the concept of self-control training (Brown, Campione, & Day, 1981; Brown & Palinscar, 1982) and the validation of the learning strategies model for learning-disabled adolescents (Schumaker *et al.*, 1983). First, a variety of basic principles from cognitive-behavior modification training were incorporated into our training procedures, including: (1) the emphasis on interactive learning between teacher and student, with responsibility for recruiting, applying, and monitoring the target strategy eventually placed on the student; (2) the use of sound instructional procedures such as initial teacher direction and modeling, feedback, reinforcement, and individualization; (3) the inclusion of the student as an active collaborator; and (4) the modeling and development of self-statements designed to assist the student in comprehending the task, producing appropriate strategies, and using these strategies and verbalizations to mediate behavior. Second, self-control training emphasizes that exceptional students not only should receive training in the use of task-appropriate strategies but also should receive instruction in the self-regulation of these strategies and training in the significance of such activities. Thus, our training regime includes self-regulation components such as self-determined criteria (goal-setting), self-assessment, and self-reinforcement. Third, the well-validated strategy acquisition steps developed by Deshler and his colleagues (Schumaker *et al.*, 1983) have been incorporated into our training program.

Self-instructional strategy training includes eight basic components: pretraining, review of current performance level, description of the strategy, modeling of the strategy and self-instructions, memorization of the strategy and self-verbalizations, controlled practice, independent practice, and procedures for promoting maintenance and generalization. Each of these components is illustrated in Table 11-1. Students initially receive instruction on any preskills necessary for learning and deploying the strategy to be taught (Step 1). The student and the teacher examine current performance on the skill of interest, and any existing negative or ineffective self-statements or strategies are identified and discussed (Step 2). Students are also made aware of the goals and significance of training. The target strategy is described and an examination of when and how to use the strategy is conducted (Step 3). The teacher then models the strategy and important self-statements (including problem definition, self-evaluation, coping and correcting, and self-reinforcing), and the student is asked to generate and record self-statements of each type that he or she would like to use (Step 4). Next, the student memorizes the steps of the strategy and examples of each of the types of self-statements generated (Step 5). The self-regulation components (goal-setting, self-assessment, and so forth) are then introduced, and the student practices the strategy and self-instructions under the guidance of the teacher (Step 6). Once students are able to apply the strategy successfully and without teacher assistance, they are instructed to use the strategy independently, and self-regulation procedures are faded gradually (Step 7). Procedures designed to promote maintenance and generalization are embedded throughout training.

Self-instructional strategy training has been used successfully with both small groups of students and individually (cf. Graham & Harris, in press a; Harris & Graham, 1985). Students are provided with external support through expert guidance and scaffolding until they can run the strategy autonomously; thus, ultimate responsibility for strategy use is assumed by the student. Training is criterion-based, and students progress to the next level of training only after mastering the previous level.

TABLE 11-1. Self-Instructional Strategy Training Steps for a Prewriting Vocabulary Enrichment Strategy

---

Step 1: Pretraining. In this step, one of the targeted parts of speech (action words) was introduced and its meaning mastered. A small chart was introduced which provided a definition and examples. After discussion, the student suggested further examples independently and used at least three examples in sentences. The student then practiced generating action words suggested by looking at a picture. (After the student completed each of the following steps for action words, instruction began again at Step 1 for action helpers. Describing words were taught last.)

Step 2: Review current performance level. The instructor and student examined the student's baseline performance on action words. The number of different action words used in each baseline story was depicted on a graph. The instructor and student then discussed the goal of training (to write better stories), why this is important, and how action words improve a story.

Step 3: Describe the composition strategy. A five-step strategy for writing good stories was introduced on a small chart. After discussing the five-step strategy, the instructor modeled several creativity self-instructions that she had found helpful in thinking of good words (i.e., "Let my mind be free . . . think of new words for old ideas"). The student was then asked to make up two or three creativity self-statements he or she would like to use; these were recorded on paper. The student practiced using these self-statements, generating several more action words for the stimulus picture.

Step 4: Model the composition strategy and self-instructions. The two charts, the list of creativity self-statements, and a new stimulus picture were set out. The instructor modeled the composition strategy, writing a story, and "thinking aloud." In addition to the creativity self-statements, the instructor modeled four types of self-instructions as she wrote: (1) problem definition (e.g., "What is it I have to do? I have to write a good story. Good stories make sense and use many action words"), (2) planning (including the five strategy steps), (3) self-evaluation, and (4) self-reinforcement. After completing the story, the instructor discussed with the student the importance of what we say to ourselves while we work. The student was asked to identify the self-instructions the instructor used (1) to get started, (2) to help write the story, and (3) to evaluate the story. The student then recorded on paper examples of each of the four types of self-instructions in his or her own words.

Step 5: Mastery of the composition strategy. The student was required to memorize the five-step strategy for writing good stories. Examples of each type of self-instruction were also memorized.

Step 6: Controlled practice of strategy steps and self-instructions. Criterion setting, self-assessment, and self-recording were introduced. The instructor and student determined the average number of action words written in baseline. After setting an initial goal, the student practiced the learning strategy and self-instructions, "thinking aloud" as he or she wrote a story in response to a new stimulus picture. Positive and corrective feedback was provided as needed. The two charts and self-instruction list were initially available as prompts, when necessary, then faded. This step was repeated, using new stimulus pictures, until the student became proficient in the use of the strategy and the overt self-instructions. Transition to covert self-instructions was then encouraged. After each practice story was completed, the student and instructor independently counted the number of different action words, compared counts, graphed the number on the student's chart, and compared performance to the criterion. As the use of action words improved, the goal became "to do as well as or better than I have been doing."

Step 7: Independent performance. The student wrote stories in response to novel stimulus pictures without instructions or feedback. After the student completed each story, the student and instructor independently counted the number of different action words, compared counts, and filled in the graph.

TABLE 11-1. (*continued*)

Step 8: Generalization and maintenance components. In addition to the criterion-setting and self-assessment components, other recommended procedures for generalization and maintenance were included. Students kept a notebook with copies of all training materials, all stories, and their graph. They were asked to share what they were learning with their teachers and their parents, and the resource teacher was asked to initial the graph each time the student discussed training. Number of teacher initials was checked during each training session. In addition, students were told to think of what they were learning while in the resource room, and to be prepared to use what they had learned during resource and regular classroom activities.

Source: Data from "Improving learning Disabled Students' Composition Skills: Self-Control Strategy Training" by K. R. Harris and S. Graham, 1985, *Learning Disability Quarterly*, Vol. 8, pp. 27–36.

Written Expression Strategies

Currently, we have developed four specific writing strategies. These strategies have been designed to enable students to activate independently a search of appropriate memory stores for writing content, plan a composition in advance of writing, and/or edit and revise texts. Each strategy consists of a series of explicit rules or steps for completing a specific writing task, either a creative story or an argumentative essay. The strategies provide the student with a procedure for directing attention and resources during composing. This may ease the executive burden of writing by minimizing the attention that students must devote to carrying out a particular process—for example, searching memory for content relevant to a particular type of genre.

In our first study (Harris & Graham, 1985), the effects of strategy plus self-regulation training on the number of action verbs, adverbs, and adjectives included in LD students' compositions was investigated. Strategy training included mastery of a five-step strategy and self-instructional statements designed to increase the diversity of each of the aforementioned vocabulary items in students' written stories. The strategy, illustrated here with verbs, directed the student to:

1. Look at the picture (stimulus item) and write down good action words (verbs).
2. Think of a good story idea in which to use my words.
3. Write my story—make sense and use good action words.
4. Read my story and ask, "Did I write a good story."
5. Fix my story—"Can I use more good action words?"

The self-instructional prompts included statements designed to facilitate generation of stimulus items (e.g., action words) through brainstorming, problem definition (e.g., "What is it I have to do?"), self-evaluation, and self-reinforcement. In addition, once students become familiar with the strategy and self-instructional prompts, self-regulation procedures were introduced. Before writing a story, students set specific goals related to the amount and types of vocabulary items they would include in their composition. When the story was completed, they graphed their performance, evaluated their success in reaching their goals, and established a new goal for their next story.

Training resulted in substantial increases above baseline levels in the number of different action verbs, adverbs, and adjectives, as well as an increase in the mean number of words written per story. Furthermore, stories written after training received substantially higher quality ratings than those written during baseline. It is important to note that increases in each of the targeted vocabulary items were not of sufficient magnitude to account for increases in story length. Thus, training procedures stimulated more than the generation of the target vocabulary items. It is possible that the process of listing words to use in advance of writing may stimulate content gneration by providing students with an executive procedure for carrying out a self-directed memory search. Furthermore, improvement in story quality may have been due to the observed increases in story length and vocabulary diversity; both of these indices have been found to be related to the quality of stories written by LD students (MacArthur & Graham, 1987).

Harris and Graham (1985) also reported that generalization from the training setting to the students' resource room was obtained and that training effects were maintained for up to 6 weeks. Nevertheless, the results of a follow-up probe collected at the start of a new school year, 3½ months following treatment, revealed that the training effects had dissipated. The students, however, remembered the five-step strategy and the three different vocabulary items. It appears, therefore, that the problem is one of rusty application; a booster session would probably have returned performance rates to their initial posttreatment level.

In two other studies (Graham & Harris, in press a; Graham & Harris, in press b), we attempted to affect what students do in advance of writing and during the act of composing. As indicated in an earlier section of this chapter, LD students do little planning in advance, have difficulty generating content, and often develop written products that are not reflective of the genre under consideration. As a result, we have directed much of our effort toward designing strategies to increase advanced planning and content generation, with the stipulation that the search for writing content be guided by the basic structural characteristics representative of specific literary types—narrative, argument, and so forth.

In the study by Graham and Harris (in press a), 22 fifth- and sixth-grade LD students were taught to use independently a strategy designed to direct the process of writing a narrative story. The strategy consisted of five steps:

1. Look at the picture (stimulus item).
2. Let your mind be free.
3. Write down the story part reminder (w-w-w-: What = 2; How =2).

4. Write down story part ideas for each part.
5. Write your story—use good parts and make sense.

The mnemonic in the second step reminded students to generate content in response to self-generated questions concerning the setting of the story, the main character's goals and efforts to achieve those goals, the ending, and the main character's reactions or emotional responses. Specifically, "w-w-w" stood for: *Who* is in the story? *When* does the story take place? *Where* does the story take place? The students also determined *what* the main character wants to do and *what* happens when he or she tries to do it. Finally, the students considered *how* the story ends and *how* the main character feels. The students were directed to use the generated information as a blueprint for their story. In addition, students generated and practiced using self-instructional prompts for promoting brainstorming, problem definition, self-evaluation, and self-rein-forcement. In addition, half of the subjects were taught to use the self-regulation procedures of goal-setting, graphing, and evaluation of success.

Following training in the use of the strategy and self-instructions, the schematic structure of stories written by LD students evidenced considerable improvement, 86% of the stories written immediately following training included all but one of the elements commonly found in narrative stories, whereas only 36% of baseline stories met this same criterion. Students also became more confident of their ability to write a "good" story, as evidenced by self-efficacy ratings. More important, the stories written immediately after training received higher quality ratings than pretest stories. The efficacy of the training procedures was further highlighted by evidence that the students used the strategy and that, following training, LD students were as effective as normally achieving students in incorporating story elements into their writing. The training was well received by both students and teachers. The observed effects also generalized to a new setting and were maintained 2 weeks after the termination of treatment. Finally, the self-regulation procedures had no cumulative effect on performance.

In the second study (Graham & Harris, in press b), we further refined our basic strategy for facilitating advanced planning and content generation and moved the focus of our investigation to argumentative essays. Although students still generated writing content in relation to genre-specific, self-directed prompts, they were further asked to evaluate possible writing content and consider who would read what they had written and why they were writing a particular composition. Also, in the Graham and Harris (in press a) study, we had informally observed that some students' advanced planning could best be described as rehearsal; what was written in advance was in sentence form and either closely or exactly resembled the eventual product. Consequently, in the second study, students were strongly encouraged to generate notes during the planning process and were directed to expand on their basic blueprint while writing their essay.

The basic strategy in the Graham and Harris (in press b) study involved three steps:

1. Think: Who will read this and why am I doing this?
2. Plan what to say, using TREE (note *topic* sentence, note *reasons*, examine *reasons*, note *ending*).
3. Write and say more.

As in the other studies, students generated and practiced using self-instructional prompts for brainstorming, problem definition, self-evaluation, coping and correcting, and self-reinforcement. Self-regulation procedures, however, were not taught.

Results from this study were very positive. Following training, sixth-grade LD students' essays have evidenced a substantial increase above baseline levels in the number of elements (premise, reasons, elaborations, examples, and conclusion) included in each composition. Similarly, essays became longer and were judged to be qualitatively better following training. These results generalized from the resource room to the students' regular classroom and were maintained over a 6-week period. Furthermore, we examined whether or not training would have a positive transfer effect to a second genre, narrative stories. At the conclusion of training, students had discussed with the examiner how to use the three-step strategy (minus the mnemonic TREE) to write a story. For one student, no transfer effects were noted; for a second student, narrative stories improved following training, but the compositions lacked many of the structural elements commonly included in short stories. Finally, a third student evidenced successful transfer across genres. Consequently, the first and second students participated in a booster session in which they received practice in using the mnemonic SPACE (note *setting, purpose, action, conclusion,* and *emotion*) during the second step of the strategy. Following the booster session, the first student's stories improved dramatically, and the second student's story contained all but one of the elements commonly associated with narrative stories. These findings provide some tentative support for our emphasis on framing the type of content that LD students generate.

The final study that we have conducted involved teaching sixth-grade LD students a strategy for revising essays written on a microcomputer (Graham & MacArthur, 1988). As was indicated earlier, LD students' revisions rarely have an impact on the meaning of what they initially write, and, when using the word processor, LD students frequently add material to their text. With these points in mind, a six-step strategy was developed:

1. Read your essay.
2. Find the sentence that tells what you believe—is it clear?
3. Add two reasons why you believe it.
4. SCAN each sentence—Does it make *sense*? Is it *connected* to my belief? Can I *add* more? *Note* errors.

5. Make changes on the computer.
6. Reread the essay and make final changes.

Writing probes were collected both during baseline and following training. Students were directed to write an initial draft and were then asked to revise it the following day. During baseline, students averaged about two to three between-draft revisions per essay, and the majority of these modifications involved surface-level and/or word changes. Only a small percentage of the revisions (average range 14% to 31%) affected the meaning of what was written, and revising had virtually no impact on the quality of students' essays. Following training, students' revising behavior was radically altered. They averaged 6 to 10 revisions per essay, the majority of which involved phrase and T-unit changes. A sizable percentage of their revisions affected textual meaning (average range 41% to 83%), and the process of revising an essay resulted in improvements in overall quality. Furthermore, essays written following training became considerably longer and all of the noted effects were well maintained over time.

While the Graham and MacArthur (1988) study demonstrated that instruction in the revising strategy had a positive affect on the number and types of revisions made by students, as well as a significant impact on the quantity and quality of what they wrote, it is instructive to examine the individual performance of the three LD students participating in this study. The first student evidenced almost a fivefold increase in the number of revisions following training; revisions were equally balanced between meaning and nonmeaning changes and surface/word and phrase/T-unit level revisions. Training resulted in approximately three times as many revisions for the second student; most of the changes, however, affected the meaning of what was written and primarily involved phrase and T-unit revisions. Moreover, training appeared to have a transfer effect to this student's initial drafts; first-draft essays written after training were more than 30 words longer than those composed before training. For the third student, number of revisions following training more than doubled, the majority of changes affected textual meaning, and T-unit revisions were very common. In contrast to the second student, the third student's initial drafts became shorter following training. It is also important to note that for the first two students it was necessary to conduct a booster session within a week to 2 weeks following the completion of training. They both evidenced a drop in number of revisions; surface level changes had been spontaneously discontinued, and only T-unit and/or word/phrase revisions were continued. Finally, two of the steps in the revision strategy were particularly salient. A majority of the students' revisions were directed at "adding two more reasons" (Step 3) and "Can I add more?" (the third step in SCAN). The data from this study demonstrate that instructors need to pay careful attention to what is internalized and how a student will initially use and modify a strategy over time.

Summary

The writing strategies and corresponding training model that we have developed provide an effective mechanism for affecting what students write and what they do during the process of composing. Learning-disabled students in the upper elementary grades were able independently and successfully to use strategies designed to facilitate content generation, textual framing, advanced planning, and revising. Our investigations have made us sensitive to four issues that need to be considered when designing and teaching writing strategies to LD students. First, careful attention must be paid to the integrity of the strategy intervention. Inadequate conceptualization and construction of strategy intervention can lead (and has led) to ineffective interventions, as can inadequate task and learner analyses (Harris, 1985). Both knowledge and application of the guidelines available in the cognitive-behavior modification literature are essential (cf. Graham & Harris, 1987a; Harris, 1982). Second, attention must be directed at what is internalized and how students use a strategy. Certain steps may be ignored, others overemphasized, and individual students may use the same self-directed prompts in totally different ways. In addition, strategies may be reconstructed by students in either efficient or ineffective ways. Third, careful consideration must be given to promoting and monitoring generalization and maintenance. Finally, the effectiveness of a strategy must be determined in terms of multiple outcomes; e.g., social validation and evidence of strategy usage as well as affective, behavioral, and cognitive measures are necessary (Harris, 1985).

CONCLUSION

The focus of this chapter has been on the use of cognitive-behavioral approaches as a means for improving the writing performance of students who receive school psychology or special-education services. The cognitive operations underlying effective composing, the writing behavior of poor writers (e.g., the learning-disabled), and the application of self-regulation and strategy training in the treatment of writing difficulties was reviewed. Taken as a whole, the available evidence indicates that cognitive-behavior modification is a viable approach to written language instruction. Conceptually, the characteristics and components of cognitive-behavioral training are a good match to the characteristics of students with writing problems. For example, LD students have difficulty with the mental operations underlying effective writing and are characterized by a lack of active task engagement. Cognitive-behavioral approaches are designed to promote active participation on the part of the learner and to alleviate deficiencies in strategic performance. Empirically, it has been shown that cognitive-behavioral approaches can be used to help students develop important writing skills and/or to promote the utilization of previously learned skills. Self-regulation training was found to be effective in increasing task engagement during writing, raising productivity, and shaping what students write. Strategy training has been successfully used to promote the generation of writing content, advanced planning, revising and editing, and intentional control over sentence and paragraph production.

Although the use of cognitive-behavioral approaches in the area of writing problems is promising, conceptual and methodological issues remain. First, almost all of the cognitive-behavioral studies conducted in the area of writing have involved learning-disabled students. Additional research is needed with other populations. Second, teachers' willingness and/or ability to use cognitive-behavioral procedures to alleviate writing problems in the context of their classrooms has yet to be adequately investigated. Third, the cost-effectiveness of cognitive behavioral approaches in writing has not been addressed. It is not clear if a cognitive-behavioral approach is more appropriate than other instructional methods for training certain kinds of skills or if cognitive-behavioral procedures are effective with all types of writing skills (Wong, 1985). Fourth, more attention needs to be directed at determining the training components necessary for promoting acquisition, maintenance, and generalization. Fifth, additional research needs to be directed at helping students develop more mature cognitive and metacognitive processes by promoting self-regulatory functions that enable students to acquire strategic behaviors as a result of their own activity.

REFERENCES

Algozzine, B., & Korinek, L. (1985). Where is special education for students with high prevalence handicaps going? *Exceptional Children, 51*, 388–396.

Alley, G., & Deshler, D. (1979). *Teaching the learning disabled adolescent: Strategies and methods.* Denver: Love.

Ballard, K., & Glynn, T. (1975). Behavioral self-management in story writing with elementary school children. *Journal of Applied Behavior Analysis, 8*, 387–398.

Beaugrande, R. de (1984). Text production: Toward a science of composition. Norwood, NJ: Ablex.

Bereiter, C. (1980). Development in writing. In T. Gregg & E. Steinberg (Eds.), *Cognitive processes in writing* (pp. 73–93). Hillsdale, NJ: Lawrence Erlbaum.

Bereiter, C., & Scardamalia, M. (1982). From conversation to composition: The role of instruction in a developmental process. In R. Glaser (Ed.), *Advances in instructional psychology* (Vol. 2, pp. 1–64). Hillsdale, NJ: Lawrence Erlbaum.

Bereiter, C., & Scardamalia, M. (1983). Does learning to write have to be so difficult? In A. Freedman, I. Pringle, & J. Yolden (Eds.), *Learning to write: First language, second language* (pp. 20–33). London: Longman's International.

Bereiter, C., & Scardamalia, M. (1985). Cognitive coping strategies and the problem of "inert knowledge." In S. Chipman, J. Segal, & R. Glaser (Eds.), *Thinking and learning skills: Current research and open questions* (Vol. 2, pp. 65–80). Hillsdale, NJ: Lawrence Erlbaum.

Bridwell, L. (1981). Rethinking composing. *English Journal, 70*, 96–99.

Blair, T., & Crump, D. (1984). Effects of discourse mode on the syntactic complexity of learning disabled students' written expression. *Learning Disability Quarterly, 7*, 19–29.

Brown, A., Campione, J., & Day, J. (1981). Learning to learn: On training students to learn from texts. *Educational Researcher, 10*, 14–21.

Brown, A., Day, J., & Jones, R. (1983). The development of plans for summarizing texts. *Child Development, 54*, 968–989.

Brown, A., & Palincsar, A. (1982). Inducing strategic learning from texts by means of informed, self-control training. *Topics in Learning and Learning Disabilities, 2*, 1–17.

Craighead, W., Wilcoxon-Craighead, L., & Meyers, A. (1978). New directions in behavior modification with children. In M. Hersen, R. Eisler, & P. Miller (Eds.), *Progress in behavior modification* (Vol. 6, pp. 159–201). New York: Academic Press.

Deno, S., Marston, D., & Mirkin, P. (1982). Valid measurement procedures for continuous evaluation of written expression. *Exceptional Children, 48*, 368–371.

Englert, C., & Raphael, T. (1988). Constructing well-formed prose: Process, structure and metacognition in the instruction of expository writing. *Exceptional Children, 54*, 513–520.

Englert, C., Raphael, T., & Anderson, L. (1986). *Metacognitive knowledge and writing skills of upper elementary and student with special needs: Extensions of text structure research*. Paper presented at the National Reading Conference, Austin, TX, December.

Englert, C. S., & Thomas, C. C. (1988). Sensitivity to text structure in reading and writing: A comparison of learning disabled and non-learning disabled students. *Learning Disability Quarterly, 11*, 18–46.

Flower, L., & Hayes, J. (1980). The dynamics of composing: Making plans and juggling constraints. In L. Gregg & E. Steinberg (Eds.), *Cognitive processes in writing* (pp. 31–50). Hillsdale, NJ: Lawrence Erlbaum.

Flower, L., & Hayes, J. (1981). Plans that guide the composing process. In C. Frederiksen & J. Dominic (Eds.), *Writing: Process, development, and communication* (pp. 39–58). Hillsdale, NJ: Lawrence Erlbaum.

Flower, L., Hayes, J., Carey, L., Schriver, K., & Stratman, J. (1986). Detection, diagnosis, and the strategies of revision. *College Composition and Communication, 37*, 16–55.

Graham, S. (1982). Composition research and practice: A unified approach. *Focus on Exceptional Children, 14*, 1–16.

Graham, S. (1989). *The role of production factors in learning disabled students' compositions*. Paper presented at the annual meeting of the American Educational Research Association, San Francisco, April.

Graham, S., & Harris, K. R. (1987a). Improving composition skills of inefficient learners with self-instructional strategy training. *Topics in Language Disorders, 7* 66–77.

Graham, S., & Harris, K. R. (1987b). Writing remediation. In C. Reynolds & L. Mann (Eds.), *Encyclopedia of Special Education* (pp. 1676–1677). New York: Wiley.

Graham, S., & Harris, K. R. (1988a). Instructional recommendations for teaching writing to exceptional students. *Exceptional Children, 54*, 506–512.

Graham, S., & Harris, K. R. (1988b). Written language instruction and research [Special issue]. *Exceptional Children, 54*(6).

Graham, S., & Harris, K. R. (in press a). A components analysis of cognitive strategy training: Effects on learning disabled students' compositions and self-efficacy. *Journal of Educational Psychology.*

Graham, S., & Harris, K. R. (in press b). Improving learning disabled students' skills at composing essays: Self-instructional strategy training. *Exceptional Children.*

Graham, S., Harris, K. R., & Sawyer, R. (1987). Composition instruction with learning disabled students: Self-instructional strategy training. *Focus on Exceptional Children, 20,* 1–11.

Graham, S., & MacArthur, C. (1987). Written language of the handicapped. In C. Reynolds & L. Mann (Eds.), *Encyclopedia of Special Education* (pp. 1678–1681). New York: Wiley.

Graham, S., & MacArthur, C. (1988). Improving learning disabled students' skills at revising essays produced on a word processor: Self-instructional strategy training. *Journal of Special Education, 22,* 133–152.

Graham, S., & Miller, L. (1979). Spelling research and practice: A unified approach. *Focus on Exceptional Children, 11,* 1–16.

Graham, S., & Miller, L. (1980). Handwriting research and practice: A unified approach. *Focus on Exceptional Children, 12,* 1–16.

Graves, D. (1983). *Writing: Teachers and children at work.* Exeter, NH: Heineman Educational Books.

Hallahan, D., Kneedler, R., & Lloyd, J. (1983). Cognitive behavior modification techniques for learning disabled children: Self-instruction and self-monitoring. In J. McKinney & L. Feagans (Eds.), *Current topics in learning disabilities* (Vol. 1, pp. 207–244). New York: Ablex.

Harris, K. R. (1982). Cognitive-behavior modification: Application with exceptional students. *Focus on Exceptional Children, 15,* 1–16.

Harris, K. R. (1985). Conceptual, methodological, and clinical issues in cognitive-behavioral assessment. *Journal of Abnormal Child Psychology, 13,* 373–390.

Harris, K. R. (1986a). The effects of cognitive-behavior modification on private speech and task performance during problem solving among learning disabled and normally achieving students. *Journal of Abnormal Child Psychology, 14,* 63–67.

Harris, K. R. (1986b). Self-monitoring of attentional behavior versus self-monitoring of productivity: Effects on on-task behavior and academic response rate among learning disabled children. *Journal of Applied Behavior Analysis, 19,* 417–423.

Harris, K. R., & Graham, S. (1985). Improving learning disabled students' composition skills: Self-control strategy training. *Learning Disability Quarterly, 8,* 27–36.

Harris, K. R., & Graham, S. (1988). Self-instructional strategy training: Improving writing skills among educationally handicapped students. *Teaching Exceptional Students, 20,* 35–37.

Hayes, J., & Flower, L. (1980). Identifying the organization of writing processes. In L. Gregg & E. Steinberg (Eds.), *Cognitive processes in writing* (pp. 31–50). Hillsdale, NJ: Lawrence Erlbaum.

Hayes, J., & Flower, L. (1986). Writing research and the writer. *American Psychologist, 41,* 1106–1113.

Hemereck, L. (1979). *A comparison of the written language of learning disabled and non-learning disabled elementary children using the inventory of written expression and spelling.* Unpublished manuscript.

Hillocks, G. (1984). What works in teaching composition: A meta-analysis of experimental treatment studies. *American Journal of Education, 93*, 133–170.

Humes, A. (1983). Research on the composing process. *Review of Educational Research, 53*, 201–216.

Kaufer, D., Hayes, J., & Flower, L. (1986). Composing written sentences. *Research in the Teaching of English, 20*, 121–140.

MacArthur, C., & Graham, S. (1987). Learning disabled students' composing under three methods of text production: Handwriting, word processing, and dictation. *Journal of Special Education, 21*, 22–42.

Meichenbaum, D. (1977). Cognitive behavior modification: An integrative approach. New York: Plenum Press.

Moran, M. (1981). Performance of learning disabled and low achieving secondary students on formal features of a paragraph-writing task. *Learning Disability Quarterly, 4*, 271–280.

Moran, M. (1988). Improving students' contextual writing. *Exceptional Children, 54*, 552–558.

Moran, M., Schumaker, J., & Vetter, A. (1981). *Teaching a paragraph organization strategy to learning disabled adolescents.* Research Report No. 54. Lawrence: University of Kansas Institute for Research in Learning Disabilities.

Morris, N., & Crump, D. (1982). Syntactic and vocabulary development in the written language of learning disabled and non–learning disabled students at four age levels. *Learning Disability Quarterly, 5*, 163–172.

Nodine, B., Barenbaum, E., & Newcomer, P. (1985). Story composition by learning disabled, reading disabled, and normal children. *Learning Disability Quarterly, 8*, 167–179.

O'Leary, S., & Dubey, D. (1979). Applications of self-control procedures by children: A review. *Journal of Applied Behavior Analysis, 12*, 449–465.

Poteet, J. (1979). Characteristics of written expression of learning disabled and non–learning disabled elementary school students. *Diagnostique, 4*, 60–74.

Rumsey, I., & Ballard, K. (1985). Teaching self-management strategies for independent story writing to children with classroom behavior difficulties. *Educational Psychology, 5*, 147–157.

Scardamalia, M., & Bereiter, C. (1985). Fostering the development of self-regulation in children's knowledge processing. In S. Chipman, J. Segal, & R. Glaser (Eds.), *Thinking and learning skills: Current research and open questions* (Vol. 2, pp. 563–577). Hillsdale, NJ: Lawrence Erlbaum.

Scardamalia, M., & Bereiter, C. (1986). Written composition. In M. Wittrock (Ed.), *Handbook of research on teaching* (3rd ed.) (pp. 778–803). New York: Macmillan.

Scardamalia, M., Bereiter, C., & Goelman, H. (1982). The role of production factors in writing ability. In M. Nystrand (Ed.), *What writers know: The language, process, and structure of written discourse* (pp. 173–210). New York: Academic Press.

Scardamalia, M., & Paris, P. (1985). The function of explicit discourse knowledge in the development of text representations and composing strategies. *Cognition and Instruction, 2*, 1–39.

Schumaker, J., Deshler, D., Alley, G., & Warner, M. (1983). Toward the development of an intervention model for learning disabled adolescents: The University of Kansas Institute. *Exceptional Education Quarterly, 4*, 45–74.

Schumaker, J., Deshler, D., Alley, G., Warner, M., Clark, F., & Nolan, S. (1982). Error monitoring: A learning strategy for improving adolescent performance. In W. M.

Cruickshank and J. W. Lerner (Eds.), *Best of ACLD* (Vol. 3, pp. 170–183). Syracuse, NY: Syracuse University Press.

Schumaker, J., Nolan, S., & Deshler, D. (1985). *The error monitoring strategy.* Lawrence: University of Kansas.

Schumaker, J., & Sheldon, J. (1985). *The sentence writing strategy.* Lawrence: University of Kansas.

Seabaugh, G., & Schumaker, J. (1981). *The effects of self-regulation training on the academic productivity of LD and NLD adolescents* (Research Report No. 37). Lawrence: University of Kansas Institute for Research in Learning Disabilities.

Stone, I. (1978). *The origin.* New York: Doubleday.

Thomas, C., Englert, C., & Gregg, S. (1987). An analysis of errors and strategies in the expository writing of learning disabled students. *Remedial and Special Education, 8,* 21–30.

Voss, J., Greene, T., Post, T., & Penner, B. (1983). Problem-solving skills in the social sciences. In G. Bower (Ed.), *The psychology of learning and motivation: Advances in research and theory* (Vol. 17, pp. 165–213). New York: Academic Press.

Wallace, L., & Pear, J. (1977). Self-control techniques of famous novelists. *Journal of Applied Behavioral Analysis, 10,* 515–525.

Wong, B. (1985). Issues in cognitive-behavioral interventions in academic skills area. *Journal of Abnormal Child Psychology, 13,* 425–442.

12
COGNITIVE TRAINING: IMPLICATIONS FOR ARITHMETIC INSTRUCTION

CLAYTON E. KELLER
University of Minnesota, Duluth

JOHN WILLS LLOYD
University of Virginia

Two lines of educational research—behavioral approaches to instruction and the effective teaching literature—have laid the foundation for how content in any domain, including mathematics, can be presented effectively and efficiently. These two research traditions have identified not only teaching behaviors that are generally important but also combinations and sequences of such behaviors that have proved effective for arithmetic instruction.

These two approaches to research on instruction, however, have not taken into account much of the recent work by cognitive psychologists and mathematics educators on the nature, acquisition, and use of mathematics knowledge and skills (e.g., Carpenter, Moser, & Romberg, 1982; Ginsburg, 1983; Hiebert, 1986; Lesh & Landau, 1983; Pellegrino & Goldman, 1987; Resnick & Ford, 1981; Romberg & Capenter, 1986; Schoenfeld, 1987). Recent research from both disciplines indicates that there is often much more involved in solving, for instance, computation or word problems than simply reading the problem and writing the answer. For example, Mayer (1985) suggests that there are four steps and types of knowledge required to solve simple word problems. The problem solver needs to (1) translate linguistic and factual information in a word problem into an internal representation, (2) use knowledge of problem types to integrate the components of the problem, (3) plan how to solve the problem using strategic knowledge, and (4) carry out the plan through algorithmic knowledge.

This research suggests a more refined and complete body of content for mathematics instruction to be presented through the behavioral and effective teaching approaches. Indeed, the emphasis by cognitive psychologists and mathematics educators on both declarative—conceptual and factual—and procedural knowledge involved in the solution of arithmetic problems meshes well with the task analysis component of the behavioral approach to teaching. In a manner similar to task analysis, cognitive psychologists and mathematics educators determine the procedural steps needed to accomplish an arithmetic or mathematical task. They also examine, however, both the sequence of declarative knowledge involved in the task and the ways declarative knowledge and procedural knowledge interact during the task.

Combined cognitive-behavioral approaches to mathematics instruction, whether purposively or coincidentally, have started to tap this body of knowledge of mathematics learning by emphasizing the use of various cognitive and metacognitive strategies while performing arithmetical and mathematical tasks. Though standing with a foot in each camp—by developing out of the behavioral tradition and by using cognitive strategy as content—such approaches to date have tended to neglect either one or both of these sources of strength. In some research the cognitively oriented material has not been effectively presented, but more frequently the potential of cognitive strategies in mathematics instruction has not been incorporated into instruction.

In this chapter we first review the instructional variables from the behavioral approach and the effective instruction literature, which we consider to be important to both mathematics instruction in general and the implementation of cognitive training in particular. We then discuss some of the recent research on mathematics knowledge and performance, focusing on theoretical frameworks for differences in mathematics abilities and the development and use of addition strategies, to suggest what can serve as the cognitive content of mathematics instruction and why it should. Next we discuss research on cognitive-behavioral approaches to mathematics instruction, to show how cognitive training in this domain has been used and to what results so far. Finally, we include some summarizing remarks and suggestions for implementing cognitive-behavioral interventions in arithmetic and mathematics.

VARIABLES IMPORTANT FOR
MATHEMATICS INSTRUCTION

An important aspect of a combined cognitive and behavioral approach is the incorporation of concepts from the study of cognitive and metacognitive processes into behaviorally organized and implemented instruction. We focus here on such aspects of instruction, and particularly, of the many factors that influence the success of instruction, on several that have to do with teacher actions. Although they may do many other things, in general, teachers must present a fact, concept, or procedure in some way. They usually do this by telling students about the fact, concept, or procedure or by *modeling* it. Then, as the pupils practice using the fact, concept, or procedure in some way, the teacher must provide consequences, particularly *reinforcement*, related to their performance. The effects of modeling and reinforcement have been studied extensively. In addition, the effects of *combinations of teacher behaviors* have also been studied.

Modeling

Modeling has long been a staple of teaching. Demonstrations may occur in many different forms. The teacher may use modeling by:

Telling the students a fact or rule (e.g., "Anything times zero is zero").

Performing a task him- or herself (e.g., "Watch how I do this long division problem. First, I estimate how many times this will go into this. Let me see, 87 [pointing to divisor] is almost 90 and 90 will go into 400 [pointing to dividend] about 4 times . . .").

Directing students to observe another student answer a question (e.g., "I bet Jack knows this one. Jack, what is three plus five?") or perform a task (e.g., "Watch Jill. She's going to show how to factor this polynomial").

Studies of the effects of modeling have revealed that careful employment of this procedure sometimes will strongly influence student performance. For example, Smith and Lovitt (1975) studied modeling with learning-disabled boys learning arithmetic skills. They found that supplying a demonstration and a permanent model (a problem with the solution for it written on the boys' worksheets) markedly improved the boys' performance. Furthermore, the students' performance also improved on other problems for which they had not received training.

Modeling can easily be incorporated into instruction designed to have a cognitive-behavioral flavor. This is particularly true when teachers model their own thinking as they solve a problem, providing students with a window on their usually covert cognitive processes. The second modeling example of the three just given illustrates this idea.

Reinforcement

As in most learning, operant reinforcement plays an important role in the development of arithmetic skills and knowledge. In the acquisition of a skill, correct responses that are reinforced will be more likely to recur. In later stages of skill development, when students answer at too slow a pace (i.e., not automatically) or with inconsistent accuracy, reinforcement of a faster rate of responding or more accurate responding can have substantial beneficial effects on performance (e.g., Hasazi & Hasazi, 1972; Smith, Lovitt, & Kidder, 1972).

Reinforcement need not necessarily take the form of praise or tangible rewards. In fact, Fink and Carnine (1975) reported that having students maintain graphs of their progress led to increased levels of performance in arithmetic. Also, Lovitt and Hansen (1976) found that simply providing the opportunity to progress to later parts of an assigned book was reinforcing.

It is important to note, however, that reinforcement is of lesser value when students do not know *how* to perform a task. Smith and Lovitt (1976) demonstrated that the effectiveness of reinforcement contingencies depends on students being capable of performing the target response. Grimm, Bijou, and Parsons (1973) showed that when intensive reinforcement schedules did not produce acquisition, teaching a student a system for deriving answers did. Thus, we should eschew the use of reinforcement to "motivate" learners; instead, we should teach them how to perform the skill and provide reinforcement for its correct performance.

Combinations of Teacher Behaviors

Researchers, particularly from the process–product or effective-teaching tradition, have also studied other teacher behaviors (see Brophy & Good, 1986, for a comprehensive review) and combinations of behaviors respresenting functions of teaching (Rosenshine & Stevens, 1986) related to student achievement. Rosenshine and Stevens provide a concise description of nine important teaching functions:

> In general, researchers have found that when effective teachers teach well structured subjects, they:
> * Begin a lesson with a short review of previous, prerequisite learning.
> * Begin a lesson with a short statement of goals.
> * Present new material in small steps, with student practice after each step.
> * Give clear and detailed instructions and explanations.
> * Provide a high level of active practice for all students.
> * Ask a large number of questions, check for student understanding, and obtain responses from all students.
> * Guide students during initial practice.
> * Provide systematic feedback and corrections.
> * Provide explicit instruction and practice for seatwork exercises and, where necessary, monitor students during seatwork. (p. 377)

The relationship between teaching behaviors and student achievement in mathematics has also been studied specifically. For example, in the Missouri Mathematics Effectiveness Study, Good and Grouws (1979) examined the effects of a set of teaching behaviors on fourth-grade pupils' mathematics performance. The teaching behaviors (review of previous work, development of new material, provision for guided practice and independent practice, and assignment of homework) were developed on the basis of previous correlational research. Teachers who implemented the procedures had students who gained more on a test of mathematics achievement than did the students of teachers who were not trained to use the procedures.

The Good and Grouws study bolsters the case for the importance of the behavioral aspects of teaching, but these data provide no information about the content of instruction. That so much can be accomplished simply by having teachers present instruction in a certain way is encouraging not only because of the gains that can be attained but also because of the hope that far greater gains can be obtained if content variables are also manipulated.

Summary

The research reviewed describes how instruction in arithmetic and mathematics can be effectively provided through the use of modeling, reinforcement, and combinations of teaching behaviors. With a few exceptions, however (e.g., Silbert, Carnine, & Stein, 1981), the role of content in such effective instruction has not been exploited to improve instruction.

There is, however, a growing body of research on how mathematical knowledge and procedures develop in and are used by individuals. By focusing on individual differences in mathematics, this research suggests content that could contribute to improved performance. By studying cognitive and metacognitive processes, one can also derive suggestions about content appropriate to cognitive-behavioral approaches to arithmetic and mathematics instruction. We now turn to this research.

RECENT RESEARCH ON MATHEMATICS KNOWLEDGE AND PERFORMANCE

Cognitive psychologists and mathematics educators have made the domain of mathematics a focus of attention in recent years (cf., Carpenter, Moser, & Romberg, 1982; Ginsburg, 1983; Lesh & Landau, 1983; Resnick & Ford, 1981; Romberg & Carpenter, 1986; Schoenfeld, 1987). Although many aspects of mathematical knowledge and development have been investigated, we focus on two in particular. First, we consider theoretical frameworks for individual differences in the mathematics domain. Such frameworks provide a rationale for including various cognitive and metacognitive components as part of the content for mathematics instruction. The frameworks also suggest possible relationships among these various components, which are often manipulated separately in cognitive-behavioral approaches. Second, by reviewing research on children's development and use of addition strategies, we present an example of the types of results that have been found and that can serve as models for the content of cognitive-behavioral approaches.

Theoretical Frameworks

Why do individuals seem to have different abilities in mathematics? Why can some people solve mathematics problems more quickly and accurately than others? Are the answers to these questions educationally useful? At one level of abstraction, early research used factor analyses and found broad cognitive factors structuring the nature of mathematical ability. Such factors included, for example, intelligence, verbal ability, spatial ability, and a speed component (Wrigley, 1958). At another level of abstraction, a neuropsychological approach considers constructs of more specific abilities or aptitudes. This perspective considers such constructs as visual memory, auditory closure, and perceptual-motor skills as possible factors responsible for differences in mathematical performance (Strang & Rourke, 1985).

Although answers for each of these levels of analysis may hold some explanatory power, they are not sufficient explanations. Too many mechanisms must intervene between such factors and constructs and mathematical performance in order for performance to be adversely affected by deficits in the factors (Briars, 1983). The factors and constructs do not address what is occurring cognitively while an individual performs mathematical tasks. That is, they do not consider what an individual is doing to solve the tasks beyond any observable behaviors that can be noticed.

Also, such factors and constructs are not especially useful educationally. Broad cognitive factors are not easily, if at all, amenable to educational intervention. Interventions that train more focused perceptual and cognitive abilities, like those studied by neuropsychology, do not automatically produce improvements in academic performance (Arter & Jenkins, 1979; Lloyd, 1984).

Research from an information-processing perspective in cognitive psychology does consider the cognitive mechanisms responsible for performance. These mechanisms, because of their specificity and closer connection to performance, may be better targets for educational interventions. An information-processing approach focuses on an individual's internal representations of information or knowledge and the strategies or processes that the person uses on the representations to meet the cognitive demands of life. Researchers taking this approach are especially concerned with explaining how the individual overcomes limitations on the amount of information that can be processed at any given point in time relative to the large amounts of information that must be processed (Flavell, 1985; Siegler, 1986).

Literature reflecting the information-processing approach to individual differences in cognitive performance, sometimes known as the expert/novice literature, investigates the component cognitive processes involved in performance as sources of differences within the domain. Researchers from this approach have developed theoretical frameworks of these processes for several domains, including mathematics. For example, Sternberg (1984, 1985) presented a subtheory of the cognitive processes, which he calls components, as part of his triarchic metatheory of intelligence. Resnick and Neches (1984) suggested a framework of factors responsible for individual differences in learning ability. Briars (1983) reviewed research on individual differences in mathematical ability from an information-processing perspective. And

Schoenfeld (1985) suggested a theoretical framework to explain differences in mathematical problem-solving performance.

Because there is great similarity among these frameworks in how the cognitive processes are categorized, we collapse our discussion of these frameworks across the categories and, for simplicity, generally use Briars's (1983) terms (with references to others' analogous terms) for the categories.

Information-Processing Skills

Information-processing skills, also referred to as "capacity differences" (Resnick & Neches, 1984) or "performance components" (Sternberg, 1984, 1985), are the processes that manipulate information coming in from the environment and representations of previously stored information. Such processes might encode new information into representations, combine or compare information, or just respond within a task (Sternberg, 1985). These processes are content-independent (Briars, 1983); that is, they are used whenever cognition takes place, regardless of the domain. Certain constraints on these skills are said to exist for all individuals, particularly for short-term or working memory, one's cognitive workspace. Thus, as a source for individual differences in performance, this category of factors is possibly not as important as the others (Sternberg, 1985).

Resnick and Neches (1984) suggest three capacity differences in information-processing abilities may be responsible for some of the individual differences in learning. Small differences in the speed at which information is processed may have cumulative effects on the amount of information processed and the efficiency with which it is processed. The amount of exposure to stimuli needed before information from the stimuli can be encoded in some relevant way might also affect learning. The capacity difference that has been most widely studied, however, is the amount of space in short-term or working memory. Briars (1983) has noted that memory span tasks and processing-speed tasks are two of the basic information-processing skills that have been studied in relation to mathematics achievement.

The ability to automatize information-processing tasks whenever possible is another important factor in individual differences in performance (Sternberg, 1984). Processing that takes place on an automatic level, besides being smooth and efficient, allows the individual to devote conscious effort to other components or aspects of the tasks, thus improving performance. If an individual cannot process certain kinds of information automatically, he or she must process them consciously. This slower process prevents effort from being used for other aspects of the tasks.

Content Knowledge

Content knowledge is another category of cognitive processes and representations that plays an important role in individual differences in intelligence, learning, and other domains. Content knowledge is also known as "domain-specific knowledge" (Resnick & Neches, 1984), "knowledge-acquisition components" (Sternberg, 1984, 1985), and "resources and heuristics" (Schoenfeld, 1985).

This category includes:

Specific knowledge (both declarative—concepts and facts—and procedural) an individual has about the domain (Resnick & Neches, 1984; Schoenfeld, 1985).

How the individual organizes the knowledge (Briars, 1983; Resnick & Neches, 1984).

Accessibility of the knowledge to the individual (Resnick & Neches, 1984; Schoenfeld, 1985).

The use of information-processing skills to acquire new knowledge for the domain (Sternberg, 1984, 1985).

The types and amount of content knowledge needed for competent performance within a domain such as mathematics may be greater than is at first realized. For example, in analyzing the demands of algebra story problems, Mayer, Larkin, and Kadane (1984) identified four types of knowledge needed to solve them. *Linguistic and factual knowledge* is necessary to translate the words of the problem appropriately into component internal representations. These representations can later be combined by *schematic knowledge* to represent the relationships stated and implied in the problem. *Strategic knowledge* determines a plan to solve for the missing components in the relationships. Finally, *algorithmic knowledge* executes the plan.

There are also some common ways of deductively organizing content knowledge in mathematics, as opposed to the idiosyncratic ways individuals inductively organize their knowledge of mathematics. These organizations may be useful to remember when considering the content of cognitive-behavioral approaches to instruction. One long-standing organization of mathematics knowledge is a dichotomy between *declarative knowledge* about mathematics, such as the base systems and properties of numbers, and *procedural knowledge*, which allows a person to solve mathematical tasks, such as computational algorithms (Hiebert, 1986; Resnick & Ford, 1981). Another way of organizing mathematics knowledge is to make a distinction between formal and informal knowledge (Russell & Ginsburg, 1984). *Informal knowledge* is composed of mathematical concepts and arithmetic skills such as counting that children tend to acquire through normal, everyday experiences before they start school. *Formal knowledge* includes concepts and skills such as place value and the base systems that are usually only acquired through formal instruction in school.

Metacognition

The third category of cognitive processes falls under the rubric of "metacognition" ("control" for Schoenfeld, 1985; "metacomponents" for Sternberg, 1984, 1985). These are processes that organize, control, and monitor the other cognitive processes that actually deal with the information of tasks encountered. For example, in Sternberg's subtheory (1985), only the metacomponents can directly activate or receive feedback from the other types of components. However, those performance and knowledge acquisition components can indirectly, through the metacomponents, activate and receive feedback from each other.

Using one of Sternberg's listings (1985), these executive processes can include:

Deciding what the problem is in a task
Selecting performance or knowledge acquisition components to use in the task
Selecting representations or organizations for information in the task
Selecting strategies for combining components
Allocating attentional resources
Monitoring the solution process
Evaluating external feedback

In comparison to performance components (basic information-processing skills), Sternberg believes "that metacomponential processes are more fundamental sources of consequential individual and developmental differences. Changes in metacomponential functioning lead almost inevitably to changes in the functioning of performance components . . ." (1985, p. 107).

Despite what seems to be the importance of metacognition for individual differences in mathematics performance, there has been little research on the topic (Briars, 1983). Some work, however, has been done on knowledge of general strategies for solving mathematics problems, awareness of problem-solving strategies, and belief systems about mathematics and problem solving in mathematics (Briars, 1983; Schoenfeld, 1985).

Summary

Information-processing psychology's three-part theoretical framework for individual differences in mathematics performance is important for cognitive-behavioral approaches in two major ways. First, the framework provides a rationale for considering and targeting cognitive and metacognitive processes in arithmetic and mathematics instruction. Also, by examining the relationships among the processes, one can assess the importance of each type of process relative to arithmetic and mathematics performance.

Second, the framework provides implications for the cognitive content or purposes of cognitive-behavioral interventions. The previous discussion suggests that information-processing skills may not be suitable content for such interventions, although there may be a place for interventions to overcome or override deficits in such skills. Content knowledge, its organization, and its accessibility, however, may provide valuable cognitive content for interventions because of its specificity to a domain. Indeed, this cognitive component is being tapped by interventions (as a later section shows). Also, the framework suggests that metacognitive processes, because of their controlling functions, can play an important part in improved arithmetic and mathematics performance. Again, we discuss later how researchers are targeting these processes.

The previous section has been mainly theoretical. We now turn to research that has investigated these cognitive processes within the context of a particular portion of arithmetic content.

The Development and Use of Addition Strategies

Researchers in cognitive psychology and mathematics education have not only considered theoretical reasons for differences in mathematics performance. Also, using the methods of interview, analysis of error patterns, computer modeling, and measurement of response time, they have investigated the interface between the cognitive demands of mathematical tasks and the cognitive and metacognitive processes individuals use to handle those demands. One of the most thoroughly studied areas concerns the strategies children use to solve simple addition problems. These researchers have considered (1) the different strategies children use, (2) the underlying knowledge structures concerning numbers and addition needed to use the strategies, and (3) the use of strategies (see also Pellegrino & Goldman, 1987, for another review on this topic).

Different Addition Strategies

Carpenter and Moser (1983) have divided the normal development of addition strategies into three levels. The first level, called *counting all with models*, contains strategies that directly model the addends of the problem with physical objects or fingers. Each addend is modeled, the models are combined either physically or conceptually, and then the combination is counted, starting from one.

Several strategies using *counting sequences without models* make up the second level (Carpenter & Moser, 1983). The first strategy at this level, called *Sum* (Groen & Parkman, 1972), is like counting all with models but involves no physical models of the addends. The second strategy is called *counting on from first*. The child uses the name of the first addend as the starting point of the counting sequence, then counts the second addend. For example, to solve the problem 2 + 3, the child would say 2, then count 3, 4, 5. The third strategy at this level is *counting on from larger* or *Min* (Groen & Parkman, 1972). This strategy is similar to the previous one except that the child first determines which addend is larger, names that addend, and counts the smaller addend. (It is called Min because it requires the minimum number of counting steps.)

Strategies at the third level use *number facts* that are known (Carpenter & Moser, 1983). Children rapidly recall some facts, such as doubles or ties (e.g.,

1 + 1), at a relatively early age (Groen & Parkman, 1972). Facts that have already been learned, such as doubles and combinations with sums of 10, are sometimes used to solve other problems. Eventually, most children will solve the basic addition facts just by recalling the answers; the predominant use of this strategy begins around the third grade in normal development (Ashcraft, 1982).

Some generalizations can be made about the development of addition strategies through the course of these levels (Carpenter & Moser, 1983). Each succeeding strategy the child learns or develops builds on the previous strategies used. The further along the child is in the levels of strategies, the more flexible he or she is in the use of strategies to solve various kinds of addition problems. The strategies increase in abstraction and efficiency as well.

Underlying Knowledge Structures

In addition to looking at the procedures of addition strategies, researchers such as Resnick (1983) and Fuson (1982; Secada, Fuson, & Hall, 1983) have also focused on the underlying understanding of numbers and addition. Children must manipulate the parts of arithmetic problems and numbers when using Min and some other addition strategies. Resnick notes that these strategies "provide evidence that children understand the compositional structure of numbers and are able to partition and recombine with some flexibility" (1983, pp. 121–122). She suggests that such understanding and ability are possible because of the presence of a schema or representation that organizes the child's knowledge about numbers; the child, however, does not need to be able to express such understanding or describe his or her representation.

Resnick points out that such a representation could develop out of a young child's everyday experiences, such as counting things and noticing the relationships between parts and wholes. Numbers need not be involved in the origin of the representation. However, numbers structured in simple forms of the representation could be connected to simple procedures, such as counting up from a given number, for solving problems involving numbers. Such experiences with numbers could lead to further development of the representation and of new procedures.

The Use of Addition Strategies

Even though efficient addition strategies develop over time, children do not always use the most efficient strategies available to them (Carpenter & Moser, 1983). They use a variety of methods, often depending on the particular addition problems they encounter (Houlihan & Ginsburg, 1981; Russell, 1977; Siegler & Robinson, 1982). In a longitudinal study of the strategies children use to solve addition and subtraction word problems from first through third grade, Carpenter and Moser (1984) found much variability in the use of strategies both between and within testing sessions. Some children who were capable of efficient counting strategies would use less efficient strategies if manipulatives were available. Usually, however, as a consequence of word problem type or number size, there were no clear patterns in the use of strategies.

Siegler and Shrager (1984) posit a strategy choice model that might account for such findings. Their model, which they call the *distribution of associations model*, explains how and why a child uses different strategies to solve particular problems. Possible answers to simple addition problems are associated with different probabilities of being the correct answer. For example, 3 would have a higher probability of being the correct answer for $1 + 2$ than would 9. The probabilities are the associative strengths between the problems and the possible answers. When approaching a problem, the child sets two parameters. One, a confidence criterion, determines what level of associative strength is needed before a child will accept a generated answer as a solution to the problem. The second parameter determines how many times the child will try to use a particular strategy to generate an answer. The model suggests that the strategies available to the child are tried hierarchically, with the most efficient strategies tried before the least efficient. The model also predicts certain relations among the associations between problems and possible answers, errors produced, time needed to solve problems, and use of observable strategies. The predictions were met in two experiments (Siegler & Robinson, 1982; Siegler & Shrager, 1984).

Summary

We think some salient points appear in the research considering cognitive processes within the context of addition strategies, and that these points have implications for selecting the content of cognitive-behavioral interventions for mathematics. As addition strategies develop, later strategies (1) develop from previous strategies, (2) are more efficient than previous ones, and (3) tend to follow similar patterns of development across individuals. In choosing strategies to teach through cognitive-behavioral approaches, then, one should probably choose the strategies that are the most efficient. But can the most efficient strategies be taught without previous exposure to the preceding sequence of less efficient strategies? This is a question that needs investigation. The research reviewed also shows that conceptual or declarative and procedural knowledge are linked and change together. Thus, cognitive-behavioral approaches may also need to target declarative knowledge as they attempt to change procedural strategies.

The research on addition strategies does not relegate much of a role to metacognitive processes. Researchers simply may not be considering metacognition in relation to the task of solving basic addition facts. Alternatively, the steps involved in addition strategies may be too automatized to make use of metacognitive processes. One implication of all this, however, is that metacognition may not be appropriate content for cognitive-behavioral interventions focusing on some types of mathematics content. The first set of studies we review in the next section shows that interventions without a metacognitive component can be useful for some arithmetic tasks.

COGNITIVE-BEHAVIORAL INTERVENTIONS

We organize this section by focusing on the cognitive content the instruction addresses and the cognitive purpose the instruction serves. The mathematics content targeted in these studies consists mainly of basic number facts and computational algorithms. Although some of the studies try to improve performance in these areas by focusing solely on matters of content knowledge (to use the information-processing framework), others address metacognitive processes in addition to content knowledge.

Content Knowledge as Cognitive Content

Studies focusing on content knowledge through their interventions seem to serve two cognitive purposes: (1) facilitating access to the appropriate content knowledge for a task and (2) increasing content knowledge, both declarative and procedural. Table 12-1 summarizes the studies in this section by listing the mathematics content, interventions, and cognitive content and purposes of the studies.

Two interventions studied cuing students' access to the appropriate procedural knowledge for computation problems. Parsons (1972) examined the effects of having pupils both circle and name the operation symbol ("a plus" or "a minus") prior to performing an arithmetic operation. He observed that this technique resulted in increased accuracy among students who often performed the wrong operation. Lovitt and Curtiss (1968) reported that requiring a student to read each problem aloud before beginning to solve it produced beneficial effects on the student's arithmetic performance.

Haupt, Van Kirk, and Terraciano (1975) described a simple method for increasing declarative knowledge and automatic recall of number facts. They gradually obscured the answer to simple subtraction problems by covering each answer with cellophane. This condition was contrasted with a control condition in which the student worked on addition problems in a traditional drill-and-practice fashion with teacher corrections for errors. Haupt and colleagues found that this fading procedure, in combination with a reinforcement contingency, resulted in the child reaching criterion (correctly answering each of the seven problems in a set within 2 seconds of presentation of each) after 34 trials. The pupil took 64 trials to reach criterion in the control condition. Furthermore, in the experimental condition the child made 28 errors, but in the control condition she made 149 errors. Finally, a follow-up examination one week later revealed that 5 of 7 subtraction facts were correctly recalled after one trial and 7 of 7 on a second trial; in contrast, none of the addition

TABLE 12-1. Cognitive-Behavioral Studies Focusing on Content Knowledge

Study	Math Content	Intervention	Cognitive Content/Purpose
Parsons, 1972	Addition, subtraction	Circle and name.	Cue access to procedural knowledge.
Lovitt & Curtiss, 1968	Computation problems	Read problem aloud.	Cue access to procedural knowledge.
Haupt, Van Kirk, & Terraciano, 1975	Subtraction facts	Cover answers with cellophane.	Increase declarative knowledge, automaticity.
	Multiplication facts	Cover answers with tracing paper.	Increase declarative knowledge.
Strategy training (e.g., Lloyd, 1980)	Any procedural knowledge	Task analysis, test for requisite skills, teach steps/sequence through modeling.	Train procedural knowledge.

facts were correctly recalled. In a second study, Haupt and co-workers (1975) had a young boy trace answers to multiplication problems but gradually introduced additional thicknesses of tracing paper so that the correct answer was gradually obscured. Results from this examination of fading were similar to those observed in the first study.

The results of these studies describe several components of arithmetic instruction that are often included in cognitive-behavioral interventions. First, the Parsons (1972) and Lovitt and Curtiss (1968) studies illustrate the use of self-verbalization in training. Although these studies have often been cited as indicative of the importance of self-verbalization (e.g., Hallahan & Reeve, 1980), additional work is needed to ascertain its role in skill acquisition and maintenance. Second, the Haupt *et al.* (1975) studies illustrate the application of the fading of prompts in learning: Cognitive interventions routinely incorporate a gradual diminution of teacher prompts of performance. Although such prompts in cognitive-behavioral programs often are delivered verbally, the Haupt *et al.* studies show how fading can be accomplished inexpensively even when the teacher is not immediately available to control them.

Unless an intervention is designed to repair a faulty algorithm (and often even when the goal is remediation), it is usually necessary to teach students the steps in a strategy or algorithm for solving problems. That is, it is often important to teach procedural knowledge. In one model of how to teach procedural knowledge—strategy training—teachers may model the steps of a strategy that students may use to solve a specific type of problem (Cullinan, Lloyd, & Epstein, 1981; Lloyd, 1980; Lloyd & deBettencourt, 1982). According to this approach, a task analysis of the skills needed to solve a class of problems is completed. Then students are tested to ascertain which, if any, of the requisite skills they have. Finally, they are taught the unknown skills and how to link them together to solve the problems. A common example of the use of a strategy of this sort is the FOIL method for multiplying binomials (multiplying in order the *first* terms, the *outside* terms, the *inside* terms, and the *last* terms and writing the answers in order as each step is completed). Research has revealed that

> Strategies for such simple tasks as number–numeral equivalences (Grimm *et al.*, 1973) and more complex tasks such as long division (Smith & Lovitt, 1975) can even be taught to atypical learners.
>
> Mastery of the component skills prior to learning how to use the skills in concert leads to greater generalization (Carnine, 1980).
>
> Failure to teach component skills prior to teaching the students how to use the strategy will result in an absence of generalization (Lloyd, Saltzman, & Kauffman, 1981).
>
> Students can be taught closely related strategies for closely related tasks (e.g., multiplication and division) without confusing the strategies (Lloyd *et al.*, 1981).
>
> Early in the acquisition of strategies, it is important for teachers to prompt the use of each step in the algorithm; but as the pupils develop facility with the algorithm, teachers should decrease the level of prompting until the students are functioning independently (Paine, Carnine, White, & Walters, 1982).

Summary

Earlier we discussed content knowledge as a source of individual differences in mathematics performance. Although successful studies using cognitive-behavioral interventions focused on content knowledge—its accessibility and increase—do not prove this component of the theoretical framework, they do suggest the efficacy of this component as the cognitive content of mathematical instruction.

Metacognitive and Content Knowledge as Cognitive Content

Some cognitive-behavioral approaches train combinations of content knowledge—usually in the form of the procedural knowledge of an algorithm's steps—and metacognitive processes. In some situations, it is difficult to separate these two components precisely. For example, one can legitimately view some of the steps involved in solving word problems (e.g., locate the information, identify the question, plan how to answer the question) as procedural knowledge for the task, although they also resemble metacognitive processes. Also, in some studies it is difficult to tell how the researchers are using the metacognitive processes. Are they training procedural knowledge and metacognitive processes separately, or are they training metacognitive processes to guide the use of procedural knowledge? Table 12-2 lists the studies reviewed in this section along with their mathematics content, interventions, and cognitive content and purposes.

Montague and Bos (1986) studied the effects of what they also called a strategy training program on adolescents' performance on two-step word problems. The training program incorporated many components—"paraphrasing, visualization, detecting relevant information, locating the question, hypothesizing, estimating, labeling, and checking" (p. 26)—and was evaluated using a multiple-baseline design. Assuming that the dependent measures were trustworthy (no data were provided about their reliability), the results indicate that the training program had beneficial effects on the pupils' performance.

Davis and Hajicek (1985) also termed one of their treatment conditions "strategy training" in their study of the arithmetic performance of pupils with

TABLE 12-2. Cognitive-Behavioral Studies Focusing on Metacognition and Content Knowledge

Study	Math Content	Intervention	Cognitive Content/Purpose
Montague & Bos, 1986	Two-step word problems	Paraphrase, visualize, detect information, locate question, hypothesize, estimate, label, check	Train procedural knowledge, metacognitive strategies.
Davis & Hajicek, 1985	Decimal multiplication	Teacher model, attention to task, self-reinforcement	Train procedural knowledge, metacognitive strategies.
Schunk, 1981	Division	Teacher model, corrective feedback	Metacognition to guide procedural knowledge
Schunk & Cox, 1986	Subtraction	Students verbalize aloud, attribution training	Metacognition to guide procedural knowledge
Johnston, Whitman, & Johnson, 1981	Addition and subtraction	Self-instructional training	Metacognition to guide procedural knowledge
Whitman & Johnston, 1983			
Leon & Pepe, 1983	Computational algorithms	Self-instructional training	Metacognition to guide procedural knowledge
Albion & Salzberg, 1982	Addition	General and task-specific self-instructional training	Metacognition to guide procedural knowledge
Cameron & Robinson 1980	Addition and subtraction	Task-specific self-instructional training	Metacognition to guide procedural knowledge
Thackwray, Meyers, Schleser, & Cohen, 1985	Addition	General or task-specific self-instructional training	Metacognition to guide procedural knowledge

behavior disorders. In this condition the teacher modeled the solution of multiplication problems involving decimals and then prompted students to imitate this strategy. Later, in the second condition the teacher repeated the modeling of the strategy and added to it a combination of steps that were designed to promote attention to task and self-reinforcement. Davis and Hajicek reported that the initial training resulted in increased performance on problems testing multiplication of decimals but had little influence on attention to task. The second intervention had greater effects on both measures. The treatments were, however, introduced in succession within the context of a multiple-baseline design. Thus, it is not possible to know whether the increases observed under the second treatment are directly attributable to the qualities of the second training procedure. It may be, for example, that the additional quantity of training provided by use of the second procedure was responsible for the improved performance.

Schunk (1981) investigated the effects of teaching low-achieving pupils a systematic approach to solving division problems. During the training phase of his study, some students observed a trainer solving division problems while verbalizing the strategy steps; in practice sessions they received corrective feedback that included additional modeling of cognitive steps. Other students were provided with explanatory materials and directions to refer to the appropriate parts of them for assistance but were not provided with cognitive models of use of the strategy steps. Schunk found that the modeling of usually covert cognitive steps significantly improved performance in comparison to the other treatment and a no-treatment control condition. Furthermore, the addition of attributional training (children were told that their successes depended on high degrees of effort and their failures depended on low degrees of effort) did not exert any influence over the performance. In a later study, Schunk and Cox (1986) found that requiring learning-disabled children to verbalize as they solved problems produced higher scores on similar tasks. Additionally, telling the students during the first half of training that their degree of effort was related to their success led children to believe that the amount of effort they expended was an important factor in their success.

Johnston, Whitman, and Johnson (1981) and Whitman and Johnston (1983) evaluated the effects of self-instructional programs on mentally retarded children's arithmetic competence. Self-instruction usually includes self-verbalization of a procedural algorithm for approaching certain kinds of problems and may also include components of self-monitoring and self-reward. The programs Johnston *et al.* and Whitman and Johnston used included instruction in using procedural algorithms for solving specific types of arithmetic problems. In both studies the results indicated that this intervention had clear and substantial effects on the students' arithmetic performance.

Similarly, Leon and Pepe (1983) used self-instructional principles (based on Mcichenbaum & Goodman, 1969, 1971) in teaching learning-disabled and educable mentally retarded pupils procedural algorithms for solving arithmetic problems. They found that this procedure was more effective than a control procedure consisting of students working through the same materials without the self-instructional training.

Albion and Salzberg (1982) used similar procedures with mentally retarded pupils. Their treatment program consisted of two main components: a general set of self-instructions and a task-specific set of self-instructions. The general self-instructions were designed to help the pupils attend to their assigned work. The task-specific self-instructions were designed to help the pupils use a self-guiding strategy for solving the arithmetic problems that had been assigned. The introduction of the combined self-instructional procedures resulted in improvement in the rate of accurate answering for some of the students. Because the two sets of self-instruction were introduced simultaneously to each of the participants in the study, the design of this study does not permit one to assess the relative contributions of the two procedures independently. Similar results were reported by Cameron and Robinson (1980), although their self-instructional procedure did not include task-specific self-instruction that was as explicit as that used by Albion and Salzberg.

Thackwray, Meyers, Schleser, and Cohen (1985) examined the relative effectiveness of general and specific self-instructional training with children identified as low-achieving and impulsive. Children in the specific self-instruction group were given a model of the cognitive steps that would lead to the solution of arithmetic problems; the trainer demonstrated self-instruction steps that were specifically related to the task of adding. Children in the general self-instruction group were given a model of cognitive steps that could help solve arithmetic and other problems; although all examples used during training were arithmetic problems, during training the trainer did not refer to specific steps in an algorithm for solving addition problems. Children in a control group were given directions about how to solve arithmetic problems; the trainer simply told them how to proceed without including all of the components of the self-instructional training. Training and practice time were equated for the groups. Thackwray and colleagues reported that although there were no significant differences on an experimenter-developed test of addition skill, there were significant differences favoring the specific self-instruction group over both other groups on a standardized achievement test of arithmetic skills and over the general self-instruction group on a standardized achievement test of general knowledge. In addition, a significant interaction effect between time of testing and groups was found favoring the general self-instruction group on a standardized achievement test of spelling.

Summary

Although the results of these studies suggest that cognitive-behavioral approaches targeting metacognitive processes in cognition with procedural knowledge can be effective in improving arithmetic and mathematics performance, the studies contain some problems regarding methodology and interventions. In some of the studies, the research designs limit the strength of the conclusions. Interventions should also be designed to fit the theoretical relationship between metacognition and content knowledge, namely, that metacognitive processes directly control access to and use of content knowledge. Interventions that train and use the components separately attempt to work counter to the theoretical framework from cognitive psychology.

RECOMMENDATIONS

To provide arithmetic and mathematics instruction that will enable students to succeed requires (1) adoption of effective teaching techniques (e.g., reinforcement for correct responding), (2) demonstrations of content and procedural algorithms for solving problems that are consistent with what we know about cognitive and metacognitive development, and (3) collection of data for monitoring student progress. In this section we make specific recommendations about each of these.

Effective Teaching

The teaching functions summarized by Rosenshine and Stevens (1986) (see page 285 of this chapter) describe the broad outlines for effective teaching. Although these functions are probably less important when instruction is focused on less arbitrary knowledge (i.e., where there are multiple correct answers) or processes (e.g., divergent thinking), we consider it quite safe to recommend them for a wide variety of arithmetic and mathematics instruction.

Teachers should organize and implement instruction along the lines of effective teaching. Supervisors and consultants should provide informative feedback to teachers about the extent to which the instruction they observe incorporates these functions. And instructional programmers should design their products so that they are consistent with these guidelines.

Broad adoption of these recommendations alone probably will not eliminate failure in arithmetic and mathematics, but it will help mightily. We consider them a necessary but not sufficient condition for effective instruction.

Inclusion of Knowledge about Mathematical Thinking and Development

Similarly, we think there is a very strong case for adjusting the content of arithmetic and mathematics instruction according to what we know and are learning about cognition and metacognition. In the past most instruction has been informed almost entirely by opinion and intuition. Although our knowledge of mathematical thinking is far from complete, there are direct implications for instruction in what we now know. For example, the literature reviewed in our section on the development of addition strategies makes it clear that the time-honored approach of teaching children to use a counting-all-with-models strategy and then expecting them to begin to use a number facts strategy for all addition combinations is likely to meet with difficulty.

Instructional designers should very carefully examine this literature and incorporate its findings into their efforts to produce programs. Teachers and supervisors will have to learn to recognize places where instructional programs are inconsistent with our knowledge of the development of mathematical knowledge and skills. Furthermore, they may have to learn to adapt materials so that such inconsistencies do not increase the chances of student failure.

Progress Monitoring

To establish whether instruction is helping students, it is necessary to monitor student performance. Techniques such as *curriculum-based assessment* (e.g., Howell & McCollum-Gahley, 1986; Howell & Morehead, 1987) are the most appropriate mechanisms for such formative evaluation in arithmetic learning. These procedures require that samples of materials on which students are expected to perform well be selected and administered to students. On the basis of the data that result from this monitoring, instruction is continued or modified. Howell and McCollum-Gahley (1986) described a five-step procedure that is abstracted in Table 12-3.

CONCLUSION

Despite the limitations of the current status of cognitive-behavioral approaches in mathematics instruction we have noted throughout the chapter, we feel optimistic about the impact these approaches can have on the improvement of arithmetic and mathematics performance. One of the main reasons for our optimism is the increasing body of research on cognitive and metacognitive processes involved in mathematics tasks—their description, relationships, and development. Future work on cognitive-behavioral approaches needs to stay abreast of this literature and tie itself more closely to these findings when developing the cognitive content and purposes of the interventions.

The second main reason for optimism is the substantial body of research from the behavioral and effective teaching traditions on how to teach any content. The use of these teaching behaviors should facilitate the impact of cognitive training. The extent to which this is true with less arbitrary knowledge and skills (e.g., metacognitive processes) deserves further study. Derry and Murphy (1986), for example, suggest that metacognitive skills, because of their nature and the way they develop, may not be amenable to direct training. In the present situation, however, it is clear that both of these conclusions can help to inform recommendations about appropriate practices.

TABLE 12-3. Five Steps in Data-Based Instruction

Step 1: Select a Short-Term Instructional Objective
In this step one establishes the instructional content that is to be learned (and, therefore, assessed) and specifies the traditional components of an objective (e.g., behavior, conditions, and performance criterion).

Step 2: Select or Develop a Procedure to Measure Achievement
In this step one devises miniature tests that are representative of the tasks the students must master to achieve the objective. Usually, these probes require only about a one-minute sample of performance. Among the guidelines for creating probes that one must consider are these: (1) order problems randomly by difficulty; (2) have alternative forms to combat memorization of item answers; and (3) include more test items than the students are likely to complete.

Step 3: Set Performance and Progress Aims
Establish acceptable levels of performance according to the performance of nonhandicapped pupils, and derive desirable progress rates according to the amount of time available to move the atypical learners to those performance levels.

Step 4: Begin Instruction and Monitor Student Progress
Have instruction designed to teach to the objective provided. Measure students' performance according to the outcomes of Step 2. Three assessments of progress per week should be the minimum number of assessments completed.

Step 5: Review Student Progress and Adjust Instruction
Compare student progress to the aims established in Step 3 and decide whether it is rapid enough to meet the objective. Consider whether (1) the correct objective is being addressed; (2) the skill is being taught in context; (3) the instructional emphasis should be on *accuracy* (student is answering less than 83% of items correctly), *fluency* (student is above 83% but answers at a slow rate), *generalization* (student answers accurately and fluently), or *maintenance* (student is at or above aim); (4) the lessons should be made more interesting (previous gains are being lost); or (5) delivery of instruction should be modified.

Source: Summarized from "Monitoring Instruction" by K. W. Howell and J. McCollum-Gahley, 1986, *Teaching Exceptional Children*, Vol. 19, No. 1, pp. 47–49.

ACKNOWLEDGMENTS

We wish to thank Bernice Y. L. Wong for her comments on an earlier draft of this chapter. Support during the preparation of this chapter was provided to the first author (C. E. K.) in part by the John B. and Florence S. May Fellowship in Learning Disabilities, Curry School of Education, University of Virginia, and by a Student Initiated Research Grant (Grant No. G008630420), Office of Special Education Programs, U.S. Department of Education. The second author (J. W. L.) was supported in part by U.S. Department of Education grants G008301207, G0087C3033, and G008630227. The opinions expressed here are those of the authors and do not reflect the views of the Department of Education.

REFERENCES

Albion, F. M., & Salzberg, C. L. (1982). The effect of self-instructions on the rate of correct addition problems with mentally retarded children. *Education and Treatment of Children, 5,* 121–131.

Arter, J. A., & Jenkins, J. R. (1979). Differential diagnosis–prescriptive teaching: A critical appraisal. *Review of Educational Research, 49,* 517–555.

Ashcraft, M. H. (1982). The development of mental arithmetic: A chronometric approach. *Developmental Review, 2,* 213–236.

Briars, D. J. (1983). An information-processing analysis of mathematical ability. In R. F. Dillon & R. R. Schmeck (Eds.), *Individual differences in cognition* (Vol. 1, pp. 181–204). New York: Academic Press.

Brophy, J., & Good, T. L. (1986). Teacher behavior and student achievement. In M. C. Wittrock (Ed.), *Handbook of research on teaching* (3rd ed.) (pp. 328–375). New York: Macmillan.

Cameron, M. I., & Robinson, V. M. J. (1980). Effects of cognitive training on academic and on-task behavior of hyperactive children. *Journal of Abnormal Child Psychology, 8,* 405–419.

Carnine, D. W. (1980). Preteaching versus concurrent teaching of the component skills of a multiplication problem-solving strategy. *Journal for Research in Mathematics Education, 11,* 375–379.

Carpenter, T. R., & Moser, J. M. (1983). The acquisition of addition and subtraction concepts. In R. Lesh & M. Landau (Eds.), *Acquisition of mathematics concepts and processes* (pp. 7–44). New York: Academic Press.

Carpenter, T. R., & Moser, J. M. (1984). The acquisition of addition and subtraction concepts in grades one through three. *Journal for Research in Mathematics Education, 15,* 179–202.

Carpenter, T. R., Moser, J. M., & Romberg, T. A. (Eds.). (1982). *Addition and subtraction: A cognitive approach.* Hillsdale, NJ: Lawrence Erlbaum.

Cullinan, D., Lloyd, J., & Epstein, M. H. (1981). Strategy training: A structured approach to arithmetic instruction. *Exceptional Education Quarterly, 2*(1), 41–49.

Davis, R. W., & Hajicek, J. O. (1985). Effects of self-instructional training on a mathematics task with severely behaviorally disordered students. *Behavioral Disorders, 10,* 275–282.

Derry, S. J., & Murphy, D. A. (1986). Designing systems that train learning ability: From theory to practice. *Review of Educational Research, 56,* 1–39.

Fink, W. T., & Carnine, D. W. (1975). Control of arithmetic errors using informational feedback and graphing. *Journal of Applied Behavior Analysis, 8,* 461. (Abstract)

Flavell, J. H. (1985). *Cognitive development* (2nd ed.). Englewood Cliffs, NJ: Prentice-Hall.

Fuson, K. C. (1982). An analysis of the counting-on solution procedure in addition. In T. P. Carpenter, J. M. Moser, & T. A. Romberg (Eds.), *Addition and subtraction: A cognitive perspective* (pp. 67–81). Hillsdale, NJ: Lawrence Erlbaum.

Ginsburg, H. P. (Ed.). (1983). *The development of mathematical thinking.* New York: Academic Press.

Good, T. L., & Grouws, D. A. (1979). The Missouri Mathematics Effectiveness Project: An experimental study in fourth-grade classrooms. *Journal of Educational Psychology, 71,* 355–362.

Grimm, J. A., Bijou, S. W., & Parsons, J. A. (1973). A problem-solving model for teaching remedial arithmetic to handicapped young children. *Journal of Abnormal Child Psychology, 1,* 26–39.

Groen, G. J., & Parkman, J. M. (1972). A chronometric analysis of simple addition. *Psychological Review, 79,* 329–343.

Hallahan, D. P., & Reeve, R. E. (1980). Selective attention and distractibility. In B. K.

Keogh (Ed.), *Advances in special education: Vol. 1. Basic constructs and theoretical orientations* (pp. 141–181). Greenwich, CT: JAI Press.

Hasazi, J. E., & Hasazi, S. E. (1972). Effects of teacher attention on digit-reversal behavior in an elementary school child. *Journal of Applied Behavior Analysis, 5,* 157–162.

Haupt, E. J., Van Kirk, M. J., & Terraciano, T. (1975). An inexpensive fading procedure to decrease errors and increase retention of number facts. In E. Ramp & G. Semb (Eds.), *Behavior analysis: Areas of research and application.* Englewood Cliffs, NJ: Prentice-Hall.

Hiebert, J. (Ed.). (1986). *Conceptual and procedural knowledge: The case of mathematics.* Hillsdale, NJ: Lawrence Erlbaum.

Houlihan, D. M., & Ginsburg, H. P. (1981). The addition methods of first- and second-grade children. *Journal for Research in Mathematics Education, 12,* 95–106.

Howell, K. W., & McCollum-Gahley, J. (1986). Monitoring instruction. *Teaching Exceptional Children, 19*(1), 47–49.

Howell, K. W., & Morehead, M. K. (1987). *Curriculum-based evaluation for special and remedial education.* Columbus, OH: Merrill.

Johnston, M. B., Whitman, T. L., & Johnson, M. (1981). Teaching addition and subtraction to mentally retarded children: A self-instructional program. *Applied Research in Mental Retardation, 1,* 141–160.

Leon, J. A., & Pepe, H. J. (1983). Self-instructional training: Cognitive-behavior modification for remediating arithmetic deficits. *Exceptional Children, 50,* 54–60.

Lesh, R., & Landau, M. (Eds.). (1983). *Acquisition of mathematics concepts and processes.* New York: Academic Press.

Lloyd, J. (1980). Academic instruction and cognitive-behavior modification: The need for attack strategy training. *Exceptional Education Quarterly, 1*(1), 53–63.

Lloyd, J. W. (1984). How should we individualize instruction—or should we? *Remedial and Special Education, 5*(1), 7–16.

Lloyd, J. W., & deBettencourt, L. J. (1982). *Academic strategy training: A manual for teachers.* Charlottesville: University of Virginia Learning Disabilities Research Institute.

Lloyd, J., Saltzman, N. J., & Kauffman, J. M. (1981). Predictable generalization in academic learning as a result of preskills and strategy training. *Learning Disability Quarterly, 4,* 203–216.

Lovitt, T. C., & Curtiss, K. A. (1968). Effects of manipulating an antecedent event on mathematics response rate. *Journal of Applied Behavior Analysis, 1,* 329–333.

Lovitt, T. C., & Hansen, C. L. (1976). The use of contingent skipping and drilling to improve oral reading and comprehension. *Journal of Learning Disabilities, 9,* 481–487.

Mayer, R. E. (1985). Mathematical ability. In R. J. Sternberg (Ed.), *Human abilities: An information-processing approach* (pp. 127–150). New York: Freeman.

Mayer, R. E., Larkin, J. H., & Kadane, J. B. (1984). A cognitive analysis of mathematical problem-solving ability. In R. J. Sternberg (Ed.), *Advances in the psychology of human intelligence* (Vol. 2, pp. 231–273). Hillsdale, NJ: Lawrence Erlbaum.

Meichenbaum, D. M., & Goodman, J. (1969). Reflection–impulsivity and verbal control of motor behavior. *Child Development, 40,* 785–797.

Meichenbaum, D., & Goodman, J. (1971). Training impulsive children to talk to themselves: A means of developing self-control. *Journal of Abnormal Psychology, 77,* 115–126.

Montague, M., & Bos, C. S. (1986). The effect of cognitive strategy training on verbal math problem solving performance of learning disabled adolescents. *Journal of Learning Disabilities, 19,* 26–33.

Paine, S. C., Carnine, D. W., White, W. A. T., & Walters, G. (1982). Effects of fading teacher presentation structure (covertization) on acquisition and maintenance of arithmetic skills. *Education and Treatment of Children, 5,* 93–107.

Parsons, J. A. (1972). The reciprocal modification of arithmetic behavior and program development. In G. Semb (Ed.), *Behavior analysis and education—1972* (pp. 185–199). Lawrence: University of Kansas Department of Human Development.

Pellegrino, J. W., & Goldman, S. R. (1987). Information processing and elementary mathematics. *Journal of Learning Disabilities, 20,* 23–32, 57.

Resnick, L. B. (1983). A developmental theory of number understanding. In H. P. Ginsburg (Ed.), *The development of mathematical thinking* (pp. 109–151). New York: Academic Press.

Resnick, L. B., & Ford, W. W. (1981). *The psychology of mathematics for instruction.* Hillsdale, NJ: Lawrence Erlbaum.

Resnick, L. B., & Neches, R. (1984). Factors affecting individual differences in learning ability. In R. J. Sternberg (Ed.), *Advances in the psychology of human intelligence* (Vol. 2, pp. 275–323). Hillsdale, NJ: Lawrence Erlbaum.

Romberg, T. A., & Carpenter, T. P. (1986). Research on teaching and learning mathematics: Two disciplines of scientific inquiry. In M. C. Wittrock (Ed.), *Handbook of research on teaching* (3rd ed.) (pp. 850–873). New York: Macmillan.

Rosenshine, B., & Stevens, R. (1986). Teaching functions. In M. C. Wittrock (Ed.), *Handbook of research on teaching* (3rd ed.) (pp. 376–391). New York: Macmillan.

Russell, R. L. (1977). Addition strategies of third grade children. *Journal of Children's Mathematical Behavior, 1*(4), 149–160.

Russell, R. L., & Ginsburg, H. P. (1984). Cognitive analysis of children's mathematics difficulties. *Cognition and Instruction, 1,* 217–244.

Schoenfeld, A. H. (1985). *Mathematical problem solving.* Orlando, FL: Academic Press.

Schoenfeld, A. H. (Ed.). (1987). *Cognitive science and mathematics education.* Hillsdale, NJ: Lawrence Erlbaum.

Schunk, D. H. (1981). Modeling and attributional effects on children's achievement: A self-efficacy analysis. *Journal of Educational Psychology, 73,* 93–105.

Schunk, D. H., & Cox, P. D. (1986). Strategy training and attributional feedback with learning disabled students. *Journal of Educational Psychology, 78,* 201–209.

Secada, W. G., Fuson, K. C., & Hall, J. W. (1983). The transition from counting-all to counting-on in addition. *Journal for Research in Mathematics Education, 14*(1), 47–57.

Siegler, R. S. (1986). *Children's thinking.* Englewood Cliffs, NJ: Prentice-Hall.

Siegler, R. S., & Robinson, M. (1982). The development of numerical understandings. In H. W. Reese & C. P. Lipsitt (Eds.), *Advances in child development and behavior* (Vol. 16, pp. 241–312). New York: Academic Press.

Siegler, R. S., & Shrager, J. (1984). Strategy choices in addition: How do children know what to do? In C. Sophian (Ed.), *Origins of cognitive skills* (pp. 229–293). Hillsdale, NJ: Lawrence Erlbaum.

Silbert, J., Carnine, D., & Stein, M. (1981). *Direct instruction mathematics.* Columbus, OH: Merrill.

Smith, D. D., & Lovitt, T. C. (1975). The use of modeling techniques to influence the acquisition of computational arithmetic skills in learning-disabled children. In

E. Ramp & G. Semb (Eds.), *Behavior analysis: Areas of research and application* (pp. 283–308). Englewood Cliffs, NJ: Prentice-Hall.

Smith, D. D., & Lovitt, T. C. (1976). The differential effects of reinforcement contingencies on arithmetic performance. *Journal of Learning Disabilities, 9,* 21–29.

Smith, D. D., Lovitt, T. C., & Kidder, J. D. (1972). Using reinforcement contingencies and teaching aids to alter subtraction performance of children with learning disabilities. In G. Semb (Ed.), *Behavior analysis and education—1972* (pp. 342–360). Lawrence: University of Kansas Department of Human Development.

Sternberg, R. J. (1984). Mechanisms of cognitive development: A componential approach. In R. J. Sternberg (Ed.), *Mechanisms of cognitive development* (pp. 163–186). New York: Freeman.

Sternberg, R. J. (1985). *Beyond IQ.* Cambridge: Cambridge University Press.

Strang, J. D., & Rourke, D. P. (1985). Arithmetic disability subtypes: The neuropsychological significance of specific arithmetical impairment in childhood. In B. P. Rourke (Ed.), *Neuropsychology of learning disabilities: Essentials of subtype analysis* (pp. 167–183). New York: Guilford Press.

Thackwray, D., Meyers, A., Schleser, R., & Cohen, R. (1985). Achieving generalization with general versus specific self-instructions: Effects on academically deficient children. *Cognitive Therapy and Research, 9,* 291–308.

Whitman, T., & Johnston, M. B. (1983). Teaching addition and subtraction with regrouping to educable mentally retarded children: A group self-instructional training program. *Behavior Therapy, 14,* 127–143.

Wrigley, J. (1958). The factorial nature of ability in elementary mathematics. *British Journal of Educational Psychology, 28,* 61–78.

13
SELF-CONTROL TRAINING WITH HYPERACTIVE AND IMPULSIVE CHILDREN

SYDNEY S. ZENTALL
Purdue University

The purpose of this chapter is to provide an explanation for the self-control problems of hyperactive children that can be used in an interpretation of the cognitive treatment literature. I have proposed in this review that hyperactive children focus their attention on external stimuli at the cost of attention directed internally to monitor and direct behavioral response (meta-attention, metacognition, and self-control). I also suggest that the cognitive-process approach should be successful in the remediation of these difficulties to the extent that attention can be focused to attributes of the self (e.g., to internal processing and behavioral manifestations) and to behavioral standards using the directing functions of language.

The criteria that we use to identify children with this disorder are defined by the American Psychiatric Association's (1980) *Diagnostic and Statistical Manual of Mental Disorders* (3rd edition) (DSM-III), revised in 1987 to DSM-III-R, which places hyperactivity within the category of attention-deficit hyperactivity disorder (ADHD). This basis for identification of ADHD has been selected because it is widely accepted in the psychiatric, psychological, and education fields. Included in this chapter is a brief description of some of the measures that are used in an assessment of the associated behavior problems of ADHD (activity, impulsivity, attentional problems, and social problems). The measurement criteria for self-control disorders and the overlap between ADHD and self-control disorders are presented. This provides the basis for an examination of the theoretical and methodological approaches in the treatment of the self-control disorders of ADHD children, and for the identification of those factors that contribute to treatment success specifically with this population.

OVERVIEW OF ATTENTION DEFICIT WITH HYPERACTIVITY DISORDER (ADHD)

The primary characteristics of hyperactivity are excessive verbal and motor activity as well as impulsivity and an inability to sustain attention to activities or tasks for an equivalent length of time to that of their peers. DSM-III-R divides these three symptom classes into 14 behavioral indicators, 8 of which must be observed at a rate that is "considerably more than" that observed for other children of the "same mental age."

Identification and Assessment

Prior to DSM-III-R, the diagnosis of hyperactivity was operationalized through teacher rating scales (e.g., the 10-item Abbreviated Teacher Questionnaire, ATQ; Conners, 1973). Teacher ratings have excellent intra- and inter-rater reliability as well as concurrent and predictive validity (Zentall, 1980; Zentall & Barack, 1979; Zentall, Gohs, & Culatta, 1983). Norms are available for the 28-item Revised Conners Teacher Rating Scale (TRS) for boys and girls separately, 3 to 17 years of age (Goyette, Conners, & Ulrich, 1978). There are also factor scales for Conduct Problems, Inattention-Passivity, and Hyperactivity. Even though there is evidence suggesting that each child selected using the hyperactivity rating scales (ATQ) did not necessarily have attentional problems (Ullmann, Sleator, & Sprague, 1985), it has been demonstrated that children aggregated statistically on this basis differ from normal children in off-task attention (e.g., Zentall & Kruczek, 1988; Zentall & Shaw, 1980) and in error scores on attentional tasks (e.g., Zentall, 1985).

In an attempt to select a more homogeneous group of children to study, researchers used additional scales (e.g., the SNAP checklist; Pelham & Bender, 1982) derived specifically from DSM-III criteria that detailed attention, activity, and impulsivity characteristics. A 92% overlap between judgments on the more comprehensive rated criteria of the SNAP and hyperactivity rating scales (e.g., the ATQ), which include only one or two items on attention and impulsivity problems, indicates comparability of assessment (Pelham & Bender, 1982). With the revision in 1987 to DSM-III-R, I have adapted the $SNAP_z$ from the SNAP to include the 14 new behavioral criteria. In Table 13-1, the 14 criteria are numbered in boldfaced type. The SNAP scale already had 12 of the criteria. SNAP item #5 was subsequently replaced with DSM-III-R #9, and SNAP item #13 was extended to include criterion item #13. Additional modifications were made in the rating standard (against mental age comparisons) and in the rating point scale (3-point scale instead of the original 5) to force the rater to make clinical judgments of severity (i.e., significantly outside the normal range of behavior). Severity levels (mild, moderate, and severe) are also part of the ADHD diagnosis. I have operationalized mild levels by 8 to 10 criteria, moderate by 10 to 12, and severe by 12 to 14. Additionally, both social and academic dysfunction are now part of the severity criteria. Social dysfunc-

TABLE 13-1. SNAP$_z$

Child's name _____ Age _____ Sex _____ Race _____

Teacher's name _____ LD: yes no

_____ # months child has shown this behavior pattern compared to children of same mental age.

	Considerably Less Than	About the Same As	Considerably More Than
1. Excessive running or climbing			
2. Difficulty sitting still or excessive fidgeting			
3. Difficulty staying seated			
4. Talks excessively			
5. Has difficulty playing quietly			
6. Often fails to finish things or follow through			
7. Often doesn't seem to listen			
8. Easily distracted			
9. Difficulty sticking to an activity or task			
10. Difficulty concentrating on school work or other tasks requiring sustained attention			
11. Often acts before thinking			
12. Excessive shifting from one activity to another			
13. Has difficulty organizing work, often loses things necessary for activities at school or home (e.g., toys, pencils, books, assignments)			
14. Needs a lot of supervision			
15. Calling out in class or blurting out answers			
16. Difficulty waiting for turn in games or group situations			
17. Fights, hits, punches, etc.			
18. Is disliked by other children			
19. Frequently interrupts other children's activities			
20. Bossy; always telling other children what to do			
21. Teases or calls other children names			
22. Refuses to participate in group activities			
23. Loses temper often and easily			
24. Poor school work—has difficulty participating successfully in school work; has some specific learning difficulties or blocks (e.g., poor in arithmetic, poor in reading.)			
25. Poor visual–motor coordination (e.g., awkward gestures, messy handwriting, poor in drawing.)			

307

tion is assessed at present by SNAP items 17 to 23. Mild social dysfunction would include one item rated "considerably more than," moderate two items, and severe three. (We have previously found that teacher-rated items of social dysfunction correlate with peer sociometric ratings, $r(48) = -69$, $p < .001$; Madan-Swain & Zentall, 1988). Academic performance is assessed by the new item, #24, which we have found in previous research (Zentall, 1986b) to be a good indication of academic dysfunction. That is, children with teacher-rated performance problems are significantly more likely to be receiving special-education services than are children with low ratings; even though IQ does not differentiate between hyperactive children who receive services and those who do not.

The identification criteria are more detailed in DSM-III-R. Furthermore, differentiation among the primary characteristics has not been retained. In light of the fact that children are often identified or assessed in the treatment literature using only one subset of these characteristics, it may be important to determine the overlap among these characteristics that justifies the aggregating of behavioral indicators into one list rather than subdividing the characteristics of activity, attention, and impulsivity.

Activity

Of the three primary problems, activity is the easiest to isolate and examine empirically. Hyperactive youngsters identified by rating scales are significantly more active and talkative, as recorded by objective measures and by "blind" observers, than were their classmates (e.g., Zentall, 1980; Zentall et al., 1983). Activity differences appear stable from preschool through elementary school (Porrino et al., 1983; and for review see Zentall, 1986a). However, the gross motor activity of younger hyperactive children (out-of-seat) (Campbell, Szumowski, Ewing, Gluck, & Breaux, 1982; Schleifer et al., 1975) may be replaced with restlessness by mid-junior high (see Safer & Allen, 1976, pp. 21–22). In a study of psychiatric patients 1 to 17 years of age, Dienske, DeJonge, and Sanders-Woudstra (1985) reported that excessive activity characterized only the diagnostic categories ADD, ADD-H, and children with IQs below 71, but not other child psychiatric disorders. DSM-III-R has subsequently dropped the category ADD (attention-deficit disorder without hyperactivity) because ADD represented infrequent clinical referrals. DSM-III-R lists ADD as a separate category, undifferentiated attention-deficit disorder, which awaits future research to establish its validity.

Attention Disorders

Hyperactive children have been characterized as having difficulty coming to attention, sustaining attention, and searching a complex field (Alabiso, 1972; Douglas & Peters, 1979). The ability to come to attention and maintain attentional responses to stimuli depends on the attentional-demand characteristics of the stimuli (e.g., intensity, complexity, meaningfulness, novelty) (Berlyne, 1960) and the child's readiness to respond and maintain responsivity (i.e., alertness or arousability). Problems in coming to attention are typically assessed by physiological response to external physical stimuli. Several reports that ADHD children and LD children demonstrate lower autonomic responsivity and smaller evoked responses to critical stimuli in discrimination, reaction time, and vigilance tasks (e.g., Dainer et al., 1981; Prichep, Sutton, & Hakerem, 1976), which indicate difficulty coming to attention. Additionally, hyperactive children react to a clear physical stimulus (e.g., a light) more slowly than normal children do (Douglas & Peters, 1979; Rosenthal & Allen, 1978).

"Sustained attention" refers to the ability to maintain responsivity to simple repetitive task demands during later trials and time periods. Problems in sustained attention can be inferred from error scores on vigilance tasks. Vigilance tasks require a response to one infrequently occurring discriminative letter stimulus ("AX") among hundreds of presentations of only 12 letters. The relevant stimulus appears on random trials in one constant physical location. This task is repetitive and boring (Rugel, Cheatam, & Mitchell, 1978), especially for hyperactive children, who demonstrate attentional preferences for novel stimuli (for review, see Zentall & Gohs, 1984). Hyperactive children perform less well on vigilance tasks than their classmates, especially during later trials (see Weiss, Minde, Werry, Douglas, & Nemeth, 1971; Zentall, 1986b). For very young children, span and breadth of attentional field are demonstrated by the number of activity or toy changes or by failure to finish activities. Researchers have observed that young hyperactive children engaged in more short-duration activities (20 seconds or less), fewer long-duration activities (2 minutes or longer) (Campbell et al., 1982), and more activity changes (Schleifer et al., 1975).

Selective attention, the third type of attention, has been described as the manner in which "attention is distributed among elements of a stimulus field" (Berlyne, 1960, p. 29). The research conducted on selective attention in LD children is based largely on Hagen's (1967) modification of Maccoby and Hagen's (1965) central incidental learning task. Skill deficits in selective attention have been demonstrated for LD children using this task (e.g., Hallahan & Reeve, 1980). However, Hagen's task actually confounds the constructs of selective attention and memory such that conclusions about selective attention are not totally justified (e.g., Copeland & Wisniewski, 1981). Nevertheless, evidence has accumulated to suggest that LD and ADHD children are more likely than normal controls to exhibit a diffuse or wide focus of selective attention (e.g., Patton, Routh, & Offenbach, 1981; Radosh & Gittelman, 1981; Steinkamp, 1980). That is, they are more likely than are controls to attend to incidental task stimuli and extratask stimuli. The extent to which this wide focus of attention to noncritical stimuli will impede performance appears to depend on whether there is sufficient time for the child to attend to multiple components of both the task and the environment (Ceci & Tishman, 1984). During fast-paced tasks performance may be disrupted.

Impulsivity

Impulsivity, like sustained attention, also refers to a temporal dimension of performance, in this case to fast and inaccurate responding. Impulsivity is typically assessed on a preschool, school-age, or adult form of a task called the Matching Familiar Figures Test (MFFT) (Kagan, Rosman, Day, Albert, & Phillips, 1964). On this task, children are required to match a sample picture (e.g., a giraffe) with one of four to six variants of the picture (i.e., where there are alternative choices and it is unclear which is correct). Hyperactive children typically perform less well on this task than comparison children (Homatidis & Konstantareas, 1981; Zentall & Dwyer, in press). Similar differences are documented for young hyperactive children on related measures of impulsivity, such as early childhood versions of the Matching Familiar Figures Test, Draw a Line Slowly Test, Cookie Delay Task, and various maze tasks that require delay or inhibition of a response (Campbell et al., 1982; Cohen et al., 1981; Schleifer et al., 1975). Impulsivity can also be assessed in children's verbal behavior. These data indicate that hyperactive children use more exclamatory, commanding, and interrupting statements, as well as more questions and comments unrelated to the tasks they are performing (Zentall, 1984, 1987; Zentall et al., 1983).

Social Problems and Aggression

Most recently there has been considerable interest in the social responses of hyperactive children. This may be due to recent documentation indicating that much of their social behavior is associated with conduct disorders and peer rejection (Lahey, Green, & Forehand, 1980; Madan-Swain & Zentall, 1988; Sandberg, Wieselberg, & Shaffer, 1980). Our own work suggests that approximately 60% of hyperactive children are rejected by their peers, which we found was associated with high rates of negative and nontask behavior and with the absence of positive physical contacts (Madan-Swain & Zentall, 1988).

Aggression was not included as a characteristic in the earlier DSM-III criteria. But with an increased emphasis on the importance of social behavior, DSM-III-R included social dysfunction as an indication of severity. Our research and that of others has documented overall differences between ADHD and normal children in teacher-rated aggression or conduct disorders as assessed by subscales—for example, on the SNAP (Zentall & Meyer, 1987) or on the Conners Parent Questionnaire (Cunningham, Siegel, & Offord, 1985). The relative contribution of the primary characteristics (activity, inattention, and impulsivity) or of the secondary characteristics (aggression or noncompliance) to the self-control and social problems of hyperactive or ADHD children are, as yet, unknown.

Overlapping Constructs

DSM-III-R may have eliminated the subgrouping by major characteristics because there is so much behavioral confluence among the primary and secondary characteristics that distinctions do not appear to be meaningful. For example, attention span can be inferred from activity shifts (e.g., out-of-seat and up-and-down) (for review, see Zentall, 1985). Dienske *et al.* (1985) have suggested that whereas "activity" reflects the quantitative dimension of behavior, "inattention" refers to a qualitative dimension specifically in response to task or social stimuli.

It has also been observed that criterion scoring on one characteristic may predict behavioral deviance in a different characteristic. That is, children who are accurate on the MFFT (impulsivity measure) are independently rated by their teachers as demonstrating better attention under a variety of academic and play conditions than are inaccurate children (Ault, Crawford, & Jeffrey, 1972). There is even some indication of considerable overlap between attentional and impulsivity assessment tests. Specifically, both tasks require sustaining attention to repeated presentations of similar task stimuli (to approximately 600 presentations of 12 letters or to almost identical details in multiple sets of four to six variants of a figure). In an examination and review of the overlap between attention and impulsivity, Zentall and Dwyer (in press) concluded that impulsivity differs from sustained attention only in its requirement to deploy attention systematically in a discrimination task.

Furthermore, aggression and attention appear to be overlapping constructs. Madan-Swain and Zentall (1988) documented poorer attentional ratings for the rejected hyperactive children than for the accepted hyperactive children, who in turn had poorer attentional ratings than their normal classmates. Similar reports of inattention in children with conduct disorders have been documented (Dienske *et al.*, 1985). In addition to the overlap between aggression and inattention, there is some evidence with nursery school–aged children to suggest that high levels of activity predict inappropriate peer relations. For example, noncompliance is positively correlated with activity (Dienske *et al.*, 1985), and a high level of activity at an early age in clinical and nonclinical populations is associated with coercive peer interactions (specifically, with noncompliance, aggression, and peer domination; for review, see Madan-Swain & Zentall, 1988).

I would argue that the primary and secondary characteristics are related theoretically, thus explaining their behavioral and performance overlap. We have presented evidence that these behaviors may be functional in the moderation of arousal (Zentall, 1975; Zentall & Zentall, 1983). The optimal stimulation theory (e.g., Berlyne, 1960) proposes that all organisms will work to maintain optimal levels of stimulation or central arousal through instrumental responses. An assumption of the theory is that when there is an imbalance of stimulation for an organism (possibly due to deviations in stimulus thresholds or to environmental load or deprivation), activity serves as a homeostatic regulator of that stimulation. That is, an organism will initiate stimulation-seeking activity when there is insufficient stimulation. We have applied this theory to hyperactive children (Zentall, 1975) and extended it by proposing that verbal activity, attentional changes, attraction to environmental novelty, response variability, failure to inhibit responses (impulsivity), and provocative social responses (aggression) also function to increase or maintain adequate levels of stimulation (for review, see Zentall & Zentall, 1983). This definitional and theoretical overlap will provide some of the basis for understanding the efficacy of treatments for self-control problems.

In sum, ADHD can be identified using scales derived from DSM-III-R criteria, such as the $SNAP_2$–DSM-III-R, which was adapted for our research purposes. Children who are identified by this procedure will be equivalent to those identified by DSM-III as ADD-H and to those originally diagnosed as hyperactive using rating scales. Not only is there considerable overlap historically in the characteristics and tasks that define the disorder, but there is also evidence to indicate that the predominant characteristics have common bioregulatory functions. Only the severity criteria that have been added by DSM-III-R potentially represent a new basis for subgrouping these children.

Identification of Self-Control Disorders

Self-Control Ratings

An examination of the measures used to identify self-control disorders and monitor response to treatment also indicates considerable overlap with those measures previously discussed that assess ADHD. The major instrument used to identify self-control disorders is the Behavior Rating Scale (BRS), also called the Kendall Self-Control Rating Scale (SCRS), developed by Kendall and Wilcox (1979). Norms are available for boys and girls ages 3 to 6. The rating scale has excellent test–retest reliability and convergent validity with children's latency performance on the MFFT, and a sum score of behavioral observations including attentional, verbal, and physical off-task, out-of-seat, and interruptions (Kendall & Wilcox, 1979). Of the 33 items, 12 assess the ability to wait and act cautiously (impulsivity); 9 assess the ability to persist or follow through on self-initiated or adult-initiated activities or instructions (attention span); 8 assess the ability to inhibit aggression in favor of more cooperative and compliant responses (aggression/compliance); and 4 assess the ability to modulate activity, affect, or response variability (hyperactivity). Thus it appears that this scale also assesses the primary and secondary social characteristics of ADHD. The fact that these characteristics intercorrelate into only one factor, accounting for 72% of the variance (Kendall & Wilcox, 1979), supports DSM-III-R in its designation of a single list of characteristics rather than subgrouping characteristics.

An adaptation of the SCRS has been developed by Humphrey (1982) entitled the Teacher's Self-Control Rating Scale (TSCRS), which has been shortened to 15 items and is rated on a 5-point instead of a 7-point scale. A factor analysis yielded two factors, one of which was related to cognitive self-attributes (e.g., plans ahead, pays attention, makes careless mistakes) and the other to an interpersonal dimension of disruptiveness, excessive talking, and the like. This scale demonstrated very good test–retest reliability, with moderate correlations with observations of goal-directed independent work and with some evidence of construct validity. In this study an additional scale called the Children's Perceived Self-Control Scale (CPSCS) was also examined under the assumption that children who expect to be successful persist longer on difficult tasks. The scale was not as strong psychometrically as the TSCRS.

An alternative eight-item self-rating scale, developed by Fagen and Long (1979) and entitled the Student Rating of Self-Control (SRSC), assesses behavior that appears to be closer to what is taught in the cognitive approach to self-control training (attention persistence, memory, anticipating consequences, verbalizing feelings, generating alternative social responses, inhibiting action, and coping with error). Reliability and validity data are not available, however, to assess the potential of this scale in identifying children with self-control problems or in monitoring their responses to treatment.

Finally, global ratings of self-control have been effectively used to assess treatments with psychostimulant medication and verbal training of coping responses to anger provocations (Hinshaw, Henker, & Whalen, 1984b). Ratings are made on a scale from one (very poor self-control; e.g., physical retaliation, screaming) to 5 (exemplary self-control; e.g., no evidence of angry response plus evidence of an overt plan to promote self-control). An additional rating from 1 to 4 on response intensity was highly correlated with these self-control global ratings.

Self-Control Tasks

In addition to rating scales, there are numerous laboratory tasks used to assess self-control (for review see Craighead, Wilcoxon-Craighead, & Meyers, 1978). These tasks variously assess voluntary delay of gratification, resistance to temptation, and tolerance of an immediate unpleasant experience in anticipation of long-term gain. According to Meichenbaum (1979), a common theme in each of these self-control tasks is an attempt to place the child in a conflict situation, such that compliance with natural inclinations represents less self-control.

Summary

There appears to be considerable overlap among the defining characteristics of ADHD children and of self-control disorders. The practical implications of such overlap are that children identified by an ADHD rating scale would probably also be identified on a self-control rating scale. Given this probability, it would appear useful to use the DSM-III-R criteria to identify the children but then to use a self-control scale or task to pre- and postassess children's responses to treatment. We have previously documented that the second of two similar or identical scales administered within a relatively short interval of time (e.g., one month) will provide an excellent pretreatment measure, whereas the first is ideal for identification (Zentall & Barack, 1979). Furthermore, DSM-III-R provides more power in identification and therefore in prediction as a result of the addition of the severity criterion to the diagnosis. Severity is defined by an assessment of academic and social dysfunction, which is not assessed in self-control scales, and by the number of behavioral characteristics. Those ADHD children with greater academic and social dysfunction would appear to be most suitable for cognitive-behavioral interventions, whereas those children who manifest primarily behavioral problems may be best treated with environmental or biochemical stimulants. This recommendation is based on evidence suggesting that environmental stimulants (e.g., color) can be reliably used to decrease behavioral disruption and increase sustained attention to a task (e.g., Zentall, 1986b) but has not yet been demonstrated as effective in teaching children to deploy attention systematically to relevant features of a task. Similarly, Douglas, Barr, O'Neil, and Britton (1986) have concluded that psychostimulant medication cannot be expected to improve complex task performance, even though the primary deficits of failure to sustain attention and inhibit responses have been altered, unless remedial training is provided for the secondary academic, social, or cognitive deficits.

TREATMENT APPROACHES FOR SELF-CONTROL

Self-control problems are typified by failure (1) to modulate response intensity, (2) to time responses appropriately, and (3) to inhibit high-probability responses that promise immediate gratification in favor of more appropriate low-probability responses that promise long-term gains. Self-control may be defined broadly (i.e., across the different methodological approaches) as the voluntary regulation of behavior in relation to a standard or rule (Carver & Scheier, 1981). The voluntary nature of self-control differentiates it from the involuntary automatic control typically seen in physiological mechanisms such as the self-regulation of biophysical and biochemical phenomena (e.g., heart rate).

Meichenbaum (1977) has argued that to bring about self-control, a sequential mediating process must be established beginning with the individual becoming an observer of his or her own behavior. Self-control requires an awareness of: (1) the nonregulated behavior, (2) a conflict of the nonregulated behavior with a behavioral standard, and (3) self-controlling responses. Karoly (1977) emphasizes the need for a recognition of conflict: "Self-control begins with the recognition of a conflict, and is maintained by the persistent use of controlling mechanisms under stress" (p. 211). A conflict may be demonstrated, for example, in the need to inhibit a high-probability response (e.g., playing) in favor of a lower probability response (e.g., studying).

The timing of responses also appears crucial to self-control. Inappropriately timed responses (i.e., too fast in response to eliciting stimuli) are, as we have discussed, often classified as impulsive, especially when inadequate delay leads to social and academic errors. Alternatively, timing errors may reflect failure to sustain a response (i.e., inadequate response persistence), as reported for attention-disordered children. In addition to problems of timing are problems in the modulation of response intensity. "Intensity" refers to the excessive magnitude and frequency of verbal, motor, or affective responses (i.e., hyperactive or conduct-disordered children).

Bringing an activity under self-control requires more than an initial awareness; it requires the production of self-controlling responses. These controlling responses are defined as responses, not under immediate external control, that are incompatible with at least some element in the behavioral chain of the nonregulated behavior. Thus, for impulsive children, self-controlling responses must facilitate inhibition of a response (e.g., blurting out answers) until the social conditions and timing are more appropriate (e.g., turn-taking). For attention-disordered children, self-controlling responses must be used to ensure continued effort in boring or difficult situations.

Teaching self-awareness and self-controlling responses are the major tasks for both the operant and the cognitive approach to self-control training. These two approaches to training are detailed next so that theoretical and procedural comparisons can be made. The assumptions and treatment procedures provide the background against which to analyze factors that contribute to treatment success.

The Operant Skills Approach

Although it is relatively easy to define self-control and give examples of self-control problems as they would be seen in the populations under review, it is more difficult to explain these problems in such a way that treatments can be derived and explanations can be subsequently tested. Explanations provided by the operant approach go beyond our earliest conceptualization of self-control as will power. Prior to a conceptualization of *self*-control, the operant literature in the early 1960s focused on external control and documented that discrete disordered behavior could be brought under the control of teachers or clinicians. Treatments were directed to increasing response delay through the use of reinforcement, and decreasing response frequency or intensity through externally administered punishment or through differential reinforcement of alternative or low-rate responses.

Because of the reliability of these externally directed procedures in producing behavioral change, the use of operant techniques with atypical populations was widely endorsed and subsequently provided the basis for the majority of educational programs. By the end of the decade, however, it became clear that improved behavior typically reverted back to disturbed levels when treatment was withdrawn, that improvements did not generalize to different situations, and that academic learning did not improve simply because inappropriate classroom behavior was reduced (for review, see Friedling & O'Leary, 1979). Furthermore, in an effort to control behavior that was assumed to be incompatible with learning, the operant methodology encouraged some educators to create unnecessarily regimented classrooms, which promoted student passivity (Winett & Winkler, 1972). Specifically for hyperactive children, there is evidence as well that an attractive reinforcer can draw hyperactive children off task and that hyperactive children demonstrate an inconsistent response to consequences (for review, see Zentall & Zentall, 1983).

These problems, especially those associated with poor maintenance of behavioral change, led behaviorist investigators away from external control to self-control. The change was designed to encourage children to take responsibility for their own behavior and become active participants in the behavior change program. By the early 1970s, it seemed clear that the best behavioral maintenance system would be a self-control system (Graziano, 1975). Specifically, the operant approach describes self-control as a learned set of responses or acquired skills in manipulating antecedent stimuli and consequent events. In essence, self-control is self-behavior modification, but instead of the teacher controlling antecedent discriminative stimuli, the child is taught self-cueing; and instead of the teacher arranging external consequences, the child is taught self-reinforcement and self-punishment. With this change from external to self-control, it became possible to use not only observable behavior but also internal events (e.g., expectations, self-statements, images) as the antecedent cues and targets of self-administered consequences. Thus, both internal and external behavior were the targets of treatment. Examples of self-controlling responses derived from this definition include individual efforts to alter non-regulated responses (sleeping late) through a manipulation of antecedent stimuli, such as alarm clocks and self-statements ("get up") (Skinner, 1953).

Although there were high expectations for improving behavioral maintenance through self-control as defined by the operant methodology, an examination of the effectiveness of external versus self-control indicates that self-reinforcement is equivalent or only somewhat superior in effectiveness to externally delivered reinforcement (Craighead et al., 1978; Marholin, Siegel, & Phillips, 1977). The equivalence may be attributed in part to the fact that most self-control techniques use external reinforcement prior to self-reinforcement, thereby confounding conditioned reinforcers (e.g., teacher attention) with self-reinforcement.

The failure of the operant skills approach in effecting long-term social, behavioral, or academic change has led to a more process-oriented approach. It was hoped that the cognitively regulated approach would be less situation-specific in its effects.

The Cognitive-Process Approach

In contrast to the operant approach and its clear conceptualization of self-control as learned skills, cognitive self-control applications are less explicit in their conceptual underpinnings. The self-control problem is thought to be cognitive, but "the exact nature of the underlying cognitive deficit eludes us" (Kendall, 1981, p. 83). The way self-control is conceptualized should determine how it is studied and subsequently taught. Most of the literature in this area, however, suggests that the opposite is true—that the practical problems and successes in teaching self-control determine the way it is conceptualized (Meichenbaum, 1979). Thus, an understanding of self-control problems from this perspective is derived from an analysis of the cognitive-process approach to treatment.

A number of treatment components are common to the different applications of this approach. Some of these components have been passed down from the operant methodology (e.g., self-reinforcement, self-monitoring). Additional components (e.g., modeling) have been derived from social learning theory (e.g., Bandura & Walters, 1963) and from the verbal mediation hypotheses of Soviet psychologists (Luria, 1961; Vygotsky, 1962). Extrapolations we have made from these components and from self-monitoring and self-instruction, to be described, indicate that self-control problems could be attributed to attentional, strategy, and verbal production deficits.

Treatment Components

Self-monitoring   This is a process by which a child becomes aware of unregulated behavior and of the cues that precipitate that behavior. The child is taught to assess whether he or she is exhibiting the behavior. The steps are (1) defining the target behavior for the child, (2) teaching the child how to record instances of the presence or absence of the behavior on a tally sheet at a time signaled by a tape recorder, (3) modeling the use of the signal and tallying procedure, and (4) having the child repeat the definitions and instructions (e.g., Hallahan & Sapona, 1983).

Self-instruction   This is a process by which a child attempts to bring a nonregulated behavior under self-control through *standard setting* and the use of verbal strategies that describe these standards, as well as to provide an analysis of performance in relation to the standards (*self-evaluation*). Training programs generally include (1) the use of a cognitive model who overtly verbalizes strategies and (2) a gradual fading program in which the child acquires the modeled strategies (Craighead *et al.*, 1978). An excellent elaboration of a self-control program is provided by Kendall (1981, pp. 59–60).

In an examination of the foregoing components, it is apparent that self-monitoring involves focusing the child's attention to a target behavior and its contiguity with environmental cues, and maintaining that attention over time. The second component (self-instruction) focuses the child's attention to a standard and to the target behavior in an attempt to match the standard. The self-instructional component also focuses on the decision-making strategies required to bring the target behavior in line with standards of performance accuracy. Decision-making strategies are particularly important during the performance of tasks that are novel or complex and hence provide greater response latitude.

Both self-monitoring and self-instruction, as components of the cognitive-process approach, can be differentiated from the operant approach by an emphasis on directing the child's attention via language to aspects of the self (Craighead et al., 1978). Both approaches may target within-person variables (attitudes, images, expectations). The operant approach to self-control may apply behavior modification principles (e.g., shaping, positive and negative reinforcement, extinction) to these within-person variables or to their cue determinants (Thoresen & Coates, 1986). In this approach, it is the rearrangement of cues and contingencies that effects behavioral change. The process approach, however, emphasizes self-attention (meta-attention, metacognition, "metabehavior") and strategy use as a means of accomplishing self-control. Thus, internal behavior is not the target or "object" of control but, rather, the "subject" of control. In this approach, it is the arrangement and use of internally directed cognitive and affective strategies that effect behavioral change. However, "from a practical (in contrast to a theoretical) viewpoint, it makes little sense merely to pit CBT programs against those based on traditional behavior therapy. Their elements commingle so naturally that one rarely finds an effective treatment protocol that does not include components of each" (Whalen, Henker, & Hinshaw, 1985, p. 405).

Treatment Factors

Verbal mediation   Attention is directed to critical components of the task or setting, the standard, one's own behavior, cognitive strategies, and attentional processes by means of language. The examiner or teacher verbally models approaches for problem definition, strategy selection, focusing attention, and reinforcement (Kendall, 1981). The child is taught to imitate these attention-directing and response-guiding verbalizations at successively reduced volumes until eventually the child whispers and then subvocalizes responses (i.e., from overt to covert verbal responses). These techniques may be taught using a "mastery model," who demonstrates ideal performance, or a "coping model," who occasionally makes mistakes but successfully corrects errors and copes with failure (Kendall, 1981).

The assumption behind language as a mediator of behavioral control is derived from Soviet psychology, wherein thinking is described as a product of social activity that was initially shared by two people (i.e., originated in conversation) and, later on in development, became internalized within one person. The Soviet psychologists Luria (1961) and Vygotsky (1962) proposed a developmental theory to explain how the initiation and inhibition of voluntary motor responses are initially controlled by parental verbal statements. The child imitates this control and, in the second stage, learns to initiate his or her own actions through similar overt speech and still later, to inhibit action. It is only in the third stage that this overt speech "folds up" and, first passing through a stage of whispered speech, becomes inner or covert speech. As covert speech, however, it continues to play the role of behavioral regulator.

It has been demonstrated that overt self-speech increases as a function of task difficulty (Vygotsky, 1962) and that the manifestation of self-speech is related to improvements in memory and performance for adults as well as for children (see Copeland, 1981; Kendall & Finch, 1979). The controlling aspects of language over social behavior have also been demonstrated empirically. For example, Combs and Slaby (1977) reported that a group of schoolchildren trained to speak aggressive words emitted stronger aggressive and fewer altruistic responses than did the group of children trained with neutral words, whereas those children trained with helpful words used more altruistic and fewer aggressive responses. Luria expanded the hypothesized controlling functions of language to include not only motor response but also cognitive and perceptual processes (i.e., planning and attention regulation).

Because of the range of control possible, Luria proposed that the incorporation of speech in planning for tasks had particular importance for hyperactive children. That is, speech could facilitate the cognitive organization of their activities and limit their immature "talkativity." A decrease in talkativity would also reduce their opportunities for disruption of goal-directed behavior (Luria, 1961). An inference of Luria's was that the verbalizations produced by hyperactive children are not self-controlling. That hyperactive children do not produce self-controlling verbalizations indicates that they are "production-deficient" but not that the self-controlling verbalizations that they do produce fail to alter their behavioral response (i.e., a "mediational deficit"; see Reese, 1962).

Related literature with aggressive boys provides some support for a mediational-deficiency hypothesis. Camp (1977) found that aggressive boys had adequate verbal production skills (vocabulary development and use of overt self-guiding speech). However, although aggressive boys demonstrated the ability to inhibit responses, they did so only under an overt self-regulation condition and not under a covert condition, which involved whispering "slower" during a finger-tapping task. The extent to which hyperactive children may be similarly deficient is reviewed next.

Verbal production deficits   ADHD children are more talkative than their peers in classroom settings (e.g., Whalen *et al.*, 1978; Zentall, 1980), in task settings with adult examiners (Copeland & Weissbrod, 1978; Zentall *et al.*, 1983), with peers (Madan-Swain & Zentall, 1988), and even in solitary play or task settings (Copeland, 1979; Cunningham *et al.*, 1985). Similarly, aggressive boys talk a great deal more than normal boys, and their verbalizations are less mature ("word play and outer-directed speech") (Camp, 1977). From an assessment of the conditions that set the occasion for the excessive talking of hyperactive children, it appears that they talk more than their peers in contexts that do not specifically elicit talking (e.g., during transitions and nonverbal tasks) but talk less than their classmates when they are individually asked to talk (i.e., to tell stories; Ludlow, Rapoport, Bassich, & Mikkelsen, 1980; Zentall, in press) or when asked to respond to requests or questions (Dienske et al., 1985).

It is not clear how commenting on nonverbal tasks was used by hyperactive children (in other words, whether it helped to guide attention and performance or was used to maintain environmental contact and express affect). Mead (1934, cited by Copeland, 1983, p. 247) suggested that children learn about their own behavior by talking about it, even when they are alone. Initially children describe their own activities to themselves; later they provide both sides of dialogues, and finally they externalize only the self-guiding parts of dialogues. In addition to this early phase of self-descriptive speech, which we documented as differentiating hyperactive children from their peers, hyperactive children also attempted to guide their own performance somewhat more (e.g., "Wait a minute, whoa," "Now I need to . . . "). Five percent of hyperactive children's statements were self-guiding, relative to 3% for their peers, although these differences did not reach statistical significance ($p = .10$) (Zentall et al., 1983). Copeland (1979) reported that during free play hyperactive children did not differ from controls in their use of self-reinforcement and planning. However, there is some indication in the literature that the effectiveness of verbal solutions that hyperactive children apply to learning tasks drops rapidly over time or in response to failure (Rosenbaum & Baker, 1984).

Taken together, these data indicate that hyperactive children spontaneously do use verbalizations to describe and enhance the stimulus value of tasks and perhaps to evaluate their concurrent responses (e.g., repeating cues, commenting on the materials, and verbalizing their choices; Zentall et al., 1983). Because hyperactive children use self-guiding statements at least as much as and perhaps more than controls, there is no support for the premise that hyperactive children are deficient in the production of overt verbal self-controlling responses, at least in initial stages of task performance. Nor were there differences in the frequency of task-related statements (Zentall et al., 1983). However, normal children did display more inaudible mutterings than hyperactive children during task performance. Copeland (1983) described inaudible mutterings as the external manifestations of covert speech, which precedes silent inner speech. Thus, it may be that hyperactive children are developmentally delayed in the *internalization* of verbal self-control. Camp (1977) also reported that aggressive boys demonstrate an inconsistent response to covert commands but were superior to normal boys in responses to overt self-verbalizations.

The use of and better response to overt self-statements reported for hyperactive and aggressive youngsters is a parallel finding to recent data we have collected suggesting that the verbalizations of hyperactive children are tied to external, not internally represented, stimuli. That is, hyperactive children were as verbally proficient as their classmates when telling stories from picture stimuli, but less proficient in the absence of external stimuli (Zentall, in press). When they were asked to project from the past (story retelling) or into the future (story telling) their stories were production-deficient. Both of these latter conditions require directing attention to internal processing (memory, cognition, organization). And although hyperactive children can recall and reason about external stimuli as well as their classmates, they can do this only when the executive functions of metamemory and metacognition are not required (Douglas, 1980). The executive functions require "self-conscious" effort applied to analyze and characterize the task, reflect on prior related knowledge, plan an approach, and monitor progress (see Douglas, 1980).

These executive functions are also necessary in social situations. Weiss & Hechtman (1986) have documented that hyperactive children are unable to respond verbally to a described social situation as well as normal children in the absence of written alternatives or of a preexisting beginning and ending structure to their social response. Similarly, when asked to respond verbally in an open-ended format (but not when given a forced-choice task), hyperactive aggressive boys were more likely than controls to attribute hostile intentions to an ambiguous provocation of a hypothetical peer (Milich & Dodge, 1984). These findings suggest that structured alternatives or preset sequences of events normalize the social/verbal responses of hyperactive children. These alternatives and sequence cues reduce the need for organization, recall, or planning.

It is also possible that the problems hyperactive children experience with open-ended verbal tasks are attributable to differences in the type of stimuli to which hyperactive children ordinarily attend. For example, hyperactive children attend to global cues more than to detailed cues in communication and nonverbal tasks (Zelniker & Jeffrey, 1976; Zentall & Gohs, 1984). It has also been documented that hyperactive, aggressive boys recall fewer cues that are neutral (i.e., less sensational) than hostile or benevolent cues (Milich & Dodge, 1984). Differences in information perceived may influence what is recalled (in the absence of specific alternatives or cue reminders) and may form the basis for social expectations (i.e., attributional biases).

Summary In summary, the cognitive approach to training is derived from the premise that children with self-control problems do not produce internal strategies to regulate their own behavioral responses in relation to behavioral standards. Self-verbalizations are viewed as the means by which implicit social information, task information, and behavioral standards can be made explicit and by which the regulation of attention and response in relation to these standards can be accomplished. Self-control training uses language as the attentional mediator between internal and external standards and aspects of the public and private self (meta-attention, metamemory, metacognition, and behavior). Thus, the success of this methodology could be attributed to its application with children who typically fail to employ covert self-guiding verbalizations or who fail to direct attention to all of the setting cues, to behavioral standards, or to themselves and their own cognitive processing. Hyperactive children do use overt self-statements to control their behavior, but mainly in response to the immediate cues in the external environment. Furthermore, they exhibit production deficiencies only when they must respond in the absence of alternative cues or a response structure.

Thus, it would appear that self-statements that focus attention to internal events, especially those related to the past and the future, and to nonsalient cues would be useful. Because self-attention is the goal, the extent to which this model succeeds may be attributed to its emphasis on self-attention and the relationship of the past and of future planning to present performance. However, the extent to which it overemphasizes an external verbally mediated methodology or a scaffolding of external cues may also predict its failure to generalize beyond the immediate setting or task.

General Factors Contributing to Treatment Success

Cognitive-process training, based on the work of Luria and Vygotsky and applied by Bem (1967); by Palkes, Stewart, and Kahana (1968); and by Meichenbaum and Goodman (1971) has been more successful on posttest performance measures and less successful on follow-up tests or on generalization probes (Craighead et al., 1978). "Present results suggest that self-control training results in relatively short-term changes in the children's behavior, the changes typically do not endure beyond treatment termination and are not generalized beyond the situation in which the procedures are taught" (Barkley, 1981, p. 261). Examples of failure to find setting transfer include Barkley, Copeland, & Sivage's (1980) failure to document transfer from individual seatwork to group work and Varni and Henker's (1979) failure to document transfer from adult-supervised to unsupervised settings. The disadvantages summarized by Barkley include the fact that (1) external consequences are necessary to get children to maintain self-control procedures; (2) therapists have been used primarily as trainees, which has not been very cost-effective; and (3) the procedures cannot be taught to very young children.

Instructional factors   There are, however, a number of training factors that contribute to the successes of the cognitive-process approach. For example, strategy training programs are more effective than simple delay training programs in the moderation of performance accuracy (Finch, Wilkinson, Nelson, & Montgomery, 1975); and strategy training used with tasks that require sequential cognitive strategies is also more effective (Meichenbaum, 1979). Craighead et al. (1978) concluded that self-verbalizations were useful to teach children better control over responses already in their repertoire (e.g., to go slower, to review responses). This may be due to the fact that self-verbalizing itself is an additional task, which slows performance. Directing attention through verbalizations disrupts the smoothness of an ongoing behavioral chain. This deautomatization may then make it possible to alter that automatic response chain.

Additionally, it should be noted that performance that is timed or requires complex processing may be disrupted by overt and covert verbalizations (Meichenbaum, 1979). It is clear why self-verbalizations would disrupt timed performance and performance that is already at a certain level of proficiency, but it is less clear why verbal strategies do not facilitate at least the initial learning of novel or complex tasks. In initial learning trials, it would appear that there are no strategies or motor plans that would need to be deautomatized. Nevertheless, if performance disruption does occur, it could be explained by the increased stimulation and/or information load provided by self-verbalizations. It may be that, besides its attentional-focusing function, overt self-speech also provides additional stimulation that increases arousal (Smith, Malmo, & Shagass, 1977). Increased arousal improves the performance of familiar material (because familiar material is less stimulating) but disrupts the performance of novel tasks (see Eysenck, 1976). Alternatively, it may be that the informational load of the additional stimulation (e.g., complex verbal strategies), especially during the performance of auditory processing tasks, may produce information overload.

Self-instructions are more readily internalized by children if the model is viewed as effective, successful, responsive, reinforced, or enthusiastic (Copeland, 1983; Meichenbaum, 1979). Furthermore, the perceived similarity between the model and the child in age, race, and sex also appears to increase the salience of the model (standard). Alternatively, external standards can be made clearer by having students write essays defining behavior (appropriate and inappropriate to a setting) and its consequences. This is a more effective punishment condition than writing irrelevant essays (Blackwood, 1970). Similarly, Spates and Kanfer (1977) reported that self-instructional training that included criterion setting was the most significant factor in the arithmetic performance of first-graders; self-reinforcement and self-evaluation yielded no further reduction in errors. The importance of attention to the standard (model or criterion) is addressed in greater detail in a subsequent section.

Developmental and other child-specific factors   In addition to the instruction- and task-specific factors described here, there are also child-specific factors that are predictive of the success of the cognitive-process approach. For example, there is evidence that younger children respond better to specific self-instructional strategies (e.g., "I need to start at the top"), whereas older children benefit from more general strategies (e.g., "I should plan out exactly what I need to do") (Copeland, 1981, 1982). Meichenbaum (1979), however, warns against using self-instructions that are mechanical in nature. This has particular relevance for hyperactive children, for whom repetitive stimulation has been demonstrated to exacerbate behavioral problems (e.g., Zentall, 1986a, 1986b).

Intelligence is another indicator of cognitive level and, as such, also predicts the effectiveness of specific types of self-instruction. In higher IQ children, multiple strategies (i.e., both verbalizations and scanning) may be more disruptive than single strategies. This is apparently due to the fact that higher IQ children are already employing their own strategies. Lower IQ children, on the other hand, are assisted by multiple strategies (e.g., Ridberg, Parke, & Hetherington, 1971). These findings are similar to those reported in strategy training to facilitate memory. As individuals become increasingly proficient in using their own strategies, the externally imposed strategy becomes detrimental to their memory performance (Hagen, Barclay, & Schwethelm, 1982).

Because the cognitive-process approach places responsibility for control with the child, children who would accept this internal locus of control should improve more than children who believe predominantly in external control factors such as luck. In general, this hypothesis has been supported in the literature (for review, see Copeland, 1982). It is also possible, however, that cognitive training may increase children's feelings of personal control (Whalen et al., 1985).

Although there are a number of child-specific and instructional factors that interact to improve the immediate and long-term success of the approach, its potential has not been realized. Abikoff (1985), who has reviewed the efficacy of cognitive training with hyperactive children, concluded that the development of self-regulation skills has not facilitated generalization or maintenance. Karoly (1977) has summarized a number of these general problems.

> It is probably a fair characterization of the field to assert that self-control training has (1) been conducted mainly in laboratory settings, (2) employed non-clinical populations, (3) neglected individual differences and cognitive developmental variables, (4) failed to apply systematic pretreatment assessment, (5) operated under the assumption of a general skills deficiency (as opposed to possible perceptual, decisional or motivational deficiencies), (6) attempted to demonstrate the efficacy of a singular (or limited) intervention strategy, (7) focused on a narrow range of self-control responses. . . . (pp. 30–31)

Although there may be many reasons for the failure of an intervention, it is perhaps of greater theoretical interest to understand the factors that contribute to its success. From an examination of these factors, an underlying component appears to be focusing attention to aspects of the self (standards, strategies, planning, organization, behavior). Subsequently, a child must become aware of and identify with standards. An awareness of standards will produce a comparison of the self with the standard (self-evaluation), which in turn will result in the need for self-controlling responses to facilitate the match between self and standard. Treatment, then, would need to follow a similar sequence. Treatment will be described initially from a theoretical perspective and subsequently with specific methods that correspond to the sequence outlined here.

SELF-CONTROL AND SELF-ATTENTION

Self-Focus

The importance of self-attention in self-control treatment has been previously suggested by Meichenbaum (1977), who stated that an individual must initially become an observer of his or her own behavior. For many individuals, however, self-observation must be learned. Carver and Scheier (1981) have indicated that attention can be directed either internally or externally. Furthermore, as attention outward to the environment increases, attention to the self decreases. Attention to the self includes an awareness of sensory and perceptual stimuli and of conceptual schema (self-concept, strategies). Focusing attention inwardly increases awareness of the private self (thoughts, attitudes, feelings, values, cognitions). Thus, awareness of one's own behavior and cognizance of oneself as an individual are overall indicators of self-focus. Self-focus, however, can also increase extant subjective feelings of depression or anger (Carver & Scheier, 1981).

Increased attention to the self can be brought about by high physiological arousal (e.g., emotion), but it does not appear to lead to increased arousal; and it can also be produced by an audience, observer, mirror, or camera (Carver, 1979; Carver & Scheier, 1981). Meichenbaum (1979) has also suggested that fantasy, and the imagery that accompanies fantasy, can also be used to increase self-focus. The mechanism by which this may be accomplished, according to Meichenbaum, is that fantasy frees the child from the control of external stimulation, allowing attention to be directed to internal representations.

Self-focus may become too narrow when physiological arousal becomes too intense (Carver & Scheier, 1981). At these times, attention will be drawn into lower levels of the self (i.e., areas that are typically automatically regulated). This will produce behavior that is physiologically based, stereotypic, or dictated by emotion (statements indicative of such occurrences are, for example, "I lost my head"). Self-focus may thus occur at the expense of any attention to the environment.

Environmental Focus

Attention to the environment is mediated by environmental novelty and by increased information-processing demands (i.e., through rapid pacing and increased task complexity) (Carver & Scheier, 1981). Attention to the environment occurs at the relative expense of attention to the self. For example, redirecting attention to some novelty in the environment can "distract" a person's self-focus away from a physiological state (e.g., reducing pain). Attention can also be drawn away from self-standards and from internalized, dominant-culture social standards. For example, in groups, where there is a diffusion of personal responsibility, antinormative behavior and poor self-control are more readily observed (Carver & Scheier, 1981). In such contexts individuals are more impulsive in their responsiveness to external cues from the immediate environment. Although attention to the perceptually salient features of a context draws attention away from the self, an adequate response to that context requires some self-focus. For example, task performance requires attending to an external stimulus field but also requires concentration, memory, and performance regulation (i.e., self-focus). These requirements would be accomplished easily for most individuals, in that attention normally shifts back and forth between self and environment (Carver, 1979).

Standard Setting

For self-attention to lead to self-control, standards must also become salient. Focusing on the self may increase the salience of one's own attitudes as standards or of previously encoded rules. Standards can also be derived from social comparison data available in the context. Seeking out information about what others are thinking, feeling, and doing increases the salience of external standards and also increases the probability of comparisons of one's own behavior with these standards, as well as the probability of self-control. According to Carver and Scheier, there are some individuals who are more likely to be guided by personal standards, whereas others are guided by the implicit public demands of the situation. Those individuals guided by a public self-consciousness make frequent social comparisons, are aware of the impressions they make on others, and are particularly concerned about facilitating social exchanges.

Even though some individuals are naturally more attentive to personal standards and others to the requirements of the social context, Carver and Scheier have documented that an audience, especially an evaluative audience, will increase the salience of public standards and subsequently of behavioral regulation in line with public standards. Thus, experimentally manipulated self-focus can increase attention to self-defined standards or to social standards, depending on whether the public or private aspects of the self are accentuated.

Summary

Carver and Sheier have clearly documented the empirical relation between self-focus and self-control. The environmental factors that promoted this self-focus (e.g., mirrors, audiences, physiological arousal) were also documented.

In addition to a lack of self-focus, certain self-control problems may be produced by an expectancy that one is unable to match one's behavior to a standard. This results in withdrawal and negative affect (Carver, 1979). Self-control problems may also be due to inappropriate public standards (e.g., where subculture norms differ from the majority culture, as with socialized delinquents) and by inaccurate standards (e.g., social perception problems). Kendall (1981) has labeled inaccurate standards "cognitive errors." Adults with cognitive errors have "illogical interpretations of the environment, irrational beliefs about personal performance abilities, and inaccurate perceptions of everyday demands" (p. 56). Kendall considers interventions with individuals with cognitive errors to be difficult because the inaccurate thinking must first be removed. Other types of self-control problems may be due to cognitive deficits such as (1) the ability to store and represent experience to be used as internal standards of reference, (2) time perception, (3) the integration of internal with external standards, and (4) the ability to use language as a mediator between standards and behavior (Karoly, 1977).

Nevertheless, the overriding conclusion from Carver and Scheier's extensive review of research was that the relative absence of self-focus resulted in the relative absence of self-control. They do not discuss what may be responsible for individual differences in biasing the direction of attentional focus. However, the data that indicate that physiological arousal increases self-focus provide a link between the self-control model proposed by Carver and Scheier and the homeostatic model (the optimal-stimulation theory) presented earlier to explain hyperactivity, impulsivity, and attentional disorders.

We have proposed that hyperactive children have a greater need for stimulation, which they self-generate through instrumental activity and attention focused outward to environmental novelty. We have attributed their greater need for stimulation to the fact that they may be inadequately physiologically aroused. Thus, increased physiological arousal, which, according to Carver and Scheier (1981) precipitates self-focusing of attention, would occur less frequently for hyperactive children. In addition to failure to focus on their own behavior or cognitive processing, hyperactive children fail to observe the social behavior of their peers (Cunningham et al., 1985); and, when they do attend, it is selectively to salient social stimuli (e.g., hostile cues) rather than to cues that may contain more information (i.e., neutral ones) (Milich & Dodge, 1984). This would limit their exposure to appropriate external standards of comparison.

SELF-CONTROL TREATMENTS FOR ADHD CHILDREN

The specific characteristics of ADHD children that contribute to their self-control problems are a lack of self-focus, standard awareness, or standard setting, and a reliance on overt but not covert verbalizations in self-guidance. Furthermore, the overt verbalizations that they do use are tied primarily to an external-stimulus environment and are insufficiently related to internal representations, especially of the future (planning) or of the past. These ADHD-specific factors have implications for treatment that go beyond the instructional factors (e.g., task complexity, model salience) and child factors (e.g., age, IQ, locus of control) that have already been described as general moderators of treatment success. Furthermore, it may be that failure to account for these disorder-specific factors contributes to the fact that only about half of the cognitive-training studies with ADHD children yielded significant changes in some measure of social-behavioral functioning (8 of the 16 studies reviewed by Abikoff, 1985).

The following will be a selective reporting of the treatment literature. Treatment studies have been selected for their significant effects and measurement of social behaviors (e.g., activity, on-task attention, aggression) and of cognitive style (attentional and impulsive laboratory performance tasks). The methods that have been validated in the literature have been divided into (1) those that promote self- and standard awareness, such as self-monitoring, videotape playback, modeling, and cue recognition/anger inoculation, and (2) those that facilitate the development of specific verbal or motor (self-controlling) responses, such as the Turtle technique and the Think-Aloud program. The techniques have been divided in this way in an attempt to understand the contribution of attentional strategies versus response strategies, even though in practice these techniques may be combined.

Methods to Promote Self- and Standard Awareness

Self-Attention

Studies in the cognitive-training literature that propose to increase self-focus are primarily the self-monitoring and self-reinforcement studies (e.g., Barkley *et al.*, 1980; Cameron & Robinson, 1980; Varni & Henker, 1979). These studies typically present a production cue to a child at random intervals, which signals the child to attend to his or her own behavior (i.e., self-monitor). Some studies also train the matching of this behavior to a prespecified behavioral standard (i.e., a self-evaluation process). (Self-evaluation will be described further in a subsequent section.)

Visual production cues   Some of the production cues that prompt self-monitoring are visual. For example, in an early study by Palkes, Stewart, and Kahana (1968), hyperactive children were trained to verbalize "stop," "look," "listen," and "think," using four visual-aid card prompts. Following two 30-minute training sessions, children were assessed on the Porteus mazes. The experimental group made fewer impulsive errors after training than did an attention control group. The experimental group cut fewer corners, crossed over fewer lines, lifted their pencils less often, and threaded the map with fewer erratic lines than did the controls. Because these test behaviors had not been specifically taught, such findings indicated that the children had learned to perform more carefully in general.

Unfortunately, many of the visual production cues that prompt self-attention and self-control are unwanted attributes of the training setting. Such discriminative stimuli contribute to a lack of generalization to settings that do not contain these cues. For example, the use and effectiveness of self-reinforcement as a means to increase the number of academic problems attempted and number correct was dependent on trainer presence (Varni & Henker, 1979).

Nevertheless, this study and others (e.g., Cameron & Robinson, 1980) provide some support for the use of cued self-monitoring and self-reinforcement to improve children's tasks persistence (motivation or attention span) and hyperactivity ratings; whereas the use of cognitive self-instructional strategies in this study with this behavior was not supported (Varni & Henker, 1979).

A nonspecific technique to increase self-awareness and self-control through visual production cues is fantasy play (Meichenbaum, 1979). The visual cues that elicit self-dialogues include instructional toys, props, story enactments, or thematic play (Saltz, Dixon, & Johnson, 1977; Singer, 1977).

Auditory production cues Similar findings of increased task persistence or productivity and decreased misbehavior have been reported with taped signals, which signal time to self-monitor, self-record and self-reinforce on-task behavior for hyperactive children (Barkley *et al.*, 1980) and for several distractible children (Osborne, Kosiewicz, Crumley, & Lee, 1987). The fact that the changes in the Barkley *et al.* study were found only in individual work but not in group time or in the regular classroom again indicates the importance of programming production cues that are used in training into alternative settings.

Because of the prepotence of production cues for task persistence and for monitoring attention and interfering behavior over time, it may be essential to (1) train for cue generalization; (2) teach children to carry with them task persistence discriminative stimuli, such as timers or self-recording cards; or (3) teach children how to self-arrange ideal study conditions (for review, see Kurtz & Neisworth, 1976).

Emotional and cognitive production cues An alternative to these approaches to transfer training is to select naturally occurring production cues that are found across settings. For example, several studies have employed production cues that are internal to the child or are readily available in problematic social environments. These studies that focus on teaching children to recognize and define interpersonal problems and their emotional and cognitive precursors are within the domain of the social problem-solving literature (e.g., Hinshaw *et al.*, 1984b). The programmatic basis for this work was designed by Spivack and Shure (1974) for impulsive and aggressive preschoolers. Some of the program components involve recognizing when self-controlling responses will be necessary. These include recognizing the emotions of others and differentiating between the self and others. Self-awareness and awareness of others is facilitated through the use of picture cards depicting simple social situations. Children are encouraged to examine these pictures for relevant cues and emotions and to make inferences from these cues about the nature of the situation and what is required in response. Bibliotherapy is an alternative method of presenting problems useful for an examination of relevant social cues.

An analysis of the effectiveness of these techniques, specifically with hyperactive children, was accomplished by Hinshaw *et al.* (1984b) in two studies with similar findings. Study 2, which was the more definitive of the two, required that each boy identify his own visceral and cognitive signs of anger and recognize anger and threats as cues indicating the need for self-control. Each child in the experimental group also rehearsed a strategy of his own choosing. The findings were that self-awareness and strategy training increased the child's self-control and use of strategies in an anger-provoking situation (i.e., with peer taunters), whereas psychostimulant medication only reduced the intensity of their responses. It is probable that these findings would have considerable generality in that (1) the children were taught to self-monitor production cues, and (2) the strategies used were specific to each child but were also generalizable across settings.

Standard Awareness

Peer models   There are a number of studies within the cognitive literature and within the social modeling literature indicating that awareness of appropriate behavior is often sufficient for improved responding. For example, Brown (1980b, Study 1, cited in Abikoff, 1985) demonstrated improved scoring on the MFFT after the children viewed reflective peer models during task performance one month earlier. Subsequently, Brown described the use of puppets as models for planning, going slowly, and attending to details; although the effectiveness of just the modeling component of that study was not evaluated. There is evidence, however, that hyperactive children are more likely than controls to imitate video models (Copeland & Weissbrod, 1980) and that modeling is more effective than direct instruction in communicating standards (Esveldt, Dawson, & Forness, 1974). Similarly, an adventitious finding of the Hinshaw et al. (1984b) study was that a number of the children in the empathy and perspective-taking trained control group also demonstrated better self-control (i.e., only those who had the opportunity to observe a peer in the strategy-trained group demonstrate a preferred strategy).

Even though hyperactive children readily copy models, a comparison of the relative effectiveness of reflective/nonactive models with impulsive/active models demonstrated that the hyperactive-like model was more effective in facilitating imitation (choice of games, activity level) than was the slow model (Copeland & Weissbrod, 1980). The authors concluded that the fast model may have been a more attractive stimulus in terms of pace and complexity for the hyperactive children.

Videotaped self-observations   Overall, the aforementioned literature suggests that ADHD children are more likely to imitate children most like themselves. For this reason, videotaped self-observations would appear to be a useful treatment for ADHD children. Videotaped recordings of a child can be played back with feedback about appropriate/inappropriate behavior (i.e., with standards) or with the tape edited such that only appropriate behavior is depicted. For the most part, research findings have relied on single-subject methodology, and thus problems are encountered in assessing significant change, as well as in determining the generality of observed effects. Neverthe-less, video self-observation produces consistent behavioral gains when the tapes include both positive and negative instances of appropriate behavior with social feedback (Booth & Fairbank, 1983; Spiegel, 1977) and without feedback (Esveldt et al., 1974) and when the tapes are edited with only positive behav-ioral exemplars but without feedback (Kehle, Clark, Jenson, & Wampold, 1986) or without feedback but with medication (Dowrick & Raeburn, 1977). In all cases videotaped self-observation reduced disruptive behavior or improved classroom behavior, self-directed play, or on-task behavior.

Even though an unedited tape without feedback does not indicate appro-priate behavioral standards, if the recording is made with a wide-angle lens, comparisons can be made by the target child with others. Furthermore, if the tapes include both positive and negative behavior, within-child comparisons can be made. However, lack of feedback may not provide for behavioral gains to the same extent that tapes with feedback do. For example, Esveldt et al. (1974) found that videotaped self-observation with feedback increased the amount of appropriate behavior in one of the two inattentive disruptive boys over that produced by video playback alone.

This indicates that the opportunity to make an attentional match between one's own behavior and a standard does not always produce a comparison (i.e., self-evaluation or a determination of a discrepancy between a standard and the the self). This may be especially true for hyperactive children, who, for exam-ple, are less likely than their peers to pay attention to comparison peer behavior (Cunningham et al., 1985). For this reason, hyperactive children may need to be taught to self-evaluate, especially when the behavior to be matched is more complex than behavior such as on-task.

Self and Standard Comparisons

A study by Cameron and Robinson (1980) used self-evaluation prompts (an answer key and recording posters paired with tokens) in addition to cognitive training to produce math accuracy and on-task changes for several behavior-disordered, hyperactive children. Self-evaluation has also been taught using a Match Game (Hinshaw, Henker, & Whalen, 1984a). In this study hyperactive children learned through a modeling procedure a behavioral standard (e.g., paying attention, doing work). They also self-monitored and specifically at-tempted to match the trainee's evaluations to obtain reinforcement (reinforced self-evaluation or RSE group). Findings were that the RSE group of hyperac-tive boys displayed fewer negative behaviors and more appropriate social behavior on the playground than did the comparison group of hyperactive boys who received points for their trainer ratings (extrinsic reinforcement). A 40% to 45% increment in success rate with the self-evaluation procedure was documented. "Because the two reinforcement conditions were closely equated for incentive value, administration procedures, and adult feedback, the superiority of the RSE treatment can be attributed specifically to the act of self-evaluation: monitoring one's behavior and comparing it with preestablished standards" (Hinshaw *et al.*, 1984a). Self-evaluation was not superior to extrinsic reinforcement only when the latter was paired with stimulant medication; but when self-evaluation was paired with stimulant medication, the negative social behavior of hyperactive boys was reduced to levels below those of normal controls.

More recently, self-evaluation has been taught in an applied setting (Fowler, 1986). In this study the teacher demonstrated criterion behavior in transition settings with follow-up role-playing examples. Instant camera pictures of appropriate behavior of various children were also posted at various locations. Knowledge of the behavioral standards was ensured by a quiz requiring 90% correct response. Prompting and praising correct responses *in situ* were assigned to team captains, who also used report cards as self-evaluation prompts (i.e., points assigned by the team captain had to match those of team members). Points were cashed for activity rewards and for the chance to be team captains. In the final phase, self-monitoring, the children self-assigned points but matching was no longer required. For the three target "disruptive" boys, inappropriate behavior during transitions was reduced significantly and maintained during self-monitoring.

Methods to Promote Self-Controlling Responses

A child must first be made aware of his or her own behavioral, cognitive, or affective response. Standard awareness training may subsequently require methods to increase identification with the standard (e.g., using similar models or self standard setting) and to assess the disparity between the behavior and the standard through self-evaluation. The next step, if necessary, is to break into a dysfunctional behavioral chain with an alternative motor or verbal self-controlling response. This final stage may only be necessary when the targeted behavior is complex or requires a sequence of skills or strategies that are not readily modeled, or when a dysfunctional habit preempts new learning. Keogh and Glover (1980) have articulated the distinction between attention and skill training in a discussion of interventions designed to elicit skills that the child already possesses, in contrast to those designed to develop skills (i.e., to promote self-controlling responses). Thus, when awareness of the standard and of the discrepancy between the standard and self fail to alter behavior, it may then be necessary to determine whether the child has the prerequisite skills. If the child already has the skill but isn't using it, however, response interventions are less efffective and more costly than interventions designed to increase self- and standard awareness (e.g., Friedling & O'Leary, 1979; Varni & Henker, 1979).

Self-Controlling Verbal Responses

In the cognitive-training literature, there are a number of general verbal statements that children are taught, such as "How am I doing?" or "Am I following my plan?" These function to interrupt ongoing performance and redirect present behavior. There is some evidence to indicate that it is the overt verbalizations that are responsible for changes in behavior. As previously discussed, visual cue cards are sometimes used to prompt production of these verbal reminders (e.g., "stop, think") (Palkes *et al.*, 1968). Palkes, Stewart, and Friedman (1971) demonstrated that reading these cue cards silently was ineffective to alter performance during training sessions. Similarly, Camp (1977) demonstrated that aggressive boys respond to overt but not covert verbalizations. In an application of her Think Aloud program, Camp (Camp, Blom, Herbert, & van Doorninck, 1977) further demonstrated that 30 half-hour sessions in overt verbal cognitive training and problem solving with aggressive boys resulted in better ratings on prosocial behaviors (but not on aggression) and reduced impulsive performance.

A similar approach is found in social problem-solving training. What is taught through direct instruction, modeling, and games is the vocabulary necessary to express thoughts and emotions (e.g., and/or, if/then, happy/mad/sad). Thought generation that is useful in the development of alternative solutions, consequential thinking, and cause–effect reasoning is practiced with puppets and picture cards (Spivack & Shure, 1974).

The importance of practicing verbal coping responses has also been documented (Goodwin & Mahoney, 1975). In this study, observations of a 3-minute videotape of a boy being taunted by his peers but coping well by making statements such as "I won't get mad" was ineffective in generating coping responses in three impulsive boys. A subsequent training session was provided in which the self-statements of the model were made explicit and the impulsive children were asked to verbalize as many of these coping responses as possible. Although practice effects in tape viewing were not controlled in this study, it appears that the verbal standard (i.e., the verbal coping responses) had to be made salient and had to be practiced.

There is further evidence to suggest that alterations in overt verbal social responses may lead to modifications of related physical responses. As discussed earlier in the chapter, children who were trained to speak altruistic words used more altruistic and fewer aggressive responses than children trained with neutral words. The opposite pattern was observed for children trained with aggressive words (see Combs & Slaby, 1977). Thus, children who present disorders in social problem solving, aggression, or social coping may be targeted for training sessions that require practicing verbally appropriate statements and responses.

Several other good studies have used a complex of verbal techniques directed toward social, academic, and attentional/impulsivity task performance.

Multiple procedures make it difficult, however, to determine the individual contribution of specific techniques. Among these is a study by Douglas (Douglas, Parry, Marton, & Garson, 1976) which employed academic, auditory, and visual tasks with perceptual-motor or memory requirements, as well as social interaction tasks, in a 3-month training program. Training was implemented by teachers and parents who used self-instruction, attention-training, cognitive-modeling, and role-playing techniques. This multicomponent study yielded changes in the errors and latency impulsivity scores of the MFFT, the time scores on the Bender, and listening comprehension on the Durrell. Changes in the impulsivity measures were maintained at a 3-month follow-up. There was also some indication in this study of changes in aggressive and realistic coping responses on a Story Completion Test (a measure of response to frustration). Hyperactivity ratings were, however, unaffected by the cognitive treatments employed.

Other studies directed toward general cognitive strategies appear to have limited success. Verbalizations that prompt children's attention to details, to sequencing, and to strategy use were cued by superhero thinking cards (Brown, Wynne, & Medenis, 1985)). This 3-month training program that also involved strategy training generalization to teachers and parents found no gains in impulsivity or attentional performance for cognitive training alone. The main findings were in listening comprehension on the Durrell. Thus, it may be that the verbal strategies employed in training improved verbal information processing (i.e., the teaching process was related to the learning outcome).

In sum, there clearly is some potential in the use of verbal mediators, especially when children demonstrate inappropriate social responses and for which appropriate statements are infrequently observed in their natural environments. These responses, however, must be practiced. Verbal mediators are effective if they are relatively short (e.g., "stop and think"), are directly related to a standard situation (i.e., response to provocation or the failure to stop and think), or are chosen by the target child for that situation. Less validated in the literature are the more general and verbally complex cognitive strategies designed to affect a wide variety of performance measures, although listening comprehension may be improved. It may be more difficult to shape and maintain hyperactive children's use of these general cognitive self-instructions (for review see Whalen *et al.*, 1985) because verbal self-instruction "fits more easily into the existing behavior of reflective children; impulsive children are being asked to alter their behaviors in a more profound way" (Copeland, 1982, p. 232). Thus, at this time, direct instruction of cognitive strategies is less likely to be successful than practice with specific social coping responses and appropriate vocabulary.

Self-Controlling Motor Responses

An alternative to teaching verbal self-controlling responses is the use of motoric self-controlling responses. These responses may fit better into preexisting responses of ADHD children in that 90% of hyperactive boys demonstrate observable physical mediating behavior (e.g., leg swinging) during delay intervals, in comparison with 45% of normal boys. In contrast, nonobservable (cognitive) mediators are self-reported in 80% of normal boys but in only 30% of hyperactive boys (Gordon, 1979). The importance of programming simple motor responses into tasks with response delays has recently received support (Zentall & Meyer, 1987). Findings from this study demonstrated that hyperactive children derived greater performance and behavioral gains than normal children did from a simple motor response that was available in one task (pressing a slide advance button) and required in the other (flipping flash cards).

A motor technique that prevents hasty selection of responses and thus interrupts an aggressive, impulsive response chain has been labeled the Turtle technique (Schneider, 1974). Children listen to a story about a young turtle who didn't want to pay attention to his teacher until a wise old turtle teaches the young turtle to draw into his shell when he feels angry and until his anger goes away. The young turtle tries the technique and it produces admiration from all the turtle's classmates. The children are then taught a behavioral facsimile of a turtle enfolding its body into an imaginary shell. This motoric response is prompted by a one-word production cue—"turtle." This total program is taught with reinforcement, relaxation, and social skills as alternatives to aggression. A 40% reduction in the frequency of aggression has been documented using this program with aggressive children (Robin, Schneider, & Dolnick, 1976). Nevertheless, it is not clear which component is responsible for the effects demonstrated. Furthermore, it appears clinically advisable to withdraw under threat only as a temporary response (i.e., to break an impulsive aggressive chain).

In addition to the function of interrupting a behavioral chain or preempting sensation-seeking or impulsive responses, a motor plan can also be taught for skill development. Miyakawa & Obnogi (1979) reported that a combined eye and hand motor response were more effective in improving impulsive performance than just the visual attention strategy alone. Children were taught to visually scan the standard in detail from top to bottom and left to right, and to compare each detail of the alternatives to that detail in the standard. The motor response involved eliminating an alternative (by crossing it out) each time a nonmatching detail was found. This visual-motor approach to training was developed because it was clear that modeling only demonstrated a model taking his or her time but didn't demonstrate how the model used that time. Increasing latency alone is insufficient in its effects on error rate (for review, see Messer, 1976).

More elaborate self-controlling motor responses can be trained in role-playing simulations. Possibly, because of the motor component in role playing, it appears to be a relatively effective technique for hyperactive children. For example, Brown (1980b, Study 2, cited in Abikoff, 1985) had hyperactive learning-disabled children reenact a puppet show that demonstrated planning and attending to details in situations. Significant improvements were demonstrated in MFFT errors and latency scores and on a sustained visual attention subtest of the Detroit, compared with an attentional control group. In this particular study, however, it is not clear to what extent the motor enactment improved responding over that produced by cognitive modeling alone (i.e., standard awareness). Addressing this issue, Staub (1971) presented some data to indicate that role playing may enhance generalization. In this study a comparison was made between teachers' prompting of alternative social problem solutions and role-playing solutions. The results suggested that only role playing produced generalization of helping and sharing behaviors to a naturally occurring situation.

In summary, self-controlling motor responses can be divided into those that interrupt an inappropriate habit (e.g., aggressive reactions to apparent provocations) and those that replace inappropriate responses (e.g., excessive activity elicited by boring tasks or delay intervals) with incompatible structured motor responses. These relatively simple motor responses are presented in contrast to those described previously that detail a sequence of motor operations necessary to perform a task efficiently (e.g., MFFT performance) or respond to a complex social situation. These motor plans are important for teaching academic or social problem solving for which the child has no apparent strategy.

CONCLUSION

"Self-control" was defined broadly as the voluntary regulation of behavior in relation to a standard, criterion, or rule. The process of bringing an unregulated behavior under self-control is initiated by self-observation (i.e., of the unregulated behavior, of an appropriate standard for that behavior, and of the discrepancy between the two) and executed by self-control responses.

A number of steps from the identification of ADHD children with self-control disorders to training of appropriate response have been suggested in this chapter. These steps can be used to generate the following list of clinically relevant questions:

1. Is the child ADHD, indicating the need for stimulant therapy (biochemical or environmental) and/or cognitive training?
2. Does the child have significant academic or social dysfunction, indicating the appropriateness of cognitive training?
3. Does the child exhibit correct responding under some conditions, even though infrequently or at a low level, which would indicate that self-awareness, standard awareness, or self-evaluation training would produce behavioral increments?
4. Does the child fail to produce the desired behavior, motor plan, or strategy in all contexts, indicating the need for verbal or motor response training?
5. Does the child demonstrate academic dysfunction, indicating the viability of motor plan training?

6. Does the child demonstrate disruption and sensation-seeking activity during delay times or during rote (boring) task performance, indicating that structured motor responses could be used as substitute responses?
7. Does the child demonstrate inappropriate social reactions triggered, for example, by perceived threats, indicating the usefulness of a response training sequence of cue recognition, habit interruptions (e.g., "turtle"), followed by practice with overt verbal coping responses?

Identification of ADHD children has been operationalized through the SNAP-DSM-III-R scale. Criterion scoring on such a scale requires some indication of social and academic dysfunction and of the severity of that dysfunction. Dysfunctional children would appear to be the best candidates for cognitive-behavioral interventions, whereas those problems restricted to the modulation of activity or attention (i.e., as indicated by the 14 behavioral criteria) may be better treated with environmental novelty or biochemical (drug) stimulant therapy. When on-task behavior, task persistence, and impulsive or disruptive classroom behavior represent the type of self-control problem identified, self-monitoring and standard awareness training would be particularly effective. This is explained by the fact that attentional deficiencies contribute significantly to the self-control problems and production deficiencies of ADHD children. Attention that is directed selectively to external environmental novelty and to emotionally salient social cues restricts input and awareness about the self (e.g., meta-attention, metamemory, metabehavior, and metacognition, including the executive functions of planning and organization) and restricts neutral and informational cues from the behavior of peers, which would contribute to the development of appropriate behavioral standards.

The attentional biasing that results in insufficient attention to aspects of the self or to the standard can be remediated through video self- and other observation or by signaling to the child when to self-observe. The effectiveness of these attentional techniques may depend in part on the salience of appropriate behavior. However, some attempts to make the standards salient (e.g., through distracting reinforcers) may be counterproductive. Furthermore, ADHD children become dependent on the presence of visual and auditory production cues, which are used to signal self-observation. Thus, maintenance of self-monitoring in the absence of these cues is difficult to obtain. For this reason, more general techniques that gradually train self-observation may be useful, such as fantasy play or the use of mirrors, audiences, or diaries. Additionally, videotaped playback and cue recognition have been specifically validated with ADHD children. Cue recognition training has considerable potential for generality in that the production cues are internal to the child (i.e., cognitions or emotions) or are found in those contexts that require self-control (e.g., in the presence of threats). There may be other cues that have some setting or task generality (e.g., response delays, study environments) and for which cue recognition could be taught.

Self-, other, or standard awareness may in itself produce a change in behavior (e.g., in on-task responses), which explains why it is the first step to take in training. ADHD children, however, may need additional training in self-evaluation (i.e., in matching the standard) or in setting their own standards, especially when the behavior to be matched is more subtle or complex than on-task behavior. Reinforcement for matching a standard or for criterion setting is effective, perhaps because it increases (1) accuracy in the perception of the standard, (2) planning and goal setting, or (3) the personal relevance of the standard.

Even though most self-control problems are due to inattention to the self and the standard, a number of ADHD children must still be specifically taught self-controlling responses. As previously noted, however, beginning with response training is inefficient and ineffective when the problem is lack of awareness of the discrepancy between self and standard.

Self-controlling responses must be taught to those children who have skill deficits (i.e., who have not demonstrated the criterion response in any context). For example, on the MFFT, ADHD children fail to deploy attention systematically and must be taught specific visual-motor self-controlling responses. Self-controlling responses may also need to be trained when observation alone produces inadequate knowledge of the standard (i.e., when the responses are covert or nonsalient). Even for those skills that can be observed directly (e.g., verbal coping statements in response to peer provocations) many ADHD children need to role-play self-controlling responses before they can produce them in an experimental context (Hinshaw et al., 1984b) or generalize them to other contexts (Staub, 1971). Finally, self-controlling responses must be taught when a habit response preempts an appropriate response to be learned. Thus, motor response training could involve teaching responses that interfere with or replace established behavioral habits or teaching a motor plan necessary for a skill. Motor self-controlling responses have been demonstrated to be particularly effective with ADHD children in producing performance and behavioral gains.

Verbal self-controlling (stopping) responses appear to be effective in habit reversal (e.g., "stop," "turtle"). However, complex verbal statements, thought to improve general strategies, produce poor compliance and interfere with auditory processing (thinking) during learning tasks and with speeded performance on practice tasks. There is evidence that when task performance is not assessed but social performance is, verbal social response training and altruistic vocabulary training are effective. Due to the production deficiencies that characterize ADHD children, certain training conditions should be observed in verbal self-control training. Verbal production deficits are seen when an attempt is made to elicit social and verbal responses from these children. Under these conditions, they can be as responsive as normal children only when there is external structure and stimulation as a part of the response format (e.g., pictures, written alternatives, beginning and ending cues). That is, social-verbal deficiencies are noted when the children are required to introspect and create their own internal response structure from nonimmediate cues (e.g., of the past or the future). For this reason, we cannot expect these children to plan responses or strategies unless we provide some external guidance or training in planning or strategy generation.

In summary, ADHD children demonstrate a number of problems in self-control due to their sensation-seeking responses and their attraction to salient stimuli. Because of their need for external stimuli, they are less likely to attend to their own internal dialogue, to processing of information, or to behavioral referents. For these reasons, cognitive interventions that focus their attention to the self, to internal processing, and to behavioral standards are effective to the extent that the children are not made dependent on situation-specific production cues or reinforcers. Thus, when the children are trained to recognize internal cognitive and emotional cues, social cues that indicate impending danger, or task and situational cues that require alterations in the timing of responses, their training should achieve some generality. The attentional explanation proposed in this chapter for self-control problems does not, however, account for those problems attributable to cognitive errors (e.g., irrational beliefs) often seen in emotionally disordered individuals, or for cognitive deficits often seen in LD and retarded children. It can explain lack of exposure to appropriate models, as well as attributional biases (e.g., children who misread neutral social stimuli or attend to hostile rather than neutral aspects of social stimuli; Milich & Dodge, 1984), and is generalizable to those children who apparently have self-control skills but don't use them (Hagen, Barclay, & Schwethelm, 1982; Karoly, 1977; Kendler, 1972; Torgeson, 1977). In addition to attention and self-evaluation training for ADHD children with performance deficits, response training is effective with ADHD children who have skill deficits or interfering behavioral habits. Verbal self-controlling responses appear to have the greatest potential in social skill development, whereas motor self-controlling responses are effective in cognitive and academic performance tasks.

REFERENCES

Abikoff, H. (1985). Efficacy of cognitive training interventions in hyperactive children: A critical review. *Clinical Psychology Review, 5*, 479–512.

Alabiso, F. (1972). Inhibitory functions of attention in reducing hyperactive behavior. *American Journal of Mental Deficiency, 77*, 259–282.

American Psychological Association. (1980). *The diagnostic and statistical manual of mental disorders* (3rd ed.). Washington, DC: Author.

Ault, R. L., Crawford, D. E., & Jeffrey, W. (1972). Visual scanning strategies of reflective, impulsive, F/A, and S/I children on the MFFT. *Child Development, 43*, 1412–1417.

Bandura, A., & Walters, R. H. (1963). *Social learning and personality development*. New York: Holt, Rinehart & Winston.

Barkley, R. A. (1981). *Hyperactive children: A handbook for diagnosis and treatment.* New York: Guilford Press.

Barkley, R. A., Copeland, A. P., & Sivage, C. (1980). A self-control classroom for hyperactive children. *Journal of Autism and Developmental Disorders, 10,* 75–89.

Bem, S. (1967). Verbal self-control: The establishment of effective self-instruction. *Journal of Experimental Psychology, 74,* 485–491.

Berlyne, D. E. (1960). *Conflict, arousal and curiosity.* New York: McGraw-Hill.

Blackwood, R. (1970). The operant conditioning of verbally mediated self-control in the classroom. *Journal of School Psychology, 8,* 257–258.

Booth, S. R., & Fairbank, D. W. (1983). Videotaped feedback as a behavior management technique. *Behavior Disorders, 9,* 55–59.

Brown, R. T., Wynne, M. E., & Medenis, R. (1985). Methylphenidate and cognitive therapy: A comparison of treatment approaches with hyperactive boys. *Journal of Abnormal Child Psychology, 13,* 69–87.

Cameron, M. I., & Robinson, V. M. J. (1980). Effects of cognitive training on academic and on-task behavior of hyperactive children. *Journal of Abnormal Child Psychology, 8,* 405–420.

Camp, B. W. (1977). Verbal mediation in young aggressive boys. *Journal of Abnormal Psychology, 86,* 145–153.

Camp, B. W., Blom, G. E., Herbert, F., & van Doorninck, W. J. (1977). "Think aloud": A program for developing self-control in young aggressive boys. *Journal of Abnormal Child Psychology, 5,* 157–169.

Campbell, S. G., Szumowski, E. K., Ewing, L. J., Gluck, D. S., & Breaux, A. M. (1982). A multidimensional assessment of parent-identified behavior problem toddlers. *Journal of Abnormal Child Psychology, 10,* 569–591.

Carver, C. S. (1979). A cybernetic model of self-attention processes. *Journal of Personality and Social Psychology, 37,* 1251–1281.

Carver, C. S., & Scheier, M. F. (1981). *Attention and self-regulation: A control therapy approach to human behavior.* New York: Springer-Verlag.

Ceci, S. J., & Tishman, J. (1984). Hyperactivity and incidental memory: Evidence for attentional diffusion. *Child Development, 55,* 2192–2203.

Cohen, N. J., Sullivan, J., Minde, K., Novak, C., & Helwig, C. (1981). Evaluation of the relative effectiveness of methylphenidate and cognitive behavior modification in the treatment of kindergarten children. *Journal of Abnormal Child Psychology, 9,* 43–44.

Combs, M. L., & Slaby, D. A. (1977). Social skills training with children. *Advances in Clinical Child Psychology, 1,* 161–201.

Conners, C. K. (1973). Rating scales for use in drug studies with children. *Psychopharmacology Bulletin, 9,* 24–84 (Special issue).

Copeland, A. P. (1979). Types of private speech produced by hyperactive and nonhyperactive boys. *Journal of Abnormal Child Psychology, 7,* 169–177.

Copeland, A. P. (1981). The relevance of subject variables in cognitive self-instructional programs for impulsive children. *Behavior Therapy, 12,* 520–529.

Copeland, A. P. (1982). Individual difference factors in children's self-management: Toward individualized treatments (pp. 207–239). In P. Karoly & F. H. Kanfer (Eds.), *Self-management and behavior change: From therapy to practice.* New York: Pergamon Press.

Copeland, A. P. (1983). Children's talking to themselves: Its developmental significance, function, and therapeutic promise. *Advances in Cognitive-Behavioral Research and Therapy, 2,* 241–278.

Copeland, A. P., & Weissbrod, C. S. (1978). Behavioral correlates of the hyperactivity factor of the Conners Teacher Questionnaire. *Journal of Abnormal Child Psychology, 6*, 339–343.

Copeland, A. P., & Weissbrod, C. S. (1980). Effects of modeling on behavior related to hyperactivity. *Journal of Educational Psychology, 72*, 875–883.

Copeland, A. P., & Wisniewski, N. M. (1981). Learning disability and hyperactivity: Deficits in selective attention. *Journal of Experimental Child Psychology, 32*, 88–101.

Craighead, W. E., Wilcoxon-Craighead, L., & Meyers, A. W. (1978). New directions in behavior modification with children. In M. Hersen, R. M. Eisler, & P. M. Miller (Eds.), *Progress in behavior modification* (pp. 159–197). New York: Academic Press.

Cunningham, C. E., Siegel, L. S., & Offord, D. R. (1985). A developmental dose-response analysis of the effects of methylphenidate on the peer interactions of attention deficit disordered boys. *Journal of Child Psychology and Psychiatry, 26*, 955–971.

Dainer, K. B., Klorman, R., Salzman, L. F., Hess, D. W., Davidson, P. W., & Michael, R. L. (1981). Learning-disordered children's evoked potentials during sustained attention. *Journal of Abnormal Child Psychology, 9*, 79–94.

Dienske, H., DeJonge, G., & Sanders-Woudstra, J. A. R. (1985). Quantitative criteria for attention and activity in child psychiatric patients. *Journal of Child Psychology and Psychiatry, 26*, 895–915.

Douglas, V. I. (1980). Higher mental processes in hyperactive children: Implications for training. In R. M. Knights & D. J. Bakker (Eds.), *Treatment of hyperactive and learning disabled children* (pp. 65–91). Baltimore, MD: University Park Press.

Douglas, V. I., Barr, R. G., O'Neill, M. E., & Britton, B. G. (1986). Short term effects of methylphenidate on the cognitive, learning and academic performance of children with attention deficit disorder in the laboratory and the classroom. *Journal of Child Psychology and Psychiatry, 27*, 191–212.

Douglas, V. I., Parry, P., Marton, P., & Garson, C. (1976). Assessment of a cognitive training program. *Journal of Abnormal Child Psychology, 4*, 389–410.

Douglas, V. I., & Peters, K. G. (1979). Toward a clearer definition of the attentional deficit of hyperactive children. In G. A. Hale & M. Lewis (Eds.), *Attention and the development of cognitive skills* (pp. 173–247). New York: Plenum Press.

Dowrick, P. W., & Raeburn, J. M. (1977). Video editing and medication to produce a therapeutic self-model. *Journal of Consulting and Clinical Psychology, 45*, 1156–1158.

Esveldt, K. D., Dawson, P. C., & Forness, S. R. (1974). Effect of videotaped feedback on children's classroom behavior. *Journal of Educational Research, 67*, 453–456.

Eysenck, M. W. (1976). Arousal, learning, and memory. *Psychological Bulletin, 83*, 389–404.

Fagan, S. A., & Long, N. J. (1979). A psychoeducational curriculum approach to teaching self-control. *Behavior Disorders, 4*, 68–82.

Finch, A., Wilkinson, M., Nelson, W., & Montgomery, L. (1975). Modification of an impulsive cognitive tempo in emotionally disturbed boys. *Journal of Abnormal Child Psychology, 3*, 45–52.

Fowler, S. A. (1986). Peer-monitoring and self-monitoring: Alternatives to traditional teacher management. *Exceptional Children, 52*, 573–581.

Friedling, C., & O'Leary, S. G. (1979). Effects of self-instructional training on second and third grade hyperactive children: A failure to replicate. *Journal of Applied Behavior Analysis, 12*, 211–219.

Goodwin, S. E., & Mahoney, M. J. (1975). Modification of aggression through modeling: An experimental probe. *Journal of Behavior Therapy and Experimental Psychiatry, 6*, 200–202.

Gordon, M. (1979). The assessment of impulsivity and mediating behaviors in hyperactive and nonhyperactive boys. *Journal of Abnormal Child Psychology, 7*, 317–326.

Goyette, C. H., Conners, C. K., & Ulrich, R. F. (1978). Normative data on revised Parent and Teacher Rating Scales. *Journal of Abnormal Child Psychology, 6*, 221–236.

Graziano, A. (1975). *Behavior therapy with children.* Chicago: Aldine.

Hagen, J. W. (1967). The effect of distraction on selective attention. *Child Development, 39*, 687–694.

Hagen, J. W., Barclay, C. R., & Schwethelm, B. (1982). Cognitive development of the learning-disabled child. In N. R. Ellis (Ed.), *International Review of Research in Mental Retardation* (pp. 1–41). New York: Academic Press.

Hallahan, D. P., & Reeve, R. E. (1980). Selective attention and distractibility. In B. K. Keogh (Ed.), *Advances in special education* (Vol. 1, pp. 141–181). Greenwich, CT: JAI Press.

Hallahan, D. P., & Sapona, R. (1983). Self-monitoring of attention with LD children: Past research and current issues. *Journal of Learning Disabilities, 16*, 616–620.

Hinshaw, S. P., Henker, B., & Whalen, C. K. (1984a). Cognitive-behavioral and pharmacologic interventions for hyperactive boys: Comparative and combined effects. *Journal of Consulting and Clinical Psychology, 52*, 739–749.

Hinshaw, S. P., Henker, B., & Whalen, C. K. (1984b). Self-control in hyperactive boys in anger-inducing situations: Effects of cognitive-behavioral training and methylphenidate. *Journal of Abnormal Child Psychology, 12*, 55–77.

Homatidis, S., & Konstantareas, M. (1981). Assessment of hyperactivity: Isolating measures of high discriminant ability. *Journal of Consulting and Clinical Psychology, 49*, 533–541.

Humphrey, L. L. (1982). Children's and teachers' perspectives on children's self-control: The development of two rating scales. *Journal of Consulting and Clinical Psychology, 50*, 624–633.

Kagan, J., Rosman, B. L., Day, D., Albert, J., & Phillips, W. (1964). Information processing in the child: Significance of analytic and reflective attitudes. *Psychology Monographs, 78* (1, Whole No. 578).

Karoly, P. (1977). Behavioral self-management in children: Concepts, methods, issues, and directions. In M. Hersen, R. M. Eisler, & P. M. Miller (Eds.), *Progress in Behavior Modification* (pp. 197–251). New York: Academic Press.

Kehle, T. J., Clark, E., Jenson, W. R., & Wampold, B. E. (1986). Effectiveness of self-observation with behavior disordered elementary children. *School Psychology Review, 15*, 289–295.

Kendall, P. C. (1981). One-year follow-up of concrete versus conceptual cognitive-behavioral self-control training. *Journal of Consulting and Clinical Psychology, 49*, 748–749.

Kendall, P. C., & Finch, A. J. (1979). Analyses of changes in verbal behavior following a cognitive-behavioral treatment for impulsivity. *Journal of Abnormal Child Psychology, 7*, 455–463.

Kendal, P. C., & Wilcox, L. E. (1979). Self-control in children: Development of a rating scale. *Journal of Consulting and Clinical Psychology, 47*, 1020–1029.

Kendler, T. S. (1972). An ontogeny of meditational deficiency. *Child Development, 43*, 1–17.

Keogh, B. K., & Glover, A. T. (1980). The generality and durability of cognitive training effects. *Exceptional Educational Quarterly, 1*, 75–88.

Kurtz, P. D., & Neisworth, J. T. (1976). Self-control possibilities for exceptional children. *Exceptional Children, 42*, 212–217.

Lahey, B. B., Green, K. D., & Forehand, R. (1980). On the independence of ratings of hyperactivity, conduct problems, and attention deficits in children: A multiple regression analysis. *Journal of Consulting and Clinical Psychology, 48*, 566–574.

Ludlow, C. L., Rapoport, J. L., Bassich, C. J., & Mikkelsen, E. G. (1980). Differential effects of dextroamphetamine on language performance in hyperactive and normal boys (pp. 185–205). In R. M. Knights & D. J. Baker (Eds.), *Treatment of hyperactive and learning disordered children*. Baltimore, MD: University Park Press.

Luria, A. R. (1961). *The role of speech in the regulation of normal and abnormal behavior* (J. Tizard, Trans.). New York: Liveright.

Maccoby, E. E., & Hagen, J. W. (1965). Effects of distraction upon central versus incidental recall: Developmental trends. *Journal of Experimental Child Psychology, 2*, 280–289.

Madan-Swain, A. J., & Zentall, S. S. (1988). *Behavioral comparisons of accepted and rejected hyperactive children and their matched controls in play settings*. Manuscript submitted for publication.

Marholin, D., II, Siegel, L. J., & Phillips, D. (1977). Treatment and transfer: A search for empirical procedures. In M. Hersen, R. M. Eisler, & P. M. Miller (Eds.), *Progress in behavior modification* (pp. 293–342). Beverly Hills, CA: Sage Publications.

Meichenbaum, D. (1977). *Cognitive behavior modification: An integrative approach*. New York: Plenum Press.

Meichenbaum, D. (1979). Teaching children self-control. *Advances in Clinical Child Psychology, 2*, 1–27.

Meichenbaum, D. H., & Goodman, J. (1971). Training impulsive children to talk to themselves: A means of developing self-control. *Journal of Abnormal Psychology, 77*, 115–126.

Messer, S. B. (1976). Reflection–impulsivity: A review. *Psychological Bulletin, 83*, 1026–1052.

Milich, R., & Dodge, K. A. (1984). Social information processing in child psychiatric populations. *Journal of Abnormal Child Psychology, 12*, 471–490.

Miyakawa, J., & Ohnogi, H. (1979). The effect of strategy training on the modification of cognitive impulsivity. *Japanese Psychological Research, 21*, 139–145.

Osborne, S. S., Kosiewicz, M. M., Crumley, E. B., & Lee, C. (1987). Distractible students use self-monitoring. *Teaching Exceptional Children, 19*, 66–69.

Palkes, H., Stewart, M., & Friedman, J. (1971). Improvement in maze performance in hyperactive boys as a function of verbal training procedures. *Journal of Special Education, 5*, 337–343.

Palkes, H., Stewart, M., & Kahana, B. (1968). Porteus maze performance of hyperactive boys after training in self-directed verbal commands. *Child Development, 39*, 817–826.

Patton, J. E., Routh, D. K., & Offenbach, S. I. (1981). Televised classroom events as distractors for reading-disabled children. *Journal of Abnormal Child Psychology*, *9*, 355–370.

Pelham, W. E., & Bender, M. E. (1982). Peer relationships in hyperactive children: Description and treatment. *Advances in Learning and Behavioral Disabilities*, *1*, 365–436.

Porrino, L. J., Rapoport, J. L., Behar, D., Sceery, W., Ismond, D. R., & Bunney, W. E. (1983). A naturalistic assessment of the motor activity of hyperactive boys. *Archives of General Psychiatry*, *40*, 681–687.

Prichep, L. A., Sutton, S., & Hakerem, G. (1976). Evoked potentials in hyperkinetic and normal children under certainty and uncertainty: A placebo and methylphenidate study. *Psychophysiology*, *13*, 419–428.

Radosh, A., & Gittelman, R. (1981). The effect of appealing distractors on the performance of hyperactive children. *Journal of Abnormal Child Psychology*, *9*, 179–189.

Reese, H. W. (1962). Verbal mediation as a function of age level. *Psychological Bulletin*, *59*, 502–504.

Ridberg, E. H., Parke, R. D., & Hetherington, E. M. (1971). Modification of impulsive and reflective cognitive styles through observation of film-mediated models. *Developmental Psychology*, *5*, 369–377.

Robin, A., Schneider, M., & Dolnick, M. (1976). The turtle technique: An extended case of self-control in the classroom. *Psychology in the Schools*, *13*, 449–453.

Rosenbaum, M., & Baker, E. (1984). Self-control behavior in hyperactive and nonhyperactive children. *Journal of Abnormal Child Psychology*, *12*, 303–313.

Rosenthal, R. H., & Allen, T. W. (1978). An examination of attention, arousal, and learning dysfunctions of hyperkinetic children. *Psychological Bulletin*, *85*, 689–715.

Rugel, R. P., Cheatam, D., & Mitchell, A. (1978). Body movement and inattention in learning disabled and normal children. *Journal of Abnormal Child Psychology*, *6*, 325–337.

Safer, D. J., & Allen, R. P. (1976). *Hyperactive children: Diagnosis and management*. Baltimore, MD: University Park Press.

Saltz, E., Dixon, D., & Johnson, J. (1977). Training disadvantaged preschoolers in various fantasy activities: Effects on cognitive functioning and impulse control. *Child Development*, *48*, 367–380.

Sandberg, T., Wieselberg, M., & Shaffer, D. (1980). Hyperkinetic and conduct problem children in a primary school population: Some epidemiological considerations. *Journal of Child Psychology and Psychiatry*, *21*, 303–311.

Schleifer, M., Weiss, G., Cohen, N., Elman, M., Cvejic, H., & Kruger, E. (1975). Hyperactivity in preschoolers and the effect of methylphenidate. *American Journal of Orthopsychiatry*, *45*, 38–50.

Schneider, M. R. (1974). Turtle technique in the classroom. *Teaching Exceptional Children*, *7*, 22–24.

Singer, J. (1977). Imagination and make-believe play in early childhood: Some educational implications. *Journal of Mental Imagery*, *1*, 127–144.

Skinner, B. F. (1953). *Science and human behavior*. New York: Macmillan.

Smith, A. A., Malmo, R. B., & Shagass, C. (1977). An electromyographic study of listening and talking. *Canadian Journal of Psychology*, *8*, 219–227.

Spates, C. R., & Kanfer, F. H. (1977). Self-monitoring, self-evaluation, and self-reinforcement in children's learning: A test of a multistage self-regulation model. *Behavior Therapy*, *8*, 9–16.

Spiegel, E. D. (1977). The effects of self-observation on the social behavior of hyperactive children. *Dissertation Abstracts International, 38*, 6061.

Spivack, G., & Shure, M. D. (1974). *Social adjustment of young children.* San Francisco: Jossey-Bass.

Staub, E. (1971). The use of role play and induction in children's learning of helping and sharing behavior. *Child Development, 42*, 805–816.

Steinkamp, M. W. (1980). Relationships between environmental distractions and task performance of hyperactive and normal children. *Journal of Learning Disabilities, 13*, 209–214.

Thoresen, C. E., & Coates, T. J. (1986). Behavioral self-control: Some clinical concerns. In M. Hersen, R. M. Eisler, & P. M. Miller (Eds.), *Progress in behavior modification* (pp. 307–352). New York: Academic Press.

Torgeson, J. K. (1977). The role of nonspecific factors in the task performance of learning disabled children: A theoretical assessment. *Journal of Learning Disabilities, 10*, 33–40.

Ullmann, R. K., Sleator, E. K., & Sprague, R. L. (1985). A change of mind: The Conners Abbreviated Ratings Scales reconsidered. *Journal of Abnormal Child Psychology, 13*, 553–565.

Varni, J. W., & Henker, B. (1979). Self-regulation approach to the treatment of three hyperactive boys. *Child Behavior Therapy, 1*, 171–192.

Vygotsky, L. S. (1962). *Thought and language* (E. Hanfmann & G. Vaker, Eds. & Trans.). Cambridge, MA: MIT Press.

Weiss, G., & Hechtman, L. T. (1986). *Hyperactive children grown up.* New York: Guilford Press.

Weiss, G., Minde, K., Werry, J., Douglas, V., & Nemeth, E. (1971). Studies of the hyperactive child: VII. Five-year follow up. *Archives of General Psychiatry, 24*, 409–414.

Whalen, C. K., Collins, B. E., Henker, B., Alkus, S. R., Adams, D., & Stapp, J. (1978). Behavior observations of hyperactive children and methylphenidate (Ritalin) effects in systematically structured classroom environments: Now you see them now you don't. *Journal of Pediatric Psychology, 3*, 177–187.

Whalen, C. K., Henker, B., & Hinshaw, S. P. (1985). Cognitive-behavioral therapies for hyperactive children: Premises, problems, and prospects. *Journal of Abnormal Child Psychology, 13*, 391–410.

Winett, R. A., & Winkler, R. C. (1972). Current behavior modification in the classroom: Be still, be quiet, be docile. *Journal of Applied Behavior Analyses, 5*, 499–504.

Zelniker, T., & Jeffrey, W. E. (1976). Reflective and impulsive children: Strategies of information processing underlying differences in problem solving. *Monographs of the Society for Research in Child Development, 41*, 1–46.

Zentall, S. (1975). Optimal stimulation as theoretical basis of hyperactivity. *American Journal of Orthopsychiatry, 45*, 549–563.

Zentall, S. S. (1980). Behavioral comparisons of hyperactive and normally active children in natural settings. *Journal of Abnormal Child Psychology, 8*, 93–109.

Zentall, S. S. (1984). Context effects in the behavioral ratings of hyperactive children. *Journal of Abnormal Child Psychology, 12*, 345–352.

Zentall, S. S. (1985). Stimulus-control factors in search performance of hyperactive children. *Journal of Learning Disabilities, 18*, 480–485.

Zentall, S. S. (1986a). Assessment of emotionally disturbed preschoolers. *Diagnostique, 11*, 154–179.

Zentall, S. S. (1986b). Effects of color stimulation on performance and activity of hyperactive and nonhyperactive children. *Journal of Educational Psychology, 78,* 159–165.

Zentall, S. S. (in press). Production deficiencies in elicited language but not in the spontaneous verbalizations of hyperactive children. *Journal of Abnormal Child Psychology.*

Zentall, S. S., & Barack, R. S. (1979). Rating scales for hyperactivity: Concurrent validity, reliability, and decision to label for the Conners and Davids abbreviated scales. *Journal of Abnormal Child Psychology, 7,* 179–190.

Zentall, S. S., & Dwyer, A. M. (in press). Color stimulation and its effects on the impulsive errors and activity of hyperactive children. *Journal of School Psychology.*

Zentall, S. S., & Gohs, D. E. (1984). Hyperactive and comparison children's response to detailed vs. global cues in communication tasks. *Learning Disability Quarterly, 7,* 77–87.

Zentall, S. S., Gohs, D. E., & Culatta, B. (1983). Language and activity of hyperactive and comparison preschoolers in a listening task. *Exceptional Children, 50,* 255–266.

Zentall, S. S., & Kruczek, T. (1988). The attraction of color for active attention problem children. *Exceptional Children, 54,* 357–362.

Zentall, S. S., & Meyer, M. J. (1987). Self-regulation of stimulation for ADD-H children during reading and vigilance task performance. *Journal of Abnormal Child Psychology, 15,* 519–536.

Zentall, S. S., & Shaw, J. H. (1980). Effects of classroom noise on performance and activity of second-grade hyperactive and control children. *Journal of Educational Psychology, 72,* 830–840.

Zentall, S. S., & Zentall, T. R. (1983). Optimal stimulation: A model of disordered activity and performance in normal and deviant children. *Psychological Bulletin, 94,* 446–471.

14
COGNITIVE TRAINING: IMPLICATIONS FOR SPELLING INSTRUCTION

ROBERT J. HALL
Texas A&M University

MICHAEL M. GERBER
University of California, Santa Barbara

ANDREW G. STRICKER
Air Force Academy

The Japanese-American semanticist S. I. Hayakawa once said that a dictionary was a history book, not a law book. The newest edition of the *Random House Dictionary of the English Language* (Second Edition Unabridged) is a good example. Its 315,000 entries reportedly include 50,000 new entries, such as "tofu," "byte," and "Reaganomics," and 75,000 *new* definitions of *old* words (Hacker, 1987). If one spent 10 minutes memorizing each word, it would take over 2 years to complete the project. Of course, by that time it is highly likely that the language would have been reshaped by thousands of new additions and by assignment of seldom used forms to the lexical trash heap of history. No one ever learns or uses all of these words, but it is an intriguing characteristic of our language that most normally achieving children, by the time they complete formal schooling, will be able to spell the vast majority of these words, excluding perhaps only those words of foreign origin that attempt to preserve either original spelling (e.g., "*burrito*") or pronunciation (e.g., "*Beijing*"). Over time, however, even the spelling of these words will become part of most children's store of spelling knowledge, just as present-day students have learned word forms that originally derived from various Latin, Greek, French, or Scandinavian sources.

Hayakawa's comment calls attention to the fact that the development of word spelling, as well as word meaning, is not entirely arbitrary, but reflects and records an active history of human thought, choice, and usage. His observation should make us mindful that students are not passive receptacles that are "filled" by language instruction from teachers. In fact, the contemporary perspective on acquisition of basic academic skills is quite different. Exciting theoretical and empirical developments in educational psychology and special education over the past two decades have tended to support the view that normally achieving students interact with their learning tasks. This view has important implications for teaching students in regular classes but perhaps has special significance for school personnel concerned with teaching slow or generally unsuccessful learners.

This chapter concerns applications of cognitive-behavioral training approaches to assessment of and intervention with students experiencing difficulty in learning how to spell. It is the thesis of this chapter that in confronting and trying to master the spelling system, students naturally engage in forms of active problem solving. In our view, each particular need to spell reflects not only specific knowledge and suitable problem-solving tactics and strategies, but also a generic set of cognitive processes directed toward collecting usable information and reducing uncertainty. Reduction of uncertainty here refers to overt actions predicated on decisions about which responses will be considered appropriate or satisfactory in given problem-solving situations.

PLAN FOR THIS CHAPTER

In this chapter, we first present background information about the American English spelling system and how it is taught in schools. Second, we argue that, for students experiencing difficulty learning to spell, there are instructional advantages gained by focusing evaluative judgments on evidence of problem-solving competence rather than on categorical incompetence. Third, we describe how careful observation and interpretation of students' attempts to spell can lead to instructionally useful developmental models of students' ability to solve spelling problems. In addition, we show how such models can be used to suggest appropriate cognitive-behavioral training (CBT) interventions, and we describe how a cognitive approach to problem-solving assessment and instruction might be implemented in applied settings by school psychologists. Finally, we extend our suggestions concerning CBT interventions to a discussion about how microcomputer technology might be linked with CBT intervention strategies to produce intelligent computer-assisted instructional (ICAI) programs in spelling.

BACKGROUND ON SPELLING INSTRUCTION

The Structure of Spelling

For schoolchildren, the American English system of spelling is a minefield of unexpected variations. Consider the following. English orthography contains seemingly irrelevant "silent" letters, such as the "gh" in "right" or the "b" in "doubt." The language also includes numerous instances of apparently random, if not chaotic, assignments of spoken sounds to written symbols, such as the six different pronunciations of "ough" in "bough," "cough," "thorough," "thought," "through," and "rough," or the 14 different spellings for /sh/. Moreover, there is a perplexing lack of correspondence between the 26 alphabet letters and the more than 40 phonemes that make up the language's basic speech sounds. Finally, there is special confusion over how five letters ("a," "e," "i," "o," and "u") can be used to represent eight basic and four glide, or diphthong, vowels. It is no wonder that one learning-disabled student, when asked by the authors why spelling included unprounounced letters and different sounds for the same letter, commented, "Because they're trying to trick you."

In fact, the spelling system is not arbitrary—it only seems that way. Rather, it contains a subtle but understandable order at the levels of phoneme representation, grapheme patterns, grammatical marking, and semantic relationship. Both its subtle orderliness and its frustrating difficulty are the fascinating result of dramatic historical events involving mass migrations and integrations of different cultural–linguistic communities. For example, so-called silent letters were once articulated, and many spelling conventions in words of foreign origin have been retained in spite of their anglicized pronunciations. Overall, the system reflects the historical fact that pronunciation has shifted and changed faster than print.

The general outline of this history is familiar, but we will sketch it briefly to make a point about cognitive training as it applies to spelling diagnosis and instruction. The Germanic-derived Old English language of the ancient Anglo-Saxons (which itself evolved from admixtures of many contributing tongues) confronted the Norman French language beginning in 1066 and became Middle English. The political consequence of the violent conquest and forced merger of these two cultures eventually brought about not only England's departure from the Catholic Church, but also a departure from written Latin as the language of official preference in the publication of documents. This search for ethnolinguistic identity was abetted by the growing importance of the printing press in a country poised for explosive cultural and economic expansion.

Over this latter period of time, from about 1350 to 1550, a series of language changes occurred that have such singular importance in the history of English orthography that linguists have given them a name: the Great Vowel Shift. This period was marked by a rapid homogenizing of spoken dialects. What resulted was a gradual and irreversible change in the "map" of articulation positions by which the Old English mouth pronounced 18 of 20 distinctive English vowels. The /a/, once pronounced as the "a" in "father," evolved into the long "a" as in "fate." The /e/ that once sounded like the long vowel "a" in "fate" began to be pronounced as the long "e" in "feat." The /i/, which was once pronounced like the long "e," shifted to become like "i" in "fine," and so on. While these dramatic changes were occurring in speech, however, spelling remained the same.

To make matters worse for modern American schoolchildren, the process of linguistic evolution continued unabated through the American colonial period. Ethnolinguistic groups continued to mix, and an enormous vocabulary of foreign and newly coined words entered both spoken and written language. This resulted in new grammatical conventions, many of which are represented in contemporary spellings. Meanwhile, with the influx and mix of accented speakers, pronunciation of vowels in unstressed syllables continued to be reduced to the lowest common denominator, the "schwa" sound. During these tumultuous years, English spelling was tolerant of pronunciation shifts, even though literate individuals debated different proposals for resolving the pronunciation/representation dilemma. The arguments centered on the desire to make spelling conform to the new tenets of pronunciation while preserving the historical, semantically relevant information contained in older spellings. Interestingly, many of the older spellings merely reflected decisions of early foreign typesetters.

By the beginning of the 19th century, the fate of American schoolchildren was sealed. When Noah Webster published his first "blue-backed speller," his aim was to define a distinctively American form of English, but his effect was to declare an end to tolerance and to create a spelling standard for American English that elementary school children still puzzle over today. For many years, code emphasis reading instruction began with drill of spelling patterns. In the late 19th century, however, reformists called for meaning emphasis reading instruction, opening the great debate between phonics-oriented and whole-word-, whole-language-oriented instructional approaches to beginning reading. While this debate continued to rage until the early 1960s, spelling gradually came to be viewed as a highly circumscribed mechanical skill that constituted an entirely separable, relatively minor part of the language arts curriculum.

Spelling Instruction in the Curriculum

When students finish elementary school, they have been formally taught only a few thousand spellings and perhaps a dozen rules. By that time, however, most normally achieving students are capable of spelling most words in the language, and can spell better than a computer programmed to apply hundreds of phoneme-to-grapheme translation rules (Hanna, Hanna, Hodges, & Rudorf, 1966; Simon & Simon, 1973). This impressive achievement, however, is not typical of all students. Some students—whether we call them "educationally handicapped," "learning disabled," or "slow learners"—must be instructed across a much greater variety of spelling variants or there is no expectation that they will attain the same level of achievement.

Although teachers apparently understand the importance of promoting skillful spelling, formal spelling instruction is assigned a relatively low priority in the curriculum. Mirkin (1981), for example, reported that teachers she observed provided less than 10 minutes of direct spelling instruction per day.

In an earlier study, Fitzsimmons and Loomer (1977) surveyed teachers to find out how familiar they were with empirically supported instructional approaches (e.g., test, self-correction, retest) and how likely they were to use such approaches. They found that teachers were generally familiar with but surprisingly unlikely to use empirically valid instructional techniques. Similar results were found in a comparable study, using special-education teachers, conducted by Vallecorsa and Zigmond (1985). Thus, although little research has been directed toward assessing the effectiveness of instructional procedures used by teachers, available data present a rather disappointing picture.

In most classrooms, spelling instruction appears to be informal, almost incidental, and heavily dependent on independent study of commercial or teacher-prepared materials. In an exploratory study, Hammill, Larsen, and McNutt (1977) investigated possible relationships between third- through eighth-grade students' tested spelling (dictation) performance and the type of formal spelling program to which they had been exposed in school. In their sample, 57% of students surveyed used one of three linguistically organized commercial spelling programs, 30% used one of seven additional commercial programs, and 13% received no specific spelling instruction. Although *some* formal system of instruction in third and fourth grades seemed to be superior to none, results were generally mixed and inconclusive, with post-fourth-grade spelling achievement sometimes favoring no specific instruction over formal commercial materials.

The evident lack of classroom implementation of valid approaches to spelling instruction must be seen in contrast to evidence that significant numbers of students experience enormous difficulty in becoming fluent spellers. Students who are classified as learning-disabled (LD), for example, represent a group of learners who characteristically have had difficulty learning to spell. Compared to their normally achieving peers, these students often exhibit chronic and steadily worsening deficiencies in all aspects of writing, particularly spelling (Cone, Wilson, Bradley, & Reese, 1985; Poplin, Gray, Larsen, Banikowski, & Mehring, 1980).

For example, we recently asked all second- through sixth-grade students in a small, middle-class school district (i.e., about 2,000 students) and all students identified as severely learning-handicapped (i.e., about 60 students assigned to self-contained classroom programs) to write a composition (Gerber, in preparation). The students were instructed to take no more than 20 minutes to produce a first draft. After all regular classroom compositions were completed and coded to identify school, grade, teacher, and student status, we drew a random sample equal to about 25% of the population and stratified by grade level. We then looked at a number of objective measures of spelling performance related to the composition task.

The number of words produced by normally achieving (NA) students during the 20-minute composition task increased steadily from about 100 to over 160 words between second and sixth grade. Over this grade span, NA students' spelling error rates decreased from about 10 misspelled words per 100 to about 4 words per 100. For learning-disabled students, however, the cross-sectional profile was dramatically different. They produced, on average, only about 20 words (i.e., about one word per minute) in second grade and not more than 90 words by sixth grade. As disappointing as these numbers are, the data on spelling errors are far worse. LD second-graders produced misspelled words at the rate of about 35 words per 100, and LD sixth-graders demonstrated an error rate of about 18 words per 100, over four times greater than the misspelling rate of their normally achieving peers.

Caution must be exercised in interpreting these data. They dramatize, but they do not clarify. Further analysis, however, indicated that there were important *qualitative* as well as quantitative differences in the performances of LD and NA students. If the cross-sectional data represent a reasonable prediction of within-child, longitudinal outcomes, then vocabulary, sentence length and grammatical complexity, sophistication of style, and specific types of spelling errors all improve faster and to higher levels for NA than for LD students.

Although spelling ability represents only a portion of the picture, it is probable that emergence of a large, reliably accurate spelling vocabulary, beyond its obvious importance as a tool for writing effectively, also indicates integration of various processes that subserve all higher order language use. However, even a relatively straightforward assessment of spelling ability proves difficult. There is ample evidence that LD students differ from their normally achieving peers on standardized measures of spelling and writing achievement, but it is difficult to know what are appropriate inferences to draw from these data. In fact, there are good reasons not to assume that standardized indicators of spelling achievement provide an unambiguous picture of spelling ability (Croft, 1982; Gerber & Cohen, 1985; Gerber & Hall, 1982; Goetz, Hall, & Fetsco, in press; Shore & Yee, 1973). Likewise, standardized measures of cognitive ability (e.g., tests of intelligence) provide little insight into capacity to perform in particular task domains (Goetz & Hall, 1984). Neither type of measure is designed to provide information that permits us to gauge the practical consequence of current level of performance or the likely responsiveness of individual students to alternative instructional approaches. The main point is that most standardized tools for measuring spelling achievement are not conceptualized or constructed so as to yield specific guidelines for developing instructional interventions in spelling. To assist teachers, therefore, school psychologists require a new set of developmentally sensitive assessment concepts that can guide them in estimating how well students can or will respond to instruction in specific academic domains such as spelling. In addition, assessment and intervention should be related explicitly via effective design and implementation procedures.

Summary

In summary, there are three compelling reasons for school psychologists to reorient their thinking and learn about the acquisition of spelling. First, despite the high regard historically expressed for good spellers (Madsen & Gould, 1979), spelling is not one of the best understood, best developed, or most successful parts of the school curriculum. Second, there is clear and consistent evidence that failure to learn to spell accurately and rapidly is one of the most common and persistent characteristics of children labeled as LD (Gerber, 1984a; Poplin *et al.*, 1980), as reading-retarded (Rutter & Yule, 1973), and as dyslexic (Boder, 1973; Nelson, 1980; Nelson & Warrington, 1974; Sweeney & Rourke, 1978). Finally, spelling represents a unique academic problem-solving task in that each phonemic element is related to previous and subsequent elements such that skilled spellers may recognize errors only when the complete product is finished (i.e., when the word doesn't look right) or when contextual information is present (i.e., in the case of homophones).

Like reading and mathematics, spelling provides the problem solver with numerous decision points, at each of which potential uncertainty must be resolved before the problem is judged complete. Unlike reading problems, however, spelling problems have clearer, better demarcated beginnings and endings; hence, completion on the spelling task is less formidable and more likely to occur. Relative to mathematics, spelling is not totally rule-driven. To produce correct spelling variants, therefore, spellers are often forced to resort to external sources such as dictionaries and/or to try to generate alternative variants. If all spelling attempts are preserved, variants can be systematically compared for the type and amount of processing that has occurred, resulting in a rich informational base. For many problems in mathematics, however, especially those that involve straightforward calculation, there is less potential information-processing variance to be analyzed. Spelling also differs from reading and mathematics in that spelling products must be generated totally by the speller. No information exists on the page or on the board to constrain initial attempts at problem solving. And, like the circumscribed task of mathematics (especially for clearly defined tool skill problems), spelling results in orderly, permanent products that can be analyzed and reproduced exactly after the speller has completed the task.

A PROBLEM-SOLVING PERSPECTIVE ON SPELLING ACQUISITION AND PERFORMANCE

Motivated problem solvers—generally those who have been successful in solving difficult problems in the past—labor to impose order, and ultimately an orderly rule system, on problems that have no simple or apparent structure. Effort to perceive a rule-governed system helps learners make decisions and guide responses under conditions that otherwise would be intolerably uncertain. The effortful process of search and construction involves a number of discernibly practical, goal-oriented tactics. These include creation of classification taxonomies, formation and testing of working hypotheses, evaluation of feedback, and search for problem components and strategies. Taken together, these tactics can be construed as analogous to those experienced in prior, perhaps unrelated, problem-solving contexts.

Search and construction processes are initially effortful because they require concentrated, self-monitored attention. That is, learners must closely monitor selection, examination, and/or mnemonic decisions (i.e., "save or discard" memory by-products) concerning any aspect of a task that might potentially lead to a problem solution or any other information that might help the learner more easily to map (i.e., give structure to) the problem. Normally achieving students seem to whittle away at problems by systematically scanning, coding, imposing schema, and developing and storing partial steps or routines so that each attempt at isomorphic problem solving is not newly begun at ground zero. With repeated attempts, retrieval of information pertinent to previous experience with the problem becomes faster, as does the execution of subroutines that have been developed for sorting, comparing, and structuring this information. With ever greater amounts of information structured and stored, and ever greater speed of subroutine operation, attentional capacity, a scarce resource, becomes available and can be deployed to help organize aspects of the problem that have yet to yield their secrets.

It is becoming increasingly fruitful for researchers, school psychologists, and teachers to view the acquisition of academic skills as the solving of problems in this way (Farnham-Diggory & Nelson, 1984; Gagne, 1985). Viewing acquisition as problem solving demands several things from us. First, it makes us appreciate and appraise students in terms of their activity and level of competence, rather than in static terms relative to their incompetence. Second, it forces us to understand what types of knowledge and procedures for applying that knowledge each academic domain requires. That is, it causes us to conduct or adopt a deep analysis of learning tasks in terms of the knowledge domain to which they apply. Third, we learn to locate a range of teachable concepts and strategic behaviors by measuring the "distance" between what students can do on their own and what they can do with various degrees of assistance (Goetz, Hall, & Fetsco, in press). Fourth, viewing acquisition as problem solving causes us to think through, to compare, and to create instructional means for bridging the differences between the tactics and strategies used by novices (i.e., students) and those used by experts (i.e., teachers). In fact, the power of this general approach to assessing and planning interventions is based on the notion that it leads to a class of very promising instructional principles, which, broadly defined, involve some type of cognitive-behavioral training.

For normally achieving students, acquisition of basic skills like spelling is generally so fast that it seems effortless, and typically requires only exposure to exemplar problems and a satisfactory model of solution processes. In these children, much of the cognitive structure required to make the academic problem meaningful, understandable, and solvable is already present in the child's existing declarative (i.e., "what") and procedural (i.e., "how") knowledge (Anderson, 1982). Moreover, many of the developmental changes in knowledge that facilitate acquisition of spelling, such as learning to classify speech sounds and to map these sounds onto the alphabet, take place rapidly and out of sight, as it were, creating the illusion of effortless acquisition.

Naturally, these children are perceived as easy to teach because they require so little external structure in order to learn (e.g., see Hall, 1980).

With learning-handicapped students (whatever their formal classification), the opposite is true (e.g., see Gerber, 1986a). The process of acquiring sufficient and relevant domain-specific and general knowledge is slowed down. Moreover, the internal cognitive structure that instruction geared to normally achieving students takes for granted is lacking or insufficient. The net effect of these crucial differences is not only below-average performance, but also cumulatively reduced capacity to benefit from instruction and consequently, cumulatively deteriorating achievement. These children are perceived as very difficult to teach because teachers are forced to expand much time and effort to extract reliable gains in achievement.

Development of Spelling Ability as Problem Solving

Commenting on the development of spelling skill from an information-processing perspective, Gerber and Hall (1987) point out that

> while several attempts have been made to model spelling by mature, skilled individuals, more satisfactory models are needed to guide research on learning disabilities, especially for studying how spelling ceases to be an effortful end in itself and begins to be an effective tool that is subordinate to higher order tasks requiring written exposition and communication. (p. 35)

Much of the contemporary theoretical work in spelling is based on a two-channel (i.e., auditory or visual) processing model (Farnham-Diggory & Nelson, 1984; Frith, 1980). Stored knowledge about spelling is presumed to represent either word-specific knowledge (i.e., morphemic information about irregular words, homophones, etc.) or knowledge of grapheme–phoneme correspondence rules (i.e., relationship between graphemic patterns and pronunciation). Spellers must select either a lexical or a nonlexical processing system to recognize or to generate English words. Within each of the processing systems, specific models (1) direct attention to the relevant stimuli to be encoded, (2) search and retrieve from memory useful information, and (3) assemble or cue programs of molecular responses.

Although the precise relationship between the two information-processing systems is unresolved and subject to theoretical debate (Gerber & Hall, 1987), spelling errors, viewed in this context, are generally characterized as one of two types. First, errors can occur when the processing system or channel responsible for selecting, encoding, examining, manipulating, or deciding about available stimuli breaks down. Second, errors can be the consequence of inadequately organized or stored knowledge about spelling. Thus, errors are considered to be static, simple functions of a global failure in the visual or auditory processing channels. Researchers and clinicians operating from this theoretical perspective, such as Boder (1973), Fox and Routh (1983), Seymour and Porpodas (1980), and Sweeney and Rourke (1978), place enormous importance on the readability, rather than the logic, of students' errors when judging whether children's processing problems are primarily auditory (i.e., phonetic or nonlexical) or visual (i.e., lexical).

Read's 1975 monograph on how children categorize speech sounds in English has primed movement away from static processing characterizations of errors toward a view that spelling errors are dynamic indicators of children's abilities to represent orthographic information. Research efforts over the past decade have been interpreted to show that errors, as produced by both normally achieving and learning-disabled students, follow a developmental course and are logical products of problem solving, given spellers' imperfect levels of knowledge (e.g., see Bookman, 1984; Englert, Hisbert, & Stewart, 1985; Gentry, 1984; Gerber, 1984a, 1985, 1987; Gerber & Hall, 1982; Henderson & Beers, 1980; Nulman & Gerber, 1984; Read, 1986). Dynamic interpretation of errors, however, means that a more complex system of relationships needs to be considered if we are to fully understand spelling as a problem-solving task.

In summary, recent empirical work in the area of spelling, indicating contingent use of general word knowledge, purposeful invention and application of rule systems to govern choices, and overt error monitoring, makes it clear that spelling skill acquisition, in both normally achieving and learning-disabled children is not solely a function of intact, well-developed data-driven processes. Rather, spelling ability is best characterized by an efficiency-seeking, qualitative reorganization of data-driven processes, wherein process and knowledge structures are mutually dependent and mutually defining (i.e., interactive–compensatory models; Stanovich, 1980).

We are not arguing here for the introduction or addition of complexity for complexity's sake. It is understood that because of constraints of time and training, many practitioners are reluctant to engage in post hoc applications of relatively well-defined but time-consuming systems for interpreting performance. By our willingness to acknowledge and to try to represent the complexity, however, we come closer to understanding the process. Thus, efficient, specifically targeted instructional programs can be developed that take into account the effects of the interaction of individual differences with task demands.

Assessment and the Analysis of Error

In our view, effective cognitive-training interventions do not result from simply acknowledging or documenting that children have difficulty in one or more academic or behavioral areas (Hughes & Hall, 1987). That is, general problems do not immediately suggest specific treatment plans. What might be effective remedial instruction for one student may be ineffective or sluggish instruction for another. All this is to say that learners have different amounts of declarative, transitional, and procedural knowledge that combine to interact with overt features of static intervention programs. If the current level of a child's acquired skill has already developed beyond entry-level intervention activities, then the program requirements may slow processing to a point where the child loses interest in participating or even begins to question what previously was understood. In either case the result can be a decrement rather than an increment in performance. If, on the other hand, the child's entering skill level is too low for the remedial program, then the potential power of the intervention to clarify and promote skill development translates into confusion and frustration. The point is that for instruction to be effective, it cannot be separated from assessment. As in the game of chess, a response occurring in a specific context must be analyzed and interpreted before a course of action is inaugurated with the next move. In this section, therefore, we turn our attention to different aspects of data gathering that have potential to affect the package of "next moves" that become the substance of cognitive-behavioral interventions.

Error analysis and the cognitive approach to diagnostic assessment are both derived from the task analytic model (see Howell, 1986, for a discussion of this model relative to school-based assessment). In general, error analysis procedures like the one used in the Kaufman Test of Educational Achievement (K-TEA) (Kaufman & Kaufman, 1985) break the targeted task into discrete components. The presence or absence of errors associated with the individual components is then interpreted as an indicator of strength or weakness in performance. Factors influencing the goodness of fit between actual performance levels and interpretive profiles are such things as how well component errors represent critical task variance, whether the number of errors in a specific category can be interpreted as a function of developmental level, and whether performance profiles lead to effective instructional plans.

The information-processing or cognitive approach to assessment is much more ambitious and detailed in its attempt to provide information about current levels of performance. Like error analysis, the cognitive approach breaks a task into component parts. It differs from error analysis, however, in that an attempt is made to model the flow of information from input to output—that is, to describe how individuals identify constraints associated with particular problems and then use those constraints to develop strategic plans. From this perspective, not only is the type of error important but so also are the speed and fluency with which cognitive resources are integrated into organizational plans. Moreover, by continuing to monitor performance into the implementation phase where plans are transferred into actions, the relative effectiveness of metacognitive instructional approaches can be evaluated against the acquisition and control of strategies, keynotes of metacognitive instruction for children with learning problems (Palinscar & Brown, 1987). In general, cognitive approaches to assessment are based on the analysis of consistent errors made in specific situational and interpersonal contexts (Messick, 1984), influenced by the presence or absence of elaborative cues (DiBello & Orlich, 1987; Rogoff & Wertsch, 1985). Thus, aggregating errors within a category such as "vowel digraphs and diphthongs" provides information that is not specific enough to drive interpretations in an information-processing analysis.

In an error analysis, the evaluator potentially knows whether the number of errors a child made in a broadly defined category compares favorably or unfavorably to the number of errors made by children in a relevant peer group. Instructionally, this allows the evaluator to generate additional hypotheses about the nature of a child's specific difficulty or difficulties or to risk time and resources on a broader based intervention that may not adequately address the balance between aptitude and treatment. As Snow and Peterson (1985) have pointed out, our past inability to identify appropriate aptitude/treatment interactions is likely due to the use of gross performance indicators in conjunction with gross measurement indicators. Hence, broad-based problem identifications like those resulting from categorizing and aggregating errors lead to interventions that confuse what needs to be learned with what the learner has already accomplished. Confronted with this type of instruction, learners are often encouraged, in the context of the instructional program, to be too careful or reflective about problems that at some earlier point had been resolved. Thus, using vowel digraphs as an example, a child may understand the notion that two adjacent vowels combine to produce the name of the first vowel in the context of one-syllable /ai/ words such as "hail," "fail," and "rail," but may fail to produce the appropriate digraph for the /o/ sound in one-syllable words such as "road" and "toad" or in multisyllabic /ai/ words such as "painting," "maintain," and "mailman."

Isolating specific problems allows the instructor to make certain that emerging skills are firm before new skills are introduced. This has the effect of reducing the probability of errors due to confusion because skills that have newly attained procedural status (i.e., facts available for interpretive procedures) can now be compared and contrasted with information that is already fine-tuned (i.e., skill at a procedural stage of acquisition; see Anderson, 1982). In other words, for some vowel digraphs a child will produce a correct response spontaneously, whereas for others the child may need to remind her-or himself about rules that govern how tense vowels are produced or that the sound being searched for is similar to one already known through familiarity with another word. By being sensitive to the level of skill acquisition that a child has attained, we appropriately develop different aspects of the overall skill.

Failure to take into account current levels of skill development may lead to programs that interrupt automatized processing. When automatized processing results in incorrect responses, then it is necessary to try to deautomatize the process and rebuild using a corrected algorithm. When only parts of an automatized process result in faulty responses, however, our surgical procedures need to separate what works from what doesn't work and concentrate instructional effort on correcting and developing aspects of the process that have led to inaccurate responding. In that way, children are encouraged to question and closely monitor only those things that were not clear to them in the first place. As already suggested, we would caution that being too considered or too reflective about what one already knows can lead to decrements rather than increments in performance (Gerber & Hall, 1982).

Development of Spelling Ability

Gerber and Hall (1982) provide an applied definitional framework for characterizing the development of spelling ability. In their view, spelling represents, for both normally achieving and learning-disabled children, a concept-driven as well as a data-driven process, indicated by the contingent use of general word knowledge, rule systems to govern choices, and overt monitoring of errors. Following is a general description, based on the presentation of Gerber and Hall (1987), outlining the current perspective on the development of spelling ability in young children.

For novice spellers and for older children with learning problems, spelling attempts may contain few letters (e.g., "p" for "pecked," "u" for "human," "ksd" for "closed," or "sm" for "swimming"). These prephonetic spellings represent only partial encoding or phonemic streams in short-term memory and remind one of typical performance on serial-recall tasks. Primacy can be seen in the clear, quick responses to the production of the first phoneme and recency in the production of highly salient stop or hard consonant sounds appearing generally at the end of a word or syllable. Often children are aware that these spellings are incorrect; sometimes they will even leave blank spaces to indicate missing parts. Once children learn to encode the entire sound stream (through repeated verbalizations of the word), phonemes are often compressed into more economical bundles that capture the most salient features of digraphs, blends, or nasalized consonants (e.g., "j" for "dr" in "dressing," "s" for "sw" in "swimming" or sig" for "sing"). Somewhat later, the opposite occurs, and phoneme strings may be expanded to include additional unstressed vowels after tense vowels (e.g., TIUP for "type") or between consonant blends (e.g., KOLOZ for "close").

Children's implicit understanding of rules governing the assignment of letters to sounds is the next phase to evidence systematic development. Initially, novice spellers try to match target phonemes with letter names. Tense vowels are represented by the letter name (e.g., CAM for "came," TOD for "toad") without apparent awareness of the permissible ways in which words must be orthographically marked to produce tense vowels (i.e., vowel pairing, silent "e"). R-controlled and L-controlled vowels are also simplified, as in BRD for "bird" and LUVATR for "elevator." For lax vowels and for vowels that are unstressed, the graphemic representation usually is carried by a vowel whose articulation position is close to that of the targeted phoneme (e.g., SWE-MENG for "swimming" or FLEPR for "flipper"). Once spellers are able to differentiate lax from tense vowels but are still not certain how to use conventional marking systems in the form of rules, a simple pattern is adopted that produces phoneme–grapheme correspondence. For tense vowels, then, lax vowels whose articulation position is close to the desired sound (e.g., PIKT for "peeked") are used. In this example, the articulation position for "i" as in "fix" is close to the articulation of the targeted tense "e."

Finally, as spellers come to understand how rules govern the production of certain sounds, their spelling attempts begin to make the transition from phonetic to correct. In these spellings (e.g., EAGEL or EAGUL for "eagle," AFFRADE for "afraid"), vowels have been appropriately marked and are legal (i.e., appropriately represented sound–symbol correspondences), although incorrect letter sequences are used to produce the desired sound. As children build larger known-word corporas for spelling and for reading, these transitional spellings are replaced by correct spellings. Even with correct spellings, however, there is considerable variance in quality of the spelling product, expressed in the overall time it takes children to produce the correct spelling and in the component or pause times needed to produce specific phonemes or letter sequences (blends, affixes, etc.). In sum, understanding the course of development for problem-solving problems such as spelling allows us to interpret more precisely the performance of a given child and to provide more specific indications of where to begin and what to include in instructional programs.

Summary

Teachers who refer children for testing are generally not ignorant of what those children typically can produce. What they lack is the time and expertise to collect systematically data that can be interpreted against a developmental theory of performance or integrated with other data to provide information about how individual children define and access generalized problem-solving algorithms.

Broadly defined, the goal of educational assessment is to collect enough interpretable information about individual performances so that evaluators can make informed statements about eligibility, placement, strengths, and weaknesses. In this chapter we have not been concerned with eligibility or placement decisions but, instead, have tried to focus on those factors that might influence how we determine what children know and what they need to learn. The emphasis to this point has been on collecting and interpreting performance data rather than on simply describing a myriad of cognitive-behavior training studies that are directly or tangentially related to spelling. This represents a conscious decision on our part as we feel that training programs can only be as good as the data used to inform those programs. Thus, we have provided in this chapter a general context for understanding what might be important considerations for data collection and analysis. In the following sections, we will continue this general theme by focusing specifically on the Spelling subtest of the K-TEA. We have chosen the K-TEA Comprehensive Form because it is new and psychometrically elegant. Moreover, by design of the authors, the K-TEA attempts to package an error analysis overlay with a measure of standardized academic achievement. The error analysis purportedly allows practitioners to generate specific hypotheses about the nature of children's problems in areas such as reading, spelling, and mathematics. Using the Spelling subtest and a sample case study, the K-TEA affords us the opportunity to illustrate how an information-processing analysis of performance might differ from the built-in error analysis. (For a detailed discussion of some implications of cognitive psychology for assessment of academic skill, and for a more complete analysis of the K-TEA spelling subtest, see Goetz, Hall, & Fetsco, in press.) The following sections will also include suggestions about enhancing the usefulness of the K-TEA by including information-processing markers in the data collection process. In sum, we hope to develop a rationale and a general procedure for collecting information that will make an important contribution to the efficient design of academic interventions.

CBT-ORIENTED SPELLING ASSESSMENT AND INTERVENTION: A CASE STUDY AND SOME EXAMPLES

In the Comprehensive Form Manual for the K-TEA, Kaufman and Kaufman (1985) present evidence for the psychometric integrity of the achievement test. As would be expected for any good, contemporary standardized test, rigorous standards for selection and inclusion of items were followed. Spelling items included high-frequency words of social utility introduced at specific grade levels. Words were referenced across several graded spelling series and checked to ensure that they contained a variety of potential spelling errors. Once a pool of items was generated, national tryouts were conducted, resulting in the computation of frequency distributions, coefficient alphas, conventional item statistics, and Rasch-Wright latent trait statistics for each age group. All this is to say that items used in each of the subtests were not chosen in an autocratic or serendipitous fashion. Nonetheless, we would point out that items chosen on this basis, though satisfactory for answering some questions, may be inappropriate for answering questions related to specific strengths or weaknesses in performance.

The K-TEA Spelling subtest contains 50 words that are administered to children in a standard dictation format. Children write their responses on a separate spelling sheet that is part of the individual test record. After the testing session, the examiner analyzes spelling attempts for errors. Given the ceiling rule (5 consecutive misses within a block) and the steeply graded word list, children are likely to produce between 5 and 9 incorrect spellings, although idiosyncratic knowledge of words may produce many more misspellings. For most children, however, the pool of possible errors to be analyzed is small. The error analysis categories for spelling include prefixes and word beginnings, suffixes and word endings, closed syllable (short) vowels, open syllable (long) and final "e" pattern vowels, vowel digraphs and diphthongs, "r"-controlled patterns, consonant clusters and digraphs, single and double consonants, and whole-word error type. The whole-word error type category is used to "indicate that the error is most accurately described as one that involves more than word part errors" (McCloskey, Kaufman, Kaufman, & McCloskey, 1985, p. 104).

For spellers, the most difficult graphemic representations to master involve the production of correct letter sequences to represent unstressed vowels (Read, 1975, 1986). The course of skill development in this area is too complex to deal with in this chapter. Tense or long vowel sound representation, however, develops early, is relatively predictable, and is generally rule-based. Thus, young children encounter many opportunities in writing and spelling to generate regular words with long vowel sounds. For these reasons, we have chosen for analysis the K-TEA category Vowel Digraphs and Diphthongs. A "digraph" refers to a pair of letters representing a single speech sound. For the vowel digraphs "ai," "ea," "oa," "ee," and "ay" occurring in a single syllable, the general rule is that the vowel pair will assume the long vowel sound of the first vowel, as in "deep" or "reach." For the vowel digraphs "ie," and "ei," the most common, hence predictable, sound is the tense /e/ as in "believe" or "receive." Because the usual spelling for the tense /e/ is "ie," the speller must note that this digraph departs from the general rule but represents a regular spelling. In contrast, diphthongs, or glided vowels, are two vowels in a syllable that assume a blended sound (e.g., "oi" and "oy" correspond to the /oi/ sound as in "oil," and "boy" and "ou" and "ow" correspond to the /ow/ sound as in "out" and "cow").

Development of skill involving representation of vowel digraphs and diphthongs occurs relatively early. Thus, young children should be afforded many opportunities to spell words containing these phonemic elements. On the K-TEA, 9 of 15 words containing vowel digraphs or diphthongs (60%) occur in the first 20 words, and 12 of 15 (80%) within the first 25 words. Given the nature of the stopping rule for the K-TEA (testing stops when all words in a block of five are misspelled), a raw score of 15 ensures that at least 20 words would be attempted. From the standard scores by grade tables in the K-TEA manual, this would mean that an average second-grader (standard score of 100) in the spring semester or a below-average (standard score of 85) fourth-grader in the fall semester would be exposed to at least 20 items on the Spelling subtest. Moreover, by the spring semester of the second grade, 7 of 10 children correctly spell the first word in the third block ("bring"). Practically speaking, then, most second-graders demonstrate enough ability to attempt at least 9 words with digraphs or diphthongs. We would judge this category, therefore, to be consistent with developmental theory in that opportunities to observe performance coincide with the approximate age at which skill in this area is being acquired. What, then—if anything—is problematic about this category?

A Case Study

Let us look at the spelling performance of a male child, Edwin, 7 years 8 months old, in the fall semester of the second grade. Referred for testing because of poor performance in reading, this child scores an 85 (age norms) on the Reading Composite and a 96 (age norms) on the Spelling subtest of the K-

TEA. With an IQ of slightly more than 100, this child would qualify for special-education services on the basis of an IQ–reading achievement discrepancy. An evaluator recommending placement, therefore, might be interested in reviewing error analyses for both Reading Decoding and Spelling, given the overlap between the analyses for these two subtests. As illustrated in case studies presented in the K-TEA manual, information from the Spelling and Reading Decoding subtests can be used in a corroborative fashion to help generate hypotheses about students and to develop instructional approaches that support and extend knowledge in both academic areas.

On the Spelling subtest, Edwin reached a ceiling item of 20 and produced the following spelling attempts. (*Legend*: "PDI" contains predictable vowel digraphs; "UDI" contains unpredictable vowel digraphs; "PDP" contains predictable vowel diphthongs; "UDP" contains unpredictable vowel diphthongs.

Word	Attempt	Word	Attempt
1. and	and	11. bring	bie
2. dog	dog	12. said (UDI)	said
3. big	big	13. wagon	woain
4. on	on	14. reach (PDI)	rec
5. she	sey	15. does (UDP)	does
6. blue (PDP)	blue	16. color	clre
7. came	kam	17. friend (UDI)	firnd
8. mother	mothe	18. because (UDP)	bucs
9. school (PDP)	school	19. ocean (UDI)	osn
10. went	whnt	20. afraid (PDI)	ofade

Edwin related to the examiner that the words "school," "said," and "does" had recently appeared on his spelling lists. Of the 12 words that Edwin misspelled, 5 contained vowel digraph or diphthong errors. Turning to the Error Analysis Summary in the K-TEA, Edwin's performance across all error categories can be summarized as follows:

Word Part	Average Number of Errors	Student's Number of Errors
1. Prefixes and word beginnings	—	2
2. Suffixes and word endings	—	2
3. Short vowels	0	3
4. Long vowels and final "e"	0–1	3
5. Vowel digraphs and diphthongs	1–4	5
6. R-controlled patterns	—	1
7. Consonant clusters and digraphs	0	5
8. Single and double consonants	1	5

According to instructions in the manual, a designation of "average" skill status is given to a student when the number of student errors is at or within the range specified by the tabled value corresponding to the Average Number of Errors. A child is designated "strong" in skill status within a category if her or his number of errors is below the tabled average value and "weak" if his or her error total exceeds the tabled average value. Tabled values allow the examiner to compare a target child's performance to the standardized performance of children in the same grade attempting the same number of items. Where tabled values for average number of errors are not given (i.e., in categories 1, 2, and 6), the authors suggest that no comparisons be made because there were too few opportunities to observe.

Considering Edwin's performance, he evidenced "skill status" weaknesses in all categories for which there were analyzable comparisons. The error analysis might be interpreted to suggest that this child has difficulty generating appropriate graphemes for a wide range of phonemic elements or, conversely, that his skill development is generally acceptable given his age-referenced standard score (96) and consistent performance across all error categories. In either case, Edwin spelled correctly only those words that were monosyllabic or recently studied. Moreover, given his difficulty in decoding letter sequences into correct sounds and blends, he is not likely to be able to use reading recognitive skills to help him distinguish between correct and incorrect spelling variants. His skill development in spelling, though average now, probably reflects knowledge of specific words and thus might begin to show sharp declines as spelling words become longer and more complex and as the demands on working memory become greater. An evaluator, noting the foregoing, might suggest a program of reading and spelling instruction that emphasizes (1) knowledge of phonic definitions and generalizable phonetic rules, (2) practice in segmenting words into phonemes and syllables, and (3) drill and rote memory practice. Improvements in reading performance should also have an impact on Edwin's spelling skill by giving him more opportunities to see grade-appropriate high- and low-frequency words.

Beyond Reliance on Formal Tests

The tentative hypotheses outlined in the preceding paragraph do not exhaust the possible interpretations that a good evaluator might generate following additional word sleuthing. These hypotheses are consistent, however, with the type and level of case study response summarized in the K-TEA manual (see especially the Howard H case in Kaufman & Kaufman, 1985 pp. 133–144). It is impressive that, in a relatively short time span, the evaluator can elicit hypotheses that reflect overall academic goals for individual children. This, we would argue, represents a step forward for standardized testing and for school psychology. Equally important is the realization that hypotheses directed at summative goals often tend to confirm teacher judgments rather than to provide the specific instructional information that teachers seek when referring children for testing. In other words, an error analysis used in this fashion tends to be more confirmative than directive.

As good as the K-TEA appears to be, we are concerned that this test, like any other measure using a similar error analysis technique, may not be good enough. As the field of school psychology moves more toward academic consultation (Stewart, 1987), psychologists, in collaborating with teachers about curriculum and educational programming decisions, will need to extract more from the assessment process. For example, looking at Edwin's performance in the category Vowel Digraphs and Diphthongs, it would appear that he is confused about how to represent these phonemic elements. Nine of the 20 words he attempted contained vowel digraphs or diphthongs. On 5 of those words, Edwin failed to produce the correct marking for the vowel sound. He also reported that 3 of the 5 correctly spelled words in this category—"school," "said," and "does"—had appeared on recent spelling lists. In addition, Edwin initially started to spell the word "said" with "si" before spontaneously amending his response to the correct variant and first represented the word "does" as "dos" before erasing and correcting. A good clinician might also note that Edwin demonstrates some ability to spell correctly words that are overlearned (e.g., "blue" and "school") and some ability to monitor his own performance for the purpose of adjusting the final product (i.e., "said" and "does"). A surface analysis, therefore, might lead us to conclude that our job is nearly complete. Permanent product data plus careful observation have provided the substantive information to develop a sound instructional program. Or have they?

If we look carefully at Edwin's performance in this category, what we see is a nonexhaustive search that results at best in the possible identification of a problem. To form instructional objectives, we need specific information about the extent of the problem. Reviewing Edwin's work, we find that three of the five misspellings in this category were for words that have unpredictable vowel digraphs or diphthongs. For the two misspelled words listed as predictable, both contained vowel digraphs. Edwin provided no marking for the long vowel sound in "reach" but did provide a VCe (silent "e") ending to mark the digraph in the word "afraid." By breaking all of the attempted words, predictable and unpredictable, into their component phonemes and then analyzing each phoneme for the presence or absence of legal graphemic markers, we might be able to give a teacher instructionally relevant information pertaining to Edwin's abilities to segment words into phonemes, to use rule-based information to guide the production of phonemes, and to use recognitive information gained through reading to help his spelling. With the addition of interletter latency and confidence interval data to help establish the precise location and extent of Edwin's uncertainty, we might provide still further information that would constrain and focus hypotheses about the child's academic difficulty. We would point out, however, that it is difficult to make statements about the presence, absence, or status of some skilled orthographic behavior by analyzing unpredictable letter sequences or by analyzing one instance each of two different vowel digraphs.

An information-processing analysis of skill in this area would seek systematically and separately to establish the level of skill development for vowel digraphs and vowel diphthongs. Moreover, care would be taken to demonstrate whether digraph or diphthong problems were specific to certain exemplars, whether there was a relationship between the level of representation and the length or complexity of the word to be spelled, and whether the time taken to produce correct letter sequences indicated pauses or hesitations that could be interpreted to reflect uncertainty. In the latter case, interletter latencies can inform the investigator about automaticity (Anderson's procedural level of skill development) (Gerber, 1987) or about how information is being clustered, without having to ask students what they were thinking about during problem solving. Given Skinner's (1987) recent admonitions to the field of cognitive psychology for *asking about* rather than *observing* behavior, it is timely to remind school psychologists that one key to interpretable observation is the systematic presentation of problems designed to cumulate information about what has been achieved. In sum, we would argue that the Spelling subtest from the K-TEA offers too few opportunities to observe how children respond to different phonemic elements within varied orthographic environments. Too much emphasis has been placed on evaluation performance that is tied to idiosyncratic understanding of unpredictable letter sequences, and not enough emphasis has been given to generating corroborative evidence useful for informing instructional programs. "Where to begin" and "how to implement" are questions that teachers want answered. Substantive responses to these questions come from systematic data collection informed by theory and from clear understanding of the cognitive requirements necessary for competent performance on a given task.

Uncertainty and Speed

We recognize that the preceding statements may represent a level of performance that is not attainable for most school psychologists given the nature of their preservice training, the constraints imposed by too little time, and the number of referrals that must be considered for assessment. Nonetheless, we would argue that some modifications in the data collection process are do-able, informative, and consistent with an information-processing analysis of behavior. In effect, we would like to suggest that certain information-processing markers be included in the data collection process. Although attention to these markers will not offset many of the problems attendant to standardized tests, we maintain that extended analysis of existing data may help school psychologists to develop a perspective on what we view as the preferred way to ask questions about skill acquisition.

In most information-processing analyses of behavior, the two elements that stand out as important to interpretation of skill acquisition are uncertainty and speed of processing. First, we are interested in the level of uncertainty associated with complex responses. If students are aware that their responses may not be correct and if they can pinpoint their uncertainty within the problem, we then have a basis for determining the point in the process where the learner is confused or not equipped to complete the problem successfully. This information can be useful if we are concerned about providing instruction that minimally overlaps with what the child already knows how to do. In this regard, the elaborated cueing technique associated with the zone of proximal development and dynamic assessment outlined in Goetz, Hall, and Fetsco (in press), provides a means for establishing the level at which a child's performance is tentative or uncertain. This technique, however, conflicts with the goals of standardized testing and hence may not be acceptable across all testing situations.

. For any problem-solving exercise that involves the production of permanent products, such as spelling, mathematics, or written composition, insight into how confident children are about their products can be obtained by asking them to rate their performance. Using spelling as an example, children can be asked, following each spelling response, whether they think their attempt is correct, incorrect, or in doubt by using a three-point scale (1 = "I'm sure," 2 = "Maybe," 3 = "No way"). To document shifts in confidence that may reflect the gradual process by which knowledge is converted from declarative to procedural, children might also be asked to rate their confidence before they begin to spell a targeted word. For example, Edwin was asked to rate his performance subsequent to spelling each of the K-TEA words. He rated his performance on the words "and," "dog," "big," "blue," "school," and "friend" as "I'm sure"; on the words "on," "wagon," and "does" as "Maybe"; and on the remaining words as "No way." Thus, for the 8 words that he spelled correctly, he was confident about 5 of his spellings; for the 12 words he spelled incorrectly, he rated 10 as "No way." He was unsure about two words that were correctly spelled and one word that was incorrectly spelled. For only two spellings, "firnd" and "said," were his ratings completely askew.

Edwin's willingness to reflect on his work and his ability to identify accurately most of his correct and incorrect spellings reiterates that he has developed some ability to monitor his own performance. An instructional program, then, might train him to react to low-confidence words by first identifying exactly where in the word he thinks his performance is confused. He should come to understand that precisely sequenced responses resulting from the application of trained problem-solving strategies need be overt only when performance is doubtful or uncertain. Training designed with the idea that all behavior in a given content area is problematic forces children to respond publicly in ways that may deautomatize or interrupt well-established problem-solving routines. The next phase of training should focus on developing his ability to generate alternative letter sequences that conform to rules or relationships (e.g., homophonic, syntactic, or semantic) that are already familiar to him. Finally, instruction should attempt to extend and expand extant knowledge corporas by introducing additional phonic generalizations that can be paired with spelling clues. For example, a preferred sequence for teaching phonics in reading would introduce vowel digraphs in the order "ai," "ea," "oa," "ee," and "ay" (Spache & Spache, 1986). In spelling, a similar sequence could be followed, separately introducing the child to a series of single syllable words that illustrate each of the phonemic elements to be taught. This minimizes confusion for the child, provides the child with breadth of understanding about rule-based digraphs, and immediately informs the teacher about any difficulties that the child might have with a particular digraph. As the child learns the most common way to represent the core set of digraphs, instruction proceeds by presenting (1) contrast lists constructed to solidify basic understanding of trained concepts or rules ("ai" with "ay," "ea" with "ee," etc.), followed by (2) lists of more complex, multisyllabic words featuring each of the core digraphs (knowledge extension), and ending with (3) word lists containing problematic and irregular digraphs (e.g., "ea" as in "head," "ie" as in believe," or "ie" as in "friend") (knowledge extension and generalization). From an information-processing perspective, the data collection process and the instructional program become inseparable. In sum, treatments that seek to maximize a child's efficiency by providing a guide for how and when to use particular cognitive resources help to avoid the aptitude/treatment problems emanating from static instructional programs that were outlined by Snow and Peterson (1985).

For many children, global judgments about response uncertainty may be inaccurate or, if accurate, may not be subject to articulation by the child. In response to questions like, "Where in the word do you think the letters are incorrect or not quite right?" a child might simply answer, "I don't know," or, "It just doesn't look right." To pinpoint a child's uncertainty within a word, therefore, a second element of information processing may be necessary. Speed, expressed as (1) the length of time taken by a child to respond, (2) the time taken before a child responds, or (3) the time taken between responses within words, can give the clinician useful, directly interpretable information regarding uncertainty. This is not always the case, however. Children who spell words quickly, with no pauses or hesitations, and who are not accurate in rating their performance are communicating something about their level of involvement in the problem-solving process. In these cases, examiners need to determine whether or not all phonemes in a word have been rendered and how well legal graphemic markers have been used to represent the individual component sounds. Unmotivated or unwilling problem solvers present a special challenge for those attempting to document level of skill development; thus in cases where nonintellective factors are suspected of suppressing performance, examiners are advised to focus their data collection efforts on determining the level of spelling development that is typical of a given child's spelling attempts. Lack of interest in problem solving is often related to large gaps in basic knowledge germane to a particular content area. Palmer and Rholes (Chapter 8, this volume) provide an in-depth discussion of issues related to the assessment of children's attributions.

Most school psychologists, however, are able to respond to potentially unmotivated behavior by providing children with supportive, nonthreatening contexts that tend to engender the best possible individual performance. Thus, the problem-solving difficulties that these children experience are different. They may not be able to articulate where in a word they are having difficulty, but they may leave other clues that point to problem areas.

In information-processing research, speed is generally thought of in millisecond increments. Without sophisticated timing equipment, however, school psychologists are unlikely to be sensitive to differences in performance that are best interpreted at the millisecond level. We would suggest, nonetheless, that practitioners can collect nonintrusive data about the speed of processing that may be very useful to describing the boundaries of individual performance. For instance, approximately how long does it take a child to begin her or his response to a particular word? Are there noticeable hesitations or pauses between letters or groups of letters? Where pauses occur, are there corresponding subvocalizations of troublesome phonemes? Does another word with a sound structure similar to that of an incorrectly spelled word produce the same pattern of hesitations for shared letter sequences? For words that are spelled correctly, are there pauses or hesitations that appear to be associated with specific phonemic elements or letter sequences? Answers to questions like these can signal the examiner about where in a word a child is uncertain, and thus can serve to guide the development of self-questioning strategies that (1) can be easily transferred to and controlled by the child, (2) will help the child to do a better job of monitoring and articulating his or her performance, and (3) will help facilitate the transition from declarative to procedural knowledge for skills being acquired.

Repeated Trials and Generalization

It is clear that variations in error quality, interpreted within a developmental framework, can provide a basis for interpreting cognitive status vis-à-vis spelling skill. We have also cautioned against "one-shot" assessments. The process of learning is dynamic. Therefore, it follows that assessment and instructional intervention must likewise be dynamic. To make the effort manageable, it is convenient to "fix" either content to be taught, assessment to be conducted, or instruction to be delivered, while allowing the others to be free to vary. Thus, we can hold instructional items (e.g., a spelling list) constant, but vary the amount and level of explanation, procedural modeling, prompts, and feedback (i.e., structure) with the aim of estimating the learning "distance" that might be achieved with differing degrees of instructional effort. Similarly, we can vary instructional items to assess transfer and generalization while holding instructional effort relatively constant. Or we can select a criterion of interest, like verbalized level of uncertainty, level of phoneme representation, speed of performance, or number of bigrams (i.e., two letter sequences) present to assess the measure's sensitivity and stability over a range of content and instructional conditions.

In any case, to assess natural changes and shifts in performance over time and to interpret these as developmental changes in cognitive status, it is convenient to create an instructional standard and pacing against which to form judgments about students' spontaneous (i.e., unassisted) ability to organize and generalize their attempts to solve spelling problems.

We have tried to do this in a series of studies using LD spellers (Gerber, 1984b, 1986b, 1987; Nulman & Gerber, 1984) in which students were asked to make repeated attempts to spell a difficult list of words. These studies were motivated by our earlier observation that not only did LD students demonstrate cross-sectional profiles of development that were similar to those of normally achieving students, though lagged, but also that qualitative improvement in errors could be observed within the same students on the same words over time (Gerber & Hall, 1982). That is, retesting LD students after a delay of several months showed strong evidence of shifts in developmental level of spelling attempts, even in the absence of a formal program of spelling instruction. We interpreted this shift to mean that there was a natural baseline rate of acquisition even for learning-disabled students. Clearly, assessment aimed at designing appropriate cognitive-behavioral training interventions needed to take this baseline into account.

To verify our longitudinal observations, we adopted a minimal approach to instruction whereby instructors provided students who had misspelled on a dictation task with a contingent imitation of their error followed by a model of the correct spelling. For example, if a child spelled "belive" for "believe," the teacher would say: "No, that is not correct. This is how you spelled the word." The instructor would then write the misspelling as it was produced by the child and then say, "This is the correct spelling for the word," and write the correct spelling beneath the modeled error.

In each of our studies, a striking phenomenon became evident. First, each repeated spelling attempt tended to produce a qualitatively better spelling. Significantly, these attempts improved gradually by modifying specific orthographic features, not by producing longer and longer strings of correct letters. For example, the student who misspelled "believe" took eight trials before the word was spelled correctly. The eight errors were: BELIVE, BEALIVE, BEELEVE, BEELIVE, BEELIVE, BELIVE, and BELEVE. The specific errors produced, along with the corresponding sequence, given the controlled instruction, can be interpreted to show something of the child's state of phonetic and orthographic knowledge, as well as something about the student's cognitive processes in response to distinct (and controllable) instructional factors. Examination of the errors reveals that there are really only two features within the word that are troublesome, the two different spellings for the long vowel / E / in the first and second syllables. All other phonetic representations are remarkably stable—for example, first consonant, medial consonant, final consonant, and final silent "e."

The instructional contingencies may have disrupted a known spelling by artificially increasing global uncertainty, but this is unlikely because there was no specific correction involving the first vowel that might have cast doubt. Moreover, consonant and final silent "e" spellings remained unaffected. It is more reasonable to suppose that the error imitation, correct modeling procedure made visible those spelling elements about which the student was still significantly uncertain. That is, although the spelling for the first vowel is nominally correct and would pass as such in a cursory inspection of the attempt, its "correctness" must not be interpreted as evidence that the student "knows" how to spell tense vowels in similar syllabic environments in light of the student's revealed propensity to change. Experienced teachers and school psychologists will recognize the similarity of this effect with that which occurs when correct answers are questioned in classrooms. Students who shift their answers obviously possess the necessary information to produce correct responses but are not yet confident that they indeed have arrived at the correct answer.

In the case at hand, it is likely that the student was applying the same misleading spelling strategy for the first and second vowels, based on the immature supposition that letter names are determinants of the speech sounds they represent. Notice the apparent matches in both sound and articulation. Thus, "e" can be regarded as a logical choice for most tense vowel /E/ sounds. The misspelling of "i" for "ie," on the other hand, represents a late stage in using this same phonetic strategy, although again it is not obvious on superficial inspection. Thus, "i" is selected to represent the tense vowel /E/ in the second syllable because the student has learned that vowel spellings have lax as well as tense forms, and pronunciation of lax /i/ is close in articulation to the speech sound intended, namely tense /E/ (i.e., "i" as in "it" and "e" as in "be*lieve*"). In other words, previous instruction, word experience, and perhaps visual memory give the student enough evidence to conclude that the spelling of the second vowel in "believe" is not simply "e." Rather, the student reasons, there is a rule (i.e., procedural knowledge) that dictates this decision. But a search for suitable algorithms retrieves a not fully understood rule pertaining to the use of nonobvious vowel graphemes to represent lax vowel speech sounds. Hence, because the student's understanding is still rather immature, he or she disregards (or does not know) the pronunciation marking function of the final "e." The result is a decision based on a comparison of articulation positions and not on a correct execution of the rule. Appropriately applied, the rule would have required a different syllabic structure and disallowed the final "e." In the ensuing trials, the confusion between the two vowel spellings not only is interpretable but also has clear instructional implications. This would not be so, of course, if older, simplistic diagnostic categories based on notions of visual discrimination or visual memory were invoked.

The second striking aspect of the results we observed in these studies was the tendency, *even under these very minimal instructional conditions,* for successful spelling of features to generalize to new lists of words. Using the imitation/

modeling format, when LD students, regardless of age, were permitted repeatedly to attempt a given list of words until all were spelled correctly, they nearly always spelled better on their first trial of a new, phonetically similar list, and reached criterion of 100% correct in fewer trials. Moreover, when given a third list and the explicit verbal instruction to "use what you've learned on previous lists to help you spell these words," LD students spelled even more words correctly on the first trial and reached criterion sooner (Gerber, 1986b). For example, the student who first took eight trials to spell "believe" needed only five trials to spell the word "relief" (RELIVE, RELEF, RELIFE, RELEIF). Inspecting only those features that were difficult in "believe," it is notable that the vowel digraph was also attempted sooner on this list and that the first vowel was never in doubt.

Repeated Trials and Automaticity

Students who experience difficulty in learning to spell not only exhibit problems in producing accurate spellings, but also often spell too slowly and laboriously for spelling to serve its natural purpose of facilitating expressive writing. In our work with LD students over several years, we have noticed that students vary not only in the quality or developmental level of their spelling errors, but also in the time and tempo associated with correct spellings. For example, consider two students asked to spell the word "theater." The first student pauses only a second, places pencil to paper and, without pause or hesitation, writes each letter—T, H, E, A, T, E, R—correctly. Now consider the second student who, while ultimately producing a correct spelling, exerts observably different effort to achieve it. This student's spelling behavior might be as follows:

Pause several seconds	
Write	F
Pause	
Write with inserted space	F AE
Pause	
Write	F AETR
Pause	
Erase, write	THAETR
Pause	
Write, insert	THAET^{E}R
Pause, cross out, rewrite	~~THAETER~~ THEATER

Conventional approaches to spelling assessment would tend to regard these very distinct performances as equivalent. Given the alternative, information-processing-oriented, more dynamic assessment approach urged in this chapter, it should be clear that potentially useful information is lost by attending to the equivalence of spellings and ignoring the important cognitive differences suggested by observation of actual behavior (e.g., see Gerber & Hall, 1987).

Theoretically speaking, attentional capacity is limited. How much knowledge we possess, and how much experience we have in using that knowledge, help us to be efficient in using that limited capacity. In problem-solving situations, repeated attempts to solve spelling problems lead not only to acquisition of pertinent spelling knowledge, but also to dynamic reorganization of that knowledge in ways that support ever faster search and retrieval of problem-related information (e.g., see Gerber & Hall, 1987). Thus, various invented, discovered, or learned subroutines become incrementally faster with repeated problem-solving attempts. It is a matter of some theoretical debate how fast normally achieving students must become before their performance can be considered "automatic," but the notion that with practice information-handling routines become automatic—that is, relatively attention-free—is generally accepted in principle by most investigators.

It is not at all clear if students with learning problems ever become as fast as their normally achieving peers, or even if they have that capacity. From a practical point of view, it is sensible to expect skillful spelling to be reliably accurate *and* fast enough so that it facilitates translation of ideation into written expression. If teachers and school psychologists assess and train only with respect to accuracy, they will have failed to recognize this important aspect of what constitutes skillful behavior.

Because cognitive events occur in periods measured in milliseconds, teachers and school psychologists must observe performance carefully to note features of overt behavior that can be interpreted as an indication that spelling is effortful and attention-demanding. Cognitive-behavioral training, like the spontaneously arising cognitive self-regulation it is meant to supplement, essentially gives students *more*, not less, cognitive work to do. Therefore, in early stages of training, as in early stages of problem solving, the effort and time required to produce partial responses both increase. The ultimate gain in decision speed that underlies observable performance is achieved because systematic and controlled development of knowledge about tasks, task requirements, and one's own capacity occurs during training and repeated practice.

To study this phenomenon, we have used microcomputers to administer repeated spelling dictation trials to LD students. Microcomputers not only help standardize elements of the task, they also permit measurement of millisecond differences in letter decision production time as a function of repeated instructional trials. In one recent study, Gerber (1987) looked at the spelling attempts of 15 LD students. Decreases in mean spelling time (in seconds) for 10 intentionally difficult words were observed over the first six trials. During the same time period, the mean percentage of correctly spelled bigrams (i.e., two-letter sequences) increased from 52% to 64%. In addition, there was an increasing negative correlation between spelling time and degree of spelling accuracy (i.e., bigrams), ranging from −.29 to −.61. One way of interpreting the relationship represented by these data is to suggest that students gradually acquire "accuracy," as seen in our earlier examples, and, moreover, that accuracy is achieved with increasing speed. Whether or when this increase in speed becomes sufficient to have a facilitating effect on writing is not currently known. It is clear from these studies, however, that CBT interventions, to the extent that they are applied in a systematic and sustained manner, hold promise for promoting spelling automaticity as well as accuracy in students who are poor spellers.

From Assessment to Training

Referring back to our example, Edwin, let us look at his spelling for the word "because." First, however, let us review the word for content and for problems that might limit interpretation of performance. "Because," the eighteenth word on the K-TEA Spelling subtest, is listed as having an unpredictable "au" diphthong. We find this somewhat puzzling. An "au" diphthong is predictable when sounded as /o/, as in the words "paw," "gaunt," "daughter," and "caught." Acceptable pronunciations for the word "because" include both "bi-koz" and "bi-kuz." If pronounced using the lax vowel /u/ sound, then the diphthong is not expressed in its most common form. If, however, the word is pronounced using the glided /o/ or "aw" sound, then the diphthong would be considered regular. We would note, too, that in the word part analysis, the "be" is listed as belonging to the Prefixes and Word Beginnings category. The correct pronunciation for the word "because" (*American Heritage Dictionary*, Second College Edition, 1982) does not recognize the open syllable "e" as representing the long vowel sound typical of the prefix "be." Since the test does not incude a guide for pronouncing this word, pronunciation problems, which may include confusing acoustic markers for the child, cannot be reconciled. We would judge this word, therefore, not to provide a good illustration for unpredictable "au" diphthongs. Nevertheless, noting the potential for misinterpretation to exist, let us review Edwin's spelling and the associated observations for this word.

   The examiner pronounced the word "because" as "bi-koz," thus not invoking the unpredictable diphthong sequence in the oral presentation of the word. Edwin paused briefly before spelling the word, during which time he repeated the word to himself, and then produced the response pattern "bu"—long hesitation (three counts), subvocalization of /k/ sound—"c"—hesitation (one count), subvocalization of /s/ sound—"s." The final spelling, therefore, with no attempt at self-correction, was "bucs." When asked to rate his spelling for correctness, Edwin glanced at his attempt and responded immediately with a rating of 3 ("No way"). What has been learned from his performance on this spelling problem?

   On first impression, Edwin's spelling attempt does not appear too sophisticated. It is not easily readable; a parent or teacher might regard "bucs" as a crude spelling variant. But let us look more closely. The first thing that might be noted about this word is that, though highly familiar to most children, it represents a relatively complex spelling word for young children. Analyzing Edwin's performance on a phoneme-by-phoneme basis using a version of the spelling quality rating (SQR) developed by Gerber and Hall (1982), we find that he correctly represented the first and third phonemes, /b/ and /k/; produced a transitional representation (legal and plausible but incorrect) for the second phoneme, /i/; represented the fifth phoneme, /z/, phonetically ("s" must be accompanied by an "e" to generate a /z/ sound unless used to indicate the plural form of a word, as in "hers"); and was given a prephonetic rating for the absent vowel diphthong. Averaging across phonemes, this spelling would be viewed, using the SQR rating system, as a good-quality phonetic spelling. Applying the same rating procedure to the five K-TEA word part categories to which this word belongs, we would rate the single consonants "c" and "s" as correct, the prefix "be" as phonetic, and the vowel diphthong and final "e" as prephonetic. Again, the overall evaluation would classify Edwin's attempt as a solid phonetic spelling.

The phoneme-by-phoneme analysis is best interpreted in conjunction with other words having similar phonemic patterns. We would point out, however, that Edwin attempted to problem-solve throughout the entire word and was able to generate logical graphemic markers for most of the phonemes or word parts. The hesitation pattern in his spelling may be interpreted to suggest that his response to the first two phonemes was automatic or nearly automatic, whereas strategic searching of known sound–symbol correspondences characterized the last three phonemes. It would appear that his greatest difficulty came at the end of the word and that his uncertainty about how to represent the space between the third and fifth phonemes (i.e., the "au" diphthong) resulted in a relatively long pause followed by markings for the most salient acoustic features. The fact that there were subvocalizations suggests to us that he attempted to guide his performance. But his quick acknowledgment that his spelling was incorrect, after his failure to make any attempt to self-correct his work, indicates to us that he struggled to apply known sound–symbol information and was unable or did not think to use recognitive-processing strategies to improve his spelling attempt. The use of recognitive information (e.g., knowledge of what certain letter patterns or words look like) is, in large measure, a function of reading ability. Words that are automatically decodable provide acoustic and visual guidelines that children can use first to detect errors given uncertainty and then to generate other spelling variants of improved quality.

Certainly, we are left with a sense that this child may have a problem representing "au" diphthongs, which is not too different from where we started with the K-TEA error analysis. What benefits, then, are derived from our attempts to identify uncertainty and to characterize speed of processing? First, the extended data collection is neither time-consuming nor especially obtrusive and does not interfere with the interpretation of standardized test results. Second, although analysis of the additional data can be time-consuming and tedious beyond what school psychologists are willing to undertake, the result is a richer informational base from which to interpret a given child's performance. Third, the resulting information directly reflects both the problem-solving process and the demands presented by the task. Thus, this information can be translated directly into instructional programs that focus on strategic solutions for specific problems in context and on generalizable strategies for guiding children's performance in the presence of uncertain responses. Finally, and maybe most important, the need from an information-processing perspective to engage in content analysis helps the practitioner to develop a clinical sense for what it takes to perform competently on the different K-TEA tasks. This, we would argue, tends to elevate school psychologists beyond the role of testers and classifiers to the level of problem solvers and experts.

TEACHING, INTELLIGENT TUTORING, AND TECHNOLOGY

The final area to be addressed in this section is how computers might be helpful to the assessment/instruction process. Certainly the use of computers does not ensure that tests will be better or that information collected by the computer will be more easily or clearly interpretable. The capability of the computer to track and to preserve accurately individuals' responses has much to offer the field of school psychology. Computerized adaptive testing (e.g., Green, 1983), in which item selection is based on the test-taker's previous responses, is but one area that is made feasible by computers. Computers would make it possible, by some estimates, to reduce testing time by as much as 50% to 60% (Ward, 1984) relative to conventional testing by reducing standard errors of measurement at the extreme ends of the ability distribution (Linn, 1986a). The result is precision with fewer items. The greatest advantage, however, may be in the area of diagnostic testing. As Linn (1986b) points out:

> Like the adaptive test, a computerized diagnostic test would be tailored to the individual test taker based on earlier responses. However, the choice of questions would be driven by substantive hypotheses regarding the person's misconceptions or the desire to probe the depth of his or her understanding, rather than by the psychometric criteria of difficulty and discriminating power of the item on a unidimensional scale. (p. 1159)

This notion of testing, blending a theory of knowledge with a theory of instruction, is consistent with the view presented in this chapter. Cumulating children's responses into data bases that preserve the order, speed, and confidence associated with those responses, and then linking the data bases by algorithms, allow children's changing learning histories to determine the level, type, and amount of support given by the computer. In sum, by using the computer to take advantage of the multifaceted nature of cognitive tasks, the result should be sharper diagnostic distinctions coupled with clearer programmatic implications.

CBT as Intelligent Tutoring

Microcomputer technology can be viewed as a potential supplement to or locus of cognitive-behavioral training interventions in spelling. Just as early computers once provided psychologists with a new, albeit limited, model of the components of human cognition, so recent developments in both computer technology and software engineering have generated exciting new levels of interdisciplinary exchange. On one hand, for example, school psychologists are beginning to seek understanding of computers as potentially powerful tools for influencing students' ability to profit from instruction. On the other hand, computer specialists and engineers, interested in building "intelligent tutoring systems," are beginning to realize their need to have better models that describe how real teachers and learners think. Moreover, through computerized formative assessment of learners, it may be possible to gain insight into the strategic and tactical decisions used by individuals within and across problem-solving environments (Wenger, 1987). As of this writing, however, educational professionals are in no immediate danger of being replaced by computers. The range and subtlety of good clinical interview and instructional skills by far surpass what engineers can recreate electronically. Nonetheless, as people from various fields and perspectives continue to work on problems using computers, there is a sense that a more powerful understanding of teaching/learning processes will emerge to assist educators.

Intelligent tutoring, as opposed to so called computer-assisted instruction, refers to a teaching system designed to communicate a body of knowledge, not merely to administer and monitor opportunities to practice simple responses. "Knowledge," in the sense it is used here and has been used throughout, means not only possession of specific facts, but also possession of information about how to use those facts. Thus, spelling knowledge includes not merely a set of sound–symbol translation rules, or a corpus of words one can spell, but also a set of procedures, tactics, and strategies for using such information in the service of written communication.

School psychologists and teachers, no less than computers, also aspire to be intelligent tutors for those students who seem most to require such deliberate instruction. Therefore, cognitive-behavioral training should not be seen as merely a repetoire of related techniques. To be "intelligent," the use of these techniques requires a nontrivial amount of cognitive effort. The barriers, however, are formidable. For example, school psychologists and teachers must possess *expertise* in the domain they wish to train. Being able to spell well, however, is not the same as being able to communicate one's expertise, as should be apparent to many who struggle to follow the psycholinguistic arguments contained in this chapter. But it is this requirement to be able to externalize one's expertise and communicate that expertise that makes a tutoring system "intelligent."

Teaching normally achieving students—those who bring significant knowledge and skill, preorganized, as it were, to be optimally receptive to available modes of instruction—is not difficult. In fact, these students could be characterized by their reliable ability to demonstrate achievement gains in response to short verbal explanations, abbreviated demonstrations and models, outlines of general strategies, disclosure of useful rules and algorithms, or simple instructions or inducements to perform. Although the success of these students is usually taken as evidence of good teaching, we should frankly admit that the observed outcomes are at least as much the result of a good student. That is, normally achieving students possess knowledge to be built on, but also exhibit knowledge about knowledge—what it is, why one needs it, who has it, how to acquire it, when it is sufficient for some specific purpose, and so forth.

Part of what makes these students "normally achieving" is their ability to use their well-integrated knowledge of language, not only for speaking, reading, and writing, but also for communicating effectively with teachers *about* speaking, reading, and writing. They have and easily use the capacity to recognize uncertainty, ambiguity, insufficient and irrelevant information, and error. Moreover, they also have the ability to prompt for additional data, to frame questions, and to understand even relatively abstract explanations. Thus, when teaching these students, teachers can communicate only, we might say, on one channel. That is, teachers need only to transmit basic information in the form of general explanations because the teacher's language maps onto an internal language and knowledge base that normally achieving students already possess.

Students experiencing learning difficulty, however, require teaching communications on two channels—one that transmits the elemental facts and another that models a structure for relating and using those facts. That is to say, teachers must make effective thinking in a domain transparent so that students can observe the thinking as well as its content. Use of this second channel of teaching communication is inherently difficult for teachers because it is cognitively demanding and time-consuming. Therefore, students who require such teaching communication are rightly viewed as difficult to teach.

Teaching spelling, for example, requires communicating a letter sequence or a rule for generating a letter sequence, but it also requires teaching language that explicitly probes what internal understanding the student possesses about spelling that will permit the student to remember and appropriately use knowledge of specific letter sequences or spelling rules. Moreover, based on iteratively derived models of the learner's current status, this second channel of teaching communication must also consist of a teaching language that is deliberately and economically constructed *as it is being used* to model for students a way of thinking and talking about logical or empirical relationships that exist among different spelling sequences or rules.

Thus, intelligent tutoring, whether incorporated in hardware and software or embodied in professionals, is quite complex. Beyond expert knowledge, it requires the ability to communicate that knowledge in an orderly and applied fashion when confronted by domain-related problems. In addition, the knowledge to be communicated must include standards for regulating and evaluating its use so that students internalize *how*, not just *what*, to learn.

Preliminary Investigations

For the present, stand-alone computer technology and software capable of intelligent tutoring of spelling is not available. However, the availability of microcomputer technology in the schools gives teachers and school psychologists a great opportunity to learn how to be intelligent tutors themselves. If computers and software are seen as tools, not substitutes, professionals will find they have increased ability to design and implement a successful CBT program in spelling. For example, one of the problems in providing intelligent tutoring is the complexity of data handling when one is forced to interpret, plan, and communicate instructional information rapidly in a dynamic transaction with students. If the computer and a reasonably "intelligent" spelling program are available as a teaching partner however, then many of the chores related to problem generation (i.e., what spelling word to use next), error detection, measurement (e.g., interletter latencies), provision of feedback (i.e., type and mode of reinforcement or correction), and attention control can be handled by the computer, leaving the tutor free to observe, assess, and respond formatively to qualitative aspects of performance that are inferred to be related to the cognitive status of the learner.

SPELLDOWN: A Pilot Illustration

The work of Varnhagen and Gerber (1984) represents an early attempt to construct a computer-assisted spelling program. Their program, SPELL, was modeled, in part, in a CBT intervention developed by Gerber (1981). Among the noteworthy features programmed into SPELL was the ability (1) to start and stop a tape recorder, (2) to adjust feedback based on the presence of certain child responses, (3) to capture the sequence of keystrokes used by children to represent words, and (4) to preserve latencies associated with each keystroke. Although the program was marginally successful in terms of improved spelling quality and children's perception of performance, the authors noted that even after 16 trials of spelling the same words, there was little improvement in search speed for children with learning problems. In reviewing their work, Varnhagen and Gerber cautioned that keyboards were likely to create special problems for children relying on computers for instruction. Because children had to concentrate on communicating with the computer through the keyboard, attention was drawn away from the central problem-solving activity. In other words, the keyboard was an obstacle to the instructional process.

In contrast, pencils are efficient, psychologically transparent tools. That is, the focal point of the pencil is the same as that for the eye, hence, workspace does not shift from one place to another. The pencil moves and makes a mark at the slightest inclination of the child, and with practice children can reliably produce marks that are easily understood by others without having to allocate any significant amount of attention to the letter production process. For unskilled or even marginally proficient keyboard users, the same constraints do not hold true. The eye, rather than being focused on the evolving problem-solving product depicted on the monitor, is subservient to the search process being conducted by the child to find the appropriate key. This results in an attentional drain, as the object of the search process is one and only one letter embedded in an unfamiliar and confusing array of letters, numbers, and symbols.

The keyboard presents a special problem when children are trying to produce sequences of letters before memory traces decay, as might be the case when spelling words or writing sentences. With a pencil, even if the child is uncertain about the proper orientation for a letter, letter variations often adequately communicate the child's intended response; thus, young children may not feel compelled to divert attention away from the phoneme translation process to the letter production process. The keyboard, then, because of its potentially disruptive effect on the problem-solving process, was viewed by Varnhagen and Gerber as a major stumbling block to using the computer as an effective tutor.

Because computers must be told precisely what to do, the development of instructional software can provide a detailed illustration for how to teach. For a computer program to serve as a useful metaphor for teaching, however, the program must be effective and the instructional environment created by interacting with the computer must be comparable to that of the classroom. Program developers often try to minimize the need to use the keyboard by presenting learners with prepackaged alternatives that can be selected by moving the cursor or by pressing one key. Contexts created by using limited or extended keyboards for communication with the computer potentially develop narrow aspects of problem solving or alter the learning process to such a degree that classroom and computer learning environments are not comparable. Thus, to consider a program as a template for teaching, our first concern is to eliminate or reduce keyboard problems.

A program called SPELLDOWN currently under development by Hall and Stricker (1988) and Stricker and Hall (1988) has attempted to address some of the keyboard problems. These researchers have taken the keyboard and graphically represented it, alphabetically, on the screen. The workspace for generating word variants is directly above the keyboard, and cursor movement among the rows of letters is accomplished via a mouse. Data already collected from children with spelling problems have been interpreted to indicate that, following short training periods, children have little trouble using the mouse. In addition, the alphabetic order of the letters is familiar to children, hence, the search process becomes less cognitively demanding over time. It would also appear that having the workspace close to the keyboard and in the same visual plane helps children to stay better attuned to the phoneme translation process. In a 26-week tryout with one child, spelling performance went from between 25% and 30% correct (based on a 20-word list) to between 95% and 100% correct, with approximately a 50% reduction in the total amount of time spent interacting with the program. Although much of the time reduction can be attributed to increased spelling skill, a sizable portion is a direct result of on-screen keyboard mastery. In sum, although we would not claim to have solved the problem of "keyboard transparency," we have certainly created a less taxing and less frustrating means for children to communicate with the computer. We feel, therefore, that the unique instructional features programmed into SPELLDOWN will serve as a guide for the development of efficient CBT problem-solving procedures in spelling.

SPELLDOWN was designed as a 5-day, self-contained tutorial system for teaching and evaluating performance in spelling. The 5-day package corresponds to the amount of time allocated in most classrooms for presenting, practicing, learning, and testing lists of words. General formats for the 5-day program are as follows:

Day 1: Presentation of tape-recorded words and corresponding sentences
Day 2: Tachistoscopic presentation of words
Day 3: Presentation of sentences with spelling words missing
Day 4: Competitive spelling (child versus computer) to foster development of spelling fluency
Day 5: Standard spelling test format (e.g., word, word used in sentence, word)

On Day 1 and 3, error prediction and detection data are collected for each word. In addition, the program is designed to preserve, for each spelling variant, (1) interletter latencies, (2) time to initial response, (3) total time, and (4) letter sequence. For words spelled incorrectly, scaffolded problem-solving cues are introduced to (1) guide children's responses; (2) provide a general model for problem solving in spelling; (3) provide extended practice in how to spell words correctly; and (4) teach phoneme–grapheme correspondence rules through systematic introduction of phonetically similar, regular words. Design features such as branching and faded cueing are used to customize feedback for children who need more elaborate constraint-seeking information. Speed and accuracy data collected by the computer are stored in a series of relational data bases linked via algorithms. These mathematical, decision-making formulas help the computer to determine the type and extent of assistance needed by children. Correct and incorrect response feedback, level of help available for any given word, and length of tachistoscopic presentation are determined by the teacher at the time spelling words are entered into the program.

Given this brief introduction to the program, how does it work and how might an intelligent computer-assisted program inform the teaching/learning process captured in CBT programs?

The first thing one might notice about SPELLDOWN is that the program changes from day to day. That is, there are slight variations in the program format on different days. We feel that instructional programs need to have indentifiable consistency so that children can predict what will happen next and thus become comfortable with the learning environment. It is also important, however, to vary, in systematic ways, how information is presented to and requested from children. This tends to lessen the effects of context-dependent learning and to increase the probability that a broader range of cues will be available to children faced with spelling problems. From the direct instruction literature, we have adopted that notion that errors must be corrected immediately and that, in correcting errors, the process of producing a correct variant should be modeled for the child. Like the SPELL program, SPELLDOWN gives children opportunities to view their own work and to compare their spelling attempts against correct standards. In that way, children can see immediately and precisely if and where errors have occurred. Let us now look more closely at how instruction proceeds using the Day 1 program as an illustration.

The initial task facing a teacher using SPELLDOWN is to enter words, sentences, and correctional and reinforcing feedback into the program and/or onto a cassette tape. This affords the teacher the opportunity to think carefully, in advance, about the pronunciation for individual words, the sentence content that will best illustrate the word's meaning, and the substance of the printed feedback that will be given to the child once the child enters a correct or incorrect spelling into the program. Our first recommendation for creating CBT interventions, then, is to plan in advance how information is to be presented and how correct or incorrect student responses will be addressed.

What are the child variables to which an information-processing-based computer program needs to be sensitive, and how does SPELLDOWN incorporate those variables into the fabric of the program? As we have already argued, the crucial information-processing indicators are uncertainty, speed, order, and type of response. On Day 1, SPELLDOWN first presents to the child, via a tape recording of the teacher's voice, the word, the word used in a sentence, and the word repeated. At this point, a message appears on the monitor requesting the child to THINK. This is followed by a message asking the child to predict, using a graded ruler line, whether the child thinks that he or she can spell the word correctly. We are attempting here to get the child to consider his or her performance before engaging in the problem-solving process. In our view, problem solving should begin with considered rather than impulsive responding. In addition, the teacher is given some sense about uncertainty as the child is queried about confidence in her or his ability to produce an accurate response. To refocus problem solving on the word to be spelled, the word is then repeated, followed by the on-screen appearance of the keyboard and a banded workspace. The child is then asked to spell the word. After a word variant is entered into the computer, the child is asked if he or she would like to go on or to spell the word again. If the child chooses to spell the word again, the keyboard and workspace reappear, along with a window containing the first spelling variant. Thus, the child does not have to struggle to recall how he or she produced a previous spelling attempt. Attention can be directed at the troublesome part of the word without regard for those letters or letter sequences viewed as satisfactory. Once the child has produced either a variant that she or he finds acceptable or has exhausted the fund of information that might inform a spelling attempt, the option to "Go on" is selected. At this point, each of the spelling variants appears in a menu on the screen, and the child is asked to pick the variant that best represents the requested spelling. Our intent here is to develop the recognitive aspect of information processing. Essentially, at this point in the teaching sequence, the child is being asked, "Which variant, if any, looks correct?"

Once the child has chosen a variant, he or she is asked to look at her or his spelling and rate the quality of what has been produced. Ratings range from "No way" to "I'm sure." Here again we focus on uncertainty but also on getting the child to understand the importance of proofreading his or her work. SPELLDOWN then gives feedback as to whether the spelling was correct or incorrect. If the spelling is correct, the child moves to the next word and the process just described is repeated. Thus, if a child evidences no problem, the program is designed to move rapidly through the spelling list so as to match the problem-solving pace of the child. If the spelling is incorrect, however, the child moves directly into a correction subroutine.

Amount and type of spelling instruction and practice are determined based on the quality of a child's misspelling, the amount of time taken to produce incorrect letter sequences, and how a child has previously performed on words containing problematic phonetic features. In the most elaborate case, the child is first presented with the correct spelling and then asked to copy the spelling. This serves to minimize memory demands, familiarize the child with the spelling, and provide the opportunity for close scrutiny of the word. Next, the child is presented with a scrambled version of the word. It is important here that all the letters needed to spell the word are present and visible so that memory demands are constrained to mapping appropriate graphemes to phonemes. As letters are chosen, they are stripped from the scrambled spelling, leaving only those letters that have yet to be used. In addition, to aid the child further, teachers can select a help option that will provide letter-by-letter feedback. Thus, children are informed after each letter whether or not they have produced a correct choice. Following the successful unscrambling of the spelling, the child is asked to produce, from memory, the correct spelling. In this phase, teachers can opt to include the help option so that after each letter the child is given feedback about how well she or he is doing. The help option has also been designed to be instructive. For example, if a child enters a letter that is not in the word, he or she is told that "Letter _____ is not in the word." If a child follows with another letter that is not in the word, the message is repeated. A third attempt to enter a letter not in the spelling is accompanied by a message, "Wrong letter, put _____ in now." In effect, we allow and encourage a child to attempt a spelling, but if a child has no clue as to what letter should be entered, the program requests a specific response. This reduces frustration and exacts a positive response from the child to conclude that phase of problem solving. If a child enters an incorrect letter that is out of position, the computer first responds, "Letter _____ is in the wrong place." If another incorrect letter is entered, the computer prompts with "May I suggest a consonant" or "May I suggest a vowel," at which point a window containing all the vowels or consonants in the current word, appears above the workspace. If a child is still unable to identify the correct letter, the computer responds with "Wrong letter, put _____ in now." Finally, to exit the correction subroutine, the word must be correctly spelled from memory with no help. In sum, the correction subroutine is designed so as not to give children more information than is necessary to evoke a correct response. If a child is successful after the initial prompt, more explicit cues are not seen. If, on the other hand, a given cue fails properly to constrain a child's response, feedback to the child is increasingly more detailed but not so annoying as to engender frustration.

Days 2 through 4 of SPELLDOWN differ from Day 1 in how information is presented. Days 2 and 3 do not use a tape recorder and prediction and detection data are collected on some days and not others. Fundamentally, however, the program proceeds at a pace that parallels a child's current level of understanding, thus maintaining a balance between instruction and correction across each of the tutorial days. In other words, the program is designed to be informative, instructive, and supportive while at the same time being systematic and consistent.

In our view, SPELLDOWN represents a method of data collection and customized feedback that is illustrative of good teaching and therefore illustrative of what should be included in any CBT instructional program. Preliminary analysis of data using the intelligent CAI spelling tutorial system (SPELL-DOWN) resulted in improved quality of children's spelling as well as increases in the number of words spelled correctly relative to performance attained using more conventional drill and practice methods. Students using SPELLDOWN correctly represented approximately 27% more bigrams per day than did students using the control version of the program. Given the ceiling effects present for nearly all students using SPELLDOWN, the relative advantage of this instructional program, and hence of this method of instruction, is probably underestimated.

CONCLUSION

In this chapter, we have expressed concern about how school psychologists collect and interpret child data. Fundamentally, when a teacher refers a child for special services, she is acknowledging that she cannot accommodate that child in her classroom given her present resources and understanding of the child's problem(s). To continue with this child, she needs qualitative information that leads directly to a plan of instruction that has a definite starting point, is sequenced to build on what a child already knows, and can be paced in such a way that the child is stimulated and challenged in all aspects of skill acquisition. Not all of these requirements can be met all of the time for all children experiencing difficulty. For instructional purposes, information about "how much" is not satisfactory. Quantitative information summarizes individual performance relative to aggregated performance and thus tends to be nonspecific with respect to the type of problem a child is experiencing and nondirectional in terms of where to begin instruction or how to elaborate feedback for incorrect responses. Error analysis, where errors are typed or categorized, offers a more well rounded picture of a child's skill development but can provide misleading information when the types or categories are too broad to specify precisely which skills are fluent, which are operative but not firm, and which are dysfluent.

Work in academic areas such as spelling, math, and reading (Benton & Kiewra, 1987) have made us aware of the sensitive relationship that exists between assessment and instruction. Elaborated instruction that becomes too cumbersome for marginally proficient children may render them uninterested or unmotivated and lead to performance decrements. Instruction that is not elaborated enough for those same children may fail to provide enough constraining information to allow them to improve their skills. Ideally, the relationship between assessment and instruction should be mutually informative, with assessment serving to shape instruction while cognitive analysis of instructional responses helps to determine what, when, how, and how much to assess. In our view, then, cognitive training efforts need to go beyond development of simple mediators that check for the presence or absence of certain behavioral responses in particular orders to programs that base feedback and presentation of stimuli on detailed analyses of children's present and past responses. How these training programs might work is nicely illustrated by intelligent computer-assisted instructional programs such as SPELLDOWN.

REFERENCES

Anderson, J. R. (1982). Acquisition of cognitive skill. *Psychological Review, 89,* 369–406.

Benton, S. L., & Kiewra, K. A. (1987). The assessment of cognitive factors in academic abilities. In R. R. Ronning, J. A. Glover, J. C. Conoley, & J. C. Witt (Eds.), *The influence of cognitive psychology on testing* (pp. 145–189). Hillsdale, NJ: Lawrence Erlbaum.

Boder, E. (1973). Developmental dyslexia: A diagnostic approach based on three atypical reading–spelling patterns. *Developmental Medicine and Child Neurology, 15,* 663–687.

Bookman, M. O. (1984). Spelling as a cognitive-developmental linguistic process. *Academic Therapy, 20,* 21–32.

Cone, T. E., Wilson, L. R., Bradley, C. M., & Reese, J. H. (1985). Characteristics of LD students in Iowa: An empirical investigation. *Learning Disability Quarterly, 8,* 211–220.

Croft, A. C. (1982). Do spelling tests measure the ability to spell? *Educational and Psychological Measurement, 42,* 715–723.

DiBello, L., & Orlich, F. (1987). How Vygotsky's notion of "scientific concept" may inform contemporary studies of theory development. *Laboratory of Comparative Human Cognition, 9,* 96–99.

Englert, C. S., Hiebert, E. H., & Stewart, S. R. (1985). Spelling unfamiliar words by analogy strategy. *Journal of Special Education, 19,* 291–306.

Farnham-Diggory, S., & Nelson, B. (1984). Cognitive analyses of basic school tasks. *Applied Developmental Psychology, 1,* 21–74.

Fitzsimmons, R. J., & Loomer, B. M. (1977). *Spelling: Learning and instruction—research and practice.* Iowa City: University of Iowa.

Fox, B., & Routh, D. K. (1983). Reading disability, phonemic analysis, dysphonetic spelling: A follow-up study. *Journal of Clinical Child Psychology, 12,* 28–32.

Frith, U. (1980). *Cognitive processes in spelling.* London: Academic Press.

Gagne, E. D. (1985). *The cognitive psychology of school learning.* Boston, MA: Little, Brown.

Gentry, J. R. (1984). Developmental aspects of learning to spell. *Academic Press, 20,* 11–19.

Gerber, M. M. (1981). *Effects of self-monitoring training on the spelling performance of LD and normally achieving students.* Unpublished doctoral dissertation, University of Virginia, Charlottesville.

Gerber, M. M. (1984a). Orthographic problem-solving ability of learning disabled and normally achieving students. *Learning Disability Quarterly, 7,* 157–164.

Gerber, M. M. (1984b). Techniques to teach generalizable spelling skills. *Academic Therapy, 20*(1), 49–58.

Gerber, M. M. (1985). Spelling as concept-governed problem solving: Learning disabled and normally achieving students. In B. Hutson (Ed.), *Advances in reading/language research.* (Vol. 3, pp. 39–75). Greenwich, CT: JAI Press.

Gerber, M. M. (1986a). Cognitive-behavioral training in the curriculum: Time, slow learners, and basic skills. *Focus on Exceptional Children, 18*(6), 1–12.

Gerber, M. M. (1986b). Generalization of spelling strategies by LD students as a result of contingent imitation/modeling and mastery criteria. *Journal of Learning Disabilities, 19*(9), 530–537.

Gerber, M. M. (1987). *Acquisition and automaticity of spelling in learning-handicapped students.* Paper presented at the annual meeting of the American Educational Research Association, Washington, DC, April 22.

Gerber, M. M. (in preparation). *Spelling in compositions by learning disabled and normally achieving students.*

Gerber, M. M., & Cohen, S. B. (1985). Assessment of spelling skills. In A. F. Rotatori & R. Fox (Eds.), *Assessment for regular and special education teachers* (pp. 249–278). Austin, TX: PRO-ED.

Gerber, M. M., & Hall, R. J. (1982). *Development of spelling in learning disabled and normally achieving children.* Unpublished monograph, University of California, Santa Barbara.

Gerber, M. M., & Hall, R. J. (1987). Information processing approaches to studying spelling deficiencies. *Journal of Learning Disabilities, 20*(1), 34–42.

Goetz, E. T., & Hall, R. J. (1984). Evaluation of the Kaufman Assessment Battery for Children from an information-processing perspective. *Journal of Special Education, 18,* 281–296.

Goetz, E. T., Hall, R. J., & Fetsco, T. G. (in press). Implications of cognitive psychology for assessment of academic skill. In C. R. Reynolds & R. W. Kamphaus (Eds.), *Handbook of psychological and educational assessment of children: Vol. 1. Intelligence and achievement*. New York: Guilford Press.

Green, B. F. (1983). Adaptive testing by computer. In R. B. Ekstrom (Ed.), *Measurement technology and individuality in education: New directions for testing and measurement* (pp. 5–12). San Francisco: Jossey-Bass.

Hacker, K. (1987). For dictionary, wordiness no defect. Knight-Ridder News Service. *Santa Barbara News-Press*, November 27.

Hall, R. J. (1980). Cognitive behavior modification and information-processing skills of exceptional children. *Exceptional Educational Quarterly, 1*(1), 9–15.

Hall, R. J., & Stricker, A. G. (1988). *Intelligent computer-assisted instruction (ICAI) in spelling: Effectiveness of scaffolded and faded cueing on the performance of learning disabled students*. Paper presented at the annual meeting of the Southwest Educational Research Association, San Antonio, Texas, January.

Hammill, D. D., Larsen, S. C., & McNutt, G. (1977). The effects of spelling instruction: A preliminary study. *Elementary School Journal, 78*, 67–72.

Hanna, P. R., Hanna, J. S., Hodges, R. E., & Rudorf, E. H. (1966). *Phoneme-grapheme correspondences as cues to spelling improvement*. Washington, DC: U.S. Government Printing Office.

Henderson, E. H., & Beers, J. W. (Eds.). (1980). *Developmental and cognitive aspects of learning to spell—a reflection of word knowledge*. Newark, DE: International Reading Association.

Howell, K. W. (1986). Direct assessment of academic performance. *School Psychology Review, 15*, 324–335.

Hughes, J. N., & Hall, R. J. (1987). Proposed model for the assessment of children's social competence. *Professional School Psychology, 2*, 247–260.

Kaufman, A. S., & Kaufman, N. L. (1985). *Kaufman Test of Educational Achievement: Comprehensive form manual*. Circle Pines, MN: American Guidance Service.

Linn, R. L. (1986a). Barriers to new test design. *The redesign of testing for the 21st century: Proceedings of the 1985 ETS Invitational Conference* (pp. 69–79). Princeton, NJ: Educational Testing Service.

Linn, R. L. (1986b). Educational testing and assessment. *American Psychologist, 41*, 1153–1160.

Madsen, S., & Gould, B. (1979). *The teacher's book of lists*. Glenview, IL: Scott, Foresman.

McCloskey, G. M., Kaufman, A. S., Kaufman, N. L., & McCloskey, L. K. (1985). Clinical analysis of errors. In A. S. Kaufman & N. L. Kaufman, *The Kaufman Test of Educational Achievement: Comprehensive form manual* (pp. 85–162). Circle Pines, MN: American Guidance Service.

Messick, S. (1984). The psychology of educational measurement. *Journal of Educational Measurement, 21*, 215–237.

Mirkin, P. (1981). *Opportunity to learn as a function of what your teacher thinks of you*. Paper presented at the annual meeting of the Council for Learning Disabilities, Houston, Texas, October.

Nelson, H. E. (1980). Analysis of spelling errors in normal and dyslexic children. In U. Frith (Ed.), *Cognitive processes in spelling* (pp. 475–493). London: Academic Press.

Nelson, H. E., & Warrington, E. K. (1974). Development of spelling retardation and its relation to other cognitive abilities. *British Journal of Psychology, 65*, 265–274.

Nulman, J. H., & Gerber, M. M. (1984). Improving spelling performance by imitating a child's errors. *Journal of Learning Disabilities, 17*, 328–333.

Palinscar, A. S., & Brown, D. A. (1987). Enhancing instructional time through attention to metacognition. *Journal of Learning Disabilities, 20*, 66–75.

Poplin, M., Gray, R., Larsen, S., Banikowski, A., & Mehring, T. (1980). A comparison of components of written expression abilities in learning and non-learning disabled children at three grade levels. *Learning Disability Quarterly, 3*, 46–53.

Read, C. (1975). *Children's categorization of speech sounds in English.* Urbana, IL: National Council of Teachers of English.

Read, C. (1986). *Children's creative spelling.* London: Routledge & Kegan Paul.

Rogoff, B., & Wertsch, J. V. (Eds.). (1985). *Children's learning in the zone of proximal development.* San Francisco: Jossey-Bass.

Rutter, M., & Yule, W. (1973). Specific reading retardation. In L. Mann & D. Sabatino (Eds.), *The first review of special education* (pp. 1–50). Philadelphia: Buttonwood Farms.

Seymour, P. H. K., & Porpodas, C. D. (1980). Lexical and non-lexical processing of spelling in dyslexia. In U. Frith (Ed.), *Cognitive processes in spelling* (pp. 443–473). London: Academic Press.

Shore, J. H., & Yee, A. H. (1973). Spelling achievement tests: What is available and needed. *Journal of Special Education, 7*, 301–309.

Simon, D. P., & Simon, H. A. (1973). Alternative uses of phonemic information in spelling. *Review of Educational Research, 43*, 115–137.

Skinner, B. F. (1987). Whatever happened to psychology as the science of behavior? *American Psychologist, 42*, 780–786.

Snow, R. E., & Peterson, P. L. (1985). Cognitive analyses of tests: Implications for redesign. In S. Embertson (Ed.), *Test design: Contributions from psychology, education, and psychometrics* (pp. 149–166). New York: Academic Press.

Spache, G. D., & Spache, E. B. (1986). *Reading in the elementary school* (5th ed.). Boston: Allyn and Bacon.

Stanovich, K. E. (1980). Toward an interactive–compensatory model of individual differences in the development of reading fluency. *Reading Research Quarterly, 16*, 32–71.

Stewart, K. J. (1987). *Academic consultation: Differences in doctoral and non-doctoral training and practice.* ERIC Document Reproduction Service No. ED 268 453.

Stricker, A. G., & Hall, R. J. (1988). *Application of an intelligent CAI tutoring system to spelling instruction for learning disabled students.* Paper presented at the annual meeting of the American Educational Research Association, New Orleans, Louisiana, April.

Sweeney, J. E., & Rourke, B. P. (1978). Neuropsychological significance of phonetically accurate and phonetically inaccurate spelling errors in younger and older retarded spellers. *Brain and Language, 6*, 212–225.

Vallecorsa, A. L., & Zigmond, N. (1985). Spelling instruction in special education classrooms: A survey of practices. *Exceptional Children, 52*, 19–24.

Varnhagen, S. J., & Gerber, M. M. (1984). Microcomputers and spelling assessment: Reasons to be cautious. *Learning Disability Quarterly, 7*, 266–270.

Ward, W. C. (1984). Using microcomputers to administer tests. *Educational Measurement: Issues and Practice, 3*, 16–20.

Wenger, E. (1987). *Artificial intelligence and tutoring systems.* Los Altos, CA: Morgan Kaufmann.

15
A COGNITIVE-BEHAVIORAL APPROACH TO THE TREATMENT OF CHILDHOOD DEPRESSION

KEVIN D. STARK
LESLIE R. BEST
ERIC A. SELLSTROM
University of Texas

School psychologists have become increasingly aware of the valuable role they can play in the early identification and treatment of depressed youths. Recently, a number of articles describing assessment tools and procedures that are appropriate for use in schools have appeared in school psychology journals (e.g., Reynolds, 1984, 1985). However, very little has been written about how to intervene with depressed children once they have been identified. In this chapter, we will first briefly describe the nature and incidence of depression in children. Subsequently, the discussion will turn to a review of the major cognitive and behavioral theories of depression that have both spawned effective treatment programs for depressed adults and provided the theoretical bases of the procedures that have been incorporated into the authors' treatment program. The theoretical review will cover Lewinsohn's (1974) behavioral model; Rehm's (1977) self-control model; Abramson, Seligman, and Teasdale's (1978) learned-helplessness model; and finally Beck's (1967, 1976, 1985) cognitive model of depression, as well as Kuiper and Derry's (1981) extension of Beck's model. Next, we will review the existing treatment outcome literature. Subsequently, some of the impediments to treating depressed children in the school setting that we have encountered over the last 3 years will be discussed. Finally, the treatment program will be described. Through this chapter it will become apparent that psychological treatments for depressed children are in an infantile state of development and that the existing intervention programs have borrowed heavily from the adult literature. It also will become apparent that treating depressed children is a complex process that poses a number of unique problems for the therapist.

SYMPTOMATOLOGY

The present consensus (e.g., American Psychiatric Association, 1980) is that, along with some additional "age-specific associated features," depression in children is quite similar to that in adults. The American Psychiatric Association's *Diagnostic and Statistical Manual of Mental Disorders*, third edition (DSM-III; American Psychiatric Association, 1980) reflects the prevailing view of childhood depression. The DSM-III criteria for major depressive disorder for children over 6 are identical to those for adults. Namely, dysphoric mood or loss of interest or pleasure in all or almost all usual activities must be accompanied by four of the following eight symptoms occurring almost every day for 2 weeks. The eight symptoms are: (1) poor appetite, (2) insomnia or hypersomnia, (3) psychomotor agitation or retardation, (4) loss of interest or pleasure in usual activities, (5) fatigue, (6) feelings of worthlessness, (7) difficulty concentrating, and/or (8) recurrent thoughts of death or suicide. For children under 6, dysphoric mood may be inferred from a persistently sad facial expression, and three of the first four symptoms need to be present for a diagnosis of major depression.

Along with the aforementioned essential elements which are required to make a diagnosis of depression, DSM-III also includes a discussion of "age-specific associated features" that are common accompanying symptoms, though not a part of the diagnostic criteria. These associated features are not seen as masking depression but, rather, as the depressed individual's way of expressing himself or herself. In adults, irritability, excessive concern with physical health, and phobias may be present. On the other hand, for prepubertal children, intense anxiety symptoms may be observed, whereas aggression, sulkiness, substance abuse, social withdrawal, and antisocial behavior may be common accompanying symptoms among depressed adolescents.

A second diagnosis that can be assigned when depression is present is dysthymic disorder. This diagnosis is utilized when depressed mood or loss of interest is present but is not of sufficient severity to be considered a major depressive episode. The essential characteristics for this diagnosis are the same for adults and children, with the exception of the time duration required. In adults, a 2-year chronic mood disturbance is required for this diagnosis, whereas children and adolescents need only one year. In addition, during this period of mood disturbance, the child must have three of the following 13 symptoms: (1) sleep disturbance, (2) fatigue, (3) negative self-evaluations, (4) decreased academic performance, (5) decreased concentration, (6) social withdrawal, (7) anhedonia, (8) irritability or anger, (9) inability to respond to praise or rewards, (10) mild psychomotor retardation, (11) hopelessness or self-pity, (12) excessive weepiness, (13) recurrent thoughts of death or suicide. The "age-specific associated features" for dysthymic disorder are the same as those that accompany a diagnosis of major depression.

Although childhood depression is included in DSM-III (1980), its status as a clinical syndrome of depression remains unclear. In DSM-III it is not listed in the section entitled "Disorders usually first evident in infancy, childhood, or adolescence," and the essential features of the disorder are very similar to those needed for the diagnosis of adult depression. Thus, although the existence of developmentally appropriate symptoms is generally accepted, the nature and extent of these differences is unclear; it is an empirical question that needs to be addressed. Furthermore, it appears that these differences may be more evident in younger children. The majority of the authors' investigations have been completed with children from grades 4, 5, 6, and 7. Thus, in the discussion that follows, we will be referring to youngsters who are 9½ to 13 years old. It is believed that the discussion may not be applicable to younger children.

The hypothesized similarity between the symptomatology of depressed children and that of adults is evident in Kovacs and Beck's (1977) review of the literature. These authors suggested that the symptoms of depressed youngsters can be categorized into the same four major categories of symptomatology that were delineated by Beck (1967) in his discussion of adult depression: (1) emotional, (2) cognitive, (3) motivational, and (4) vegetative and physical. Beck (1967) defined the term "emotional manifestations" as "the changes in the patient's feelings or the changes in his overt behavior 'directly' attributable to feeling states" (p. 16). The change in affective state is gauged by comparing the individual's premorbid mood with his or her present mood. Beck (1967) delineated the following six emotional manifestations of depression: dysphoric mood, anhedonia, self-dislike, crying spells, loss of attachments, and loss of mirth response. Most of these symptoms have been associated with depression among children. Dysphoric mood has been widely reported as a symptom of childhood depression (Carlson & Cantwell, 1980a; Poznanski, Cook, & Carroll, 1979; Poznanski, Cook, Carroll, & Carzo, 1983; Poznanski & Zrull, 1970; Weinberg, Rutman, Sullivan, Renick, & Dietz, 1973), as has anhedonia (Carlson & Cantwell, 1980a; Poznanski et al., 1979, 1983). Self-dislike (Kashani & Simonds, 1979; Poznanski & Zrull, 1970) and excessive weepiness (Poznanski & Zrull, 1970) have also been cited in the childhood depression literature. However, researchers have not reported the symptoms of loss of attachments or loss of mirth response in the literature.

According to Beck's cognitive theory of depression (1967), distorted perceptions in cognitive processes are the primary feature of the syndrome of depression. Beck (1967) divided these distortions into three major classes of symptoms, the first of which is the "negative cognitive triad." Specifically, the negative cognitive triad is believed to consist of negative thoughts about oneself, the world, and the future. These distortions are believed to be manifested in low self-evaluations, negative expectancies, and distortions of body image. Research has indicated that low self-evaluations (Kashani & Simonds, 1979; Kaslow, Rehm, & Siegel, 1984; Weinberg et al., 1973) and negative expectancies for the future (Kazdin, French, Unis, Esveldt-Dawson, & Sherick, 1983a) are present in the symptomatology of depressed children. The distortion of body image has yet to be systematically studied.

The second class of cognitive symptoms Beck (1967) delineated as a feature of depression was self-blame, which expresses the individual's notion of causality. Beck (1967) believed that depressed individuals are prone to blame themselves for any difficulties or problems that they might encounter. Research with depressed children has supported Beck's (1967) clinical judgments by indicating that these children tend to attribute bad events to internal, stable, and global causes (Moyal, 1977; Seligman et al., 1984). For instance, depressed children with such an attributional style might attribute a failing test score to a belief that they are stupid, and may believe that they will always fail in all kinds of endeavors. An example of an external, unstable, and nonglobal attribution for the same failure would be evident if the children thought that they were actually quite intelligent and simply failed because they had been very busy and did not have time to prepare adequately for the test. Such children would expect to do well on future tests and other endeavors if adequately prepared.

The third class of cognitive symptoms delineated by Beck (1967) as being common to depressed individuals is that of indecisiveness. Although this symptom is an item on the most commonly used measure of childhood depression, the Children's Depression Inventory (CDI; Kovacs, 1981), no research to date has directly addressed the prevalence of this symptom.

Another major category of depressive symptoms described by Beck (1967) was the motivational manifestations of the disorder. Beck (1967) stated that the depressed adult's motivation is "regressive" in nature, as he or she seems to be drawn to activities that require the least amount of responsibility, initiative, and expenditure of energy. The depressed individual "prefers passivity to activity, and dependence to independence; he avoids responsibility and escapes from his problems rather than trying to solve them; he seeks immediate, but transient gratifications instead of delayed, but prolonged satisfactions" (Beck, 1967, p. 27). By avoiding their problems, depressed individuals allow their problems to accumulate until they seem overwhelming and suicide may be viewed as the only escape. The four specific motivational symptoms that Beck (1967) discussed as being common to depressed individuals are: (1) paralysis of will, (2) withdrawal, (3) suicidal ideation, and (4) increased dependency. Although there is no specific mention in the childhood depression literature of a loss of motivation, perhaps children reflect this loss of spontaneous desire to do things in their academic performance. The depressed child may not have the energy or desire to do his or her schoolwork, as this endeavor is not something that brings immediate gratification but, rather, something that results in long-term benefits. Consequently, depressed children may not be inclined to do their schoolwork. Diminished functioning in school has been reported by Weinberg et al. (1973) and Poznanski, Cook, and Carroll (1979). Social withdrawal is also a commonly reported symptom of depressed children (Poznanski et al., 1979; Poznanski & Zrull, 1979). Although the long-term impact of this withdrawal is unclear, it is probable that delays in the development of social skills may result, which may in turn lead to social rejection. Indeed, research indicates that depressed children tend to be rejected by their peers (Jacobsen,

Lahey, & Strauss, 1983; Vosk, Forehand, Parker, & Rickard, 1982). Research in the field of childhood depression has also indicated that depressed children, like their adult counterparts, think about, attempt, and commit suicide (Carlson & Cantwell, 1980b, 1982; Kazdin, French, Unis, Esveldt-Dawson, & Sherick, 1983a). Finally while one might expect that depressed children would be more dependent on their parents and adults in general, there is no research that directly addresses this motivational symptom.

Beck's (1967) final category of depressive symptomatology consisted of the vegetative and physical symptoms of depressed adults, including loss of appetite, sleep disturbance, loss of libido, and fatigability. With the exception of loss of libido, these symptoms have been shown to occur in depressed children. The pathological extreme of loss of appetite, anorexia nervosa, has been associated with childhood and adolescent depression (Hendren, 1983), and sleep disturbance has been shown to be evident in many behavior disorders of childhood, including depression (Carlson & Cantwell, 1980b). Although fatigability has not been reported as a symptom of depressed children, our research suggests that it may be fairly common. Finally, psychomotor retardation, a behavioral symptom not included in Beck's (1967) discussion, is a commonly cited symptom of depressed adults (e.g., Rehm, 1977) and depressed children (Poznanski et al., 1979; Poznanski, Cook, Carroll, & Carzo, 1983).

PREVALENCE OF DEPRESSION AMONG CHILDREN

The majority of researchers studying childhood depression have used children between the ages of 6 and 13. Although researchers have reported depression in infants (e.g., Spitz, 1946) and children under the age of 5 (e.g., Frommer, Mendelson, & Reid, 1972), it is assumed that these children do not have the cognitive capacity to experience depression in a manner analogous to that in adults (Cole & Kaslow, in press).

The incidence of depression reported by researchers is highly variable. This variability is a function of researchers using different assessment devices and diagnostic criteria, and sampling from psychiatric and pediatric clinics as well as nonhospitalized populations. The vast majority of studies reporting on the epidemiology of childhood depression have been conducted with inpatient or outpatient samples. Another common source of subjects has been the children of parents who have been hospitalized with an affective disorder. Few studies have been completed using children from the general population. The incidence of childhood depression among inpatients at psychiatric hospitals has ranged from 15.4% (Kazdin, French, Unis, Esveldt-Dawson, & Sherick, 1983) to 40% (Poznanski et al., 1983). The incidence of depression among children who were seen on an outpatient basis was reported to be 27% (Carlson & Cantwell, 1980a), and the incidence among a group of inpatients and outpatients was 28% (Carlson & Cantwell, 1980b). Carlson & Cantwell (1982) report that 25% of the children referred to a psychiatric institute for behavior disorders were depressed. Researchers also have reported a high incidence of depression among children referred to a neuropsychiatric clinic for headaches (40%) (Ling, Oftedal, & Weinberg, 1970), among children referred to an educational diagnostic clinic (58%) (Weinberg et al., 1973), and among children with severe medical problems (26%) (Poznanski et al., 1979).

The incidence of depression among offspring of parents who have been hospitalized for an affective disorder ranges from 7% (Welner, Welner, McCrary, & Leonard, 1977) to 19.2% (Kazdin, French, Unis, & Esveldt-Dawson, 1983) to 76% (McKnew, Cytryn, Efron, Gershon, & Bunney, 1979).

Few large-scale studies of the incidence of depression in schoolchildren have been reported in the literature. The existing research varies widely in the incidence rates reported. This variance stems from a number of variables, including variation in diagnostic criteria, use of nonstandardized measures, differences in age groups, variance in assessment method utilized (self-report versus interview, child versus parent report), and failure to include either dysthymic disorder or major depression in their statistics. Kashani and Simonds (1979) interviewed 103 schoolchildren (7 to 12 years old) and their mothers and reported that 1.9% of the sample received a DSM-III diagnosis of major depression. This estimate may be lower than the actual rate of children suffering from a clinically relevant depressive disorder. First, their sample was composed of middle- to high-socioeconomic-status (SES) subjects. Depression appears to be less common among more affluent groups. Second, Kashani and Simonds did not report the incidence of dysthymic disorder. In a more recent study, Kashani et al. (1983) studied the incidence of depression in a sample of 9-year-old children from New Zealand. They reported that 6.8% of the children were classified as currently experiencing major depression or dysthymic disorder, and an additional 9.2% of the children had experienced a major or minor depressive episode in the past. Pfeffer and colleagues (Pfeffer, Zuckerman, Plutchik, & Mizruchi, 1984) studied the incidence of depression among randomly selected 6- to 12-year-old schoolchildren in New York. The authors interviewed both the children and their mothers. They reported that 13.9% of the children could be diagnosed as experiencing dysthymic disorder using DSM-III criteria. In our own research, we find that 4% to 5% of the 10- to 13-year-old schoolchildren assessed are experiencing major depression or dysthymic disorder, with an approximately equal number of children reporting a past episode of a depressive disorder.

STABILITY OF DEPRESSION

The data on the incidence of depression both among children in the general population and among children referred to psychiatric clinics indicate that it is a very serious problem, affecting a large number of individuals. An extremely important question concerns how stable or recurrent the depressive syndrome is in children. Do depressed children become depressed adults? Unfortunately, there are few systematic longitudinal studies that address these issues. There are some studies that suggest that depression is stable over a short period of time (3–6 months) (Seligman *et al.*, 1984; Tessiny & Lefkowitz, 1982). There also is some evidence that depression in children may be stable or recurrent over a long period of time. Poznanski, Krahenbuhl, and Zrull (1987) reported that 50% of the children they had diagnosed as depressed received a diagnosis of depression 6½ years later. Kovacs, Feinberg, Crouse-Novak, Paulauskas, & Finkelstein (1984) noted that the earlier the age of onset, the more protracted the illness. Furthermore, Kovacs *et al.* reported that 65% of the children diagnosed as having a dysthymic disorder still had the disorder 4 years later. However, major depression was much shorter lived, as the majority of subjects had recovered spontaneously within one year. Evidence from a more recent study indicates that some depressed children do become depressed adults. Thirty-two percent of the depressed adults participating in a treatment study reported that their depression first appeared in childhood or adolescence (Simons, Garfield, & Murphy, 1984).

MAJOR COGNITIVE AND BEHAVIORAL THEORIES OF DEPRESSION

Lewinsohn's Behavioral Model

Lewinsohn (1974) proposed a behavioral model of depression based on the notion that part of the depressive syndrome is caused by a reduced rate of response-contingent positive reinforcement. Depression is not simply due to a reduced rate of positive reinforcement; rather, it is caused by a lack of contingency between the emission of adaptive behavior and subsequent reinforcement. An individual becomes depressed when the emission of appropriate behavior is not followed by reinforcement for a prolonged period of time. Thus, the individual's adaptive behavior is placed on an extinction schedule. In addition, depression is presumed to be caused by reinforcement for not emitting adaptive behavior.

The low rate of response-contingent positive reinforcement leads to the central depressive symptom, dysphoric mood. In addition, it directly leads to fatigue and other somatic complaints. The symptom of dysphoria yields a number of secondary cognitive complaints, including decreased self-esteem, pessimism, and guilt. These secondary cognitive symptoms stem from the difficulty associated with labeling the feeling of dysphoria. The label the individual attaches to the feeling determines the nature of the cognitive symptom. A number of alternative labels are available, such as: (1) "I am sick," which leads to somatic symptoms; (2) "I am weak-inadequate," which leads to decreased self-esteem; (3) "I am bad," which leads to guilt; and (4) "I am not likable," which leads to social isolation.

Lewinsohn (1974) stated that the amount of positive reinforcement a person receives is a function of three variables. One of them is the number of events that are potentially reinforcing for the individual. This is assumed to be a variable that is subject to individual differences, which may be either biologically or experientially determined. The person who is prone to depression is assumed to have a restricted range of potentially reinforcing events. Consequently, since few things are reinforcing, the emission of behavior, even adaptive behavior, is infrequently followed by positive reinforcement.

The second variable is the availability of positive reinforcement in a person's environment. Lewinsohn (1974) hypothesized that the depressed person either has few potential reinforcements in his or her environment, or is experiencing a sudden reduction in the amount of reinforcement available in the environment. This sudden reduction could result from the loss of a loved one, a financial crisis, or social isolation.

The final variable, and the most important one according to Lewinsohn (1974), is the amount of skill the individual has to elicit positive reinforcement from the environment. In addition to possessing these skills, the person must also emit the socially skilled behaviors that elicit that positive reinforcement. Thus, depressed persons may not receive response-contingent positive reinforcement either because they don't have the skill to elicit the reinforcement or because they have the skill in their repertoire but, for some reason, fail to perform the behavior. Consequently, they are unable to elicit positive reinforcement even when it is potentially available.

Once the individual begins to exhibit depressive symptomatology, the social environment plays a role in fostering and maintaining the symptoms. Significant others in the person's social milieu inadvertently reinforce the depressive behavior by showing increased interest, concern, or sympathy for the person. Even this positive reinforcement is short-lived, however, because interactions with depressed people are aversive. Eventually, the significant others withdraw from the person, resulting in a further reduction in the amount of reinforcement available to him or her.

Rehm's Self-Control Model

Rehm (1977) extended Kanfer's model of self-control (Kanfer, 1970; Kanfer & Karoly, 1972) and applied it as a heuristic model for studying the symptoms, etiology, and treatment of depression. Rehm defines "self-control" as those processes and strategies by which individuals organize and direct their behavior toward long-range goals in the relative absence of, or in opposition to, immediate environmental controls. Within a self-control framework, depression is conceptualized as a failure to adjust to change or to an undesirable outcome. Hence, depression is conceptualized as resulting from a maladaptive coping style. The person with an adaptive coping style engages in self-regulation when he or she confronts change or a disappointing outcome. Although some depressed individuals may begin to self-regulate, the process is disengaged early in the chain. For example, the person may begin to self-monitor but then fail to self-evaluate or self-consequate. Other individuals may suffer from a deficit in self-regulation that results in maladaptive behavior. In this latter case, the individual simply doesn't know, for example, how to self-monitor.

According to Kanfer's (1970) model of self-control, an individual engages in a three-stage sequence of behaviors when confronted with change or a deficiency in an outcome. The three stages—self-monitoring, self-evaluation, and self-reinforcement—operate within a feedback loop model. Self-monitoring involves the active observation of one's own behavior and its situational antecedents and consequences. The information that is gathered about one's performance is then compared to an internal standard. This comparison results in an evaluation of success or failure. Rehm (1977) extended Kanfer's model by incorporating the attributional dimension of internality–externality at this point. Rehm argues that the person must make internal attributions of causality in order to make a personally relevant judgment. Conversely, if the cause is attributed to an external source, then the performance is not self-determined and thus is neither praiseworthy nor blameworthy. This self-evaluation serves as a cue for self-consequation. The self-administered rewards or punishments may be either overt or covert, and are assumed to affect behavior in the same manner as externally administered rewards or punishments. Self-reinforcement is assumed to supplement external reinforcement and, consequently, to maintain behavior until long-range goals are achieved.

People vary in their style of self-management. Specifically, people who are good self-managers are able to initiate, maintain, and organize their behavior in a manner that facilitates achievement of long-term goals. In contrast, poor self-management implies poor organization of goals and standards, and control by immediate, less desirable reinforcers. The behavior of depressed individuals is characterized by the latter style of self-management. Specifically, Rehm (1977) postulated six factors within the model that typify the self-management style of depressed people: (1) selective monitoring of negative events; (2) selective monitoring of immediate, as opposed to delayed, consequences of behavior; (3) stringent self-evaluative criteria; (4) inaccurate attributions of responsibility; (5) insufficient self-reward; and (6) excessive self-punishment.

As suggested earlier, Rehm characterizes the self-monitoring of depressed individuals in two ways, both of which are maladaptive. First, they demonstrate a proclivity for attending to negative events, often to the exclusion of positive events. Second, depressed people tend to attend selectively to immediate rather than to delayed outcomes of their behavior. Monitoring of negative events to the exclusion of positive events leads to pessimism and a negative view of the world, the future, and oneself. In addition, as a result of monitoring immediate consequences to the exclusion of delayed consequences, the individual lacks motivation and experiences a sense of hopelessness about the future.

Kanfer (1970) described self-evaluation as "the logical basis on which a person judges his own behavior, when no external consequences are present to permit an objective assessment of the effectiveness of one's behavior" (p. 202). Thus, self-evaluation involves comparing one's perception of the result of an act with one's internal standard of performance for that act. The performance can be judged as either meeting, exceeding, or falling short of the standard. These internal standards evolve from the person's learning history of external reinforcement and vicariously through observing the standards for performance set by significant others. The standards are relatively constant over time and across situations. Rehm (1977) hypothesized that depression may result from either of two forms of maladaptive self-evaluation. The depressed person may either (1) set excessively stringent criteria for positive self-evaluation, or (2) fail to make accurate internal attributions of causality. Self-evaluative standards may be stringent in any of three ways: (1) a high threshold requiring great quantitative or qualitative excellence for self-approval; (2) low thresholds for negative self-evaluation (so that a minimal deficiency is considered to be a total failure); and (3) stringent in the sense of excessive breadth (failure in one instance is taken as failure in an entire class of behaviors). Setting such stringent self-evaluative criteria results in poor self-esteem, negative self-evaluations, and the setting of unrealistic goals that cannot be met.

Rehm (1977) hypothesized that the helpless behavior exhibited by many depressed adults is the result of a faulty attributional style. These individuals may make excessive external attributions and consequently believe that a high degree of response–consequence independence exists. Although such individuals are passive and apathetic, because they believe there is little they can do to change or improve their situation, they do not have a poor view of themselves because they do not see themselves as responsible for their plight. A second form of helplessness results when individuals make excessive internal attributions for aversive events while perceiving that they lack the ability to obtain positive outcomes. Such individuals believe that lawful response–consequence relationships exist, but that they are too incompetent and ineffective to obtain positive reinforcement. Consequently, these individuals may exhibit poor self-esteem and guilt.

The rate of self-reinforcement for depressed persons can be characterized by the self-administration of relatively low rates of self-reward and high rates of self-punishment. The self-punishment also produces an internal dialogue that is dominated by negative self-statements. The indecisiveness of depressed persons can be accounted for by hypothesizing that such people self-punish each result early in the response chain. Thus, a response may be initiated, but it is quickly dropped and another behavior is begun.

The Reformulated Theory of Learned Helplessness

The basic premise of Seligman's (1975) learned-helplessness model of depression is that learning that outcomes are uncontrollable results in the motivational, cognitive, and emotional correlates of depression. Abramson, Seligman, and Teasdale (1978) believe that this original formulation is inadequate on the following four grounds:

1. The expectation of uncontrollability in itself is not sufficient for depressed affect.
2. The model does not address the symptom of lowered self-esteem.
3. The tendency to make internal attributions for failure is not explained.
4. The generality, chronicity, and intensity of the effects of helplessness are not accounted for.

Seligman's (1975) original model was reformulated within an attributional framework in an effort to alleviate the aforementioned inadequacies. The reformulated theory, like the original theory, holds the expectation of response–outcome independence to be the crucial determinant of learned helplessness. Abramson *et al.* (1978), however, believe that mere exposure to noncontingency is not enough to produce helplessness. Rather, the individual must first perceive the noncontingency. Subsequently, it is believed that the individual asks him- or herself "why"? The causal attribution that serves as the answer to this query determines the expectations the individual holds for the future. These expectations, in turn, "determine the generality, chronicity, and type of his helplessness symptoms" (Abramson *et al.*, 1978, p. 52).

In order to construct a comprehensive model, Abramson *et al.* (1978) had to refine attribution theory by hypothesizing the existence of three attributional dimensions that are orthogonal to each other: specificity, stability, and internality. (The dimensions are further divided into global–specific, stable–unstable, and internal–external, respectively.) The first two dimensions predict when and where the expectations of helplessness will occur. An attribution to specific factors predicts that the expectation of helplessness will occur only in situations that are very similar to the original situation. An attribution to global factors predicts that the expectation of helplessness will recur across many situations. An attribution to stable factors predicts that the expectation of helplessness will become chronic—they will recur after time lapses. An attribution to unstable factors predicts that the expectation need not recur after a time lapse.

The internality dimension does not predict the recurrence of the expectations of helplessness; rather, it determines whether the helplessness is experienced as personal or universal. Individuals who are experiencing noncontingency and make external attributions for failure are universally helpless, whereas those who make internal attributions for failure are personally helpless. This dimension has additional implications. The individuals who make internal attributions for failure will experience lower self-esteem. This dimension, however, is neutral with respect to the cognitive and motivational deficits associated with helplessness. The cognitive and motivational deficits occur in both personal and universal helplessness. It is believed that the expectation of noncontingency is sufficient to produce these deficits.

Within this model, the intensity of the cognitive and emotional deficits is believed to be dependent on the strength of the certainty of the expectation of noncontingency. The intensity of the loss of self-esteem and emotional change is dependent on the subjective certainty of the expectation of uncontrollability and the importance of the event that the person is helpless to control. These deficits will also become more intense if the attribution is to global or stable factors.

The Reformulated Learned-Helplessness Model of Depression

Abramson *et al.* (1978) hypothesized that the affective changes that accompany a depressive episode are not the direct result of the expectation of uncontrollability; rather, they result from the expectation that undesirable outcomes will occur regardless of what the person does. The affect-producing outcomes could result from either the loss of a highly desirable outcome or the occurrence of a highly aversive outcome. The intensity of the emotional response is a function of a number of factors. The emotional response increases with the desirability of the unobtainable or lost outcome, and with the aversiveness of the unavoidable outcome. The perceived strength of certainty of the expectation of uncontrollability also has an impact on the intensity of the emotional response. The more certain a person is that he or she will lose something of importance, the more depressed the individual will feel. Finally, whether the person views him- or herself as personally or universally helpless influences the intensity of the emotional response. The person who makes internal attributions and thus is personally helpless experiences a greater emotional response.

One of the hallmark symptoms of depression is lowered self-esteem. A number of authors have manipulated self-esteem and recorded the changes in depression (see Coleman, 1975; Wilson & Krane, 1980). Although Seligman's (1975) model of depression did not account for the occurrence of lowered self-esteem, the reformulated model does account for this symptom. Abramson *et al.* (1978) postulated that depressed individuals make more internal attributions following a failure and thus experience lowered self-esteem. Moreover, depressed individuals appear to make internal, global, and stable attributions for failure. Thus, they will attribute the cause of their failure to themselves across many situations and over an extended period of time. In addition, when a depressed individual experiences success, it will be attributed to external sources and to the specific situation, and will not necessarily be expected to occur in the future.

The reformulated theory of hopelessness asserts that the generality and chronicity of the depressive symptoms are dependent on the globality and stability of the attribution for helplessness. Finally, the affective and self-esteem deficits are dependent on the internality of the attribution for the helplessness.

Beck's Cognitive Model

Beck, Rush, Shaw, and Emery (1979) have developed a comprehensive model of information processing in depression. They believe that depressive cognitions, more specifically the "negative cognitive triad," are the major depressive phenomena. Beck *et al.* (1979) believe that the content of the depressed individual's cognitions is blameful and derogatory in nature and self-referent in direction. Specifically, the "negative cognitive triad" is believed to consist of negative thoughts about oneself, the world, and the future.

Beck *et al.* (1979) listed the following six information-processing errors which they have found to occur in depressed individuals, and which they believe are at the root of the "negative cognitive triad."

1. *Selective abstraction*: Focusing on only one aspect of a situation while ignoring other, more salient features, and evaluating the situation only on the basis of this limited information.
2. *Overgeneralization*: Drawing general conclusions about something on the basis of an isolated incident.
3. *Personalization*: Relating unrelated events to the self when there is no basis for making such a connection.
4. *Magnification or minimalization*: Overestimating or underestimating the importance of an event.
5. *Arbitrary inference*: Drawing conclusions without supporting evidence, or in the presence of contradictory evidence.
6. *Absolutistic or dichotomous thinking*: Thinking in which all experiences are put into one of two opposite categories. For example, the two categories might be "great" and "lousy." The depressed person would tend to choose the negative category to describe him- or herself.

Beck *et al.* (1979) employed the terms "primitive" and "mature" thinking to describe the perceptual and thinking disorders that they see in depressed individuals. As Beck states, depressed individuals are relatively primitive in their thinking as they tend to make broad judgments regarding events which happen to them. In addition, their thinking is also likely to be "extreme, negative, categorical, absolute, and judgmental" (Beck *et al.*, 1979, p. 14). On the other hand, more mature thinking is characterized by viewing situations more fully and by considering a situation on more dimensions before making an interpretation of an event.

Although Beck's (1967; Beck *et al.*, 1979) beliefs about the cognitions of depressed individuals are based on clinical impressions, empirical research indicates that the hypothesized negative biases in perception do indeed exist. Results from several studies (e.g., DeMonbreum & Craighead, 1977; Lishman, 1972) indicate that, relative to nondepressed controls, depressed adults recall more negatively toned personal information. In addition, Nelson and Craighead (1977) showed that, in addition to underestimating the amount of reward they receive, depressed adults recall more punishment than do nondepressed persons. Overall, these studies indicate that, as Beck *et al.* (1979) hypothesized, depressed individuals have a negative bias in their self-perceptions, as they tend to be very self-critical and very negative in their appraisal of their own capability.

Research indicates that depressed children have negative perceptual biases very similar to those of depressed adults. Haley, Fine, Marriage, Moretti, and Freeman (1985) and Kendall, Stark, and Adam (1987) have studied the relationship between depression and cognitive distortions in groups of in- and outpatients in a children's psychiatric unit and in a group of sixth-grade students, respectively, and have obtained results indicating that depressed children's thinking is very self-critical and negative in nature.

In another investigation, Seligman et al. (1984) found support indicating that depressed children's attributional style, like that of depressed adults, is negatively biased. Specifically, depressed children were more likely than non-depressed children to give internal, stable, and global explanations for bad events. Results also indicated that opposite styles for good events were found. Other empirical studies have found that depressed children also perceive their world in a negative way (Moyal, 1977), have negative expectancies toward the future (Kazdin et al., 1983a), and have low opinions of themselves (Stark, Kaslow, Hill, & Lux, 1988b).

Taken together, these studies indicate that depressed children, like their adult counterparts, tend to have a negative perceptual bias. We will now briefly examine Beck et al.'s (1979) theoretical framework into which these negative thought patterns may be incorporated.

Beck et al. (1979) believe that the negative thoughts of depressed individuals are incorporated into a depressed schema that distorts reality in a negative way, thereby maintaining the person's negative thoughts despite objective evidence of positive events in the person's life. They believe that the schema has both a structural and functional component. Structurally, the self-schema is believed to be an organized cluster of knowledge about aspects of the person and his or her world, which has been derived from lifetime experiences. Functionally, the schema is believed to act as a filter through which incoming stimuli are interpreted.

According to Beck (1967), when individuals encounter a situation, their conceptualization and evaluation of that situation is dependent on which of a vast array of stimuli are attended to, and it is the person's schemata that are mechanisms through which the stimuli are selectively filtered. The interpretation of any experience is then dependent on which schemata are activated and on the appropriateness of these schemata. Beck (1967) believes that in depressed individuals, conceptualizations and evaluations of situations are distorted to "fit" the person's prepotent dysfunctional schema. The depressed person may not be able to activate the appropriate schema because of the strength of the only active negative schema. The result will be a distorted perception of reality in a negative direction because, as the prepotent negative schema leads to more distortions of reality, the person will become less and less likely to believe that his or her negative interpretations are not based on reality.

Though not directly addressed by Beck et al. (1979), the idea that different levels of depression are characterized by different types of schematic processing is consistent with their theory of depression, and has been elaborated on by Kuiper and Derry (1981) in their self-schema model of depression.

The Self-Schema Model of Depression

The self-schema model of depression states that an individual's level of depression mediates both the content of the self-schema and the efficiency of self-referent processing. The model predicts that since the self-schemata of severely depressed and nondepressed individuals are, respectively, primarily negative and positive in context, they will display efficient processing of negative and positive content, respectively. On the other hand, the self-schemata of mildly depressed individuals are expected to contain both positive and negative content, and self-referent processing is expected to be marked by some uncertainty. Thus, this model of depression is simply an extension of Beck et al.'s (1979) model, as it emphasizes the effect different levels or depths of depression can have on self-perceptions. In each case, it is predicted that an individual's self-schema guides the selective processing of schema-consistent data to the relative neglect of nonschematic data.

Research with mildly depressed, severely depressed, and nondepressed adults has tended to support the self-schema model of depression. These studies have typically employed an incidental-recall paradigm to test the hypothesis that level of depression affects the processing of personally relevant information. Subjects are presented with word lists that contain some depressed-content adjectives and some nondepressed-content adjectives, and are instructed to decide whether or not the words are self-descriptive. Then, in an incidental recall task, subjects are asked to recall as many words as possible. Results have consistently shown that nondepressed adults tend to display a positive bias in their recall of personally relevant information by recalling significantly more positive information about themselves, whereas severely depressed adults tend to display a negative bias as they recall significantly more negative information about themselves. Mildly depressed adults tend to recall equal amounts of positive and negative personal information, thus indicating that their schematic processing, unlike that of severely depressed and nondepressed adults, is characterized by uncertainty (Kuiper & Derry, 1981, 1982; Kuiper & MacDonald, 1980).

To date, there have been only two published research studies (Hammen & Zupan, 1984; Zupan, Hammen, & Jaenicke, 1987) that have examined the self-referent processing of depressed children. Though methodologically flawed, these studies have given some preliminary support to the self-schema model of depression, as they have shown that depressed children display self-referent processing patterns much like those of depressed adults. Currently, additional research on the schematic processing tendencies of depressed children is underway (Sellstrom & Stark, 1987), which will, we hope, provide us with a better understanding of the etiology, nature, and maintenance of negatively biased cognitions in depressed individuals.

TREATMENT OUTCOME RESEARCH

Perhaps the most noteworthy aspect of the treatment outcome literature is the general dearth of investigations of psychological interventions for depressed youths. There also are very few articles that even offer suggestions or guidelines for treating depressed children. The majority of the treatment outcome research has been directed toward evaluating the efficacy of pharmacotherapy. This is somewhat surprising given the general success of psychological treatments, especially cognitive-behavioral treatments, with depressed adults (Reynolds & Stark, 1983). Furthermore, many of these cognitive-behavioral procedures have been successfully adapted for use with children with other disorders.

The existing research represents the initial steps in the development and empirical evaluation of treatment programs for depressed youths. Researchers have started this process by borrowing heavily from the adult literature. Several case studies (Frame, Matson, Sonis, Fialkov, & Kazdin, 1982; Petti, Bornstein, Delamater, & Conners, 1980) that employed behavioral procedures have appeared, two control group treatment outcome studies (Butler, Miezitus, Friedman, & Cole, 1980; Stark, Reynolds, & Kaslow, 1987c) that employed cognitive-behavioral procedures have been reported, and we have just completed a third study. The two case studies were conducted with inpatients at psychiatric hospitals, whereas the two control group studies were completed in schools with mildly to moderately depressed children, and our most recent investigation was completed with moderately to severely depressed school children.

Case Studies

Petti and colleagues (1980) reported on their treatment of a 10½-year-old girl who was hospitalized for depression and aggressive behavior. A multimodal treatment was employed that consisted of the following: (1) individual psychotherapy directed at understanding feelings; (2) individualized teaching and academic skills training; (3) creative dramatics group designed to improve social skills; (4) supportive family therapy and parent training in behavior management techniques; (5) imipramine; and (6) social skills training to facilitate her move back home and back to school. After 5 weeks of treatment, the first four components had not produced the desired improvement, so imipramine treatment was initiated. Following the addition of imipramine to the treatment regimen, the authors noted a marked improvement in the girl's depressive and aggressive symptoms. The final treatment component, social skills training, was then added and consisted of instruction, modeling, behavioral rehearsal, and performance feedback. The training was conducted in 15-minute sessions over a 3-week period. The targets of the skills training were eye contact, frequency of smiles, duration of speech, and requests for new behavior.

Interpretation of the results of the Petti, *et. al.* (1980) study is limited by the relative absence of a systematic assessment methodology, but anecdotal reports from the child's foster parents and ward staff suggested that she had shown general improvement in a number of areas. In addition, systematic data were kept on the efficacy of the social skills training. Significant improvement was noted for eye contact, frequency of smiles, duration of speech, and requests for new behavior. Although the conclusions that can be drawn from this study are limited by the failure to assess systematically the subjective manifestations of depression, the results do suggest that a comprehensive, multimodal approach to the treatment of depression, which combines antidepressant medication with behavior therapy, may be a viable approach.

Frame *et al.* (1982) utilized operant behavioral techniques with a 10-year-old boy who had limited intellectual ability (IQ 79) and was hospitalized for major depression. The authors targeted a number of the overt manifestations of depression, including inappropriate body position, lack of eye contact, poor speech quality, and bland affect. Skills training was conducted every day for 4 weeks in 20-minute sessions. Training consisted of instructions, modeling, role playing, and performance feedback. The treatment produced an "immediate, marked improvement" in the undesirable behaviors. Once again, although the study did demonstrate that the treatment was effective at changing these overt behaviors, the conclusions that can be drawn about the impact of the treatment on the syndrome of depression in this youngster are limited because neither the covert manifestations of depression (e.g., dysphoric mood, anhedonia) nor the other, less noticeable symptoms (e.g., sleep and eating disturbances) were assessed.

Control Group Treatment Outcome Studies

Butler and colleagues (1980) completed an investigation that yields some useful information about potentially effective procedures for treating depression in children. Subjects were 56 schoolchildren from grades 5 and 6 who reported some depressive symptomatology on the Children's Depression Inventory (CDI; Kovacs, 1981) and a number of additional self-report measures of related constructs. The investigators compared the relative efficacy of "role play, cognitive-restructuring, attention placebo, and classroom control conditions. The role play treatment was a bit of a misnomer in that it consisted of much more than simple role playing. Each session focused on a problem relevant to depressed children. At a cognitive level, the children were sensitized to their own thoughts and feelings and to those of others, and were taught to take a problem-solving approach to threatening or stressful situations. In addition, subjects were taught social skills to improve their relationships with peers. The role playing served as a medium for trying out the problem-solving and other skills. Discussions followed each role play, and homework assignments were given after each session. The cognitive-restructuring procedure consisted of a primarily educational treatment that helped the children get in touch with their feelings and thoughts. It does not appear as though their cognitive-restructuring procedure was similar to Beck's (e.g., Beck *et al.*, 1979) procedure. Students in the attention placebo condition were taught the group investigation model of teaching, and subjects in the classroom control condition simply completed the assessment measures. The treatments were conducted in groups of seven students and were completed in 10 weekly, one-hour sessions.

Results of the study indicated that the problem-solving, behavioral-rehearsal (role play) treatment was clearly the most effective procedure and that the "cognitive restructuring" procedure was moderately effective. The authors also noted that the children were not as interested in this treatment because of its heavily didactic nature. Thus, the limited showing of the procedure may be more a reflection of the investigators' construction of their cognitive-restructuring procedure than evidence for the limited efficacy of cognitive restructuring. In contrast to the results reported for the two active treatments, minimal improvement was reported by children in the two control conditions. Follow-up data were not collected, so it is not possible to evaluate whether the gains demonstrated at the end of treatment were maintained.

Stark, Reynolds, and Kaslow (1987c) evaluated the relative efficacy of a self-control treatment and a behavioral problem-solving treatment for depressed 9- to 13-year-old children. The treatments were conducted in a school setting with 29 moderately depressed children. Depression was assessed from multiple perspectives (mother's and child's) using multiple methods (interview and self-report measures). The children were randomly assigned to either a self-control, behavioral problem-solving, or waiting-list condition. The self-control treatment consisted of training in self-monitoring, scheduling activities, making more adaptive self-evaluations, self-consequating (both self-reinforcement and self-punishment), and making more adaptive attributions. The behavioral problem-solving therapy consisted of education, self-monitoring of pleasant events, and group problem solving directed toward improving social behavior. Subjects in both therapy conditions met 12 times for 45 to 50 minutes over a 5-week period. The children and their mothers completed the assessment battery prior to treatment, immediately after treatment, and 8 weeks after treatment had been completed.

Results of the study indicated that children in both active treatments reported significant improvements in depressive symptomatology immediately following treatment. In contrast, children in the waiting-list condition reported minimal change. The improvements were maintained at an 8-week follow-up assessment. In fact, children who received the self-control treatment reported continued improvement and they were significantly less depressed at follow-up compared to posttesting. The results also indicated that children in both treatment conditions reported significant improvements in anxiety, but only children in the self-control condition reported a significant improvement in self-concept.

Although the children who received treatment reported significant improvements in depression, their mothers did not report a significant improvement in their children's depressive symptomatology. It is unclear whether this reflected a failure of the treatment effects to generalize to the home environment or whether it reflected more of an assessment issue. The measure used for the mothers' assessment of their children's depression, the Child Behavior Checklist (CBCL; Achenbach & Edelbrock, 1978) has a limited response format, thus reducing the range of severity of symptomatology that can be reported. Another potential explanation for the failure to find significant differences on the CBCL may be a function of the fact that the mothers' ratings of their child's depression were uncorrelated with children's self-ratings of depression. Thus, it is unclear what mothers were rating when they rated their child's depressive symptomatology.

Preliminary results from the authors' most recent investigation suggest that an expanded cognitive-behavioral treatment program (to be described later in this chapter) may be the most effective treatment program to date. This cognitive-behavioral treatment was compared to a nonspecific therapy control condition. Preliminary results indicate that subjects in the cognitive-behavioral condition, as well as their parents, noted dramatic improvements in the children's depressive symptomatology that appear to be both statistically and clinically significant. In contrast to the cognitive behavioral condition, subjects in the nonspecific condition reported some change; but it was significantly less than that reported by subjects in the cognitive-behavioral condition.

Summary and Implications

The existing treatment outcome literature provides the interested mental health professional with some ideas about what may prove to be effective treatment procedures for depression in children. The case studies indicate that operant procedures and other more traditional behavioral procedures such as social skills training may prove useful for modifying some of the overt manifestations of depressed children. Specifically, the existing evidence indicates that instruction, modeling, behavioral rehearsal, and performance feedback are effective for increasing eye contact, frequency of smiling, quality and duration of speech, and a number of other observable behaviors. The impact of these procedures on the syndrome of depression is unclear, however, because the studies lacked an appropriate assessment methodology. The study conducted by Petti et al. (1980) also suggests that it may be the most useful to combine pharmacotherapy with psychotherapy.

The control group studies suggest that short-term, multicomponent cognitive-behavioral treatment programs may be effective for alleviating mild to moderate levels of depressive symptomatology in 10- to 12-year-old schoolchildren. The Butler et al. (1980) study indicated that a treatment program that consisted of identifying target behaviors and teaching the children to utilize problem solving as a means of coping with the situation may be an effective intervention. Problem solving also was used successfully as a major treatment component in the Stark et al. (1987c) study. A self-control treatment program

(Stark *et al.*, 1987c) based on Rehm's (e.g., Fuchs & Rehm, 1977) treatment program for depressed adults also appears to warrant further development. One of the most effective treatments for depressed adults is Beck's (e.g., Beck *et al.*, 1979) cognitive therapy. Butler and colleagues used their own version of cognitive restructuring with some success. The authors noted that this more didactic treatment failed to maintain the children's attention and involvement. These results and impressions suggest that a cognitive-restructuring procedure based on Beck's approach may prove effective but must be modified in its delivery format so as to capture and maintain the children's interest and active involvement in treatment. Such a procedure was developed and used in our most recent investigation and appeared to be extremely effective. In fact, anecdotal reports from the children's parents suggest that this may have been one of the more effective treatment components.

Despite some significant findings, the aforementioned treatment outcome research is fraught with limitations. The case studies did not include an adequate assessment methodology for assessing the syndrome of depression. This is a major limitation, which greatly circumscribes the interpretations that can be drawn from these studies. Specifically, it is unclear whether the treatments had any impact on the syndrome of depression or whether they simply changed some overt behaviors. The control group studies also were limited by their assessment methodology. The Butler *et al.* (1980) study relied on the CDI as the sole measure of depression for subject selection and as the primary outcome measure. Our own research as well as that of others (e.g., Saylor, Finch, Spirito, & Bennett, 1984) indicates that this may be problematic for a number of reasons. Specifically, as the sole assessment device for selecting subjects, the CDI overidentifies children as being depressed; it may be more of a measure of psychological distress than a measure specifically of depression. In the Stark *et al.* (1988b) article, the authors noted the limitations of the CDI as a selection device and recommended greater reliance on interview measures for selecting subjects. Thus, in our most recent investigation we have used the K-SADS interview (Puig-Antich & Ryan, 1986) for selecting subjects. The CDI also possesses a number of qualities that can contribute to spurious conclusions about the effectiveness of a treatment program. Children who complete the CDI a second time after a short interval, but with no intervention, report significantly fewer depressive symptoms. The reason for this reduction is unclear. Regardless of the underlying reason or reasons, subjects will report a significant first to second administration reduction in symptomatology. Thus, if there is only one pretreatment administration of the CDI, it ensures significant pre- to posttreatment reductions in depressive symptomatology that reflect an assessment issue and not the efficacy of the treatment program itself.

The case studies are noteworthy for their use of children from clinic populations, thus yielding some indication of the effectiveness of the treatment procedures for clinic populations. The existing control group studies are to be commended for their ecological validity for school practitioners. Both published studies and our most recent investigation were conducted in schools with public school students. The conclusions that can be drawn about the applicability of these interventions for clinic populations, however, are limited by the facts that subjects in both the Butler *et al.* (1980) and Stark *et al.* (1987c) studies did not receive DSM-III diagnoses of affective disorder and that they ranged in their severity from mild to moderate levels of depressive symptomatology. Our experiences with the CDI would indicate that the vast majority of the schoolchildren who were identified as depressed on the CDI in these studies would not have received a DSM-III diagnosis of a current affective disorder. In our most recent investigation, the subjects received DSM-III diagnoses. Thus, if the preliminary results hold up, there will be no question about the applicability of these procedures for clinic children.

The ability of the various treatment programs to promote the maintenance of treatment effects for long periods of time is unknown. This is a key consideration when treating individuals who are experiencing an episodic disorder such as depression. The only study that systematically assessed the maintenance of treatment effects was the Stark *et al.* (1987c) study. Results of this investigation indicated that subjects in both the behavioral problem-solving and self-control treatments maintained their improvements. Furthermore, the subjects who received the self-control treatment continued to improve and rated themselves as significantly less depressed 8 weeks after treatment. Thus, these preliminary results are favorable. Whether these results were an isolated phenomenon, or whether they will prove to be more generalizable, is a question that remains open to future empirical scrutiny.

Our own experience with completing empirically evaluated treatment outcome research suggests that there are a number of other important questions that need to be addressed in future investigations. The most efficacious and cost-efficient time frame for treatment needs to be identified. The existing research has employed relatively brief treatment programs. Butler *et al.* (1980) and Stark *et al.* (1987c) used 10 and 12 one-hour sessions, respectively, in their treatment programs. In our current treatment outcome research with a more severely depressed sample, we have utilized 27 50- to 60-minute sessions. It is evident to us that this time frame will produce significant changes. However, to produce even more meaningful, ingrained, essentially philosophical changes in the way these children approach their day-to-day life, a longer time frame may be necessary.

Current and past research indicates that some of the children improve dramatically, whereas others do not. Furthermore, some children work hard and conscientiously complete their behavioral homework, whereas other children do not become actively involved in treatment and fail to complete homework assignments. It would be useful to identify predictor variables for determining who is going to become involved in treatment and improve and for who is likely to do poorly in this form of treatment, which relies heavily on completion of homework assignments for its efficacy. A related treatment/ assessment issue is developing more individualized treatment programs that match the youngsters' psychological needs with specific intervention procedures. This therapeutic ideal, however, appears to be quite a way off in the future.

The dropout rate from treatment is a measure of the success of intervention programs for depressed adults (Reynolds & Stark, 1983), but this appears to be less of a concern with children, in part because the children are excused from class to attend therapy meetings. In our own research, the subjects also are rewarded on an intermittent schedule for involvement in the treatment sessions. This also appears to facilitate completion of treatment. However, we have noted a trend toward some difficulty with middle school youngsters, who appear to be under more pressure to achieve academically. Thus, missing class is aversive because attendance in the treatment group results in getting behind in schoolwork, which may lead to problems with the child's grades. In such situations, it is extremely important to consult with the child's teachers to make some special arrangements for the youngsters to make up missed assignments.

A number of our recently completed and soon-to-be-completed investigations (Brookman, Stark, & Carlson, 1987; Stark, Humphrey, Crook, & Lewis, 1988a) into the nature of the family environment of depressed children have clearly indicated the need to intervene at the family level when treating depressed youths. This is not meant to imply that all families with a depressed child are unhealthy. Many of them are, however, and family intervention appears to be a necessity. Moreover, in the healthy families, the parents can be extremely helpful therapeutic agents. None of the published studies included such a treatment component. Our most recent school-based treatment program includes monthly cognitive-behavioral family therapy sessions. Our plans are to expand this treatment component further for future research and clinical work.

CONDUCTING TREATMENT PROGRAMS IN THE SCHOOLS: THE GENTLE BALANCE

Providing group therapy for depressed children in the school setting involves a series of balances. Various elements within the group itself, within the school, and within the children's families must be carefully balanced by the therapists.

Within the group, therapists themselves need to achieve a balance between being the child's friend and being an adult whom the child respects. Therapists also need to balance between being a disciplinarian and somewhat authoritarian, and letting the group dictate its own behavior and the flow of each session. Becoming the children's trusted confidant, almost a friend, is important because if too little rapport is established, the children will not feel comfortable sharing their concerns with the therapists and will not be as engaged in treatment. This friendly and collaborative attitude is fostered by the therapists' participation in all the activities within the sessions and by his or her completion of the homework assignments. As noted, however, it is also important that the children view the therapists as adults whom they respect. This position is encouraged by the establishment of some basic rules of conduct (e.g., taking turns talking) at the outset of treatment and by the consistent enforcement of these rules by the therapists. Respect is also attained through impartial and appropriate behavior on the part of the therapists.

Therapists must also attempt to achieve an optimal working atmosphere within the group. This involves, first of all, balancing the children's desire to have fun with the therapists' need/desire to address some of the serious issues underlying the children's emotional problems. Likewise, the therapists must attempt to balance the group's desire for fun with their own need to keep the children's behavior within the normal school limits. The balance between fun and work (i.e., therapy) is a particularly difficult one to sort out given that, for depressed children, having fun can in and of itself, be therapeutic. Nonetheless, at this age, activities that are fun can quickly become chaotic; thus, some structure must be imposed. Moreover, in order to achieve ingrained, essentially philosophical changes in the way these children deal with their day-to-day lives, some serious discussion of relevant issues must be included in the treatment. During most sessions, an attempt is made to balance fun and therapeutic work by beginning the session with didactic material or discussion of individual concerns, and ending the session with an enjoyable activity. Creating an optimal therapeutic atmosphere also involves balancing the number of structured and unstructured activities in which the children are asked to engage. At times, structure must be imposed in order to expedite the procedure; at other times, the children are allowed to determine the specific content of an activity. For example, at times the therapist may decide which hypothetical situation is to be role played, whereas at other times the children may be allowed to make this decision.

Deciding on the content of each session also requires the therapists to balance several elements. They must balance the children's discussion of their individual concerns with teaching them specific skills aimed at decreasing their depressogenic symptoms. Although 50 or 60 minutes per session may seem like a lot of time, it can easily be spent discussing the children's concerns and problems. However, in the interest of providing them with the skills and insight to help them deal with their present as well as future, problems, the sessions are generally divided into two sections, with approximately 20 minutes devoted to individual issues and the remainder to broader therapeutic issues and skill development. Moreover, as implied earlier, didactic material must be balanced with activities that are fun in order to maintain the children's interest. Similarly, the amount of homework assigned must be appropriately balanced so that the children derive the most benefit from the sessions while not feeling overwhelmed or feeling that the group is just like another class with lots of homework. As discussed later, it is difficult to get the children to complete their homework, and both self-reinforcement and external contingency procedures may need to be used to encourage the children to complete such assignments.

While balancing these elements within the group, therapists working in the schools must also balance their own needs (or those of the project in which they are involved) with the needs of the schools as a whole. Likewise, the therapists' or project's needs must be balanced with those of individual administrators and/or teachers. These balances are important in order to prevent administrators and/or teachers from sabotaging the treatment program by, for example, limiting the amount of time children are allowed to miss class, or being unwilling to let them make up tests they have missed. Describing the treatment program and its value for the children, as well as involving the school staff in deciding what time of day to hold the sessions, can be helpful in preventing any problems between therapists and school personnel. In addition, therapists need to balance teachers' desire and/or need to know how their students are doing in therapy with the therapists' promise to the children that their confidentiality will not be violated. This can usually be best handled by giving the teachers general feedback about what didactic material is being discussed in the treatment sessions and how that child is performing within the group. In addition, it is useful to explain to them that, ethically, therapists are unable to give them more specific information.

As mentioned in earlier sections of this chapter, the involvement of the family is essential when treating depressed children and adolescents. Working with the children's families, however, also involves the balancing of several elements. For one, the therapists must be able to provide feedback to the family (about how specific changes within the family might have a positive effect on the depressed child and on other family members) while not being perceived by the family as threatening or controlling. Typically, adopting a consultative role can be helpful in these situations; in this role, the therapist can facilitate the family's discussion of specific issues and different ways of coping with the situation, without being perceived as an expert who is trying to tell them what to do. In addition, like teachers, therapists need to balance giving the parents some feedback on the child and his or her progress with their obligation to protect the child's confidentiality. Again, general feedback can be provided to the parents along with an explanation of why the therapist cannot provide specific information. In addition, before the family meeting, the therapist can discuss with the child whether he or she wishes to bring up any of the material discussed during the treatment sessions. If the child decides to share some information, the therapist can facilitate this discussion during the family meeting.

THE TREATMENT OF DEPRESSED CHILDREN: A PROGRAMMATIC EXAMPLE

Time Frame

The time frame for treatment that we have followed with fourth-, fifth-, and sixth-grade children has varied in both the total number of, and the spacing of, the sessions. As noted earlier, in our initial investigation, the treatment was conducted in 12 sessions over a 5-week period. Currently, we have utilized 27 sessions completed over 3½ months. The most efficient number and spacing of sessions remains an empirical question. Our experience would suggest that some children would require even more sessions to produce a more philosophical change in the way they approach life. In the ideal situation, the number of sessions provided for any client would match his or her needs. Treatment would continue until there was a clinically significant reduction in the presence and severity of symptomatology, as well as evidence that the child had mastered the cognitive-behavioral skills and could apply them to controlling symptoms.

The spacing of the sessions appears to be an important consideration. We have found that it is useful to begin with twice weekly sessions and then cut back to one session per week. This could then be reduced to one session every two weeks and finally to a check-in or as-needed basis. Twice weekly sessions are utilized in the beginning of treatment, for a number of reasons. First, the serious and destructive nature of the syndrome of depression requires that steps be taken to promote the rapid reduction of symptoms. Second, meeting twice a week with the children increases the chances that they will spend more time thinking about what they have learned during the sessions. Weekly sessions appear to be too limited in this respect, allowing too much time between sessions for the children to slip back into their old, maladaptive style of thinking and behaving, and to forget what was discussed during the previous session. Furthermore, too much time between sessions makes it less likely that the children will complete the homework assignments. A child may be successful at completing the homework assignments for a day or two, even three, and then may slip and forget. Once he or she has forgotten, it is not uncommon for the child to fail to complete any other assignments during the week. This failure does not help the child feel good about either him- or herself or the treatment program.

As the severity of symptomatology subsides, the therapists and children meet on a weekly basis. This is useful because it allows the children to try out their new skills and to see the symptom reduction that results from their use. This becomes especially true beginning with the assertiveness and social skills training sessions and continues through the self-evaluation training, where the children begin working toward self-improvement. It takes time for the children to see some measurable improvement in personally meaningful areas such as body weight or a relationship with a significant other. At this point, it may even prove useful to reduce the meetings to once every 2 weeks so that the children have plenty of time to improve through their own efforts and thereby enhance their sense of self-efficacy.

Overview of Treatment

The treatment program consists of a number of cognitive and behavioral procedures that are combined in a logical way. Cognitive restructuring is utilized throughout the treatment, and a number of sessions are specifically devoted to teaching the children to identify the thoughts that lead to sadness and other depressogenic symptomatology. Then children are taught to be "personal scientists" and investigate the evidence for the validity of these symptom-producing thoughts. Covert modeling also is used throughout treatment as a means of teaching the children an alternative way of processing information about the self, the world, and the future.

The children are taught a number of self-control skills, including self-reinforcement, self-monitoring, and more adaptive ways of self-evaluating. These skills are taught through educational and therapeutic exercises and are applied and further internalized through behavioral homework assignments.

A number of more traditional behavioral procedures also are used, including assertiveness and social skills training. Social skills are taught through education, modeling, rehearsal, coaching, and feedback. In addition, specific behavioral homework assignments are given to help the children utilize these skills to improve their lives.

The family also is involved in the treatment program. An attempt is made to change the way that family members interact, the amount of recreational activity they are involved in together, and the way that family members communicate and manage each other's behavior. Finally, the parents are taught to become therapeutic change agents who can facilitate the generalization of treatment effects.

A group treatment format is utilized. Each group consists of four children, matched in terms of social skill and social status when possible. Two therapists are used for a number of reasons. First, this is a way to have both a male and a female therapist available for the children. Second, it helps keep the sessions moving along smoothly and at a good pace. Given the need to review homework assignments, address personal issues, and teach new skills, it is crucial to use time as efficiently as possible. Finally, having two therapists present increases the likelihood that a solution will be developed for any given problem that the children may bring up.

Cognitive Restructuring

Overview

Cognitive-restructuring procedures are designed to modify the client's thinking and the premises, assumptions, and attitudes underlying the client's thoughts (Meichenbaum, 1977). They are used to change the way the individual derives meaning from the world. Three primary cognitive-restructuring procedures have emerged (Mahoney & Arnkoff, 1978), including *cognitive therapy* (e.g., Beck *et al.*, 1979), *rational-emotive therapy* (e.g., Ellis, 1962), and *self-instructional training* (Meichenbaum, 1977). We use Beck's and Meichenbaum's cognitive-restructuring procedures in our treatment program for depressed children.

The Training Procedure

Throughout the treatment program, the therapists are vigilant for opportunities to use cognitive-restructuring procedures to help the children develop a more adaptive style of processing information. During each session, the therapists listen to the children for examples of depressogenic thinking as well as overt signs of mood change. These depressive cognitions are evident in the things the children spontaneously say to one another and to the therapist, and in their descriptions of what they have done between sessions. Once a depressive cognition has been identified, the therapists identify for the child the maladaptive thought and explore the parameters of its occurrence—how often, when, where, and what is usually happening. Subsequently, the child, the child's fellow group members, and the therapists collaboratively explore alternative, more adaptive ways of conceptualizing the situation; then they explore the evidence for each alternative. Subsequently, the alternative with the most evidence is posed to the child as being the most realistic appraisal of the situation. In most cases, this is a more positive conception, and an adaptive way of processing information is accepted. In other cases, however, the most realistic and accurate way of conceptualizing what is happening is fairly disappointing and bleak. In such cases, the therapists help the child see that although the situation is disappointing, it is not the end of the world and he or she can live with it. Moreover, in these latter cases, the child, his or her fellow group members, and the therapists use problem solving to work out a plan of action that will result in an improvement in that particular area of the child's life.

As time passes, the therapists turn over more and more of the responsibility for this cognitive restructuring to the group. This gives the children the opportunity to practice the process and to learn to take a more objective, problem-to-be-solved approach to their own depressive thoughts and problematic situations.

Later in the intervention program, there are a number of sessions that are specifically designed to teach the children to identify and evaluate their depressogenic thoughts. During the first of these sessions, the children complete a depressive-cognitions questionnaire (Stark, Best, & McNitsky, 1987a), which enables the therapists to identify each child's maladaptive thoughts. These thoughts are then linked to hypothetical situations, and the children are instructed to act as investigators and go through the process of generating alternative conceptualizations of the situation and evaluating the evidence for each one. Subsequently, the children choose the one that is most adaptive and realistic according to the evidence. This process is done aloud so that each child's fellow group members as well as the therapists can coach the child through the process and provide him or her with feedback. In addition, the subjects compare their current responses to the depressive-cognitions questionnaire to their pretreatment responses. Typically, by this point in treatment, a good deal of change has been achieved. Thus, this exercise also demonstrates to each child that he or she has improved, which enhances the children's sense of self-efficacy.

To individualize the process and to help the children identify their depressogenic cognitions, the children complete thought records on a daily basis. Each time they are aware of a thought that makes them feel bad, they note it on a form that facilitates correct completion of the restructuring process. The children note what was happening, how they were feeling, and what they were thinking. Subsequently, the child generates a list of alternative conceptualizations and the evidence for them. Finally, the child notes his or her choice for the most adaptive and accurate way of conceptualizing the situation. By completing this process outside of therapy as homework, this procedure also facilitates the generalization of the process to the children's extratherapy environment.

With children who are having difficulty learning the steps of the cognitive-restructuring process, the self-instructional training procedure is also used. This procedure (see Meichenbaum, 1977, for a more detailed description) serves as the process for helping the children internalize a set of self-statements that guide cognitive restructuring. Specifically, they are taught to use low levels of dysphoric mood as a cue to say "What was I thinking?" "What are the alternatives?" "What's the evidence?" "Choose my answer," "I did a good job," or "I made a mistake, I'll try harder next time." Through practice, the children also acquire an understanding of what each self-statement means and how to use the statements to guide themselves through the cognitive-restructuring process.

Covert Modeling

Covert modeling is a procedure in which the therapists model more adaptive cognitions for the children in the group. This procedure is used throughout treatment as a means of teaching the children more adaptive cognitions. The therapists, whenever it is appropriate, model their thoughts by thinking aloud. For example, something disappointing to one of the therapists might happen during one of the sessions. The therapist verbalizes what has happened and his or her coping thoughts aloud. This procedure also is used as a way to model effective problem solving. Whenever a therapist or the group runs into a problem, the therapist thinks aloud. The number of opportunities to model adaptive thinking is surprisingly high, and the children truly remember these examples.

Self-Monitoring

Overview

Self-monitoring is the metacognitive act of observing one's own behavior (overt or covert) and making a judgment about the occurrence or nonoccurrence of the target response (the behavior, either overt or covert, that is the focus of change). We all do self-monitoring quite frequently, especially when something unexpected occurs. Individuals can be taught to self-monitor target responses as either an assessment of a therapeutic procedure. In fact, it may be difficult to disentangle the two (Gross & Drabman, 1982). In either case, it is a procedure that is appropriate for use with children older than 6 years of age (Ollendick & Hersen, 1984). It is important to note, however, that the therapist is not teaching the children the meta-cognitive process of self-monitoring; rather, the children are being taught to monitor different, therapeutically relevant responses and events.

Depressed children, like depressed adults, exhibit a propensity for self-monitoring negative events to the exclusion of positive events (Kaslow, Rehm, & Siegel, 1984). In other words, depressed children tend to pay attention to the unpleasant or negative things going on in their lives to the exclusion of the positive things. Additionally, they tend to focus on their own shortcomings to the exclusion of their strengths. Depressed children often are hypersensitive or "self-conscious," spending an inordinate amount of time thinking about themselves and their weaknesses. It is important to break this cycle of negative self-attention, and the self-monitoring procedure is one of the techniques used to do this.

In many ways, the self-monitoring procedure is central to the success of the treatment program. Initially, the procedure is used as an assessment technique that helps the therapists to create a picture of the positive and negative things going on in each child's life. Therapists can use the information gained from self-monitoring to help the youngsters identify pleasant activities to target for increase. It is especially useful for identifying activities that are associated with elevated mood. As therapy progresses and the children learn additional self-regulatory skills, the self-monitoring procedure is used as a means of assessing both the youngsters' ability to use the new skills and the change in symptomatology that results from their use. As a child demonstrates progress, he or she uses this information as a cue to self-reinforce. Later in therapy, when the youngsters have gained greater control over their mood, self-monitoring is used as the primary means for identifying negative, depression-producing cognitions.

As noted before, the training in self-monitoring is designed to direct the focus of attention rather than to teach the children the metacognitive process of self-attention itself. It is assumed that the children already have the meta-cognitive ability to self-monitor therapeutically relevant events and responses. The responses and events that are targeted for self-monitoring include: (1) depressogenic, emotionally laden, and positive thoughts; (2) pleasant events that occur in the child's daily life; (3) pleasant activities that the child engages in; (4) the acquisition and implementation of coping skills; and (5) the outcome of behavioral homework assignments. In order to facilitate the accurate self-monitoring of those responses and events, a number of record sheets were developed by the authors and their colleagues. Multiple copies of the record sheets are then compiled into booklets that the children carry with them to and from school.

The Training Procedure

The training process is rather simplistic and is modeled after the training procedures used with depressed adults (e.g., Fuchs & Rehm, 1977) and with children who have other psychological disorders (cf. Kendall & Braswell, 1982). Training the participants to self-monitor their cognitions is a prerequisite for successful use of cognitive restructuring. As a prelude to the actual training, the children are taught that the things they think about influence how they feel. This is accomplished both subtly, through completion of a number of activities, and directly, through a story and a discussion that follows it. Once the link has been made, the children are given the homework assignment to pay attention to any noticeable changes in mood. Once they notice this change, they are instructed to listen in to the thoughts they are having. Then they record the thoughts on a record sheet.

As treatment progresses, the record sheets change, and the children become more aware of the role their thoughts play in their depression, emphasis is placed on monitoring and identifying the thoughts they have when they are feeling the onset of depressed or more depressed mood. These thoughts are recorded on a second type of thought record. In addition to monitoring and recording their depressogenic thoughts, the particpants monitor their independent attempts at cognitive restructuring on these record sheets.

Another primary use of self-monitoring is designed to break the cycle of negative self-attention as well as to increase activity level, thus decreasing time spent thinking about negative, maladaptive things. To do this, children's versions of pleasant events schedules were developed (Stark, Best, & Lux, 1986). These schedules consist of lists of enjoyable activities (e.g., swimming, staying overnight at a friend's house), positive events (receiving a desirable object as a gift), and positive thoughts ("someone cares about me"). At the bottom of the list is an 11-point Likert scale on which the children rate their overall mood for the day.

The training procedure utilized to teach the children to monitor their engagement in pleasant activities and events was very similar to the one noted here. Through a Socratic process of questioning and discussion, the children are taught the relationship between mood and engagement in pleasant activities and the occurrence of pleasant events. In addition, the relationship is made more concrete through a series of cartoons illustrating this relationship. Subsequently, the children are given copies of the pleasant-events schedules and some practice in completing them. This is accomplished through a card game in which each item from the schedule is written down on a 3" × 5" card. The cards are placed in a pile in the middle of the group, and the children take turns picking cards and recording what they picked by placing a check mark in front of the same item on the list. After all the cards are picked, the children review their pile of cards and rate their mood for the hypothetical day. Subsequently, the children are given multiple copies of the measures, enough for each day until the next session. They are instructed to complete one a day by checking off the activities and events in which they engaged. This checkoff process is completed three times a day: at lunch, after dinner, and before bed. During this final time, the children rate their mood for the day.

Self-Reinforcement Training

Overview

Self-reinforcement is the process of presenting rewards to oneself contingent on performance of a desired response. It is one of the cognitive processes of self-consequation (the other being self-punishment) that are presumed to follow self-evaluation automatically. Specifically, if the child's performance meets or exceeds his or her standards, then he or she self-reinforces; if the performance is substandard, then self-punishment follows.

The process of self-reinforcement involves two major steps: (1) the child must demonstrate self-control by delaying gratification for a brief period of time; and (2) the child administers a reinforcer when the desired goal has been met. Reinforcers can be either overt (e.g., tangible objects, enjoyable or high-frequency activities) or covert in nature (e.g., thoughts).

Self-reinforcement is one of the most widely studied behavioral techniques, and research indicates that it is an effective procedure with adults (Mahoney & Arnkoff, 1978) including depressed adults (Rehm & Marston, 1968). For reinforcement (either self- or externally administered) to be effective, reinforcers must be identified and readily available for administration upon performance of the desired response. Finding effective reinforcers for depressed children is problematic because of their symptom of anhedonia. Things that once were reinforcing no longer have the same effect. As we will see, however, it is possible to find effective reinforcers for these depressed youngsters.

Self-reinforcement is an integral component of treatment for depressed youths. As noted earlier, preliminary research indicates that mildly depressed children exhibit a deficit in self-reinforcement and a propensity for self-punishment. In addition, self-reinforcement, administered contingent on emission of nondepressogenic behavior, is a means of increasing activity level. It also is a procedure that can be used to help youths acquire skills for coping with their depression. For example, it is used as a means of increasing the probability that a therapeutic task such as self-monitoring of pleasant events will be completed outside the therapist's office.

The Training Procedure

The first phase involves identifying positive reinforcers for each individual. As noted earlier, these reinforcers should be readily accessible, and it should be possible for the youngsters to self-administer the rewards with little or no help. It is also important to identify a continuum of reinforcers, varying in cost. Activities and thoughts can also serve as reinforcers and should be included in the individual's list. It is crucial to include parents in the process of identifying potential reinforcers. This is important not only because they can identify objects and activities that the youngster engaged in prior to his or her depressive episode, but also because their support (e.g., money, transportation) may be necessary for the enactment of some pleasant activities and the purchase of certain objects.

In its first application, self-reinforcement is used as a way to increase the likelihood that the youngsters will complete their homework assignments. The participants are taught to administer rewards contingent on completion of therapeutically relevant tasks such as completing the self-monitoring log sheets described earlier. Self-reinforcement also plays a key role in the last few sessions, during which the participants are taught to self-reinforce for subgoal and goal attainment as they work toward self-improvement.

Because the self-reinforcement process may feel foreign to the depressed youngsters, modeling and rehearsal are used as teaching modalities. During the initial sessions, the youngsters rehearse self-reinforcement for the completion of their therapeutic homework exercises. Later, during the self-improvement portion of the treatment, the therapists model the setting of adaptive criteria, dividing the goal into subgoals, developing an action plan, matching reinforcers to actions and subgoals, and administering the rewards. Subsequently, the children practice the self-reinforcement process in hypothetical situations, based on specific goals they have set for self-improvement. During these practice sessions, the youngsters are coached on administering rewards whose value is consistent with that of the task being completed. Thus, smaller rewards are given for completion of subgoals and larger rewards for completion of goals. During these practice sessions, the therapists may initially model appropriate behavior, but as the children progress through the hypothetical situations, the therapists gradually fade their involvement. The youngsters also are encouraged to use covert reinforcement. These positive self-statements are also rehearsed in practice sessions, with the children progressing from initially verbalizing the self-statements aloud to eventually self-verbalizing covertly.

The final phase of the self-reinforcement training is designed to ensure that the children continue to use the self-reinforcement skill. The therapists monitor the children's progress though discussions with them and with their parents, and by checking their self-monitoring log sheets.

Parental Involvement

It is very helpful to involve parents in these aspects of the training procedure. During the family meetings, a discussion about what is rewarding for each family member can be initiated, and family members are encouraged to reward each other more often. Parents, in particular, are encouraged to reward their child by spending positive time with him or her. Parents are also informed that the therapists are trying to teach their child to self-reward for accomplishments. The parents can be asked to encouarge this self-reinforcement and model the process for their child.

Activity Scheduling

Overview

Activity scheduling, the systematic planning of the youngsters' daily activities, is a collaborative process involving the therapists and the youngsters. For the children, this increase in activity level reduces the time available to ruminate about their sorry state of affairs. The therapists and the children identify activities that they find especially enjoyable through systematically reviewing the self-monitoring log sheets and graphs. Activities that are consistently associated with elevated mood are particularly important to target for increased enactment.

The Training Procedure

Self-monitoring of pleasant activities often leads to an increase in activity level, but systematic programming is a prerequisite for success. To accomplish this, the therapists work collaboratively with the children to identify activities that they would like to do more often. Subsequently, each child identifies impediments to engaging in the scheduled activities. The therapists then model the use of problem solving (identifying the problem, generating alternative actions, and projecting the outcomes of each possible action into the future) to help the children develop plans for overcoming potential impediments. Finally, the therapists encourage the children to use problem solving to overcome the impediments, and thereby increase their activity level. When working with a group of youngsters, the group members also give each other suggestions for how to develop plans that maximize their opportunity for success.

At times we have worked with children who are so seriously withdrawn that they reported doing only one or two things a day. Typically, their activities were very passive and didn't involve other people—for example, watching television or listening to the radio. In such instances, borrowing from the adult literature (Beck *et al.*, 1979), we literally helped the children plan their day on an hour-by-hour basis. This is worked out using an activity scheduling sheet. The therapists encourage the youngsters to generate a list of everything they like to do (or liked to do prior to their depression). Subsequently, the therapists and children work through the schedule for the next week, filling in activities and opportunities to interact with others. In later sessions, the youngsters keep the schedules in a folder and complete them as homework.

Parental Involvement

To help ensure that the children follow the plan, the youngsters' parents must be involved in the program and must be willing to monitor and help the children implement the actions. The best results occur when the parents work collaboratively with their youngsters to develop activity plans so that the whole family becomes involved in ensuring that they, as a group, do more enjoyable things together. Collaboration between child and parents also helps ensure that the scheduled activities are realistic in terms of the family's financial situation and the parents' work and social commitments.

In many cases, the parents are eager to help in any way they can, but the affected child simply does not want to do anything. In these cases, it is important to avoid forcing the child to do something that he or she does not want to do. The child should be informed of the therapeutic benefits of increasing activity level and should be encouraged, rather than coerced, to increase his or her activity level. The pace of the increase should be tailored to fit the youngster's comfort level. Typically, there is a snowball effect. The individual starts out doing a few activities, then a few more, and in a relatively short period of time is back to a premorbid activity level.

Assertiveness Training

Although there has been little research indicating that depressed children are less assertive than their nondepressed peers, our clinical work suggests that this is indeed the case. The reasons are unclear, but we believe that depressed youngsters either may lack the necessary skills (a skills deficit) and/or may possess maladaptive, self-defeating cognitions that interfere with performance (a performance deficit). Thus, our training procedure is designed both to teach the children assertiveness skills and to also counteract any inhibitory cognitions.

Maintaining the emphasis on increasing pleasant activity level, the focus of our assertiveness skills program is on teaching the children to (1) ask family members or peers to do more enjoyable activities with them, (2) tell people what they are doing that the child likes, and (3) tell people to stop doing something that the child does not like.

The children are taught these skills through the traditional behavioral procedures of education, modeling, coaching, rehearsal, and feedback. Initially, the therapists portray coping models as they role play an assertiveness situation that is of concern to a member of the group. A therapist verbalizes his or her apprehension about the situation as the child role plays the target individual (e.g., a parent) and tries to behave as this individual might. Following the modeling, the therapist and child switch roles and the therapist coaches the youngster through the request. Supportive feedback is provided and, once the child seems to be performing adequately, therapist and child plan a time when the child can actually speak to the target person.

Social Skills Training

The focus of the social skills training program is twofold: to teach the children (1) skills for coping with maladaptive cognitions that may be inhibiting effective social behavior, and (2) performance of some social skills. Education and cognitive restructuring are employed to dispute the irrational beliefs preventing social interactions; the skills training component is directed toward the acquisition and performance of (1) initiating interactions, (2) responding to the initiations of others, (3) maintaining interactions, and (4) dealing with disagreements.

As with the assertiveness component of the treatment program, social skills training includes education, modeling, rehearsal, coaching, and corrective feedback. We have found that the treatment group is an ideal medium for training in both assertiveness and social skills, as the children can practice in a safe and supportive environment and can receive immediate corrective feedback.

Adjunct Procedure

Videotaping equipment has been a useful addition to the assertiveness and social skills training components of our program. Role plays can be recorded and replayed to facilitate corrective feedback. In addition, we have found that most children like being videotaped, so that interest and enjoyment in these activities is high.

Self-Evaluation Training

Overview

Self-evaluation is the cognitive process of comparing one's performance to one's standards for performance. Within Kanfer and Karoly's (1972) model of self-regulation, it is hypothesized that humans automatically self-evaluate, and then self-consequate as a function of their evaluation. This is something we all do. However, it is most noticeable when we do something new or when something out of the ordinary happens. We are especially aware of this when we are in competitive or evaluative situations, such as playing tennis in front of a crowd. At these times we are constantly monitoring and evaluating our performance.

One of the hypothesized symptoms of depression in children is a distortion in the self-evaluation process that results from setting excessively stringent, unattainable standards for performance. Given these excessive standards, depressed children are typically unable to measure up to their expectations, and consequently evaluate themselves negatively.

Children can be trained to evaluate their behavior more accurately (Spates & Kanfer, 1977). Unfortunately, this training has had minimal impact on children's overt behavior when it is used as the sole intervention strategy (O'Leary & Dubey, 1979). When the procedure is used in combination with another self-control procedure such as self-reinforcement, however, it contributes to the efficacy of the combined intervention and produces a change in overt behavior

(Bandura & Perloff, 1967). Stark and colleagues (1987c) have combined training in setting more realistic standards and working toward personally meaningful goals as part of a self-control treatment for depression in children.

The Training Procedure

Standard setting   A complex and extensive training procedure has been used to teach depressed children to set realistic, attainable standards for performance as well as realistic, attainable goals for self-improvement.

Phase 1 involves setting realistic standards. The first stage of this phase is to assess the children's standards for their own performance and their evaluation of their current performance. This assessment is accomplished with a simple questionnaire entitled "My Standards." The therapists and the group then discuss discrepancies between standards and current evaluations. In the second step, the therapists help the youngsters to evaluate the rationality of their standards and then to set more realistic standards that are also acceptable to the child. These standards should be achievable, although they may require some effort. In step 4 of this phase, the therapist models the use of these new standards in hypothetical situations. Next, the children rehearse these standards while the therapists coach, model, and probe, as necessary. During the final step of phase 1, the children try out and self-monitor the use of the new standards in actual situations. The results of this procedure are discussed in subsequent therapy sessions, and any necessary revisions are worked out.

Phase 2 involves setting realistic goals that are consistent with the youngsters' standards. These goals should also involve personally meaningful areas in which the children are currently not meeting their own expectations for performance. These areas will have already been identified in phase 1 during the completion of the My Standards questionnaire. During step 1 of this second phase, the therapists and each child review, and subsequently prioritize, these goals. The children are then encouraged to pursue one of the more readily attainable goals to ensure that they experience success in their initial attempts at self-improvement. Step 3 involves ensuring that the children's goals are realistic and then dividing them into subgoals. The use of subgoals ensures more rapid success, self-reward, and the development of a sense of self-efficacy. Step 4 involves developing an action plan for obtaining the subgoals and, eventually, the long-term goal. In developing this action plan, effort is made to anticipate any potential obstacles and to develop contingency plans for coping effectively with these impediments, should they arise. Step 5 involves the therapists modeling implementation of action plan, if appropriate. The therapists use a coping model, demonstrating how they would incorporate one of the contingency plans when an obstacle arises. The children are actively involved in this step, talking the therapists through the plan and answering the therapists' questions as to how they would deal with potential problems. Step 6 involves each child carrying out and self-monitoring his or her action plan. The results of this procedure are discussed during the next session and any problems are addressed. The children continue this process until their goals have been achieved and their behavior meets their own standards. Then, each child sets and pursues another goal.

Behavioral Homework

From the previous description of the treatment program, it may be apparent that the intervention involves daily homework assignments. This poses a potential problem for the therapists because children do not enjoy completing psychologically relevant homework assignments much more than they do academic homework. Our research and clinical experience indicates, however, that completion of these homework assignments is integral to the success of treatment. It helps the children to master the skills and to change their overt and covert behavior. Furthermore, it promotes the generalization of treatment effects outside of the therapy setting.

Given the importance of the homework, steps need to be taken to ensure that the participants complete their assignments. We have used a number of procedures to accomplish this. The self-reinforcement procedure is taught first as a means of giving the children the necessary skills to reward themselves for completing their homework assignments, thus bridging the gap in time between the initial attempts at change and the symptomatic improvement that results from the changes. Another self-control procedure involves teaching the children to change their environment slightly so that they are more likely to remember to complete their assignments. This form of stimulus control involves teaching the children to place cartoons in places that would serve as cues to complete their homework and to remember to bring their practice books to and from school. The children tape the cartoons to the top of their school desks, assignment folders, and refrigerator doors. To remind them to complete their homework, they might also tape the cartoons to their bedroom desks or nightstands.

External contingency procedures also are used to help ensure that the children complete their therapeutic homework. Both individual and group contingencies are utilized. The children can earn small tangible rewards (e.g., sugarless gum) on an intermittent schedule for completion of their homework. When a group member fails to complete the homework or forgets to bring it to group, the child receives only partial reinforcement. The group also is given the opportunity to earn larger activity rewards (e.g., viewing a movie on a VCR). These larger rewards are contingent on everyone in the group completing the assignments a given number of times. For example, a pizza party might be made contingent on all of the children completing their homework 15 times.

The children's parents also are involved in helping ensure that the children complete their homework. However, discretion is necessary here. In the case of the depressed child who is continually derided by his or her parents, it may be unwise to ask such parents to remind the child to complete the homework. In such cases, this request has the potential for being highly problematic, as it may offer the parents additional opportunities to hassle the child. When there is a healthy relationship between the child and his or her parents, the parents are asked to remind the child, gently, to complete his or her homework. They also are asked to help by reinforcing their child for completing the forms. In addition, they are asked to participate in the actual homework process by doing such things as scheduling pleasant activities along with the child.

Cartoons

In order to concretize the concepts being taught, two cartoon characters were developed. The characters are depicted in scenes that illustrate the therapeutic concepts as well as the use of the coping skills being taught. Then the cartoons are compiled into booklets, which the children keep. It is common to find that the children have referred to their cartoon books between sessions. Often, they have colored in the cartoons or added in new, adaptive thought bubbles. Our experience with the cartoons has been very positive. The children have reported that it makes it easier for them to understand what we are trying to teach them. Furthermore, they report that the images created by the cartoons often serve as cues to what to do to cope with various situations that arise between sessions.

Family Treatment Component

Research (Cole & Rehm, 1986; Stark *et al.*, 1987c) indicates that there may be differences in the family environments of depressed and nondepressed children. To change this home environment and to secure the parents' help in the process, the family has also been a focus of our therapeutic efforts. It is important to note, however, that not all of the families in which there is a depressed child are unhealthy. Some of the families have very adaptive interaction patterns. Furthermore, within the distressed families, there is no single common maladaptive pattern of interaction. Rather, they are quite heterogeneous with a few overlapping or common patterns of unhealthy behavior.

The family treatment sessions have been designed to achieve a number of objectives:

1. To address any concerns the family members might have about their interpersonal relationships
2. To prime the parents for encouraging positive, nondepressogenic change in their child's behavior
3. To secure the parents' assistance with seeing that their child completes his or her behavioral homework
4. To solicit some changes in the parents' own behavior that might be supporting either depressogenic or maladaptive behavior
5. To promote accurate communication about the nature and content of the treatment program

6. To establish more active and involved forms of family recreation
7. To educate the parents so that they can serve as therapeutic change agents for their child
8. To establish a more positive and assertive style of behavior management among family members.

Participants

For a number of practical reasons, and to protect client confidentiality, most of the family meetings included the target child and his or her parent(s). Siblings were not included. The exception to this (abbreviated) family meeting was in the case in which it was apparent that a sibling was a key player in some interpersonal or other problem. In these cases, the sibling would also be included. In general, our experience with this format has been quite positive and has made scheduling of the sessions a little less difficult.

Spacing of Family Meetings

In our most recent investigation, each therapist met once a month with the same family, for a total of four meetings. Each family meeting lasted approximately 1½ hours. In the future, the number of family sessions will be expanded to a meeting once every 3 weeks. Further expansion to biweekly or weekly sessions would be ideal. When one is conducting treatment outcome research in the schools, however, a gentle balance must be struck between experimental rigor, parental support (or lack thereof) for the treatment program, and the parents' own obligations. It would be extremely difficult to get the parents to stick to a weekly or biweekly meeting schedule. Inconsistencies in the spacing of the meetings would create methodological problems. Another limiting factor is the fact that these parents did not solicit the treatment for their child; rather, the researchers have solicited the family's participation. Thus, the parents are not always willing to make the large commitment of time and energy that would be necessary for more frequent sessions.

The Treatment Program

The first meeting is devoted to interviewing the parents of the child to gain an understanding of their perspective on the child's depression. Subsequently, the parents and child are brought together and, given the child's permission, the family is directed through a discussion that leads to a consensus about the nature of the disorder. Part of the second meeting with the parents is spent establishing rapport and informing the parents in greater detail about the research project and the treatment program. Subsequently, an attempt is made to come to a common understanding about the nature of the child's depressive symptomatology, and the cognitive-behavioral perspective of depression is introduced. The parents are introduced to the concept of rewards, both self-

and externally administered, and the idea of managing behavior through the contingent administration of rewards rather than punishment alone. In addition, the parents are asked to help their child gain access to tangible and activity rewards for self-administration.

Another parallel focus of treatment is on activity scheduling. The importance of engagement in pleasant activities by all family members, and the target child in particular, is emphasized. The parents are asked to help their child both schedule and enact pleasant activities. In addition, they are encouraged to take a look at their own degree of involvement in their child's recreation. If it is limited, then the advantages of increasing their time commitment to positive activities are emphasized and a commitment is secured. Finally, an initial attempt is made to air, and work out, any interpersonal conflicts, disagreements, concerns, or misunderstandings. Behavioral homework assignments may be given at the end of the session.

The third session begins with some time spent establishing rapport. Subsequently, if a behavioral homework assignment was given, compliance with the assignment is checked, as is its outcome. In addition, the family's attempts at managing each other's behavior through positive means is reviewed, as well as their engagement in pleasant recreational activities. Successful attempts at compliance are met with social reinforcement from the therapist. Next, the target child is encouraged to show off what he or she has learned by reviewing for the parents what has been covered in the child's therapy sessions since the last family meeting. The parents are introduced to the children's pleasant-events schedules, their utility, and the fact that their child should be completing one every day. Their assistance in reminding their child to do so is secured. They are asked to remind their child gently rather than coercing the child into cooperating. They are also encouraged to reward their child for completing his or her homework.

The discussion then turns to future sessions, especially those dealing with assertiveness. The therapist emphasizes that the child will be learning to communicate more openly and directly, but with *respect*. The emphasis is on respectful assertiveness. The parents are asked to watch for examples of their child being assertive and to respond positively to them when they feel they can. Furthermore, when appropriate, they are asked to inform the child assertively why they won't respond affirmatively to a request. In these cases, they are asked nevertheless to praise their child for being assertive. The parents also are asked to point out times when their child could have behaved assertively but failed to do so.

Again, the session ends with an attempt to get the family to discuss any problems they have with one another. Since the children are often afraid to bring up their concerns about their parents, some steps are taken to help the child gain the confidence necessary to bring up such concerns. Prior to this meeting, if the child has brought up some concerns about his or her parents during the treatment, the therapist and child role play how to bring this up in the family meeting. This seems to help the child gain the necessary confidence to do so.

The fourth family meeting begins with a few minutes of rapport building, followed by a discussion of how the target child is doing in therapy and how things are going in the family. This is followed by a check of the family's compliance with therapeutic homework assignments. Subsequently, the child's attempts at being assertive are discussed. Again, with some coaching by the therapist, the child describes what he or she has learned in the sessions. Emphasis is now placed on the relationship between mood, behavior, and thoughts. The parents are shown the thought records and informed that their child is now completing one of these each night. Their assistance in seeing that their child completes his or her homework is solicited and secured.

At this time the parents play a greater role in their child's treatment. The therapist teaches the parents how to recognize overt examples of their child's depressogenic thinking. Once they have identified a statement that reflects negative thinking, they remind the child to use his or her skills for cognitive restructuring. The parents also are taught how to help their child go through the process of generating alternative constructions and evaluating the evidence for their validity.

Again, the session ends with a discussion of any concerns the family members might have about one another. These discussions tend to be quite lively and productive.

REFERENCES

Abramson, L. Y., Seligman, M. E. P., & Teasdale, J. (1978). Learned helplessness in humans: Critique and reformulation. *Journal of Abnormal Psychology*, 87, 49–74.

Achenbach, T. M., & Edelbrock, C. S. (1978). The classification of child psychopathology: A review and analysis of empirical efforts. *Psychological Bulletin*, 85, 1275–1301.

American Psychiatric Association (1980). *Diagnostic and statistical manual of mental disorders* (3rd edition). Washington, DC: Author.

Bandura, A., & Perloff, B. (1967). Relative efficacy of self-monitored and externally imposed reinforcement systems. *Journal of Personality and Social Psychology*, 7, 111–116.

Beck, A. T. (1967). *Depression: Clinical, experimental and theoretical aspects*. New York: Hoeber.

Beck, A. T. (1976). *Cognitive therapy and emotional disorders*. New York: International Universities Press.

Beck, A. T. (1985). Cognitive therapy, behavior therapy, psychoanalysis, and pharmacotherapy: A cognitive continuum. In M. J. Mahoney & A. Freeman (Eds.), *Cognition and psychotherapy* (pp. 325–347). New York: Plenum Press.

Beck, A. T., Rush, A. G., Shaw, B. F., & Emery, G. (1979). *Cognitive therapy of depression*. New York: Guilford Press.

Brookman, C., Stark, K. D., & Carlson, C. (1987). *Family interaction patterns and depression in children*. Manuscript in preparation.

Butler, L., Miezitis, S., Friedman, R., & Cole, E. (1980). The effect of two school-based intervention programs on depressive symptoms in preadolescents. *American Educational Research Journal, 17,* 111–119.

Carlson, G. A., & Cantwell, D. P. (1980a). A survey of depressive symptoms, syndrome, and disorder in a child psychiatric population. *Journal of Child Psychology and Psychiatry, 21,* 19–25.

Carlson, G. A., & Cantwell, D. P. (1980b). Unmasking masked depression in children and adolescents. *American Journal of Psychiatry, 137,* 445–449.

Carlson, G. A., & Cantwell, D. P. (1982). Suicidal behavior and depression in children and adolescents. *Journal of the American Academy of Child Psychiatry, 21,* 361–368.

Cole, D. A., & Rehm, L. P. (1986). Family interaction patterns and childhood depression. *Journal of Abnormal Child Psychology, 14,* 297–314.

Cole, P. M., & Kaslow, N. J. (in press). Interactional and cognitive strategies for effect regulation: A developmental perspective on childhood depression. In L. B. Alloy (Ed.), *Cognitive processes in depression.* New York: Guilford Press.

Coleman, R. E. (1975). Manipulation of self-esteem as a determinant of mood and of elated and depressed women. *Journal of Abnormal Psychology, 84,* 693–700.

DeMonbreum, B. G., & Craighead, W. E. (1977). Distortion of perception and recall of positive and neutral feedback in depression. *Cognitive Therapy and Research, 1,* 311–329.

Ellis, A. (1962). *Reason and emotion in psychotherapy.* New York: Lyle Stuart.

Frame, C., Matson, J. L., Sonis, W. A., Fialkov, M. J., & Kazdin, A. E. (1982). Behavioral treatment of depression in a prepubertal child. *Journal of Behavior Therapy and Experimental Psychiatry, 3,* 239–243.

Frommer, E., Mendelson, W. B., & Reid, M. A. (1972). Differential diagnosis of psychiatric disturbances in preschool children. *British Journal of Psychiatry, 121,* 71–74.

Fuchs, C. Z., & Rehm, L. P. (1977). A self-control behavior therapy program for depression. *Journal of Consulting and Clinical Psychology, 45,* 206–215.

Gross, A. M., & Drabman, R. S. (1982). Behavioral contrast and behavior therapy. *Behavior Therapy, 12,* 231–246.

Haley, G. M. T., Fine, S., Marriage, K., Moretti, M. M., & Freeman, R. J. (1985). Cognitive bias in depression in psychiatrically disturbed children and adolescents. *Journal of Consulting and Clinical Psychology, 53,* 535–537.

Hammen, C., & Zupan, B. A. (1984). Self-schemas, depression, and the processing of personal information in children. *Journal of Experimental Child Psychology, 37,* 598–608.

Hendren, R. L. (1983). Depression in anorexia nervosa. *Journal of the American Academy of Child Psychiatry, 22,* 59–62.

Jacobsen, R. H., Lahey, B. B., & Strauss, L. C. (1983). Correlates of depressed mood in normal children. *Journal of Abnormal Child Psychology, 11,* 29–40.

Kanfer, F. H. (1970). Self-monitoring: Methodological limitations and clinical applications. *Journal of Consulting and Clinical Psychology, 35,* 148–152.

Kanfer, F. H., & Karoly, P. (1972). Self-control: A behavioristic excursion into the lion's den. *Behavior Therapy, 3,* 398–416.

Kashani, J. H., & Simonds, J. F. (1979). The incidence of depression in children. *American Journal of Psychiatry, 136,* 1203–1205.

Kashani, J. H., McGee, R. O., Clarkson, S. E., Anderson, J. C., Walton, L. A., Williams, L. A., Silva, P. A., Robins, A. J., Cytryn, L., & McKnew, D. H.

(1983). Depression in a sample of 9 year old children. *Archives of General Psychiatry*, *40*, 1217–1227.

Kaslow, N. J., Rehm, L. P., & Siegel, A. W. (1984). Social-cognitive and cognitive correlates of depression in children. *Journal of Abnormal Child Psychology*, *12*, 605–620.

Kazdin, A. E., French, N. H., Unis, A. S., Esveldt-Dawson, K., & Sherick, R. B. (1983b). Hopelessness, depression, and suicidal intent among psychiatrically disturbed children. *Journal of Consulting and Clinical Psychology*, *51*, 504–510.

Kazdin, A. E., French, N. H., Unis, A. S., & Esveldt-Dawson, K. (1983). Assessment of childhood depression: Correspondence of child and parent ratings. *Journal of the American Academy of Child Psychiatry*, *22*, 157–164.

Kendall, P. C., & Braswell, L. (1982). Cognitive-behavioral self-control therapy for children: A component analysis. *Journal of Consulting and Clinical Psychology*, *50*, 672–689.

Kendall, P., Stark, K. D., & Adam, T. (1987). *The nature of the cognitive disturbance among depressed children: Cognitive deficit or cognitive distortion.* Manuscript submitted for publication.

Kovacs, M. (1981). Rating scales to assess depression in school-aged children. *Acta Paedapsychiatrica*, *46*, 305–315.

Kovacs, M., & Beck, A. T. (1977). An empirical-clinical approach toward a definition of childhood depression. In J. G. Schulterbrandt & A. Raskin (Eds.), *Depression in childhood: Diagnosis, treatment, and conceptual models* (pp. 1–25). New York: Raven Press.

Kovacs, M., Feinberg, T. L., Crouse-Novak, M. A., Paulauskas, S. L., & Finkelstein, R. (1984). Depressive disorders in childhood. I. A longitudinal prospective study of characteristics and recovery. *Archives of General Psychiatry*, *41*, 229–237.

Kuiper, N. A., & Derry, P. A. (1982). Depressed and nondepressed content self-reference in mild depressives. *Journal of Personality*, *50*, 67–79.

Kuiper, N. A., & MacDonald, M. R. (1980). *Self-reference and person perception in depression.* Unpublished manuscript, University of Western Ontario.

Lewinsohn, P. M. (1974). A behavioral approach to depression. In R. M. Friedman & M. M. Katz (Eds.), *The psychology of depression: Contemporary theory and research* (pp. 157–185). New York: Wiley.

Ling, W., Oftedal, G., & Weinberg, W. (1970). Depressive illness in childhood presenting as severe headaches. *American Journal of Diseases of Children*, *120*, 122–124.

Lishman, W. A. (1972). Selective factors in memory: Part 2. Affective disorder. *Psychological Medicine*, *2*, 248–253.

Mahoney, M. J., & Arnkoff, D. B. (1978). Cognitive and self-control therapies. In S. L. Garfield & A. E. Bergin (Eds.), *Handbook of psychotherapy and behavior change* (2nd ed.) (pp. 689–722). New York: Wiley.

McKnew, D. H., Cytryn, L., Efron, A. M., Gershon, E. S., & Bunney, W. E., Jr. (1979). Off-spring of patients with affective disorders. *British Journal of Psychiatry*, *134*, 148–152.

Meichenbaum, D. H. (1977). *Cognitive behavior modification: An integrative approach.* New York: Plenum Press.

Moyal, B. R. (1977). Locus of control, stimulus appraisal, and depressive symptoms in children. *Journal of Consulting and Clinical Psychology*, *45*, 951–952.

Nelson, R. E., & Craighead, W. E. (1977). Selective recall of positive and negative feedback, self-control behaviors, and depression. *Journal of Abnormal Psychology, 86,* 379–388.

O'Leary, S. G., & Dubey, D. R. (1979). Applications of self-control procedures by children: A review. *Journal of Applied Behavior Analysis, 12,* 449–465.

Ollendick, T. H., & Hersen, M. (Eds.). (1984). *Child behavioral assessment: Principles and procedures.* New York: Pergamon Press.

Petti, T. A., Bornstein, M., Delamater, A., & Conners, C. K. (1980). Evaluation and multimodality treatment of a depressed prepubertal girl. *Journal of the American Academy of Child Psychiatry, 19,* 690–702.

Pfeffer, C. R., Zuckerman, S., Plutchik, R., & Mizruchi, M. S. (1984). Suicidal behavior in normal school children: A comparison with child psychiatric patients. *Journal of the American Academy of Child Psychiatry, 23,* 416–423.

Poznanski, E. O., Cook, S. C., & Carroll, B. J. (1979). A depression rating scale for children. *Pediatrics, 64,* 442–450.

Poznanski, E. O., Cook, S. C., Carroll, B. J., & Carzo, H. (1983). Use of the Children's Depression Rating Scale in an inpatient psychiatric population. *Journal of Clinical Psychiatry, 44,* 200–203.

Poznanski, E. O., Krahenbuhl, V., & Zrull, J. P. (1976). Childhood depression: A longitudinal perspective. *Journal of the American Academy of Child Psychiatry, 15,* 491–501.

Poznanski, E. O., & Zrull, J. P. (1970). Childhood depression: Clinical characteristics of overtly depressed children. *Archives of General Psychiatry, 23,* 8–15.

Puig-Antich, J., & Ryan, N. (1986). *Schedule for Affective Disorders and Schizophrenia for School-Age Children (6–18 years)—Kiddie-SADS (K-SADS).* Unpublished manuscript, Western Psychiatric Institute and Clinic, Pittsburgh, PA.

Rehm, L. P. (1977). A self control model of depression. *Behavior Therapy, 8,* 787–804.

Rehm, L. P., & Marston, A. R. (1968). Reduction of social anxiety through modification of self-reinforcement: An instigation technique. *Journal of Behavior Therapy and Experimental Psychiatry, 6,* 101–103.

Reynolds, W. M. (1984). Depression in children and adolescents: Phenomenology, evaluation, and treatment. *School Psychology Review, 13,* 171–182.

Reynolds, W. M. (1985). Depression in childhood and adolescence: Diagnosis, assessment, intervention strategies and research. In T. R. Kratochwill (Ed.), *Advances in school psychology* (Vol. 4, pp. 133–189). Hillsdale, NJ: Lawrence Erlbaum.

Reynolds, W. M., Anderson, G., & Bartell, N. (1985). *Journal of Abnormal Child Psychology, 13,* 513–526.

Reynolds, W. M., & Stark, K. D. (1983). Cognitive behavior modification: The clinical application of cognitive strategies. In M. Pressley & J. R. Levin (Eds.), *Cognitive strategy research: Psychological foundations* (pp. 221–267). New York: Springer.

Saylor, C. F., Finch, A. J., Spirito, A., & Bennett, (1984). The CDI: Systematic evaluation of psychometric properties. *Journal of Consulting and Clinical Psychology, 52,* 955–967.

Seligman, M. E. P. (1975). *Helplessness: On depression, development, and death.* San Francisco: Freeman.

Seligman, M. E. P., Peterson, C., Kaslow, N. J., Tanenbaum, R. L., Alloy, L. B., & Abramson, L. B. (1984). Attributional style and depressive symptoms among children. *Journal of Abnormal Psychology, 93,* 235–238.

Sellstrom, E., & Stark, K. D. (1987). [Schematic processing and self-reference in childhood depression]. Unpublished raw data.

Simons, A. D., Garfield, S. L., & Murphy, G. E. (1984). The process of change in cognitive therapy and pharmacotherapy for depression. *Archives of General Psychiatry, 41*, 45-51.

Spates, C. R., & Kanfer, F. H. (1977). Self-monitoring, self-evaluation, and self-reinforcement in children's learning: A test of a multi-stage self-regulation model. *Behavior Therapy, 8*, 9-16.

Spitz, R. (1946). Anaclitic depression. *Psychoanalytic study of the child, 2*, 113-117.

Stark, K. D., Best, L. R., & Lux, M. G. (1986). *Development and empirical evaluation of pleasant events schedules for school-aged children.* Manuscript in preparation.

Stark, K. D., Best, L. R., & McNitsky, M. (1987a). *Development and psychometric evaluation of depressive cognitions questionnaire for children.* Manuscript in preparation.

Stark, K. D., Humphrey, L. L., Crook, L., & Lewis, K. (1988a). *Perceived family environments of depressed, depressed and anxious, anxious and nondisturbed children: Child's and mother's perspectives.* Manuscript submitted for publication.

Stark, K. D., Kaslow, N. J., Hill, S. J., & Lux, M. G. (1988b). *The assessment of depression in children: Are we assessing depression or the broad-band construct of negative affectivity?* Manuscript submitted for publication.

Stark, K. D., Rehm, L. P., Kaslow, N. J., & Linn, J. (1987b). *Social skill, social status, and childhood depression.* Manuscript in preparation.

Stark, K. D., Reynolds, W. M., & Kaslow, N. J. (1987c). A comparison of the relative efficacy of self-control therapy and a behavioral problem-solving therapy for depression in children. *Journal of Abnormal Child Psychology, 15*, 91-113.

Tesiny, E. P., & Lefkowitz, M. M. (1982). Childhood depression: A 6-month follow-up study. *Journal of Consulting and Clinical Psychology, 50*, 778-780.

Toolan, J. M. (1981). Depression and suicide in children: An overview. *American Journal of Psychotherapy, 35*, 311-322.

Vosk, B., Forehand, R., Parker, J. B., & Richard, K. (1982). A multimethod comparison of popular and unpopular children. *Developmental Psychology, 18*, 571-575.

Weinberg, W. A., Rutman, J., Sullivan, L., Renick, E. C., & Dietz, S. G. (1973). Depression in children referred to an educational diagnostic center: Diagnosis and treatment. *Journal of Pediatrics, 83*, 1065-1072.

Welner, Z., Welner, A., McCrary, M. D., & Leonard, M. A. (1977). Psychopathology in children of inpatients with depression: A controlled study. *Journal of Nervous and Mental Disease, 163*, 408-413.

Wilson, A. R., & Krane, R. V. (1980). Change in self-esteem and its effects on symptoms of depression. *Cognitive Therapy and Research, 4*, 419-421.

Zupan, B. A., Hammen, C., & Jaenicke, C. (1987). The effects of current mood and prior depressive history on self-schematic processing in children. *Journal of Experimental Child Psychology, 43*, 149-158.

16
COGNITIVE-BEHAVIORAL TREATMENT OF SCHOOL-RELATED FEARS AND ANXIETIES

REBECCA A. McREYNOLDS
Private Practice, Tucson, Arizona

RICHARD J. MORRIS
University of Arizona

THOMAS R. KRATOCHWILL
University of Wisconsin–Madison

Fear and anxiety are integral parts of normal childhood development (Morris & Kratochwill, 1983). Many children's fears and anxieties are transitory, appear in children of similar ages, and generally do not interfere with everyday functioning. Experiences and emotions associated with such "developmental" fears and anxieties often provide children with various methods for coping with life stressors. Fears and anxieties, therefore, generally involve normal reactions to stimuli that are either construed by the child as directly threatening or associated with threatening stimuli.

On the other hand, when a child or adolescent experiences a repeated fear that is not age-related in a setting where there is no obvious external danger, then the fear is irrational and intervention may be necessary. Although a variety of intervention procedures are available to mental health professionals and educators (see, for example, Kratochwill, Sanders, Wiemer, & Morris, 1987; Morris & Kratochwill, 1983), only been within the past 10 or 15 years have cognitive-behavioral approaches contributed to the treatment literature in this area (e.g., Beck, 1976; Karoly, 1981; Kazdin, 1978; Mahoney, 1974; Meichenbaum, 1977). Such approaches include Ellis's (1962) rational-emotive therapy, which has recently been used with children and adolescents (e.g., Bernard & Joyce, 1984; Ellis & Bernard, 1983), self-instructional training developed by Meichenbaum and his associates (e.g., Meichenbaum, 1977), and self-regulation procedures as advocated by Kanfer and his colleagues (e.g., Kanfer, 1975; Kanfer & Gaelick, 1986; Kanfer, Karoly, & Newman, 1975;

Kanfer & Phillips, 1970; Kanfer & Schefft, 1988). In contrast, however, to other behavior therapy approaches used with childhood and adolescent fears and related anxieties, the area involving cognitive-behavior therapy procedures contains relatively few empirical studies (see, for example, Morris & Kratochwill, 1983; Ramirez, Kratochwill, & Morris, 1987).

In this chapter, we provide an overview of the research literature regarding cognitive-behavioral interventions used to treat child and adolescent fears and anxiety disorders, with an emphasis on those cognitive-behavioral approaches that have been implemented or are potentially applicable in school and classroom settings. In reviewing this literature, we have focused exclusively on child and adolescent school-related fears and anxiety disorders, and on those interventions that practitioners in school settings may find potentially useful in their work with fearful and anxious children and adolescents. Prior to reviewing the treatment literature, we present a review of the prevalence and incidence of childhood and adolescent fears and related anxieties and a discussion of diagnostic issues and common assessment practices used in treating fearful and anxious children and adolescents.

PREVALENCE AND INCIDENCE DATA

Children and adolescents typically experience a wide variety of normatively based fears and related anxieties. For example, fears characteristic of infancy usually occur as a reaction to something specific that is taking place in the infant's environment. During the early school years, the child's fears broaden to involve such stimuli as the dark; supernatural figures; and/or particular persons, objects, or events. In the later school years, children's fears involve more imaginary figures, specific objects and events, the future, and tests in school (Jersild, 1968). During preadolescence and adolescence, typical anxieties and fears involve physical appearance, school performance, bodily injury, social rejection, death, imaginary figures, specific objects and events, and the future (e.g., Bamber, 1977, 1979; Orton, 1982; Rose & Ditto, 1983).

Several studies have been published over the past 50 years on the prevalence and incidence of children's fears and related anxieties. Many of the studies, however, are outdated and/or suffer from methodological and conceptual flaws (Graziano & Mooney, 1984). Cognizant of this limitation in the research, Morris and Kratochwill (1983) attempted to organize and systematize what is known about the developmental nature of children's fears. They listed some of the more common fears that have been reported in children at various age levels:

0–6 months: Loss of support, loud noises;
7–12 months: Fear of strangers, fear of sudden, unexpected and looming objects;
1 year: Separation from parent, toilet, injury, strangers;

> *2 years:* A multitude of fears including loud noises (e.g., vacuum cleaners, sirens, trucks, thunder), animals (e.g., large dogs), a dark room, separation from parent, large objects/machines, change in personal environment;
>
> *3 years:* Masks, dark, animals, separation from parent;
>
> *4 years:* Parent separation, animals, dark, noises (including at night);
>
> *5 years:* Animals, "bad" people, dark, separation from parent, bodily harm;
>
> *6 years:* Supernatural beings (e.g., ghosts, witches), bodily injuries, thunder and lightning, dark, sleeping or staying alone, separation from parent;
>
> *7–8 years:* Supernatural beings, dark, fears based on media events, staying alone, bodily injury;
>
> *9–12 years:* Tests and examinations in school, school performance, bodily injury, physical appearance, thunder and lightning, death, dark (low percentage). [Reprinted by permission from *Treating Children's Fears and Phobias* by R. J. Morris and T. R. Kratochwill, 1983, New York: Pergamon Press, p. 2].

Although numerous studies and reviews have been published on the developmental nature of children's fears and related anxieties, relatively few studies have been published that focus specifically on the prevalence and incidence of school-related fears (e.g., Bamber, 1977, 1979; Krans, 1973; Trueman, 1984a; Wine, 1979). Moreover, those studies that have focused on school-related fears have been concerned primarily with social withdrawal in preschool and primary-grade children and on school phobia and test anxiety in older students (e.g., Baker & Willis, 1978; Johnson, 1979; Kennedy, 1965; Sarason, 1980; Sarason, Davidson, Lighthall, Waite, & Ruebush, 1960; Trueman, 1984b). In reviewing the literature on school-related fears, Johnson (1979) listed three major fear categories that occur in the school setting. The first category, "school phobia," referred to a fear of school as well as severe associated anxiety that prevented the student from attending school. This fear can occur suddenly or can be chronic in nature (e.g., Baker & Willis, 1978; Coolidge, Hahn, & Pack, 1957; Kennedy, 1965; Trueman, 1984b), with an incidence ranging from 3.2 to 17 per 100 schoolchildren (Kennedy, 1965; Yule, 1979). Prevalence of school phobia appears to occur most often around 5 to 7 years of age (frequently associated with separation anxiety), 9 to 11 years of age (when children change to middle schools and junior high schools), and around 14 years of age (often concomitant with depression) (Baker & Willis, 1978; Chazan, 1962; Herzov, 1977). Some writers consider school phobia to occur in three girls for every two boys (e.g., Wright, Schaefer, & Solomons, 1979); others contend that there are no sex differences (e.g., Johnson, 1979; Trueman, 1984b).

The second fear category, according to Johnson (1979), was "social withdrawal," where children avoid interaction with their peers and sometimes refuse to talk in the classroom. The incidence of this fear has been estimated to range between 10% and 20% in "normal" preschool samples (e.g., Evers & Schwartz, 1973; O'Connor, 1972). On the other hand, complete mutism in school is rare (Kratochwill, 1981; Kratochwill, Brody, & Piersal, 1979).

Johnson's (1979) third fear category was "test anxiety," involving the interruption and/or prevention of taking tests as a result of such factors as excessive worry about one's test performance, sleep disruption, memory lapses, fear of failure, and/or heightened physiological arousal. Incidence figures for test anxiety vary from 10% to 30% of all students (e.g., Johnson, 1979; Kondas, 1967; Nottelmann & Hill, 1977).

Although most fear studies have found girls to have more fears than boys, this does not appear to be the case with specific school-related fears and anxieties (e.g., Croake & Knox, 1971; Staley & O'Donnell, 1984; Trueman, 1984b). There are also no clear social class differences in school-related fears and anxieties, although Lapouse and Monk (1959) found that lower-social-class students between 6 and 12 years of age reported more fears and worries about grades than did upper-class students, and Phillips (1978) found higher levels of school anxiety among lower-social-class Anglo students and middle- and upper-class minority students.

DIAGNOSIS OF CHILD AND ADOLESCENT FEARS AND ANXIETIES

Fear in children and adolescents is a strong emotion associated with behavioral, cognitive, and physiological indicators of anxiety. In general, when a child or adolescent experiences fear that is not age-appropriate and in a situation where there is no obvious external danger, the fear may be described as irrational and defined as a phobia (Morris & Kratochwill, 1983). When the child or adolescent attempts to avoid the nondangerous feared situation, even though maintaining that this behavior is "silly" or foolish, the phobia is commonly referred to as a phobic reaction (e.g., Knopf, 1979; Morris, 1986).

The classification of child and adolescent emotional and behavior disorders has typically fallen within two broad approaches. One approach has been based on the development of clinically derived categories, such as those of the various editions of the American Psychiatric Association's *Diagnostic and Statistical Manual of Mental Disorders* (DSM-I, 1952; DSM-II, 1968; DSM-III, 1980; DSM-III-R, 1987). The second approach to classification was empirically derived through multivariate statistical procedures such as factor analysis and cluster analysis (e.g., Achenbach & Edelbrock, 1978; Quay, 1979). In addition, several specific attempts at classifying child and adolescent fears and phobias have been proposed in the research literature in order to develop more behaviorally oriented approaches to the classification of these disorders.

According to the DSM-III-R classification system, three childhood disorders in which anxiety is the predominant clinical feature are proposed:

Separation anxiety disorder   "[T]he essential feature of this disorder is excessive anxiety, for at least two weeks, concerning separation from those to whom the child is attached" (American Psychiatric Association, 1987, p. 58), in which the child may experience anxiety to the point of panic. Though representing a form of phobia, it is not included in the phobic disorder category because of its unique features and its occurrence in childhood.

Avoidant disorder of childhood or adolescence   "[T]he essential feature of this disorder is an excessive shrinking from contact with unfamiliar people that is of at least six months' duration. This is coupled with a clear desire for social involvement with familiar people, such as peers the person knows well and family members. Relationships with family members and other familiar figures are warm and satisfying" (APA, 1987, p. 61).

Overanxious disorder   This disorder is characterized by excessive or unrealistic anxiety or worry that is not focused on a specific situation or object and is not due to a recent psychological stressor.

Like the earlier DSM systems, DSM-III-R adheres to a categorical, disease-entity conceptualization of child and adolescent behavior disorders and exemplifies a tradition of diagnosis, despite many basic problems in defining emotional and mental disorders. With regard specifically to the diagnosis and classification of child and adolescent fears and related anxieties, the major problem with the DSM-III-R system is the lack of adequate reliability and validity data. When clinicians are instructed to categorize various disorders, there is generally acceptable interrater agreement on major categories (e.g., discrimination between psychoses, neuroses, and conduct disorders) but less agreement when fine discriminations are required. For example, Matison, Cantwell, Russell, and Will (1979) found that anxiety disorders were diagnosed with low agreement. At present, there are few reliability and validity studies conducted with children and adolescents where anxiety disorders have been examined.

Several specific fear classification schemes have been proposed. An early effort to classify childhood fears was reported by Angelino, Dollins, and Mech (1956), who classified the fears of 1,100 students (ranging in age from 9 to 18 years) according to the following general categories: safety, school, personal appearance, natural phenomena, economical and political, health, animals, social relations, personal conduct, and the supernatural. Using a factor analysis procedure, Scherer and Nakamura (1968) identified the 10 most salient childhood fears from the 80-item Fear Survey Schedule for Children. After determination of the factor structure for these fears, the following eight factors emerged: (1) fear of failure or criticism, (2) major fears (primarily social), (3) minor fears (small animals), (4) medical fears, (5) fear of death, (6) fear of the dark, (7) home–school fears, and (8) several miscellaneous fears. A factor analysis of the Louisville Fear Survey for Children, developed by Miller, Barrett, Hampe, and Noble (1972), yielded the following three primary factors: (1) fear of physical injury (e.g., wars, food poisoning, surgery), (2) fear of natural and supernatural dangers (i.e., storms, the dark, animals), and (3) interpersonal/social fears (e.g., taking examinations, making mistakes, receiving criticism). Investigations using multivariate statistical procedures have not usually involved adolescents, which limits their generalizability for defining and identifying fears in this population (Morris, Kratochwill, & Dodson, 1986).

Kennedy (1965) proposed that a differential diagnosis between two types of school phobia can be made on the basis of any seven often differential symptoms, and employed a grade distinction in his classification system. Miller, Barrett, and Hampe (1974) incorporated school phobia within the category of social anxiety but dropped the grade distinction, finding age to be the more important variable. Marine (1968–1969) has also proposed diagnostic categories for children displaying separation anxiety and three other more severe types of "school refusal" ("mild school refusal," "chronic severe school refusal," "childhood psychosis with school refusal"). These diagnostic categories are matched with four treatment modalities and potential change agents.

Kratochwill and Morris (1985) cite several reasons for using extreme caution in drawing firm conclusions from the literature on the diagnosis and classification of child and adolescent fears and anxieties. First, there is a paucity of data related to these classification systems. Second, the literature is based on self-reports from parents and children, which are subject to considerable distortion and bias (Graziano, DeGiovanni, & Garcia, 1979). Finally, there has typically been an exclusive reliance on the feared object as a focus of classification attempts (Graziano et al., 1979), which assumes subject homogeneity within a particular fear category (Magrath, 1982). Thus, children who display a fear of school might be called "school-phobic" or further subdivided into types I and II following Kennedy's (1965) scheme. Yet, such categorical classification might actually mask the considerable variability in children's actual fears and the circumstances maintaining their fears or phobic responses.

ASSESSMENT PRACTICES

Major advances have occurred in the area of behavioral assessment, and there have been several published reviews that are specifically related to the assessment of children's fears and related anxieties (e.g., Barrios, Hartmann, & Shigetomi, 1981; Barrios & Shigetomi, 1985; Miller et al., 1974). The extensive body of research on the behavioral assessment of adult fears and anxiety disorders (e.g., Agras & Jacob, 1981; Bernstein, 1973; Borkovec, Weerts, & Bernstein, 1977; Emmelkamp, 1979) also forms an important foundation for the assessment of child and adolescent fears and related anxieties. In addition, many of the issues raised in the behavioral assessment of adult disorders are relevant for assessment of child and adolescent behavior disorders in general and specifically for the assessment of school-related fears and anxieties.

A popular conceptualization of fear or anxiety in both the child and the adult literature, formally developed by Lang (1968), is known as the "triple response mode" (e.g., Cone, 1979), "multiple response components" (e.g., Nietzel & Bernstein, 1981), or "three response system" (e.g., Kozak & Miller, 1982). This position that anxiety is a complex multichannel/response pattern of behavior is also shared by many writers (e.g., Barrios *et al.*, 1981; Graziano *et al.*, 1979; Johnson & Melamed, 1979; Phillips, 1977; Rachman, 1978).

To provide a perspective on this approach for defining child and adolescent fears and a framework for discussion of specific assessment methods applicable in school settings, we briefly review the three channels.

Cognitive Systems

One system or channel frequently used to define fears and anxieties is the cognitive or self-report system. This subjective system depends on the child or adolescent's self-report to validate the existence of a particular fear or anxiety reaction. Self-reports may consist of direct statements to another person (e.g., "I'm afraid to go to school," "I'm afraid to read out loud"), self-monitoring data, or responses to structured interviews or questionnaires.

Virtually every approach to the treatment of child and adolescent fears and related anxieties regards cognitions as an important data base for defining the concept of fear, phobia, or anxiety. Considerable variation exists, however, in the behavioral literature on the emphasis placed on this cognitive system. For example, cognitive-behavior therapists place much greater emphasis on self-report data than do proponents of applied behavior analysis (see, for example, Morris & Kratochwill, 1983).

Of particular relevance to this chapter is the increasing interest in the relation between children's observable behaviors and their cognitive processes (e.g., Kendall, Pellegrini, & Urban, 1981). In this regard, cognitions may be targeted for intervention; the trend, therefore, toward the development of multiple-method cognitive assessment techniques to supplement direct behavioral observation measures seems important (Bergin, 1971; Kazdin & Wilson, 1978). Milby, Wendorf, and Meredith (1983) have also advocated the assessment of cognitions when assessing those children exhibiting obsessive–compulsive disorders. For example, they suggested an examination of the role of children's imagery or fantasies relating to the dire or terrible consequences of their behavior.

Physiological Systems

The physiological channel (also referred to as the "somatic" or "visceral" channel) focuses on measurement of the sympathetic portion of the autonomic nervous system (e.g., Nietzel & Bernstein, 1981; Paul & Bernstein, 1973). Within this channel, anxiety and fear are assessed by a variety of measures of the auto-nomic nervous system (e.g., blood pressure, heart rate, galvanic skin response, temperature, muscular tension, respiration rate). More than one physiological measure is ideally used to define anxiety within this system because different physiological measures may not correlate highly (Haynes, 1978).

Motor System

The third channel, referred to as motor or overt behavior, focuses on assess-ment of the actual overt behavior of the child or adolescent, and has been divided into direct and indirect measures (Paul & Bernstein, 1973). Direct measures refer to overt behavioral consequences of physiological arousal. For example, the observation of a child trembling in the presence of a particular stimulus (e.g., a large group, a test, a reading assignment) would be a direct measure of the presence of anxiety. Indirect measures include escape and/or avoidance behaviors from certain stimuli (e.g., running away from school, leaving the classroom).

We believe it is necessary to define school-related fears and anxieties within the context of these three systems. Evidence for these constructs may be derived from one or any combination of the three systems. Although it is unnecessary for measures taken from the three systems to demonstrate high correlations, it can be assumed that the lack of a strong relation may be due to a variety of factors, all of which should be considered during assessment. Thus, when anxiety or a particular fear becomes a problem for a child or adolescent and his or her school personnel, the child or adolescent may exhibit problems in any one of the systems, or in all of them, which has important implications for both assessment and treatment. For example, treatment may be imple-mented for one or all of the different systems identified as problematic for the child or adolescent.

ASSESSMENT METHODS IN THE SCHOOLS

Interview Assessment

The interview assessment format is one of the most common assessment methods used with children and adolescents experiencing fears and related anxieties. Although a number of writers have reviewed this method in the behavioral literature (e.g., Ciminero, 1977; Haynes & Jensen, 1979; Meyer, Liddel, & Lyons, 1977; Morganstern, 1976; Ollendick & Hersen, 1984), only a few have specifically addressed this topic in relation to child behavioral assess-ment (e.g., Gross, 1984).

The use of interview assessment with child and adolescent fears and related anxieties may be examined along three dimensions. One dimension on which the interview may vary is the degree to which interviewer questions are predetermined. Such categories may include a standardized (structured) interview, a moderately standardized (semistructured) interview, and an unstandardized (unstructured) interview. The standardized interview consists of a list of questions or statements that are followed during the actual interview with the child or adolescent. Few standardized interview formats, however, are available for the assessment of child and adolescent fears and related anxieties (Morris & Kratochwill, 1983). Less standardized interview procedures, offering greater flexibility, can also be employed. Interview assessment strategies having no predetermined questions or format have also been used. These strategies provide much flexibility in exploring the child or adolescent's specific problem, but the format may compromise both the reliability and validity of the assessment procedure (Morris & Kratochwill, 1983).

Although Ciminero and Drabman (1977) have noted that "the data available at this time suggest that one must be very cautious, if not skeptical, of interview data for children and parents" (p. 56), there are certain advantages to interview assessment approaches. The flexibility of this approach is apparent. In addition, the assessment interview promotes the development of a therapeutic relationship with the child or adolescent (Ciminero & Drabman, 1977). The importance of the relationship in the assessment phase cannot be emphasized enough, particularly when the therapist is working with a child or adolescent experiencing a school-related fear or anxiety.

With regard to the use of teacher and/or parent interviews, motivation, cooperation, and commitment to assuming an active role in the child's treatment may also be evaluated, and the interview can be used to educate teachers and parents regarding the nature of a child's particular fear (Haynes & Jensen, 1979). With a teacher or parent interview, information may be gathered concerning their perceptions of the child's school-related fear or anxiety, as well as their personal concerns and goals.

On the other hand, certain disadvantages associated with using interviews as an assessment technique may also be identified. For example, individuals from identical theoretical orientation may be likely to obtain disparate information from the same child or adolescent with a similar problem, and thus may apply different treatment procedures (Kratochwill, Morris, & Campbell, 1985). As a result, the reliability and validity of this form of assessment are questionable. Sources of error in the interview include such variables as race, sex, social class, social sensitivity, age of the child or adolescent, content, format, and structure of the interview (Haynes & Jensen, 1979).

Self-Report Measures

Self-report measures elicit indirect samples of behavior involving a verbal representation of the fear or related anxiety occurring at a different time and in another setting (Morris & Kratochwill, 1983). In the past, self-report measures have been avoided in behavioral assessment because of perceived problems inherent in verbal reports and the subjectivity of their formats, or the lack thereof. Recently, however, there has been an increased emphasis on this type of assessment (Kratochwill *et al.*, 1985). For example, the growing emphasis on cognitive-behavior therapy has enhanced the credibility of self-reported verbalizations (e.g., Hughes, 1987; Kendall, 1981; Kendall & Finch, 1979; Kendall & Hollon, 1979). There has also been increased recognition that the operational criteria for the existence of a problem lie with the child or adolescent's self-reported verbalizations (Tasto, 1977). Some research suggests that children are able to describe their affective states and that such reports agree with other assessment measures (Carlson & Cantwell, 1980; Kovacs & Beck, 1977). In addition, self-report measures have become more acceptable as assessment has increasingly focused on the three response channels.

A variety of self-report measures have been used in the assessment of children's fears and related anxieties, although relatively few have been employed with adolescents. Some examples include the Children's Manifest Anxiety Scale (Castaneda, McCandless, & Palmero, 1956), the Test Anxiety Scale for Children (Sarason, Davidson, Lighthall, Waite, & Ruebush, 1960), the Children's School Questionnaire (Phillips, 1966), the Fear Survey Schedule for Children (Scherer & Nakamura, 1968), the State–Trait Anxiety Inventory for Children (Speilberger, 1973), the Louisville Fear Survey for Children (Miller *et al.*, 1972), and various miscellaneous self-report measures such as the Hospital Fears Rating Scale (Melamed & Siegel, 1975), the Snake Attitude Measure (Kornhaber & Schroeder, 1974), and the "faces test" (Barrios *et al.*, 1981). It is possible that many of the existing self-report scales could be adapted for the assessment of school-related fears and anxieties (Morris *et al.*, 1986). Several sources provide excellent reviews of these and other self-report measures in the area of child and adolescent fears, phobias, and anxieties (e.g., Barrios *et al.*, 1981; Johnson & Melamed, 1979; Kratochwill *et al.*, 1985; Miller *et al.*, 1974; Morris & Kratochwill, 1983).

A major reason for the potential use of self-report measures in school settings is that these measures are easy and convenient to administer and provide extensive information in a relatively small amount of time. Some of the inventories and questionnaires cited here might be more efficient than other methods (e.g., direct observation) for general screening purposes. In addition, self-report measures promote the use of a personal criterion for distress. Thus, children and adolescents could presumably report personal distress even though they exhibit little or no physiological or overt behavioral indications of fear or related anxiety.

The limitations of self-report measures have been well articulated in terms of their general use (e.g., Haynes, 1978; Kratochwill, 1982; Tasto, 1977), as well as their specific applications for children's fear and anxiety assessment (e.g., Barrios *et al.*, 1981; Johnson & Melamed, 1979; Kratochwill *et al.*, 1985). One major concern is the degree to which self-report data are an accurate reflection of the child's actual fear and anxiety. Children's reports may be inconsistent, may not correspond to other measures of fear via the three response modes, and are subject to distortions. In addition, children's responses on self-report scales may not correspond to teacher or parents reports of the child's fears.

A second concern with many self-report scales is that they were designed for purposes other than behavioral assessment. As Barrios *et al.* (1981) note, self-report inventories that assess cross-situational cognitive aspects of fear often fail to describe individual situations adequately. Such scales do not usually include items that allow for specific situational analysis, and they often fail to identify the specific nature of the cognitive problem. A third limitation of many self-report scales is the lack of descriptive detail in the items to which children and adolescents are required to respond (Barrios *et al.*, 1981). For example, it may be unclear whether children's fear inventory responses reflect a general fear of all spiders and snakes or a fear of specific types of spiders and snakes. Finally, some self-report scales lack adequate norming, reliability, and validity data, a failing that is of particular concern in light of their widespread use in research and practice. Normative data are especially important in view of the developmental nature of children's and adolescents' fear and anxiety disorders (Morris & Kratochwill, 1983).

Self-Monitoring

Self-monitoring (SM) has not been frequently employed in the assessment of child and adolescent school-related fears and anxieties. It requires the child or adolescent to discriminate and record the occurrence of his or her own behavior at the time it actually occurs. SM may be distinguished from self-report assessment in that the latter involves reporting of behavior that occurred at some other time and place. Several writers have provided an overview of SM in the area of behavioral assessment (e.g., Ciminero, Nelson, & Lipinski, 1977; Haynes, 1978; Kazdin, 1974; McFall, 1977; Nelson, 1977).

A variety of recording devices and formats tailored to the targeted fear or anxiety may be used for SM. Common methods include record booklets, checklists, forms, counters, meters, timers, measures, and scales. An example of a SM device developed by Kelley (1976), based on Walk's (1956) fear thermometer for adults, consists of a device manipulated by the child to indicate one of five fear levels, which are differentiated by color. Another SM procedure is the *in vivo* thought-sampling technique reported by Klinger (1978), which is potentially applicable with children and adolescents in fearful situations. Using this technique, the child or adolescent carries a portable beeper and records his or her cognitions or feelings at variable intervals signaled by the beeper. Shapiro (1984) suggests that counting devices, such as golf counters, grocery store counters, and wrist counters, may also be used.

Direct Observation Assessment

Much of the behavior therapy research on child and adolescent fears and related anxieties has employed direct observation of behavior in either naturalistic (e.g., home, school), contrived, or analogue (e.g., clinic, hospital) settings. Direct observational strategies include the "recording of behavioral events in their natural settings at the time they occur, not retrospectively, the use of trained observer–coders, and descriptions of behaviors which require little if any inference by observers to code the events" (Jones, Reid, & Patterson, 1975, p. 46). Three types of direct observational assessment strategies that have been used with children and adolescents are the Behavioral Avoidance Test, global behavioral ratings, and direct observation in naturalistic settings.

The Behavioral Avoidance Test (BAT) has been used frequently in child and adolescent fear assessment research (Barrios et al., 1981; Barrios & Shigetomi, 1985; Kratochwill et al., 1985) and has a long history (e.g., Jersild & Holmes, 1935), with the Lang and Lazovik (1963) technique serving as a prototype for most work in the field. This strategy consists of presenting a child or adolescent in a step-by-step format with various increasingly more anxiety-provoking stimuli, and requesting that she or he make approach responses toward the feared object while observers record the approach behaviors on a predetermined form. The BAT is tailored to the particular targeted fear or anxiety and provides a number of different avoidance measures, including response latency, number of steps completed, and distance from the feared object. A passive BAT can also be employed, whereby the feared object is gradually moved toward the child (e.g., Murphy & Bootzin, 1973).

Because BATs are not standardized, comparison across studies is difficult (Barrios et al., 1981). BATs may vary across several dimensions, such as the number of steps employed and the instructions provided before and during the BAT, thus raising questions about the external validity of results obtained across studies. Another related problem pertains to the actual "threat" posed by the feared stimulus. Some authors have suggested that reducing uncertainty with the BAT results in increased approach behavior and less physiological arousal (Lick, Unger, & Condiante, 1978). For example, the knowledge that a spider or snake will remain in a cage is likely to reduce anxiety about approaching it. Other concerns regarding the use of BATs in research on child and adolescent fears relate to the demand nature (i.e., high versus low demand) and influence of instructions for terminating approach behavior on the BAT, the presence or absence of the therapist, the variation across studies in the presentation of instructions, the lack of reliability and validity data on these measures, and their analogue nature. Despite these concerns, writers in the field have cited several reasons for continuing to use BATs in future research as well as in clinical practice with children and adolescents (e.g., Barrios & Shigetomi, 1985; Morris & Kratochwill, 1983). For example, a variety of measures, in addition to approach behavior, may be recorded, including facial expressions, trembling, time required to complete the various steps, and latency (Barrios & Shigetomi, 1985). The BAT also has direct implications for treatment and, as noted by Barrios and Shigetomi (1985), is invaluable for directly addressing the idiosyncratic nature of a child or adolescent's fear or anxiety. Thus, the BAT represents one of the few strategies in which the treatment process is linked directly to the assessment of treatment progress.

Global behavioral ratings, another direct measure of behavior, involve recording the fear behavior at the time it occurs along a dimensional scale (e.g., seldom to always, definitely negative to definitely positive). Although global ratings appear to simplify the measurement process, there is usually a corresponding loss of information, depending on the actual rating format. Kazdin (1980) maintains that these scales represent a flexible assessment method because of the many dimensions of behavior rated, provide a summary evaluation of the child's status on the problem pre-, during, and posttreatment, and provide a standardized format for soliciting judgments of therapists or others (e.g., parents, teachers) involved with the child or adolescent. One major problem, however, is that data obtained from "global" ratings are subject to ambiguity, particularly when the rating dimension is not defined operationally. Responses may also change, independent of any actual change in the fear or anxiety, across time.

A third direct observational method of assessment involves observations of the child or adolescent's behavior in natural settings (e.g., Ayllon, Smith, & Rogers, 1970; Bornstein & Knapp, 1981; Kuroda, 1969; Lewis, 1974; Miller & Kratochwill, 1979; Pomerantz, Peterson, Marholin, & Stern, 1977). Using this assessment strategy, the therapist develops a code specific to the targeted fear behaviors (e.g., crying, behavioral avoidance). For example, Neisworth, Madle, and Goeke (1975) measured "separation anxiety" by recording the duration of crying, screaming, and sobbing exhibited during daily preschool activities. However, few standardized observational manuals and recording formats applicable in naturalistic settings are available.

Two direct observational procedures developed specifically for children's school-related fears have been reported. In the Preschool Observation Scale of Anxiety, developed by Glennon and Weisz (1978), the observer rates the occurrence of 30 indicators of anxiety (e.g., rigid posture, trembling voice, trembling lips) while the children perform tasks in the presence and absence of their mothers. Wine (1979) described an observational procedure in which children varying in test anxiety were observed during a period preceding an examination and also when no examinations were scheduled. The behavior categories included attending behaviors, task-related behaviors, activity, communication, and interpersonal behaviors.

Behavior Checklists and Rating Scales

Behavior checklists and rating scale are indirect assessment strategies in which an individual rates the children or adolescent on the basis of past observations of his or her behavior. Thus, the rating occurs subsequent to the actual behavior of concern, rather than at the time of its occurrence (Cone, 1978; Wiggins, 1973). General scales or checklists usually include items within several general domains, in addition to a fear or anxiety subdomain (e.g., aggression, conduct disorder). Some examples of rating scales containing items related to children's fears include the Walker Problem Behavior Identification Checklist (Revised) (Walker, 1983), the Children's Behavior Inventory (Burdock & Hardesty, 1968), the Devereux Elementary School Behavior Rating Scale (Spivack & Swift, 1967), and the Devereux Adolescent Behavior Rating Scale (Spivack, Spotts, & Haimes, 1967). These rating scales are typically completed by a teacher or other person who is familiar with the child or adolescent, and usually have been used to form an overall index of the child or adolescent's level of adjustment. One example of a global behavior rating scale is the Child Behavior Checklist (Quay, 1979), which may be used with individuals between the ages of 4 and 16. This checklist provides both parent and teacher forms and contains separate norms for males and females at ages 4 to 5, 6 to 11, and 12 to 16. A large body of literature is available on the norming, reliability, and validity of these types of scales (e.g., Kendall *et al.*, 1981; O'Leary & Johnson, 1979).

Few formalized fear rating scales and checklists have been developed specifically for use with children and adolescents. Some examples include the Teacher Rating Scale (Sarason *et al.*, 1960), which assesses motor components of a child's anxiety or fear, the Louisville Fear Survey for Children (Miller *et al.*, 1972), the Global Mood Scale (Vernon, Foley, & Schulman, 1967), the Parent Anxiety Rating Scale (Glennon & Weisz, 1978), and the Teacher's Separation Anxiety Scale (Doris, McIntyre, Kelsey, & Lehman, 1971) in which the teacher rates the child's reaction to separation from mother or father when left at nursery school.

Rating scales and behavior checklists are economical in terms of therapist time and cost and can be easily used in school settings. In many cases, data may be obtained that would otherwise be difficult to collect. This form of assessment can also serve as a measure of social validation (Kazdin, 1977; Wolf, 1978).

Many issues, however, have been raised over the application of behavior rating scales and checklists in research and practice (e.g., Anastasi, 1976; Evans & Nelson, 1977; Kratochwill & Sheridan, in press; Spivack & Swift, 1973). Because these procedures are indirect measures of behavior, the data are gathered retrospectively, and their relation to the actual occurrence of the fear behavior is unknown. These instruments are also typically completed by the child or adolescent's care providers, and thus may be affected by situational and contextual biases and by "potential misconceptions of those individuals, resulting in an inaccurate reflection of the child's actual behavioral characteristics and tendencies" (Wells, 1981, p. 505). Finally, although there are some data suggesting that teachers can make reasonable predictions of behavior (e.g., Strain, Cooke, & Apolloni, 1976), there are virtually no data regarding the relation of ratings to actual fear and anxiety behaviors exhibited across various situations.

Psychophysiological Assessment

The use of psychophysiological assessment has increased in behavior therapy research on fears and related anxieties as a result of the increasing recognition of the complexity of these behavior disorders. In addition, with a corresponding emphasis on triple mode assessment, there has been a growing body of literature in psychophysiological assessment within the area of fears and anxiety disorders in general (e.g., Agras & Jacob, 1981; Borkovec et al., 1977; Taylor & Agras, 1981). Among the physiological measures used in research on fears are electromyography (EMG), cardiovascular measures (i.e., heart rate, blood pressure, peripheral blood flow), and electrodermal measures (i.e., skin conductance and skin resistance). However, there have been relatively few discussions of psychophysiological assessment with children and adolescents experiencing fears and related anxieties (see Barrios et al., 1981; Johnson & Melamed, 1979; Melamed & Siegel, 1980, for exceptions) and few treatment studies where such measures have been employed in school or other applied settings.

COGNITIVE-BEHAVIORAL INTERVENTIONS

In this section, we review the treatment literature on the use of cognitive-behavioral interventions with child and adolescent school-related fears and anxieties. The role of cognition and dysfunctional cognitive processes in the development of fears and anxiety disorders has been well documented (e.g., Beck, 1976; Ellis & Bernard, 1983; Sarason, 1980). Thus, cognitive-behavioral interventions, such as self-control, rational-emotive therapy, and self-instructional training procedures, would appear to hold promise for the treatment of child and adolescent school-related fears and anxieties.

Our framework for presenting these cognitive-behavior interventions consists of a description of each specific procedure, a review of the available research literature concerning the procedure, and a case example illustrating the use of each procedure with a child or adolescent experiencing a school-related fear and/or anxiety. Because of the paucity of treatment literature in this area, both empirical and case studies have been included.

Self-Control

Description

Self-control may be described as a process through which a child or adolescent becomes the primary agent in directing and regulating aspects of his or her behavior that lead to preplanned and specific behavioral outcomes and/or consequences (Goldfried & Merbaum, 1973; Kanfer & Gaelick, 1986; Richards & Siegel, 1978). Although self-control and related self-regulation processes have been included in theoretical discussions and in the research literature on learning and conditioning (e.g., Bandura, 1969; Dollard & Miller, 1950; Homme, 1966; Kanfer & Phillips, 1970; Skinner, 1953), it is only since the early to mid-1970s that these procedures have been integrated into the cognitive-behavior therapy area (Goldfried & Goldfried, 1980; Kanfer & Schefft, 1988; Mahoney, 1974; Meichenbaum & Genest, 1980). Self-control encompasses several intervention methods, each of which recognizes the contribution of cognitive processes to behavior change and views the individual as capable of regulating their behavior. According to Kanfer and his associates (e.g., Kanfer & Gaelick, 1986; Kanfer & Schefft, 1988), a common element among these intervention methods involves the therapist's role as motivator and instigator in helping the individual to initiate a behavior change program. Self-control is, thus, a treatment emphasis or strategy in which the therapist teaches the child or adolescent how, when, and where to apply various cognitions to facilitate learning new behavior patterns (Kanfer & Gaelick, 1986; Richards & Siegel, 1978).

With regard to fear and anxiety reduction methods, many writers maintain that an individual's self-statements may contribute significantly to his or her fear and anxiety (e.g., Goldfried & Davidson, 1976; Kanfer & Gaelick, 1986). Self-control procedures focus on helping individuals to develop specific thinking skills and to use these skills when confronted with a particular feared stimulus, event, or object. Therapy sessions are conducted according to a consultation/negotiation model, which is consistent with the training of many school professionals (Bergan, 1977; Conoley & Conoley, 1982; Parsons & Meyers, 1984) and conducive to application in school settings.

In applying self-control procedures to the modification of child and adolescent fears and related anxieties, it must first be demonstrated that the child is aware of his or her fear or anxiety to the extent that she or he is able to identify the various components of the specific fear or anxiety and the conditions under which he or she becomes fearful or anxious. Second, the procedures require the child or adolescent to have the verbal capacity to generate with the therapist a series of incompatible self-statements and rules, which can be incorporated, at least temporarily, into his or her verbal repertoire. Third, the child or adolescent must possess the ability to apply these self-statements and rules under those conditions in which he or she experiences the fear or anxiety (Morris & Kratochwill, 1983).

Prior to initiating a self-control program, the child or adolescent's motivation for behavior change and his or her willingness to accept responsibility for changing the behavior must be addressed (Kanfer & Gaelick, 1986; Kanfer & Schefft, 1988; Thoresen & Mahoney, 1974). The relative effectiveness of this approach with children and adolescents is closely tied to the procedure's effectiveness, the therapist's competency, and the child or adolescent's receptiveness and interest level in receiving treatment and implementing it in the natural setting. Kanfer (1980) maintains that when a client is concerned about his or her behavior problem and "can anticipate improvement by its resolution," then self-control may be used more easily and effectively.

Research Literature

Although a number of studies have been published on self-control treatment of adult fears and anxiety disorders (see, for example, Deffenbacher, 1976; Deffenbacher & Michaels, 1980; Goldfried & Davison, 1976; Morris, 1986), only a small number of studies have used this approach with fearful and anxious children and adolescents (see, for example, Genshaft, 1982; Kanfer *et al.*, 1975; Leal, Baxter, Martin, & Marx, 1981; Morris & Kratochwill, 1983, Peterson & Shigetomi, 1981; Ramirez, Kratochwill, & Morris, 1987). Even fewer studies have been reported using self-control procedures with children and adolescents who experience fear and anxiety in school settings (Morris, Kratochwill, & Aldridge, 1988). Thus, any conclusions regarding the relative effectiveness of this approach for treating child and adolescent school-related fears and anxieties should be viewed as speculative until additional research data are reported.

Most studies that have been reported on the use of self-control with fearful and anxious children and adolescents have examined the effectiveness of these procedures on modifying children's fear of the dark (e.g., Campbell, 1987; Graziano, Mooney, Huber, & Ignasiak, 1979; Kanfer *et al.*, 1975), medical fears (e.g., Peterson & Shigetomi, 1981), and dental fears (e.g., Siegel & Peterson, 1980). The few studies that have been reported on children's and adolescents' school-related fears and anxieties have focused primarily on test anxiety. For example, Leal, Baxter, Martin, and Marx (1981) compared systematic desensitization, cognitive modification, and a no-treatment control condition on reducing test anxiety in a group of 10th-grade students. A standard systematic desensitization approach was followed. The cognitive modification procedure involved informing the students that their anxiety during exams was due to self-statements and thoughts that occurred prior to and during exams. They were further instructed that an increasing awareness of these self-statements was necessary in order to learn incompatible positive self-statements. The results showed that systematic desensitization was more effective than either the cognitive modification or no-treatment control condition on a direct observation performance measure of test anxiety, whereas the cognitive modification procedure was more effective on self-report measures. It was concluded that the cognitive modification procedures were superior to systematic desensitization on self-report measures of test anxiety. No follow-up evaluation or test for generalization was conducted.

Self-Instructional Training

Description

Self-instructional training may be viewed as a specific cognitive self-control strategy. This cognitive-training strategy was originally developed for children who fail to use self-talk sufficiently and who, as a result, exhibit uncontrolled or inappropriate behavior (Kendall & Braswell, 1985; Kendall & Finch, 1979). Cognitive self-instructional interventions are based on the assumption that certain behavioral excesses or deficits reflect either a lack of appropriate verbal mediators (i.e., the failure to develop inner speech for self-regulation), or reliance on maladaptive inner speech, which may result in inappropriate emotional responses or maladaptive behavior.

Self-instructional training was initially developed by Meichenbaum and Goodman (1971) in order to teach impulsive children a reflective problem-solving approach for improving academic performance. The treatment procedure involves the therapist's modeling cognitive strategies by and helping the child answer four primary questions: "What is my problem?" "What is my plan?" "Am I using my plan?" and "How did I do?" (Meichenbaum & Goodman, 1971). The self-instructional training paradigm consists of the following steps, as outlined by Meichenbaum (1986):

1. An adult model performs a task while talking to him or herself out loud (cognitive modeling).
2. The child performs the same task under the direction of the model's instructions (overt, external guidance).
3. The child performs the task while instructing him or herself aloud (overt self-guidance).
4. The child whispers the instructions to him- or herself as she or he proceeds through the task (faded, overt self-guidance).
5. The child performs the task while guiding his or her performance via inaudible or private speech or nonverbal self-direction (covert self-instruction).

Like self-control procedures, self-instructional training procedures focus on assisting the child or adolescent to develop specific self-instructions, or self-talk, and to apply these skills whenever they are confronted with a particular fear or anxiety-provoking stimulus, event, object, or situation. According to Meichenbaum and Genest (1980), such an approach involves helping the child and/or adolescent in each of the following areas:

1. [To] become aware of the negative thinking styles that impede performance and that lead to emotional upset and inadequate performance;
2. [To] generate, in collaboration with the trainer, a set of incompatible, specific self-statements, rules, strategies, and so on, which the trainee can then employ;
3. [To] learn specific adaptive, cognitive and behavior skills. (p. 403)

Research Literature

Although primarily applied to the modification of children's impulsive behavior (e.g., Kendall & Finch, 1979) and aggressive behavior (e.g., Camp & Bash, 1981), several studies utilizing self-instructional training to treat children's and adolescents' school-related fears and anxiety disorders have been reported. For example, using a combination of procedures, Kelly (1981) assessed the effect of relaxation training and self-directed verbalizations on measures of self-monitored fear, anxiety, and academic performance in learning-disabled students. Subjects were identified from a group of learning-disabled students by administering the Test Anxiety Scale for Children (TASC) and selecting those children who scored in the highest 30%. One group was trained in relaxation and self-directed commands, a second group was trained in self-directed commands only, and a third group received counseling. Results indicated that the combination of relaxation and self-directed commands significantly reduced self-monitored fear and TASC anxiety while significantly increasing academic performance. The combined procedures were also more effective in reducing self-monitored fear than were self-directed verbalizations alone. Self-directed commands alone were as effective as the combination of procedures in reducing anxiety and increasing academic performance, with those subjects who evidenced the largest reduction in fear and anxiety showing the greatest increase in academic performance.

In another study, Genshaft (1982) implemented a self-instructional training program in order to teach 7th-grade adolescent females a strategy to control their anxiety regarding mathematics. Subjects were identified by their teachers as experiencing some degree of math anxiety and as achieving in math at least one year behind their reading achievement. The study compared self-instructional training plus tutoring, tutoring alone, and a no-treatment control condition in reducing math anxiety. The self-instructional training procedure consisted of having subjects practice overt and covert positive self-statements in relation to those mathematics situations regarded as anxiety-provoking, in addition to tutoring and regular math classes. An attempt was made to facilitate generalization of the self-instructional procedure to other anxiety-provoking situations, such as public speaking. The results showed a significant improvement in math computation for the self-instructional training plus tutoring group; all three groups were shown to improve on a test of math application. In addition, those females who received self-instructional training developed a more favorable attitude toward math. Although no attempt to facilitate generalization of the treatment procedure was reportedly made, no generalization or follow-up assessment data were provided.

Fox and Houston (1981), on the other hand, investigated the effectiveness of cognitive self-statements for reducing anxiety in children in an evaluative situation. Fourth-grade children identified as either high or low in trait anxiety were assigned to self-instructional treatment, "minimal" treatment, or a no-treatment control group. The evaluative situation involved having the children recite a poem while being videotaped with the expectation that their performance would subsequently be judged. Subjects in the self-instructional group were taught self-instructions that focused on reevaluating the aversive nature of reciting the poem—for example: "Even if I don't do this correctly, nothing terrible will happen. Doing this in front of others really won't be so unpleasant." Minimal treatment consisted of focusing self-instructions on obvious facts concerning the evaluative situation—for example, "This will just take a few minutes." Portions of the State-Trait Anxiety Inventory for Children (STAIC) were also administered prior to and immediately following subjects' recitation of the poem, with the instruction to respond according to how they felt while performing in front of a video camera. Behavioral ratings of anxiety and a measure of performance accuracy were also collected. Contrary to expectations, subjects in the self-instruction condition exhibited more behavioral signs of anxiety and spent less time reciting the poem than did subjects in the other conditions. Self-instructions had no appreciable effect on either performance state anxiety or quality of performance. Additionally, high-anxiety subjects reported more state anxiety while anticipating reciting the poem. The investigators suggest that the self-instructional treatment may have a deleterious effect when applied to stressful situations involving task performance and may be most effective in anxiety-provoking situations that children are required to endure, such as medical and dental procedures.

Commentary

Given the paucity of research in the areas of both self-control and self-instructional training, we feel unable to provide any definitive statements regarding the relative effectiveness of these interventions for reducing children's and adolescents' school-related fears and anxieties. The results of studies using self-control procedures and self-instructional training to treat behavior disorders (e.g., hyperactive behavior, aggressive behavior) as well as other types of children's fears (e.g., fear of the dark, fear of medical and dental procedures) are both encouraging and conflicting. Thus, the area is in need of additional well-controlled research similar to that reported by Kanfer *et al.* (1975). In addition, there are no studies to suggest which children and/or adolescents, with which types of fears or anxieties, and under what environmental conditions will set the occasion for the effective use of self-control procedures and self-instructional training.

Rational-Emotive Therapy

Rational-emotive therapy (RET) is perhaps the first theoretical and therapeutic approach that may be considered an example of cognitive-behavioral treatment (e.g., Ellis, 1962, 1984; Kendall & Bemis, 1983). Within this approach, Ellis (1962) articulated the notion that psychological and emotional difficulties result from irrational thoughts and beliefs. The underlying assumption of a rational-emotive theory of psychopathology is that events do not cause emotional or behavioral consequences. Instead, Ellis proposed that individuals' thoughts and beliefs about these events influence their feelings and behavior. Although individuals may be generally aware of their affective responses, Ellis maintained that they frequently do not attend to or consider the beliefs or thoughts that mediate and determine their responses. From this perspective, when these underlying beliefs or thoughts are inaccurate and are framed in absolute or imperative terms, psychological disturbances are likely to occur (Kendall & Bemis, 1983).

The primary goal of RET as developed by Ellis is to teach individuals to identify and change the irrational beliefs (IBs) that underlie their psychological difficulties. More specifically, RET emphasizes disputation of those beliefs and thoughts that are not likely to be supported empirically in an individual's environment and do not promote one's enjoyment and survival. Haaga and Davison (1986) have classified people's IBs into the following categories: (a) awfulizing statements; (b) shoulds, oughts, and musts; (c) evaluations of human worth; and (d) need statements.

RET is a structured cognitive-behavioral intervention that focuses on irrational thinking patterns rather than on specific symptoms or behaviors. According to Ellis (1984), the therapist is active and directive, often taking responsibility for most of the discussion in the early therapy sessions. The goal is to enable the individual to view him- or herself and others in a sensible and rational manner. For example, individuals are taught to replace maladaptive thoughts such as, "I can't stand it," or, "It shouldn't happen," with more rational thoughts, such as, "It is unpleasant, but I can tolerate it," or, "I wish it hadn't happened" (Lipsky, Kassinove, & Miller, 1980). In addition to discussion and disputation, RET may also include rational role reversal, rational-emotive imagery, shame-attacking exercises, *in vivo* desensitization, and flooding. Reading assignments are also often recommended in conjunction with RET (e.g., Ellis & Harper, 1975; Maultsby, 1975).

Several excellent sources are available on the use of RET with child and adolescent behavior disorders (e.g., Bernard & Joyce, 1984; Ellis & Bernard, 1983). Supportive research, however, on the use of RET with children and adolescents having school-related fears and anxieties is sparse.

Bernard, Kratochwill, and Keefauver (1983) applied RET and self-instructional training in order to reduce high-frequency, chronic hair pulling in a 17-year-old girl. From a cognitive-behavioral perspective, it was hypothesized that maladaptive thought patterns occasioned high levels of anxiety and worry during studying periods and maintained the hair-pulling behavior. During initial treatment phases, RET principles and techniques, with an emphasis on disputation of irrational beliefs, were explained to the subject. Self-instructional training, which was subsequently introduced, consisted of the therapist modeling problem-solving verbal statements that the subject imitated and progressively internalized. Data on the number of hairs pulled out and the total amount of time spent studying were recorded by the subject. Results showed that RET led to a moderate reduction in hair-pulling behavior, with the introduction of self-instructional training in addition to RET leading to a rapid cessation of all hair pulling, which was maintained at a 2- and 3-week follow-up period. The authors suggest that the relative effectiveness of RET and self-instructional training cannot be determined from this case study, and that the order in which the two treatments were introduced may have affected their findings.

Van der Ploeg-Stapert and Van der Ploeg (1986) evaluated a group treatment that incorporated various aspects of RET for reducing test anxiety in adolescents. The treatment program consisted of muscle relaxation exercises, instruction in study skills, self-monitoring procedures, hypnosis, and RET for "worry." The results demonstrated a significant reduction in anxiety, as measured by various self-report inventories, for adolescents who received the group treatment in comparison to those who received no treatment. In addition, a 3-month follow-up evaluation showed that the reductions in reported test anxiety were maintained. Because a combination of procedures was used, it is impossible to determine exactly what aspect(s) of the treatment were most effective.

Commentary

Many of the RET procedures that have been suggested for use with children and adolescents have been adapted from those that have been used with adults. Although RET has been shown to be effective for reducing adult fears and related anxieties (e.g., DiGiuseppe & Miller, 1977; Zettle & Hayes, 1980), its effectiveness with children and adolescents has not been sufficiently demonstrated to permit any conclusions at this time. One of the considerations with using RET with children, as suggested by Halford (1983), pertains to the necessity of adjusting this particular approach to an appropriate level of cognitive complexity. With younger children, RET may need to focus primarily on teaching specific skills for specific problem situations, whereas adolescents might be taught more general cognitive strategies for dealing with anxiety provoking situations. In spite of these concerns, RET appears to be a promising and potentially useful cognitive strategy for reducing children's and adolescents' school-related fears and anxieties.

CONCLUSIONS

We have presented an overview of the diagnosis, assessment, and major cognitive-behavioral treatments that have been employed with children's and adolescent's school-related fears and anxieties. Those school-related fears and anxieties that have been modified with cognitive-behavioral treatment procedures include test anxiety, math anxiety, and performance anxiety. Although the research has shown that school phobia has generally been treated with several variations of desensitization and contingency management, it seems plausible to suggest that cognitive-behavioral strategies may serve as useful adjuncts to these behavioral methods. For example, previous studies have shown that certain behavior therapy procedures, such as *in vivo* exposure (Emmelkamp & Mersch, 1982) and modeling (Tearnan, Lehey, Thompson, & Hammer, 1982), may be enhanced by the addition of a self-verbalization training component.

Although major empirical questions continue to exist regarding the various cognitive-behavior procedures discussed in this chapter, it is clear that many of these procedures, such as the self-control and self-instructional training strategies, have potential for use by school personnel. At present, however, the paucity and conflicting nature of the research in this area does not permit us to make any recommendations regarding the merits of specific cognitive-behavioral approaches for reducing particular child and adolescent school-related fears and anxieties. The area is burgeoning but is in need of additional well-controlled research.

ACKNOWLEDGMENT

Portions of this chapter were prepared under grant #G008730074 from the U.S. Department of Education, Program in Special Education and Rehabilitation.

REFERENCES

Achenbach, T. M., & Edelbrock, C. S. (1978). The classification of child psychopathology: A review and analysis of empirical efforts. *Psychological Bulletin, 85,* 1275–1301.

Agras, W. S., & Jacob, R. G. (1981). Phobia: Nature and measurement. In M. Mavissakalian & D. H. Barlow (Eds.), *Phobia and pharmacological treatment* (pp. 35–62). New York: Guilford Press.

American Psychiatric Association. (1952). *Diagnostic and statistical manual of mental disorders* (1st ed.). Washington, DC: Author.

American Psychiatric Association. (1968). *Diagnostic and statistical manual of mental disorders* (2nd ed.). Washington, DC: Author.

American Psychiatric Association. (1980). *Diagnostic and statistical manual of mental disorders* (3rd ed.). Washington, DC: Author.

American Psychiatric Association. (1987). *Diagnostic and statistical manual of mental disorders* (3rd ed., rev.). Washington, DC: Author.

Anastasi, A. (1976). *Psychological testing.* (5th ed.). New York: Macmillan.

Angelino, H., Dollins, J., & Mech, E. V. (1956). Trends in the fears and worries of school children as related to socioeconomic status and age. *Journal of Genetic Psychology, 89,* 263–276.

Ayllon, T., Smith, D., & Rogers, M. (1970). Behavioral management of school phobia. *Journal of Behavior Therapy and Experimental Psychiatry, 1,* 125–138.

Baker, H., & Willis, U. (1978). School phobia: Classification and treatment. *British Journal of Psychiatry, 132,* 492–499.

Bamber, J. H. (1977). The factorial structure of adolescent responses to a fear survey schedule. *Journal of Genetic Psychology, 38,* 229–238.

Bamber, J. H. (1979). *The fears of adolescents.* New York: Academic Press.

Bandura, A. (1969). *Principles of behavior modification.* New York: Holt, Rinehart & Winston.

Barrios, B. A., Hartmann, D. P., & Shigetomi, C. (1981). Fears and anxieties in children. In E. J. Mash & L. G. Terdal (Eds.), *Behavioral assessment of childhood disorders* (pp. 259–304). New York: Guilford Press.

Barrios, B. A., & Shigetomi, C. C. (1985). Behavioral assessment of children's fears: A critical review. In T. R. Kratochwill (Ed.), *Advances in school psychology* (Vol. 4, pp. 89–132). Hillsdale, NJ: Lawrence Erlbaum.

Beck, A. T. (1976). *Cognitive therapy and the emotional disorders.* New York: International Universities Press.

Bergan, J. R. (1977). *Behavioral consultation.* Columbus, OH: Charles E. Merrill.

Bergin, A. E. (1971). The evaluation of therapeutic outcomes. In A. E. Bergin & S. L. Garfield (Eds.), *Handbook of psychotherapy and behavior change: An empirical analysis* (pp. 1–35). New York: Wiley.

Bernard, M. E., & Joyce, M. R. (1984). *Rational-emotive therapy with children and adolescents.* New York: John Wiley & Sons.

Bernard, M. E., Kratochwill, T. R., & Keefauver, L. W. (1983). The effects of rational-emotive therapy and self-instructional training on chronic hair pulling. *Cognitive Therapy and Research, 7,* 273–280.

Bernstein, D. A. (1973). Behavioral fear assessment: Anxiety or artifact? In H. Adams & P. Unikel (Eds.), *Issues and trends in behavior therapy* (pp. 225–267). Springfield, IL: Thomas.

Borkovec, T. D., Weerts, T. C., & Bernstein, D. A. (1977). Assessment of anxiety. In A. R. Ciminero, K. A. Calhoun, & H. E. Adams (Eds.), *Handbook of behavioral assessment* (pp. 367–428). New York: Wiley.

Bornstein, P. H., & Knapp, M. (1981). Self-control desensitization with a multi-phobic boy: A multiple baseline design. *Journal of Behavior Therapy and Experimental Psychiatry, 12,* 281–285.

Burdock, E. I., & Hardesty, A. S. (1968). Psychological test for psychopathology. *Journal of Abnormal Psychology, 73,* 62–67.

Camp, B. W., & Bash, M. A. S. (1981). *Think aloud. Increasing social and cognitive skills—A problem-solving program for children.* Champaign, IL: Research Press.

Campbell, K. P. (1987). *Reducing children's fear of the dark: A comparative outcome study.* Unpublished doctoral dissertation, University of Arizona, Tucson.

Carlson, G. A., & Cantwell, D. P. (1980). Unmasking masked depression in children and adolescents. *American Journal of Psychiatry, 3,* 445–449.

Castaneda, A., McCandless, B., & Palmero, D. (1956). The children's form of the Manifest Anxiety Scale. *Child Development, 27,* 317–326.

Chazan, M. (1962). School phobia. *British Journal of Educational Psychology, 32,* 209–217.

Ciminero, A. R. (1977). Behavioral assessment: An overview. In A. R. Ciminero, K. S. Calhoun, & H. E. Adams (Eds.), *Handbook of behavioral assessment* (pp. 3–14). New York: Wiley.

Ciminero, A. R., & Drabman, R. S. (1977). Current developments in the behavioral assessment of children. In B. B. Lahey & A. E. Kazdin (Eds), *Advances in clinical child psychology* (Vol. 1, pp. 1–53). New York: Plenum Press.

Ciminero, A. R., Nelson, R. O., & Lipinski, D. P. (1977). Self-monitoring procedures. In A. R. Ciminero, K. S. Calhoun, & H. E. Adams (Eds.), *Handbook of behavioral assessment* (pp. 195–232). New York: Wiley.

Cone, J. D. (1978). The behavioral assessment grid (BAG): A conceptual framework and taxonomy. *Behavior Therapy, 9,* 882–888.

Cone, J. D. (1979). Confounded comparisons in triple response mode assessment research. *Behavioral Assessment, 1*, 85–95.

Conoley, J. C., & Conoley, C. W. (1982). *School consultation: A guide to practice and training.* New York: Pergamon Press.

Coolidge, J. C., Hahn, P. B., & Pack, A. L. (1957). School phobia: Neurotic crisis or way of life. *American Journal of Orthopsychiatry, 27*, 296–306.

Croake, J. W., & Knox, F. H. (1971). A second look at adolescent fears. *Adolescence, 2*, 459–468.

Deffenbacher, J. L. (1976). Relaxation *in vivo* in the treatment of test anxiety. *Journal of Behavior Therapy and Experimental Psychiatry, 7*, 290–292.

Deffenbacher, J. L., & Michaels, A. (1980). Two self-control procedures in the reduction of targeted and nontargeted anxieties—A year later. *Journal of Counseling Psychology, 27*, 9–15.

DiGiuseppe, R. A., & Miller, N. J. (1977). A review of outcome studies on rational-emotive therapy. In A. Ellis & R. Grieger (Eds.), *Handbook of rational-emotive therapy* (pp. 72–95). New York: Springer.

Dollard, J., & Miller, N. E. (1950). *Personality and psychotherapy.* New York: McGraw-Hill.

Doris, J., McIntyre, J. R., Kelsey, C., & Lehman, E. (1971). Separation anxiety in nursery school children. *Proceedings of the 79th Annual Convention of the American Psychological Association, 79*, 145–146.

Ellis, A. (1962). *Reason and emotion in psychotherapy.* New York: Stuart.

Ellis, A. (1984). *Rational-emotive therapy and cognitive behavior therapy.* New York: Springer.

Ellis, A., & Bernard, M. E. (Eds.). (1983). *Rational-emotive approaches to the problems of childhood.* New York: Plenum Press.

Ellis, A., & Harper, R. A. (1975). *A new guide to rational living.* North Hollywood, CA: Wilshire.

Emmelkamp, P. M. G. (1979). The behavioral study of clinical phobias. In M. Hersen, R. M. Eisler, & P. M. Miller (Eds.), *Progress in behavior modification* (Vol. 8, pp. 55–125). New York: Academic Press.

Emmelkamp, P. M. G., & Mersch, P. P. (1982). Cognition and exposure *in vivo* in the treatment of agoraphobia: Short-term and delayed effects. *Cognitive Therapy and Research, 6*, 77–90.

Evans, I. M., & Nelson, R. O. (1977). Assessment of child behavior problems. In A. R. Ciminero, K. S. Calhoun, & H. E. Adams (Eds.), *Handbook of behavioral assessment* (pp. 603–682). New York: Wiley.

Evers, W. L., & Schwarz, J. C. (1973). Modifying social withdrawal in preschoolers: The effects of filmed modeling and teacher praise. *Journal of Abnormal Child Psychology, 1*, 245–256.

Fox, J., & Houston, B. (1981). Efficacy of self-instructional training for reducing children's anxiety in an evaluative situation. *Behaviour Research and Therapy, 19*, 509–515.

Genshaft, J. L. (1982). The use of cognitive behavior therapy for reducing math anxiety. *School Psychology Review, 11*, 32–34.

Glennon, B., & Weisz, J. R. (1978). An observational approach in the assessment of anxiety in young children. *Journal of Consulting and Clinical Psychology, 46*, 1246–1257.

Goldfried, M., & Davison, G. (1976). *Clinical behavior therapy.* New York: Holt, Rinehart & Winston.

Goldfried, M. R., & Goldfried, A. P. (1980). Cognitive change methods. In F. H. Kanfer & A. P. Goldstein (Eds.), *Helping people change* (2nd ed.) (pp. 97–130). New York: Pergamon Press.

Goldfried, M. R., & Merbaum, M. A. (1973). A perspective on self-control. In M. R. Goldfried & M. Merbaum (Eds.), *Behavior change through self-control* (pp. 3–36). New York: Holt, Rinehart & Winston.

Graziano, A. M., DeGiovanni, I. S., & Garcia, K. A. (1979). Behavioral treatments of children's fears: A review. *Psychological Bulletin, 86*, 804–830.

Graziano, A. M., & Mooney, K. C. (1984). *Children and behavior therapy.* New York: Aldine.

Graziano, A. M., Mooney, K. C., Huber, C., & Ignasiak, D. (1979). Self-control instructions for children's fear reduction. *Journal of Behavior Therapy and Experimental Psychiatry, 10,* 221–227.

Gross, A. M. (1984). Behavioral interviewing. In T. H. Ollendick & M. Hersen (Eds.), *Child behavioral assessment: Principles and procedures* (pp. 61–79). New York: Pergamon Press.

Haaga, D. A., & Davison, G. C. (1986). Cognitive change methods. In F. H. Kanfer & A. P. Goldstein (Eds.), *Helping people change* (3rd ed.) (pp. 236–282). New York: Pergamon Press.

Halford, K. (1983). Teaching rational self-talk to help socially isolated children and youth. In A. Ellis and M. E. Bernard (Eds.), *Rational-emotive approaches to the problems of childhood.* New York: Plenum Press.

Haynes, S. N. (1978). *Principles of behavioral assessment.* New York: Gardner Press.

Haynes, S. N., & Jensen, B. J. (1979). The interview as a behavioral assessment instrument. *Behavioral Assessment, 1,* 97–106.

Herzov, L. A. (1977). School refusal. In M. Rutter & L. Herzov (Eds.), *Child psychiatry: Modern approaches* (pp. 455–486). Oxford: Blackwell.

Homme, L. E. (1966). Contiguity theory and contingency management. *Psychological Record, 16,* 233–241.

Hughes, J. N. (1987). Cognitive behavior therapy. In C. R. Reynolds & L. Mann (Eds.), *Encyclopedia of special education* (pp. 354–355). New York: Wiley.

Jersild, A. T. (1968). *Child psychology* (6th ed.). Englewood Cliffs, NJ: Prentice-Hall.

Jersild, A. T., & Holmes, F. B. (1935). Children's fears. *Child Development Monographs, 20.*

Johnson, S. B. (1979). Children's fears in the classroom setting. *School Psychology Digest, 8,* 382–396.

Johnson, S. B., & Melamed, B. G. (1979). The assessment and treatment of children's fear. In B. B. Lahey & A. E. Kazdin (Eds.), *Advances in clinical child psychology* (Vol. 2, pp. 108–139). New York: Plenum Press.

Jones, R. R., Reid, J. B., & Patterson, G. R. (1975). Naturalistic observation in clinical assessment. In P. McReynolds (Ed.), *Advances in psychological assessment* (Vol. 3, pp. 42–95). San Francisco: Jossey-Bass.

Kanfer, F. H. (1975). Self-management methods. In F. H. Kanfer & A. P. Goldstein (Eds.), *Helping people change* (pp. 309–356). New York: Pergamon Press.

Kanfer, F. H. (1980). Self-management methods. In F. H. Kanfer & A. P. Goldstein (Eds.), *Helping people change* (2nd ed.) (pp. 334–389). New York: Pergamon Press.

Kanfer, F. H., & Gaelick, L. (1986). Self-management methods. In F. H. Kanfer & A. P. Goldstein (Eds.), *Helping people change* (3rd ed.) (pp. 283–345). New York: Pergamon Press.

Kanfer, F. H., Karoly, P., & Newman, A. (1975). Reduction of children's fear of the dark by confidence-related and situational threat–related verbal cues. *Journal of Consulting and Clinical Psychology, 43,* 251–258.

Kanfer, F. H., & Phillips, J. S. (1970). *Learning foundations of behavior therapy.* New York: Wiley.

Kanfer, F. H., & Schefft, B. K. (1988). *The basics of therapy.* Champaign, IL: Research Press.

Karoly, P. (1981). Self-management problems in children. In E. J. Mash & L. G. Terdal (Eds.), *Behavioral assessment of childhood disorders* (pp. 79–126). New York: Guilford Press.

Kazdin, A. E. (1974). Self-monitoring and behavior changes. In M. J. Mahoney & C. E. Thoresen (Eds.), *Self-control: Power to the person* (pp. 218–224). Monterey, CA: Brooks/Cole.

Kazdin, A. E. (1977). Assessing the clinical or applied importance of behavior change through social validation. *Behavior Modification, 1,* 427–452.

Kazdin, A. E. (1978). *History of behavior modification.* Baltimore, MD: University Park Press.

Kazdin, A. E. (1980). *Research design in clinical psychology.* New York: Harper & Row.

Kazdin, A. E., & Wilson, G. T. (1978). *Evaluation of behavior therapy: Issues, evidence, and research strategies.* Cambridge, MA: Ballinger.

Kelley, C. K. (1976). Play desensitization of fear of darkness in preschool children. *Behaviour Research and Therapy, 14,* 79–81.

Kelly, M. S. (1981). The effect of relaxation training and self-directed verbalizations on measures of anxiety and learning in learning-disabled children (United States International University). *Dissertation Abstracts International, 42,* 3806B–3807B.

Kendall, P. C. (1981). Cognitive–behavioral interventions with children. In B. B. Lahey & A. E. Kazdin (Eds.), *Advances in clinical child psychology* (Vol. 4, pp. 53–90). New York: Plenum Press.

Kendall, P. C., & Bemis, K. M. (1983). Thought and action in psychotherapy: The cognitive-behavioral approaches. In M. Hersen, A. E. Kazdin, & A. S. Bellack (Eds.), *The clinical psychology handbook* (pp. 565–592). New York: Pergamon Press.

Kendall, P. C., & Braswell, L. (1985). *Cognitive-behavioral therapy for impulsive children.* New York: Guilford Press.

Kendall, P. C., & Finch, A. J. (1979). Developing non-impulsive behavior in children: Cognitive-behavioral strategies for self-control. In P. C. Kendall & S. D. Hollon (Eds.), *Cognitive-behavioral interventions: Theory, research, and procedures* (pp. 37–80). New York: Academic Press.

Kendall, P. C., & Hollon, S. D. (Eds.). (1979). *Cognitive-behavior interventions: Theory, research, and procedures.* New York: Academic Press.

Kendall, P. C., Pellegrini, D. S., & Urbain, E. S. (1981). Approaches to assessment for cognitive-behavioral interventions with children. In P. C. Kendall & S. D. Hollon (Eds.), *Assessment strategies for cognitive-behavioral interventions* (pp. 227–286). New York: Academic Press.

Kennedy, W. A. (1965). School phobia: Rapid treatment of fifty cases. *Journal of Abnormal Psychology, 70,* 285–289.

Klinger, E. (1978). Modes of normal conscious flow. In K. S. Pope & J. L. Singer (Eds.). *The stream of consciousness: Scientific investigations into the flow of human experience* (pp. 226–258). New York: Plenum Press.

Knopf, I. J. (1979). *Childhood psychopathology*. Englewood Cliffs, NJ: Prentice-Hall.

Kondas, O. (1967). Reduction of examination anxiety and "stage fright" by group desensitization and relaxation. *Behaviour Research and Therapy*, 5, 275–281.

Kornhaber, R. C., & Schroeder, H. E. (1974). Importance of model similarity on extinction of avoidance behavior in children. *Journal of Consulting and Clinical Psychology*, 43, 601–607.

Kovacs, M., & Beck, A. T. (1977). An empirical–clinical approach toward a definition of childhood depression. In J. G. Schulterbrandt & A. Raskin (Eds.), *Depression in childhood: Diagnosis, treatment, and conceptual models* (pp. 1–25). New York: Raven Press.

Kozak, M. J., & Miller, G. A. (1982). Hypothetical constructs vs. intervening variables: A re-appraisal of the three-systems model of anxiety assessment. *Behavioral Assessment*, 4, 347–358.

Krans, P. E. (1973). *Yesterday's children: A longitudinal study of children from kindergarten into the adult years*. New York: Wiley.

Kratochwill, T. R. (1981). *Selective mutism*. New York: Lawrence Erlbaum.

Kratochwill, T. R. (1982). Advances in behavioral assessment. In C. R. Reynolds & T. B. Gutkin (Eds.), *Handbook of school psychology*. New York: Wiley.

Kratochwill, T. R., Brody, G., & Piersal, W. (1979). Elective mutism in children. In B. B. Lahey & A. E. Kazdin (Eds.), *Advances in clinical child psychology* (Vol. 2, pp. 194–240). New York: Plenum Press.

Kratochwill, T. R., & Morris, R. J. (1985). Behavioral treatment of children's fears and phobias: A review. *School Psychology Review*, 14, 84–93.

Kratochwill, T. R., Morris, R. J., & Campbell, K. P. (1985). Assessment of children's anxiety-related disorders. In J. R. Bergan (Ed.), *School psychology in contemporary society: An introduction* (pp. 163–206). Columbus, OH: Charles Merrill.

Kratochwill, T. R., Sanders, C., Wiemer, S., & Morris, R. J. (1987). Fears and phobias in school age children. In A. Thomas & J. Grimes (Eds.), *Children's needs: Psychological perspectives* (pp. 214–220). Washington, DC: National Association of School Psychologists.

Kratochwill, T. R., & Sheridan, S. M. (in press). Advances in behavioral assessment. In C. R. Reynolds & T. B. Gutkin (Eds.), *Handbook of school psychology* (2nd ed.). New York: Wiley.

Kuroda, J. (1969). Elimination of children's fears of animals by the method of experimental desensitization—An application of learning theory to child psychology. *Psychologia*, 12, 161–165.

Lang, P. J. (1968). Fear reduction and fear behavior: Problems in treating a construct. In J. M. Shlien (Ed.), *Research in psychotherapy* (Vol. 3, pp. 90–102). Washington, DC: American Psychological Association.

Lang, P. J., & Lazovik, A. D. (1963). Experimental desensitization of a phobia. *Journal of Abnormal and Social Psychology*, 66, 519–525.

Lapouse, R., & Monk, M. A. (1959). Fears and worries in a representative sample of children. *American Journal of Orthopsychiatry*, 29, 803–818.

Leal, L. L., Baxter, E. G., Martin, J., & Marx, R. W. (1981). Cognitive modification and systematic desensitization with test anxious high school students. *Journal of Counseling Psychology*, 28, 525–528.

Lewis, S. A. (1974). A comparison of behavior therapy techniques in the reduction of fearful avoidant behavior. *Behavior Therapy*, 5, 648–655.

Lick, J. R., Unger, T., & Condiante, M. (1978). Effects of uncertainty about the behavior of a phobic stimulus on subjects' fear reactions. *Journal of Consulting and Clinical Psychology, 46,* 1559–1560.

Lipsky, M. J., Kassinove, H., & Miller, N. J. (1980). Effects of rational-emotive therapy, rational role reversal, and rational-emotive imagery on the emotional adjustment of community mental health center patients. *Journal of Consulting and Clinical Psychology, 48,* 366–374.

Magrath, K. (1982). *Investigating the developmental analysis of children's fears.* Unpublished doctoral dissertation, Syracuse University, Syracuse.

Mahoney, M. J. (1974). *Cognition and behavior modification.* Cambridge, MA: Ballinger.

Marine, E. (1968–1969). School refusal—Who should intervene? *Journal of School Psychology, 7,* 63–70.

Matison, R., Cantwell, D. P., Russell, A. T., & Will, I. (1979). A comparison of DSM-II in the diagnosis of childhood psychiatric disorders: II. Interrater agreement. *Archives of General Psychiatry, 36,* 1217–1222.

Maultsby, M. C. (1975). Rational behavior therapy for acting-out adolescents. *Social Casework, 56,* 35–43.

McFall, R. M. (1977). Parameters of self-monitoring. In R. B. Stuart (Ed.), *Behavioral strategies, techniques, and outcomes* (pp. 196–214). New York: Brunner/Mazel.

Meichenbaum, D. (1977). *Cognitive behavior modification.* New York: Plenum Press.

Meichenbaum, D. (1986). Cognitive behavior modification. In F. H. Kanfer & A. P. Goldstein (Eds.), *Helping people change* (3rd ed.) (pp. 346–380). New York: Pergamon Press.

Meichenbaum, D., & Genest, M. (1980). Cognitive behavior modification: An integration of cognitive and behavioral methods. In F. H. Kanfer & A. P. Goldstein (Eds.), *Helping people change* (2nd ed.) (pp. 390–422). New York: Pergamon Press.

Meichenbaum, D., & Goodman, J. (1971). Training impulsive children to talk to themselves: A means of developing self-control. *Journal of Abnormal Psychology, 77,* 115–126.

Melamed, B., & Siegel, L. (1975). Reduction of anxiety in children facing hospitalization and surgery by use of filmed modeling. *Journal of Consulting and Clinical Psychology, 43,* 511–521.

Melamed, B., & Siegel, L. J. (1980). *Behavior medicine.* New York: Springer.

Meyer, V., Liddel, A., & Lyons, M. (1977). Behavioral interviews. In A. R. Ciminero, K. S. Calhoun, & H. E. Adams (Eds.), *Handbook of behavioral assessment* (pp. 117–152). New York: Wiley.

Milby, J. B., Wendorf, D., & Meredith, R. L. (1983). Assessment and treatment of obsessive–compulsive disorders in children. In R. J. Morris & T. R. Kratochwill (Eds.), *Practice of child therapy* (pp. 1–26). New York: Pergamon Press.

Miller, A. M., & Kratochwill, T. R. (1979). Reduction of frequent stomachache complaints by time-out. *Behavior Therapy, 10,* 211–218.

Miller, L. C., Barrett, C. L., & Hampe, E. (1974). Phobias of childhood in a prescientific era. In A. Davids (Ed.), *Child personality and psychopathology: Current topics.* New York: Wiley.

Miller, L. C., Barrett, C. L., Hampe, E., & Noble, H. (1972). Factor structure of childhood fears. *Journal of Consulting and Clinical Psychology, 39,* 264–268.

Morganstern, K. (1976). Behavioral interviewing: The initial stages of assessment. In M. Hersen & A. Bellack (Eds.), *Behavioral assessment: A practical handbook* (pp. 51–76). New York: Pergamon Press.

Morris, R. J. (1986). Fear reduction methods. In F. H. Kanfer & A. P. Goldstein (Eds.), *Helping people change* (3rd ed.) (pp. 145–190). New York: Pergamon Press.

Morris, R. J., & Kratochwill, T. R. (1983). *Treating children's fears and phobias*. New York: Pergamon Press.

Morris, R. J., Kratochwill, T. R., & Aldridge, K. (1988). Fears and phobias. In J. C. Witt, S. N. Elliott, & F. M. Gresham (Eds.), *Handbook of behavior therapy in education* (pp. 679–717). New York: Plenum Press.

Morris, R. J., Kratochwill, T. R., & Dodson, C. L. (1986). Fears and phobias in adolescence: A behavioral perspective. In R. A. Feldman & A. R. Stiffman (Eds.), *Advances in adolescent mental health* (Vol. 1, Part A, pp. 63–117). Greenwich, CT: JAI Press.

Murphy, C. M., & Bootzin, R. R. (1973). Active and passive participation in the contact desensitization of snake fear in children. *Behavioral Therapy, 4,* 203–211.

Neisworth, J. T., Madle, R. A., & Goeke, K. E. (1975). Errorless elimination of separation anxiety: A case study. *Journal of Behavior Therapy and Experimental Psychiatry, 6,* 79–82.

Nelson, R. O. (1977). Assessment and therapeutic functions of self-monitoring. In M. Hersen, R. M. Eisler, & P. M. Miller (Eds.), *Progress in behavior modification* (Vol. 5, pp. 264–308). New York: Academic Press.

Nietzel, M. T., & Bernstein, D. A. (1981). Assessment of anxiety and fear. In M. Hersen & A. Bellack (Eds.), *Behavioral assessment: A practical handbook* (2nd ed.) (pp. 215–245). New York: Pergamon Press.

Nottelmann, E., & Hill, K. (1977). Test anxiety and off-task behavior in evaluative situations. *Child Development, 48,* 225–231.

O'Connor, R. D. (1972). Relative efficacy of modeling, shaping and the combined procedures from modification of social withdrawal. *Journal of Abnormal Psychology, 79,* 327–334.

O'Leary, K. D., & Johnson, S. B. (1979). Psychological assessment. In H. C. Quay & J. S. Werry (Eds.), *Psychopathological disorders of childhood* (2nd ed.) (pp. 210–246). New York: Wiley.

Ollendick, T. H., & Hersen, M. (1984). *Child behavioral assessment: Principles and procedures*. New York: Pergamon Press.

Orton, G. L. (1982). A comparative study of children's worries. *Journal of Psychology, 110,* 153–162.

Parsons, R. D., & Meyers, J. (1984). *Developing consultation skills*. San Francisco: Jossey-Bass.

Paul, G. L., & Bernstein, D. A. (1973). *Anxiety and clinical problems: Systematic desensitization and related techniques*. Morristown, NJ: General Learning Press.

Peterson, L., & Shigetomi, C. (1981). The use of coping techniques in minimizing anxiety in hospitalized children. *Behavior Therapy, 12,* 1–14.

Phillips, B. N. (1966). *An analysis of causes of anxiety among children in school*. (Final Report Project No. 2616 United States Office of Education Cooperative Research Branch). Austin: University of Texas.

Phillips, B. N. (1978). *School stress and anxiety: Theory, research, and intervention*. New York: Human Sciences Press.

Phillips, C. A. (1977). A psychological analysis to tension headache. In S. J. Rachman (Ed.), *Contributions to medical psychology* (Vol. 1, pp. 91–113). Oxford: Pergamon Press.

Pomerantz, P. B., Peterson, N. T., Marholin, D., & Stern, S. (1977). The *in vivo* elimination of a child's water phobia by a paraprofessional at home. *Journal of Behavior Therapy and Experimental Psychiatry, 8*, 417–421.

Quay, H. C. (1979). Classification. In H. C. Quay & J. S. Werry (Eds.), *Psychopathological disorders of childhood* (2nd ed.) (pp. 1–42). New York: Wiley.

Rachman, S. (1978). *Fear and courage.* San Francisco: Freeman.

Ramirez, S. Z., Kratochwill, T. R., & Morris, R. J. (1987). Childhood anxiety disorders. In M. Ascher & L. Michelson (Eds.), *Cognitive behavior therapy* (pp. 149–175). New York: Guilford Press.

Richards, C. S., & Siegel, L. J. (1978). Behavioral treatment of anxiety states and avoidance behaviors in children. In D. Marholin II (Ed.), *Child behavior therapy* (pp. 274–338). New York: Gardner Press.

Rose, R. J., & Ditto, B. (1983). A developmental-genetic analysis of common fears from early adolescence to early adulthood. *Child Development, 54*, 361–368.

Sarason, I. G. (1980). *Test anxiety: Theory, research and applications.* Hillsdale, NJ: Lawrence Erlbaum.

Sarason, S., Davidson, K., Lighthall, F., Waite, R., & Ruebush, B. (1960). *Anxiety in elementary school children.* New York: Wiley.

Scherer, M. W., & Nakamura, C. Y. (1968). *A Fear Survey Schedule for Children* (FSS-FC): A factor analytic comparison with manifest anxiety (CMAS). *Behaviour Research and Therapy, 6*, 173–182.

Shapiro, E. S. (1984). Self-monitoring procedures. In T. H. Ollendick & M. Hersen (Eds.), *Child behavioral assessment: Principles and procedures* (pp. 148–165). New York: Pergamon Press.

Siegel, L. J., & Peterson, L. (1980). Stress reduction in young dental patients through coping skills and sensory information. *Journal of Consulting and Clinical Psychology, 48*, 785–787.

Skinner, B. F. (1953). *Science and human behavior.* New York: Macmillan.

Spielberger, C. (1973). *Manual for the State-Trait Inventory for Children.* Palo Alto, CA: Consulting Psychologists Press.

Spivack, G., Spotts, J., & Haimes, P. E. (1967). *The Devereux Adolescent Behavior Rating Scale.* Devon, PA: Devereux Foundation.

Spivack, G., & Swift, U. (1967). *The Elementary School Behavior Rating Scale.* Devon, PA: Devereux Foundation.

Spivack, G., & Swift, U. (1973). Classroom behavior of children: A critical review of teacher-administered rating scales. *Journal of Special Education, 1*, 55–89.

Staley, A. A., & O'Donnell, J. P. (1984). A developmental analysis of mothers' reports of normal children's fears. *Journal of Genetic Psychology, 144*, 165–178.

Strain, P., Cooke, T., & Apolloni, T. (1976). *Teaching exceptional children: Assessing and modifying social behavior.* New York: Academic Press.

Tasto, D. L. (1977). Self-report schedules and inventories. In A. R. Ciminero, K. S. Calhoun, & H. E. Adams (Eds.), *Handbook of behavioral assessment* (pp. 153–194). New York: Wiley.

Taylor, C. B., & Agras, S. (1981). Assessment of phobia. In D. H. Barlow (Ed.), *Behavioral assessment of adult disorders* (pp. 181–208). New York: Guilford Press.

Tearnan, B. H., Lahey, B., Thompson, J. K., & Hammer, D. (1982). The role of coping self-instructions combined with covert modeling in specific fear reduction. *Cognitive Therapy and Research, 6*, 185–190.

Thoresen, C. E., & Mahoney, M. J. (1974). *Behavioral self-control.* New York: Holt, Rinehart & Winston.

Trueman, D. (1984a). Behavioral treatment of school phobia: A review. *Psychology in the Schools, 21,* 215–223.

Trueman, D. (1984b). What are the characteristics of school phobic children? *Psychological Reports, 54,* 191–202.

Van der Ploeg-Stapert, J. D., & Van der Ploeg, H. M. (1986). Behavioral group treatment of test anxiety: An evaluation study. *Journal of Behavior Therapy and Experimental Psychiatry, 17,* 255–259.

Vernon, D., Foley, J. L., & Schulman, J. L. (1967). Effect of mother–child separation and birth order on young children's responses to two potentially stressful experiences. *Journal of Personality and Social Psychology, 5,* 162–174.

Walk, R. D. (1956). Self-ratings of fear in a fear-invoking situation. *Journal of Abnormal and Social Psychology, 52,* 171–178.

Walker, H. M. (1983). *The Walker Problem Behavior Identification Checklist (revised): Test and manual.* Los Angeles: Western Psychological Services.

Wells, K. C. (1981). Assessment of children in outpatient settings. In M. Hersen & A. Bellack (Eds.), *Behavioral assessment: A practical handbook* (pp. 484–533). New York: Pergamon Press.

Wiggins, J. S. (1973). *Personality and prediction: Principles of personality assessment.* Reading, MA: Addison-Wesley.

Wine, J. (1979). Test anxiety and evaluation threat: Children's behavior in the classroom. *Journal of Abnormal Child Psychology, 7,* 45–59.

Wolf, M. F. (1978). Social validity: The case for subjective measurement or how applied behavior analysis is funding its heart. *Journal of Applied Behavior Analysis, 11,* 203–214.

Wright, L., Schaefer, A., & Solomons, G. (Eds.) (1979). *Encyclopedia of pediatric psychology.* Baltimore, MD: University Park Press.

Yule, W. (1979). Behavioral approaches to the treatment and prevention of school refusal. *Behavioral Analysis and Modification, 3,* 55–68.

Zettle, R. D., & Hayes, S. C. (1980). Conceptual and empirical status of rational-emotive therapy. In M. Hersen, R. M. Eisler, & P. M. Miller (Eds.), *Progress in behavior modification* (Vol. 9, pp. 125–166). New York: Academic Press.

17
INTERPERSONAL COGNITIVE PROBLEM-SOLVING TRAINING WITH CHILDREN IN THE SCHOOLS

EUGENE S. URBAIN
Wilder Foundation, St. Paul, Minnesota

PAULA SAVAGE
Private Practice, Minnetonka, Minnesota

The potential of schools in promoting the mental health of children has been recognized for some time (Caplan 1961; Cowen, 1973, 1977; Glasser, 1969, Long, 1970; Minuchin, Biber, Shapiro, & Zimules, 1969). Recently, longitudinal research has provided increasing empirical demonstration of the role that effective schools and teachers can play in the long-term life adjustment of individuals, including children experiencing multiple life stresses and unstable home environments during much of their childhood (Rutter, 1983). Teachers are important societal role models for children, and schools play a significant role in a child's adaptation to the broader society and culture outside the home (Goodlad, 1984; Sarason, 1971). Moreover, teachers and school staff convey to children, both explicitly and implicitly, information about societal norms for desirable and undesirable social behavior. Effective teachers may differ in methods and personal style, but in general they are able to maintain a strong academic focus in children while creating a climate of organization, reasonable behavioral order, and positive interpersonal relationships in the classroom as a group (Bickel & Bickel, 1986; Carnegie Forum on Education and the Economy, 1986; Ysseldyke, 1984). In view of the evidence of some positive relationship between children's academic and social competence (Laughlin, 1954; Muma, 1965, 1968; Northway, 1944; Porterfield & Schlichting, 1961), and of the importance of both these dimensions to a child's personal competence and self-esteem formation (Coopersmith, 1976; Gresham, 1982, 1984; Harter, 1982, 1985), it is logical to ask what methods schools and teachers might use to enhance most effectively the interpersonal as well as the academic competence of the children they serve. A variety of approaches currently exist. For example, it has been demonstrated that academic task instruction utilizing cooperative learning and grouping arrangements can facilitate cooperation and conflict resolution skills among students (Aronson, 1978, Johnson & Johnson, 1975, 1979, 1983, 1986). Consultation with teachers and teacher skills training have also been effective in assisting students with interpersonal and behavioral difficulties in the classroom (Aspy, 1972; Gordon, 1974; Meyers, 1979; Tyne & Flynn, 1979). A third approach has been the development of classroom curricula for mental health promotion in children (Cooper, Munger, & Ravlin, 1980). These include a variety of affective development and interpersonal awareness curricula, programs such as Developing Understanding of Self and Others (grades K–3) and Towards Affective Development (grades 3–6) (American Guidance Service); Lifeline (grades 7–12) (Argus Communications); Dimensions of Personality (K–12) (Pflaum); Focus on Self Development (K–6) (Science Research Associates); the self-control curriculum developed by Fagen, Long, and Stevens (1975); self-esteem approaches like that of Canfield and Wells (1976); moral development approaches (Mattox, 1975); and values clarification approaches such as that of Raths. Harmin, and Simon (1966). An earlier prototype is the causal-thinking curriculum developed by Ojemann (1961), designed to enhance children's understanding of relationship dynamics and their causal reasoning about interpersonal relationships and events. Later in the 1960s the Magic Circle curriculum (Bessell & Palomares, 1967) was developed for preschool and elementary school children, followed by a program of Human Relations Development (Gazda et al., 1973). Assertiveness training programs have also been implemented effectively in the schools (Rotheram, Armstrong, & Bodracm, 1982). Gazda and Brooks (1985) offer a useful history of the development of the social/life skills training movement in the schools.

It should be noted that there is little research demonstrating the relative effectiveness of one of these approaches over another, Moreover, common content elements often overlap across different programs. As new research data come in, what seems important from the practitioner's standpoint is to develop more awareness of the "active ingredients" or most effective program elements that cut across different intervention programs, and to retain a flexible repertoire of alternative techniques for different purposes and problems facing school decision makers.

An important recent programmatic direction over the last 10 years or so in the area of strategies for enhancing children's social competency has been the creation of a number of interpersonal problem-solving training curricula (Pellegrini & Urbain, 1985; Urbain & Kendall, 1980). A number of research and programmatic efforts have begun to look more specifically at the role of interpersonal cognitive problem solving (ICPS) skills in children's social and behavioral adjustment. Although research into human problem solving has a long and extensive history in psychology (Davis, 1966; Dewey, 1910; Duncan, 1959; Gagne, 1970), Jahoda (1953, 1958) was among the first to place explicit theoretical emphasis on the relation of effective interpersonal problem solving to social and emotional adjustment. She proposed that psychological health is related to a problem-solving sequence characterized by a person's tendency to recognize and admit a problem, to reflect on possible solutions, to make a decision, and to take action. Until recently, however, empirical research has focused almost exclusively on problem solving as it is applied to nonsocial content, such as puzzles, mazes, and anagrams. Consequently, we are just beginning to know more about the exact nature of interpersonal problem-solving skills and the process by which they are applied in social interaction (see Pellegrini, 1985, for discussion of the differences between social and nonsocial problem solving).

Essential to the interpersonal cognitive problem-solving (ICPS) approach is the emphasis on adaptive thinking processes, as opposed to an emphasis on internal psychodynamics or on specific overt behaviors per se as major factors in psychological adjustment. D'Zurilla and Goldfried (1971) define the concept of "problem" as follows:

> The term *problem* will refer here to a specific *situation* or *set of situations* to which a person must respond in order to function effectively in his environment. To point up this situational emphasis (as opposed to the traditional *intrapsychic* connotation of the word *problem* in clinical psychology), the term *problematic situation* will be used in most instances in place of *problem*. In the present context, a situation is considered problematic if "no effective response alternative is immediately available to the individual confronted with the situation." (pp. 107–108; emphasis in original)

The emphasis is on examining the internal cognitive processes that lead to successful problem solving, processes akin to "the operation of cognitive strategies or 'learning sets' . . . which enable an individual to 'create' or 'discover' symbolically solutions to a variety of unfamiliar problems" (D'Zurilla & Goldfried, 1971, p. 108).

A number of different programs have recently been devised for teaching ICPS skills specifically to children. Although programs differ in the content and number of problem-solving skills taught, there is general agreement on a number of important problem-solving thinking skills:

1. *Problem identification*: Component skills involve problem sensitivity or the ability to "sense" the presence of a problem by identifying "uncomfortable" feelings; also included are skills for identifying major problem issues as well as maintaining a general problem-solving orientation or "set" versus a tendency to deny, avoid, or act impulsively in dealing with the problem.
2. *Alternative thinking*: The ability to generate multiple potential alternative solutions to a given interpersonal problem situation.
3. *Consequential thinking*: The ability to foresee the immediate and more long-range consequences of a particular alternative and to use this information in the decision-making process.
4. *Means–ends thinking*: The ability to elaborate or plan a series of specific

actions (a means) to attain a given goal, to recognize and devise ways around potential obstacles, and to use a realistic time framework in implementing steps towards the goal.

Another significant research trend over the last decade has been the reawakening of interest in the importance of children's peer relations and the component social skills and behaviors involved in friendship formation and conflict resolution. With this renewed interest has come growing awareness of the many developmental functions that peers fulfill. For example, as agents of socialization, peers communicate and reinforce standards of behavior (Hartup, 1980, 1983). In addition, they are a major source of emotional support while also providing instruction in a variety of social, cognitive, and motor skills (Asher, 1978). Their role in shaping sexual and aggressive behavior may be especially important (Suomi, 1980).

Poor peer relations are characteristic of children demonstrating a wide variety of behavioral and emotional difficulties. Indeed, relational problems are often a major reason that children are referred for therapy (Janes, Hesselbrook, & Schectman, 1980). Given the important role that peers appear to play in development, it is not surprising that poor peer relations in childhood have been linked with maladjustment later in life as well (Cowen, Pederson, Babigian, Izzo, & Trost, 1973; Janes, Hesselbrook, Meyers, and Penniman, 1970; Janes, et al., 1980; Roff, Sells, & Golden, 1972). For example, Cowen et al. (1973) found that negative peer evaluations in third grade were superior to a variety of other adjustment indices in predicting mental health problems 11 years later. Roff et al. (1972) found that children who were disliked by their peers were more likely to engage in juvenile delinquency. Although correlational findings of this kind cannot conclusively establish that poor peer relations *cause* current or later maladjustment, they are consistent with such a relationship. Moreover, they highlight the importance of treating peer relationship difficulties directly.

Most reported ICPS interventions have focused heavily, though not exclusively, on problem situations involving peer interaction. This emphasis is not surprising given the fact that most ICPS programs have been school-based, with their major focus on the school setting. While the current review focuses specifically on attempts to improve social interaction through cognitive ICPS skill enhancement, a number of different strategies have been devised for remediating peer relationship difficulties and deserve brief mention here. Asher (1978) identified three social skills training approaches frequently adopted with children. *Contingency management* strategies teach children new ways of behaving by reinforcing desirable behaviors while ignoring or punishing undesirable ones. *Modeling* strategies teach skills by demonstrating competent performance in particular social situations. *Coaching* strategies typically involve the combined use of direct instructions, modeling, behavioral rehearsal (role play), and feedback. Discussion of the literature on behavioral social skills training is, however, outside the scope of present review. A number of reviews of this literature exist (Asher, 1978; Cartledge & Milburn, 1980; Combs & Slaby, 1978; Gresham, 1981, 1985; LeCroy, 1983; Strain & Odom, 1986; Van Hasselt, Hersen, Whitehill, & Bellack, 1979). Problem solving is a cognitive-behavioral process in that it deals with cognitive processes and their relationship to behavioral adjustment (Kendall & Hollon, 1979). ICPS interventions thus share with other behavioral interventions an emphasis on social learning principles (Bandura, 1977; Rotter, 1954). Problem-solving interventions do, however, place greater emphasis on training at the level of thinking *processes* (e.g., identifying problem issues, generating alternative solutions, evaluating consequences, etc.) in contrast to interventions designed to train more specific behavioral responses to various situations (e.g., eye contact, assertive responses, smiling, etc.). The ICPS training emphasis on cognitive *processes* (i.e., "*how* to think") also differs from the greater coaching program emphasis on training cognitive *content* ("*what* to think") in particular social situations. There is an underlying assumption in ICPS training that teaching children to evaluate problems for themselves and to make decisions more thoughtfully will increase their sense of personal effectiveness and, perhaps, their ability to solve problems more independently later in life as well (Clabby & Elias, 1986).

ICPS training appears to have another potential advantage as an intervention strategy, in that it is easily implemented by teachers in the typical classroom context. Several prevention strategists (e.g., Allen, Chinsky, Larcen, Lochman, & Selinger, 1976; Bower, 1965; Cowen, 1973, 1977) have observed that the school may be an ideal setting for therapeutic efforts (see also Chapter 19 this volume). For example, schools represent one of the few socialization systems that involve almost all children in their operations. Thus, programs geared toward promoting the psychological health of children would have enormous impact if integrated into the ongoing routine of classroom education. As training settings, schools obviate the need to separate children with problems from their peers and thus avoid the negative side effects of such stigmatization. Finally, teachers represent a readily available helping resource if therapeutic programs can be designed to take advantage of their skills, needs, and interests.

In reviewing the literature on ICPS interventions, it is evident that studies vary considerably from one to the next on a number of dimensions, making comparability across studies quite problematic. Some of these dimensions include:

Frequency and duration of training sessions.
Trainer characteristics. Some studies involve teachers as trainers, others use graduate students; trainers also differ in personal styles along such dimensions as interpersonal warmth and control.
Training content. What specific skills receive greater training emphasis?
Assessment methods. Studies vary considerably in the problem-solving assessment instruments they use; some include measures of actual behav-

ioral adjustment, but many studies confine themselves only to laboratory-type cognitive problem-solving tests.

Subject characteristics. Some studies involve children in special educational or institutional settings, some specifically select aggressive or shy children, others train normal elementary classroom groups.

Training methods. Whereas studies nearly always use verbal instruction, modeling, and reinforcement in some form, they vary in emphasis or use of role-playing techniques, video modeling/feedback, token reinforcement systems, verbal self-instruction, and perspective taking (i.e., procedures for teaching children to assume different social perspectives in an interpersonal situation; see Feshbach, 1983; Feshbach, Feshbach, Fauvre, & Campbell, 1983; Urbain & Kendall, 1980); some trainers use a small-group training format, whereas others administer training in the larger classroom setting.

School "climate" factors (Rutter, 1983). Although these issues are rarely addressed directly in the problem-solving literature, individual schools where research takes place clearly vary in the level to which school staff model positive interaction and effective interpersonal problem-solving among themselves (Urbain, 1980).

In selecting studies for review in this chapter, emphasis has been given to studies that (1) involve training in a school setting; (2) are frequently cited in the literature; (3) are fairly sound methodologically or make some methodological contribution to the literature; and (4) make some attempt to measure actual behavior outcomes beyond demonstrating outcomes on cognitive problem-solving tests alone. The studies are grouped in sections according to age of the target population—preschool, school-age, and adolescent. The discussion section examines strengths and weaknesses of the existing research and offers consideration for future studies: At the end of this chapter there is a sampling of practical ICPS training activities from our own work in this area. The reader interested in specific training activities is referred to Kendall and Braswell (1985) and Urbain (1985).

OUTCOME STUDIES

Preschool Children

The most extensive programs to date on the assessment and training of ICPS skills in children has been conducted by Spivack and Shure and their co-workers at Hahnemann University in Philadelphia (Shure & Spivack, 1978; Spivack, Platt, & Shure, 1976; Spivack & Shure, 1974). The problem-solving training programs developed by Spivack and Shure and associates are presented in the form of specific training lessons or scripts, consisting of structured daily activities and discussion to teach component ICPS skills. The training script for preschoolers (Spivack & Shure, 1974) consists of a sequence of 46 short (20–30-minute) daily lessons, activities, and games conducted by the preschool teacher. The program first involves teaching a number of skills felt (though not demonstrated) to be prerequisite for problem solving, namely, linguistic concepts such as "same–different" and "if–then," and the ability to identify basic emotions (happy, angry, scared, sad). The remainder of the program is devoted to a series of hypothetical and actual interpersonal problem situations and is divided sequentially into three parts: (1) enumerating solutions, (2) enumerating consequences, and (3) pairing specific solutions with specific consequences. Teacher demonstration and puppet play are used to illustrate the training concepts, and whenever possible that problem-solving methods are applied to actual problems that arise among the children in school through teacher–child "dialoguing" using the problem-solving model.

The results of the program indicated that the trained children improved relative to a no-treatment control group on measures of alternative and consequential thinking as well as on teacher ratings of overt behavioral adjustment. Although the teachers were aware of the experimental conditions when they rated the children at posttesting, improvement was maintained at follow-up one year later when children were rated by new teachers who were unaware of the experimental conditions. However, the absence of some type of control group procedure other than a no-treatment group makes it difficult to examine to what extent the problem-solving training itself was responsible for the outcomes, as opposed to factors that were not specific to the training, such as special attention to the children and expectancy for change.[1] It is also difficult to determine which of the specific component skills taught might have been most responsible for the observed improvements.

A classic study of the modification of dominant interpersonal behavior patterns in preschool children was reported by Chittenden (1942). Children were selected on the basis of high dominance and low cooperation scores derived from behavioral observations. Training consisted of 11 sessions during which an adult experimenter met individually with each child and worked out solutions to interpersonal problem situations presented through doll play. For example, two dolls, playing the roles of preschool children, would be faced with the problem of finding a way to play successfully with only one toy. Emphasis was placed on learning alternative responses to aggressive or dominative behaviors. Immediately following training, behavioral observations indicated a decrease in dominative and an increase in cooperative interactions. The decrease in domination scores was still evident a month later, but the increase in cooperation was no longer significant.

A technique involving instruction in alternative thinking was applied by Zahavi and Asher (1978) with aggressive nursery school children. In this study,

---

[1]Given the length of the treatment program, use of a strict attention control group might present ethical difficulties. However, other types of contrast groups can be used as alternatives to a no-treatment control group (O'Leary & Borkovec, 1978).

the preschool teacher used rational verbal instructions, explaining to the children (1) that hitting others causes hurt, (2) that other children do not like children who hit, and (3) that it is wise to think of alternatives to hitting. Modeling and role play components were specifically avoided, however, as the focus of the study was on the effect of teacher instructions on the children's behavior. The teacher instructed each child individually on one occasion for approximately 10 minutes. Posttreatment observations showed reduced aggressiveness in these children, as opposed to aggressive children who did not receive the instructions. Decreases in aggression were accompanied by increases in cooperation. Observers were blind to the experimental conditions. Subsequent training of the control children led to reduced aggression in these children as well. No follow-up assessment was reported in the study.

Unfortunately, not every ICPS-oriented intervention effort with children "at risk" has had beneficial results. One particualarly noteworthy failure was reported by Sharp (1981), who attempted to replicate the findings of Spivack and Shure (1974) while eliminating and/or controlling for earlier methodological problems. Nursery school teachers were not used as trainers. They were told only that participants would be meeting daily with project staff as part of a special program designed to enrich language, number, and thinking skills. University graduate students led the training sessions. Teachers were blind as to which children received the actual treatment program. Finally, teacher ratings of classroom behavior were supplemented by blind observers' ratings of social interaction during play periods. Fifty-four black, low-income nursery school children were assigned to one of three experimental conditions: (1) the original 46-session training program designed by Spivack and Shure (1974); (2) a modified training program that substituted games, songs, and story-telling exercises for the first 12 lessons that are concerned with language concepts in the original program; or (3) a cognitive enrichment program emphasizing language skills and number concepts. Posttesting indicated that initially maladjusted children who received the complete training program made the greatest gains in alternative thinking, although no training effects on consequential thinking were apparent. Otherwise, results differed sharply from those reported by Spivack and Shure (1974). The number of trained children who improved behaviorally did not differ significantly from the number who deteriorated over the same period. Similarly, observational findings suggested that general activity levels, as well as aggression and dominance, increased from pretest to posttest for both adjusted and aberrant children across all three conditions.

A 6-month follow-up of this sample is reported by Rickel, Eshelman, and Loigman (1983). Blind teacher ratings of behavioral adjustment and ratings by an independent classroom observer continued to show no significant training effects at the 6-month follow-up. The differential effect for generating alternatives had also disappeared by the time of follow-up. The authors suggest that sustained behavior change in young children may not be mediated through a strictly cognitive intervention, and may more logically require a better integration of behavioral and cognitive techniques.

This discrepancy in results is puzzling and may be accounted for by several factors, as Sharp (1981) herself points out. For example, Spivack and Shure (1974) may have been misled by their failure to supplement teacher reports of behavior with actual behavioral observations or other unbiased sources of data. On the other hand, the lack of behavioral improvement in the Sharp (1981) study may be attributed to the failure to provide children with *in vivo* or real-life experience and reinforcement of problem-solving strategies, because the classroom teacher was not the primary trainer (a central component of the original Spivack and Shure program). Training teachers themselves in the use of ICPS skills prior to instruction of the children may be an important factor in ensuring effective teacher modeling of skills and application to real-life problems that come up day to day with children.

Vaughn, Ridley, and Bullock (1984) found that an interpersonal problem-solving training program was successful in increasing the total number of problem solutions and cooperative responses in a group of aggressive preschoolers. Children were evaluated on the Behavioral Interpersonal Problem Solving Test, which assesses a child's ability to generate solutions to actual interpersonal problems with a peer (a confederate to the experimenter, who role plays a part in set problem situations). The experimental group received problem-solving skills training, whereas the control group had an equal amount of contact with the experimenter and peers acting out stories with puppets. Results indicated that children trained in interpersonal problem-solving skills acquired the ability not only to generate a greater number of responses but also to persist in the task and generate more relevant responses than controls. A 3-month follow-up indicated maintenance of their gains.

School-Age Children

Similar to findings using their preschool curriculum, Shure and Spivack (1979) report positive effects for ICPS training with 74 black children attending inner-city kindergartens. Prior to treatment, teachers rated 16 of these youngsters as impulsive and aggressive, 4 as inhibited, and 54 as well adjusted. Thirty-nine of the experimental children had previously participated in the nursery school training program. The concepts taught were essentially the same in both years, although the content was more sophisticated for the older children. Posttesting indicated that children trained for the first time during kindergarten improved relative to a matched no-treatment control group on tests of alternative and consequential thinking. Seventy percent of initially maladapted children were rated by teachers to be adjusted following training in kindergarten, in comparison only 6% of maladapted control children ($p < .01$). Moreover, 2 years of training generally resulted in significantly greater cognitive gains that did one year of training occurring in either nursery school or kindergarten, although 2 years of cognitive training did not appear to yield additional gains in behavioral adjustment relative to one year of training. Unfortunately, once again, no attention control group and no blind evaluation of social-behavioral adjustment was included.

Allen *et al* (1976) reported on the results of an ICPS intervention program (24 sessions of 30 minutes each) with third- and fourth-grade elementary school children in a normal school setting. The intervention made use of modeling and role play techniques. Exercises were included for teaching divergent thinking (e.g., brainstorming alternative uses for an object), problem identification (e.g., the teacher helped clarify the problem in a series of unfinished problem stories), alternative thinking, consequential thinking, and elaboration of solutions. Alternative solutions and consequences were discussed with respect to common interpersonal problems that arise in school, and children were encouraged to give one another feedback about the adequacy of various solutions. Results of the program indicated that the trained children improved over a no-treatment group on a cognitive problem-solving measure and in their number of solutions to a simulated real-life problem (the experimenter suggests playing a game with the child, but the experimental room is occupied). Trained children also improved on a locus-of-control scale in the direction of increased feelings of internal control over the environment. However, no effect of training was evident on ratings of behavioral adjustment on the Walker Problem Behavior Checklist or on a sociometric measure of peer status. Whether the lack of enhancement of adjustment following training was due to the insensitivity of the measures, to the intractability of behavior problems among the 9-year-olds, or to the weakness of the intervention is not known.

In a study by McClure, Chinsky, and Larcen (1978), an elaborated version of the same training program was evaluated. Four experimental conditions were used: (1) videotape modeling only, (2) videotape plus discussion, (3) videotape modeling plus role played exercises, and (4) a no-treatment control group. McClure *et al.* found that the training conditions generally enhanced internal locus-of-control scores on a cognitive problem-solving test, and performance on a structured group peer interaction measure, the Friendship Club Interaction (FCI). For the FCI, children where asked to participate in a Friendship Club contest, in which an award was promised to the team that gave the best answers to a series of contest questions. In addition to contest questions, the children were confronted with a number of actual problems embedded in the FCI setting. These additional problems included: (1) five chairs for six students (chair problem), and (2) five officer cards for six students (missing role problem), and (3) the problem of how to distribute officer titles (role distribution problem). The entire procedure was videotaped and scored for problem-solving responses. McClure *et al.* (1978) did not include measures of overt behavioral adjustment in their study, but the FCI would appear to be a promising analogue measure for assessing problem solving in a structured real-life situation. Results indicated that video modeling combined with role play exercises led to higher scores for the per interaction measure (FCI) than did the other three conditions. The findings thus suggested that problem-solving training that combines both observational learning (modeling) and behavior rehearsal (role play) may be more likely to transfer to everyday social interactions.

Weissberg *et al.* (1987b) devised six parent training sessions to support children's use of ICPS skills acquired in the course of a 52-lesson, school-based training program. Participants included a group of black, inner-city, lower-class third-graders, as well as a group of white, suburban, middle-class youngsters, in order to compare directly the effectiveness of such training with different socioeconomic groups. The structured curriculum was presented in lessons of 20 to 30 minutes each, four times per week, for 13 weeks. Teachers conducted the training and were assisted by undergraduate aides for two of the four lessons each week. There were 16 90-minute training workshops for teachers to discuss and role play each week's lesson. The following problem-solving steps were taught:

1. Look for signs of upset feelings.
2. Say exactly what the problem is.
3. Decide on your goal.
4. Stop and think before you act.
5. Think of as many solutions as you can.
6. Think ahead to what might happen next.
7. When you have a good solution, try it.
8. If your first solution doesn't work, be sure to try again.

Results indicated that both groups improved with training on a variety of cognitive problem-solving tests. In addition, trained children tried more solutions and persisted longer than controls in a simulated real-life problem situation. Behavioral adjustment findings, however, were more complex and disconcerting. In the suburban sample, trained children improved more than the no-treatment control group on teacher ratings of social-behavioral problems (e.g., reduced inattention and acting out) and competencies (e.g., enhanced assertiveness and frustration tolerance), although adjustment and ICPS test gains were not correlated. By contrast, teacher-rated data suggested that the same training program may have had a negative impact on the urban children, since these trained children *declined* significantly on five of nine behavior rating dimensions. Such findings were unexpected in that the urban group also acquired the cognitive ICPS skills, and previous ICPS interventions with inner-city children have yielded significant gains in teacher-rated adjustment (Elardo & Caldwell, 1979; Spivack & Shure, 1974). Teacher reactions to the training program itself help to clarify the adjustment findings. Weissberg *et al.* (1981b) report that experimental teachers in the suburban schools felt that brainstorming alternative solutions helped children to express ideas more creatively. Urban teachers, on the other hand, found that the same process produced mostly aggressive solutions and, in the process, negatively affected class discipline. One such teacher expressed her discomfort with the program at the outset and implemented it only reluctantly. Such expectations (positive and negative) may have introduced bias into teacher-based outcome ratings. Such detrimental effects were not reflected in measures of self-esteem, trait anxiety, or sociometric status, in which no experimental–control group differences were apparent.

The following studies examine more closely the complex issue of "linkage," or relationship between cognitive skills gains and actual behavioral improvement. In a subsequent study, Weissberg *et al.* (1981a) modified their ICPS curriculum in an attempt to meet the needs of urban inner-city teachers and children. For example, a stronger emphasis was placed on classroom management strategies to encourage children to apply new problem-solving concepts to everyday conflict situations. The program itself was implemented earlier in the school year, although it was trimmed to 42 lessons. Again, samples were drawn from suburban and inner-city schools, although on this occasion second-, third-, and fourth-grade classrooms participated in the training venture. This time results indicated that training improved the problem-solving skills and teacher-rated social behavior of suburban *and* urban experimental children relative to no-treatment control group. The possibility of rating bias, however, still cannot be ruled out. Moreover, no significant effects were noted with regard to peer sociometric ratings. Finally, correlations between the 6 ICPS measures and the 11 behavior change scores were either weak or nonsignificant. In other words, the children who acquired new cognitive problem-solving skills over the course of training may not have been the same children who made behavioral gains. Similar findings were reported by Winer, Hilpert, Gesten, Cowen, and Schubin (1982), who adopted Spivack and Shure's (1974) training program for use with predominantly white kindergarten children from suburban middle-class families. Program children gave significantly more, and better, solutions, and fewer irrelevant responses on cognitive ICPS assessments. They also improved more than a no-treatment group on several teacher-rated dimensions of behavioral adjustment. Direct correlations between increased ICPS skills and adjustment gains, however, were generally not found.

Alvarez, Cotler, and Jason (1984) also demonstated improved cognitive problem-solving test performance following a 10-week social problem-solving program with fourth-grade children. Relative to a no-treatment control group, the trained group learned to generate more alternative solutions to problems and to anticipate the consequences of these solutions. No training effects were found on classroom behavioral observations, or on sociometric or self-esteem measures. Since the children were trained by psychology graduate students with undergraduate assistants, it is possible that the children did not receive the necessary real-life practice and reinforcement in the classroom that the teacher might have provided as trainer. The finding is reminiscent of Sharp's (1981) results with a preschool group. It might also be unrealistic to expect meaningful and lasting changes in social behavioral adjustment with a just a 10-week training program. Urbain (1980) was also relatively unsuccessful in using a short-term (11-session) intervention to intervene with second- and third-graders identified by teachers as impulsive and aggressive with peers. In this study, a behavioral intervention procedure (contingency management) was compared with two different cognitive approaches (ICPS plus self-instructional training; social perspective taking plus self-instructional training). Training was carried out by the investigator and undergraduate psychology students in small-group setting outside the classroom. As in Sharp's (1981) study, no provision was made for *in vivo* training, and posttesting indicated little specificity of outcome. All three training conditions led to improvement on cognitive problem-solving and role-taking measures, whereas none produced overall improvement in teacher-rated behavior. Nevertheless, a moderate relationship was obsereved between behavioral improvement and improvement on the ICPS measures.

Elardo and Caldwell (1979) reported more positive findings from their multifaceted training efforts with fourth- and fifth-grade children in a predominantly middle-class school. Problem-solving components of their 56-lesson curriculum focused on formulating alternatives to social problem situations through role-play and discussion. Other facets of the program were designed specifically to enhance the children's ability to identify emotions and to foster their awareness of their own thoughts and feelings and those of others. Outcome data suggested that experimental children improved more than no-treatment controls on measures of cognitive role taking and alternative thinking, as well as on ratings of social behavior. Although once again teachers served as both program implementors and evaluators, links found between cognitive and behavioral gains suggested that the beneficial results of training were real. Unfortunately, it is not clear what specific aspects of the training curriculum itself might have been responsible for such gains.

Elias (1983) found positive behavioral changes using ICPS training combined with televised prosocial peer modeling with a group of emotionally and behaviorally disordered boys (ages 7 to 15). Despite some positive behavior adjustment changes, the intervention did not yield changes in locus-of-control or self-concept measures relative to a no-treatment control group. Elias *et al.* (1986) also recently reported on the positive impact of a preventive interpersonal problem-solving intervention, the Improving Social Awareness Social Problem Solving (ISA-SPA) project, on children coping with the stresses of transition to middle school. The following steps for critical problem-solving thinking were used.

1. Look for signs of different *feelings.*
2. Tell yourself what the *problem is.*
3. Decide on your *goal.*
4. Stop and *think of as many solutions as you can.*
5. For each solution, *think of all the things that might happen next.*

6. Choose your *best solution*.
7. *Plan* it out, make a *final check*.
8. Try it and *rethink* it.

Training was conducted by fifth-grade teachers in the classroom setting, using a curriculum consisting of 20 lessons of approximately 40 minutes each, conducted twice per week. Training also included an application phase in which teachers were provided with specific activities designed to bring problem solving into the regular classroom routine. Sample application activities included use of a classoom problem-solving chart, a student's personal problem-solving notebook, and methods for the teacher to dialogue with students to facilitate the student's own independent problem-solving thinking rather than stepping in and providing teacher solutions to the problem. Results indicated greater positive adjustment on a Survey of Middle School Stressors for the full training group compared to a no-treatment or a partial curriculum condition. There was also evidence linking adjustment to performance on cognitive problem-solving measures.

Camp, Blom, Herbert, and Van Doorninck (1977) reported on the effects of a program entitled Think Aloud (Camp & Bash, 1986), which combines self-instructional and ICPS training in a 30-session program for aggressive elementary school-age boys. Classroom teachers served both as program implementors and evaluators. Training took place in small groups. Emphasis was placed on modeling of cognitive strategies and developing answers to four basic questions: "What is my problem?" "What is my plan?" "Am I using my plan?" "How did I do?" Initially to engage the children in the process of rehearsing the self-instructions, a "copycat" game was used in which the children repeated self-statements modeled by the experimenter. The copycat procedure was gradually phased out, and the child was encouraged to verbalize his or her own strategy silently. The training content for social problem solving consisted of a sequenced series of games providing practice in identifying emotions (happy, sad, mad, scared), considering "what might happen next" in various situations (consequential thinking), and generating multiple alternatives in a given situation. The trainer also suggested that "thinking out loud" could help in the classroom, and asked the children to think of ways they could use "thinking out loud" in doing their schoolwork and in getting along with others. Role play was not used. Posttesting indicated that both trained and untrained control children decreased in aggression ratings, although only trained children showed significant increases in prosocial behavior as well. This relative behavioral advantage following training, however, occurred without demonstrable improvements in alternative thinking. The investigators noted that frequent disruptions of training sessions by experimental children may have interfered with the learning of problem-solving concepts, thereby limiting the effectiveness of the intervention program. The need for a firm behavioral control system as an adjunct to the cognitive training with aggressive children was noted.

The potential preventive impact of ICPS training is best examined when longer term follow-up data are collected. For example, Gesten *et al.* (1982) had teachers administer a 17-lesson ICPS program to suburban, middle-class second- and third-graders. Results indicated that the full training program resulted in greater ICPS gains than did either an abridged version of the same program or a no-treatment control condition. Moreover, children receiving the full program showed the greatest problem-solving persistence on a posttreatment stimulated problem situation. Gains in teacher-rated or peer-rated social adjustment were not evident immediately following treatment. Control group children, however, appeared to deteriorate over the following year in comparison to trained children. At follow-up one year later, trained children exceeded controls on 7 of 10 social competence and pathology factors, as rated by new teachers who were unaware of the previous training. In addition, sociometric findings indicated that experimental children liked their peers more and were more accepted by peers than children who were not trained.

Some additional studies also deserve mention here. Rotheram *et al.* (1982) administered an assertiveness-training program with a group problem-solving component to 343 normal fourth- and fifth-grade children. Intervention procedures were administered by graduate and upper-level undergraduate students for 2 hours per week for 12 weeks in groups of six pupils each. Assertiveness and teacher ratings of comportment and achievement were higher for the training group than for either a no-treatment group or an attention control group in which children played a modified simulation of the "College Bowl" game on TV. Trained children also showed higher quality of alternatives on an interpersonal problem-solving measure and a group decision task. Grade point averages increased for the pupils in the assertiveness group at one year following the intervention.

Lochman, Curry, Burch, and Lampron (1984), used social problem solving and cognitive-behavioral techniques for coping with anger with 76 boys ages 9 to 12. Trained children improved on parent reports of aggression and behavioral observations of disruptive and off-task behavior, but not on teacher behavior ratings or on a peer sociometric measure. A reduction in impulsive and aggressive behavior using a cognitive self-control and problem-solving approach was also reported by Pitkanen (1974), Schneider (1974), and Robin, Schneider, and Dolnick (1976).

Mannarino, Duriak, Christy, and Magnussen (1982) demonstrated improved peer sociometric status following a social problem-solving intervention with six 8-year-old children identified as at risk on the basis of teacher ratings. No measures of problem-solving ability were used, however, so it is difficult to establish the link between improved problem-solving skills and social status improvements.

Finally, a number of additional studies have demonstrated improvement on cognitive problem-solving tests following ICPS training interventions (Houtz & Feldheusen, 1976; Russell & Roberts, 1979; Stcifvater, Kurdek, & Allik, 1986; Stone, Hinds, & Schmidt, 1975). Actual behavioral adjustment, however, was not measured in the studies.

Adolescent Studies

A number of studies of ICPS training effects have also been conducted with adolescents. Social problem-solving training (recognizing and defining the problem, generating and evaluating solutions, developing a plan) was employed in conjunction with training of concrete conversational skills to improve the social skills of shy adolescents ages 12 to 14 by Christoff et al. (1985). A group training procedure was employed over eight sessions. Following intervention, the students' daily interactions with peers increased (self-recorded), reports of social interaction skill were more positive, and students displayed more positive patterns of self-evaluation. Results at a 5-month follow-up indicated that gains were maintained. However, the independent treatment effects of problem-solving training versus conversational skill training could not be determined.

Marsh, Serafica, and Barenboim (1980) studied the effect of perspective-taking training on the ability of eighth-graders to solve interpersonal problems. Subjects in the experimental group participated in role-playing experiences, including role play/role switch, videotape playback, and discussion. During training, each subject had the occasion to play two different roles and to observe other role plays. After subjects viewed the videotaped role plays, a discussion followed, centered on the thoughts, feelings, perceptions, intentions, and so forth among story characters and on the results when different people played the same roles, the same person played different roles, or the roles were played by males versus females. A control group spent a comparable amount of time in regular curriculum activities with the experimenter. Subjects were pre- and posttested on measures of means ends interpersonal problem analysis, and social and affective perspective taking. Results suggested that training had a significant positive effect on subjects' performance on the interpersonal problem analysis measure. The study thus offers evidence for a relationship between perspective-taking training and performance on a measure of interpersonal problem solving. Unfortunately, no behavioral outcome measures were included in this study.

Sarason and Sarason (1981) used live modeling (experimental group 1) or videotape modeling (experimental group 2) and role playing in an attempt to increase the cognitive and social skills of students (mean age 14.8 years) in an urban high school with high dropout and delinquency rates. Subjects tended to be low achievers with low academic motivation. Experimental groups received 13 class sessions focused on decision making, in which behavior and cognitions were modeled. Thinking about consequences, alternatives, understanding of others, and communication skills was emphasized. Trainers first determined skills their subjects lacked, than wrote scripts for role plays incorporating these skills. Models for the student roles were chosen from the school, with the graduate student experimenters playing the adult roles. Subjects watched the role play (live or video), summarized and discussed what they had viewed, and then role played the situation themselves. In addition, after each of the training sessions, subjects were required to complete a 5-minute homework assignment consisting of a problem situation and questions. Quizzes were given midway and again at the end of training. The control group participated in regular health care of discussions. Subjects in both experimental groups were able to think of more adaptive ways to respond to problem situations and were better able than controls to present themselves effectively in a job interview situation. Experimental subjects also showed lower rates of tardiness and fewer absences and behavior referrals at a one-year follow-up.

Weissberg and Caplan (1988) recently examined the effects of a social problem-solving intervention with young adolescents ($N = 421$, grades 5–8). The 16-lesson program, implemented by teachers in the normal classroom setting, emphasized application to the actual classroom environment through teacher–student "dialoguing" about real-life problems using the social problem-solving model. The teacher also stressed to the students that he or she was available to discuss problems if a student wished to do so. A problem-solving essay was used as an adjunctive measure for handling actual school problem behavior. Problem-solving steps included:

1. *Stop, calm down and think* before you act.
2. Say the *problem* and how you *feel*.
3. Set a positive *goal*.
4. Think of lots of *solutions*.
5. Think ahead to the *consequences*.
6. *Go* ahead and *try* the best *plan*.

In contrast to a no-treatment group, the trained group improved at posttesting in both number and quality of alternative solutions on cognitive problem-solving measures, as well as on teacher ratings of self-control. The trained students also showed a lower level of self-reported delinquent acts. On a sociometric measure of peer status, however, no change was found, suggesting that modification of peer status may require application of general social problem-solving skills to more specific domains of peer-related behavior (i.e., making conversation, entering a group, responding to peer provocation, etc.).

A variety of attempts have been made to teach ICPS skills to seriously disturbed or maladjusted young people. The majority of these training studies have taken place in institutional settings. For example, Ollendick and Hersen (1979) identified 36 incarcerated juvenile delinquents with an external locus of control. Subjects matched on age (age range 13–16 years) and IQ were assigned randomly to either a social skills or a discussion group. Subjects in the social skills training condition were instructed to bring to the group problems they were having with each other and with the staff. Alternative ways of responding were devised and modeled by the therapist and by other group members. After rehearsing the situation themselves, subjects received feedback on their performance as well as social reinforcement for problem-solving thinking and behavior. Members of the discussion group were also instructed to bring their problems to the group, but training was limited to discussion about ways to circumvent the problems at hand. The social skills group reported a lowered level of state anxiety following treatment, as well as a more internal locus of control. Moreover, this group demonstrated significantly greater improvement than did the discussion-only group on measures of eye contact, requests for new behavior, latency of responding, and decreased aggression in a series of role-played situations. Finally, the social skills group earned more points for appropriate behavior in the institutional token economy system. However, they showed only a nonsignificant trend toward a decrease relative to the discussion group in the number of acting-out behaviors (insubordination and fighting) observed during a 2-week follow-up period. Unfortunately, it is not possible to separate out the remedial effects of ICPS training in this study from the effects of other, simultaneously applied training strategies (e.g., social reinforcement and direct coaching of appropriate behavior). Since no attention-control group was employed, it is also unclear to what extent adjustment changes can be attributed to nonspecific treatment factors (e.g., subject motivation, exposure to multiple assessments, and therapist attention). Finally, since the investigators failed to assess ICPS abilities before and after treatment, one cannot be certain (1) that the youngsters targeted for training in fact had cognitive deficits in interpersonal problem solving underlying their obvious behavioral deficits; (2) that they acquired these cognitive skills in the course of the training; and (3) that behavioral changes actually were mediated by such cognitive skill acquisition.

Similar methodological problems characterize the efforts of Sarason (1968) and Sarason and Ganzer (1968, 1973), who incorporated a major cognitive problem-solving component in their social skills program for institutionalized delinquents (ages 15–18). Unlike Ollendick and Hersen (1979), however, these investigators found that modeling and discussion approaches had equally positive effects. Counselors' ratings of prosocial and negative behaviors similarly improved for the two treatment groups relative to a non-treatment control condition. Unfortunately, one cannot rule out the possibility of rater bias in this case, since counselors also were responsible for the implementation of training. More convincing evidence of treatment effectiveness came from improved self-descriptions and more internal locus-of-control ratings for both treatment groups relative to controls, as well as decreased recidivism a full 2 to 3 years following treatment.

Hains (1984) attempted to improve the problem-solving performance of four adolescents (ages 14–17) on hypothetical social problems and then examine generalizability of these skills to solving actual social problems encountered by the subjects during the study. The children were adjudicated delinquents living in the same group home. They were introduced to problem-solving steps and had them modeled by the experimenter during individual sessions where they had to solve hypothetical dilemmas. Each youth was encouraged to use the problem-solving steps during sessions and in solving his own social problems outside of sessions. The assessment of actual problem solving was conducted through interview and self-recording procedures. Under training conditions all four students generally showed an increase in their ability to solve hypothetical dilemmas. However, results indicated only a small amount of transfer to actual social problems for two of the youths, and this was not consistently maintained. It is possible that generalization effects were limited by the brevity of training and the lack of *in vivo* training.

DISCUSSION

The results of ICPS training studies to date should be viewed with cautious optimism. Serious methodological problems exist in the literature, such as the lack of optimal control groups, inadequate assessment of actual behavioral change, lack of blind assessment procedures, and limited availability of long-term follow-up data. Nonetheless, the available data suggest that a variety of approaches are effective for teaching ICPS skills to children. Positive results have been reported for training efforts differing broadly in intensity and complexity. Beginning as early as nursery school (Spivack & Shure, 1974), children have demonstrated the capacity to improve their performance on measures of cognitive problem solving. Moreover, both normal (Winer et al., 1982) and socially maladjusted children across a wide IQ range (Shure & Spivack, 1979) have been able to learn such skills. Classroom teachers (Allen et al., 1976), parents, (Shure & Spivack, 1978), and clinically experienced investigators (Urbain, 1980) have all been successful at fostering such cognitive gains.

Although ICPS training appears to offer a useful methodology for intervention with children and adolescents, it is nevertheless clear that newly acquired cognitive skills do not generalize automatically into more adaptive social behavior (Sharp, 1981). A number of studies have failed to find significant generalization of cognitive skill improvements to actual social–behavioral adjustment (Allen et al., 1976; Alvarez et al., 1984; Sharp, 1981; Winer et al., 1982). Taken as a whole, however, the data do suggest that ICPS training can have beneficial effects going beyond improved cognitive test performance. A number of studies report generalization of training effects to relevant behavioral situations, including associated decreases in impulsive and aggressive behavior, and increases in prosocial and cooperative behavior (Camp, et al., 1977; Elardo & Caldwell, 1979; Elias, 1983; Gesten et al., 1982; Spivack & Shure, 1974; Weissberg, 1981a). Moreover, although long-term follow-up data are sparse, some initial findings suggest significant holding power for behavioral treatment effects, at least in the early years (Gesten et al., 1982; Shure & Spivack, 1978). Some important factors in producing generalization of training probably include length/intensity of training and guided opportunity for children to practice problem-solving skills in real-life situations and to receive *in vivo* reinforcement for their problem-solving efforts. This goal might best be met by maximizing the involvement in training of significant adults in the child's life (e.g., teachers, parents) and of other peers for modeling and/or reinforcement of skills.

Also of particular importance the need for future research to identify the active ingredients of complex, multifaceted training programs that are responsible for reported treatment effects. The use of more optimal control groups is essential to demonstrate what aspects (e.g., generating alternatives, evaluating consequences, identifying emotions, social–causal reasoning, etc.) of a problem-solving training approach are truly essential. Wherever possible, the use of attention control groups to control for nonspecific treatment factors (e.g., adult attention, expectancy for change, special-group membership) is indicated. Alternative treatment or component contrast groups may be required for longer term intervention programs, in which a strict attention control group may not be possible (O'Leary & Borkovec, 1978).

Future studies would also benefit from more systematic inclusion of multiple measures (i.e., self-report, teacher and parent ratings, peer sociometrics, behavioral observations) for assessing a broader range of both cognitive and behavioral outcomes of intervention. To confirm that the cognitive components of the interventions are important in producing behavioral change, assessments and evaluations of both cognitive processes and behavior are essential (Kendall & Hollon, 1981; Kendall & Korgeski, 1979).

Significant difficulties exist, however, in the realm of social problem-solving skill assessment. Unfortunately, no problem-solving assessment device has been adequately validated to date. Current approaches are diverse, and each has its own set of advantages and limitations (for a review, see Krasnor & Rubin, 1981). Observational strategies represent a particularly promising new approach, although they are time-consuming, costly, and variable in their rate of data acquisition. In one of the few studies designed to provide normative data on naturalistically occurring social problem-solving behavior in young children, Krasnor & Rubin (1983)) observed 15 preschoolers for 5 hours each. They recorded 6,338 social problem-solving (SPS) attempts by the children and coded the attempts for target, strategy, goal, and outcome. They found that the children's SPS attempts were successful approximately 57% of the time. Sharp (1983) also used naturalistic observation methods to examine preschoolers' behavior during their attempts to gain, maintain, and regain materials, space, and peers' attention/interaction in the classroom. Results indicated that "most" and "least" socially competent preschoolers differed in the types of strategies used to solve interpersonal problems, but not in the number of ways they attempted to solve problems or in the number of times they encountered problems. "Most" competent children used more verbal and prosocial strategies, as opposed to the "least" competent children, who tended to use more nonverbal and antisocial strategies. Normative data like these can provide guidelines for ICPS training. Though probably not suitable for prevention studies, where it is generally necessary to assess large numbers of children in as efficient a way as possible, observational methods may be ideal for the periodic evaluation of randomly selected individuals in the course of training. In this way, it may be possible to determine whether newly taught cognitive skills are being implemented effectively in social interactions.

Developmental Considerations

Eisenberg and Harris (1984) discuss the importance of a developmental perspective in research focused on social competence. They review studies that indicate developmental changes in cognitive and affective role taking and in children's conceptions of friendship. Children increase in their understanding of others' intentions, motives, and thoughts from preschool through adolescence. Affective role-taking ability also increases with age. Concepts of friendship move from a self-centered outlook to a reciprocal mutual view and from momentary acts to enduring relationships. Eisenberg and Harris (1984) suggest that different skills or processes may emerge as mediators of social competence with age. Thus, developmental changes should be a major concern in interpersonal problem-solving research.

As children move through the preadolescent period, the influence of sociometric status on peer relationships seems to increase. Norms and standards of the peer group become clearer, and children become more peer-oriented (Bowerman & Kinch, 1959). Sociometric status becomes more stable, and there is greater consensus about the reputation of each group member (Horrocks & Buker, 1951). Thus, for this age agroup, a successful intervention may have to be directed at the peer group as well as the child. After treatment, peers' responses to the target child's behavior, as well as the child's behavior itself, should be measures of treatment success.

Mahoney and Nezworski (1985) challenge the theoretical status of traditional rationalistic cognitive treatments, and argue that cognitive-behavioral approaches need to move in the direction of more developmental, process-oriented conceptualizations and research. Kazdin (1982) argues that for cognitive-behavioral intervention results to be clear and unified, more information is needed about the relationship between basic cognitive processes and different behaviors at different ages. Brion-Meisels and Selman (1984) have made a start by examining developmental changes in adolescents' ability to create and use interpersonal negotiation strategies in social interactions. In their work, they describe four levels of interpersonal negotiations: (1) unreflective physical strategies, (2) one-way commands or obedience, (3) reciprocal exchanges, and (4) mutual collaboration. They propose that each new level of negotiation strategy is related to adolescents' developmental ability to view themselves in broader social contexts and relationships. Findings from their research suggest that interventions were most effective when they were designed to move a student operating at one level up to the next closest stage of interpersonal negotiation. Thus, assessment of the adolescents' developmental level was of importance to successful intervention.

Expectancies and Attributions

Sobol, Earn, Bennett, and Humphries (1983) studied three groups of elementary school–age children to assess their social attributions, social self-esteem, and expectation of social success. The groups were learning-disabled children, control children of low peer acceptance, and control children of high acceptance among peers as rated by teachers. An open-ended interview format was used in which 12 social situations were presented that varied according to outcome (success or no success) and according to who initiated the social activity (the child or a peer). The learning-disabled group used luck more frequently and personality factors less frequently than the control groups to explain outcomes. Expectations of social success were lowest in the group of learning-disabled children. Both the learning-disabled and the low-acceptance groups had lower self-esteem scores than did the high-acceptance group. An important consideration when designing a social problem-solving intervention for learning-disabled children, then, would be the advisability of addressing and attempting to modify the child's attribution of success from luck to effort. Earn and Sobol (1984) found developmental differences in the interpretation of social causes among children ages 8 to 17, with the same causes having different meanings for children of different ages. Compared with the older groups, the youngest children saw luck as more stable and more controllable, but effort as less controllable. Consideration of these developmental differences would be important when designing SPS interventions, because children's beliefs about social causes very likely will affect outcomes of treatment. For example, Bugental and colleagues (Bugental, Whalen, & Henker, 1977; Bugental, Collins, Collins, & Chaney, 1978) found that children's attributional style affected the outcomes of a cognitive-behavioral program for hyperactive children—that is, children who tended to attribute causes to internal factors such as effort or ability (as supposed to external factors such as luck or chance) also benefited more from the cognitive-training program. Children with a more external orientation benefited more from a more standard behavioral reinforcement intervention. For further discussion of attributional and expectancy effects with children, see Pearl (1985) and Braswell, Koehler, and Kendall (1985).

CONCLUSION

It should be clear at this point that numerous problems and questions have yet to be adequately addressed in the ICPS literature. Future studies will also have much to tell us about the exact nature of the relationship among the different ICPS skills, and about the antecedent life experiences crucial to their development in children. For example, initial research efforts point to an important relationship between parental problem-solving skills and child-rearing attitudes on the one hand, and the problem-solving skills and solution preferences of preschool children on the other (Jones *et al.*, 1980; Shure & Spivack, 1978; Spivack *et al.*, 1976). Clearly, many significant and possibly prototypical interpersonal problems arise in the family unit. However, Youniss (1980) has argued that fundamental differences exist in the structure of parent–child and child–child relationships and that different rules or conventions govern them. In the parent–child dyad, conflicts are frequently resolved unilaterally, with decisions emanating more often from parents. In the child–child dyad, conflicts tend to be resolved reciprocally, at least by middle childhood when friendships blossom. Thus, principles of problem solving among family members may not transfer readily to the peer group. Nevertheless, a direct comparison of the therapeutic effectiveness of peer group and family training approaches would be enlightening.

Although ICPS training is sensible and appealing as a social skills training approach, outcome data indicate that its successful application is a matter of considerable complexity. A program's content and mode of presentation may differentially affect its outcome depending on the age and sociodemographic attributes of the target population (Weissberg *et al.*, 1981b). For example, the nonevaluative approach to ICPS training may be initially (if not persistently) disruptive in inner-city school settings, where a greater premium is placed on behavioral control than on self-expression. Family-based ICPS training may be most effective in early childhood, but less effective than peer-based training in middle childhood and adolescence, when the changing nature of peer relations requires greater reciprocity. Such parameters must be better understood if the promise of this approach to remediation and prevention is to be realized.

REFERENCES

Allen, G., Chinsky, J., Larcen, S., Lochman, J. E., & Selinger, H. (1976). *Community psychology and the schools: A behaviorally oriented multilevel preventive approach.* Hillsdale, NJ: Lawrence Erlbaum.

Alvarez, J., Cotler, S., & Jason, L. A. (1984). Developing a problem-solving program in an elementary school setting. *Education, 104*, 281–286.

Aronson, E. (1978). *The jigsaw approach.* Beverly Hills, CA: Sage Publications.

Asher, S. R. (1978). Children's peer relations. In E. Lamb (Ed.), *Social and personality development.* New York: Holt, Rinehart & Winston.

Aspy, D. (1972). *Toward a technology for humanizing education.* Champaign, IL: Research Press.

Bandura, A. (1977). *Social learning theory.* Englewood Cliffs, NJ: Prentice-Hall.

Bessell, H., & Palomares, V. H. (1967). *Methods in human development.* San Diego, CA: Human Development Training Institute.

Bickel, W. E., & Bickel, D. D. (1986). Effective schools, classrooms, and instructions: Implications for special education. *Exceptional Children, 52*, 489–500.

Bower, E. (1965). Primary prevention of mental and emotional disorders—a frame of reference. In N. Lambert (Ed.), *The protection and promotion of mental health in the schools.* Public Service Publication No. 1126, U.S. Department of Health, Education and Welfare, Bethesda, Maryland.

Bowerman, C. E., & Kinch, J. W. (1959). Changes in family and peer orientation of children between the fourth and tenth grades. *Social Forces, 37,* 206–211.

Braswell, L., Koehler, C., & Kendall, P. C. (1985). Attributions and outcomes in child psychotherapy. *Journal of Social and Clinical Psychology, 3,* 458–465.

Brion-Meisels, S., & Selman, R. L. (1984). Early adolescent development of new interpersonal strategies: Understanding and interventions. *School Psychology Review, 13,* 3, 278–291.

Bugental, D. B., Collins, S., Collins, L., & Chaney, L. K. (1978). Attributional and behavioral changes following two behavioral management interventions with hyperactive boys: A follow-up study. *Child Development, 49,* 247–250.

Bugental, D. B., Whalen, C. K., & Henker, B. (1977). Causal attributions of hyperactive children and motivational assumptions of two behavior change approaches: Evidence for an interactionist position. *Child Development. 48,* 847–884.

Camp, B., & Bash, M. (1986). *Think Aloud: Increasing social and cognitive skills—A problem-solving program for children, primary level.* Champaign, IL: Research Press.

Camp, B., Blom, G., Herbert, F., & Van Doorninck, W. J. (1977). "Think Aloud": A program for developing self-control in young aggressive boys. *Journal of Abnormal Child Psychology, 5,* 157–168.

Canfield, J., & Wells, H. (1976). *100 ways to enhance self-concept in the classroom.* Englewood Cliffs, NJ: Prentice-Hall.

Caplan, G. (Ed.). (1961). *Prevention of mental disorders in children.* New York: Basic Books.

Carnegie Forum on Education and the Economy. (1986). *Report of the Task Force on Teaching as Profession,* P.O. Box 157, Hyattsville, MD 20781.

Cartledge, G., & Milburn, J. F. (Eds.). (1980). *Teaching social skills to children: Innovative approaches.* New York: Pergamon Press.

Chittenden, G. E. (1942). An experimental study in measuring and modifying assertive behavior in young children. *Monographs of the Society for Research in Child Development, 7* (1, Serial No. 31).

Christoff, K. A., Scott, W. O. N., Kelley, M. L., Schlundt, D., Baer, G., & Kelly, J. A. (1985). Social skills and social problem-solving training for shy young adolescents. *Behavior Therapy, 16,* 468–477.

Clabby, J. F., & Elias, M. J. (1986). *Teach your child decision-making.* New York: Doubleday.

Combs, M. D., & Slaby, D. A. (1978). Social skills training with children. In B. Lakey & A. Kaydin (Eds.), *Advances in child clinical psychology.* (Vol. 1). New York: Plenum Press.

Cooper, S., Munger, R., & Ravlin, M. M. (1980). Mental health prevention through affective education in schools. *Journal of Prevention, 1,* 24–34.

Coopersmith, S. (Ed.). (1976). *Developing motivation in children.* San Francisco: Albion.

Cowen, E. L. (1973). Social and community interventions. *Annual Review of Psychology, 24,* 423–472.

Cowen, E. L. (1977). Baby-steps toward primary prevention. *American Journal of Community Psychology, 5,* 1–22.

Cowen, E. L. Pederson, A., Babigian, H., Izzo, L. D., & Trost, M. A. (1973). Longterm follow-up of early detected vulnerable children. *Journal of Consulting and Clinical Psychology, 41,* 438–446.

Davis, G. (1966). Current status of research and theory in human problem-solving. *Psychological Bulletin, 66,* 36–54.

Dewey, J. (1910). *How we think.* Boston: Heath.

Dodge, K. A., & Frame, C. M. (1982). Social cognitive biases and deficits in aggressive boys. *Child Development, 53,* 620–635.

Duncan, C. P. (1959). Recent research on human problem solving. *Psychological Bulletin, 56,* 397–429.

D'Zurilla, T., & Goldfried, M. (1971). Problem solving and behavior modification. *Journal of Abnormal Psychology, 78,* 107–126.

Earn, B. M., & Sobol, M. P. (1984). *Developmental differences in the interpretation of social causes.* Paper presented at the Annual Convention of the American Psychological Association, Toronto, August.

Eisenberg, N., & Harris, J. D. (1984). Social competence: A developmental perspective. *School Psychology Review, 13*(3), 267–277.

Elardo, P. T., & Caldwell, B. M. (1979). The effects of an experimental social development program on children in the middle childhood period. *Psychology in the Schools, 16,* 93–100.

Elias, M. J. (1983). Improving coping skills of emotionally disturbed boys through television-based social problem solving. *American Journal of Orthopsychiatry, 53,* 61–72.

Elias, M. J., Gara, M., Ubriaco, M., Rothbaum, P. A., Clabby, J. F., & Schuyler, T. (1986). Impact of a preventive social problem solving intervention of children's coping with middle school stressers. *American Journal of Community Psychology, 14,* 259–275.

Fagen, S. A., Long, M. J., & Stevens, D. J. (1975). *Teaching children self-control: Preventing emotional and learning problems in the elementary school.* Columbus, OH: Merrill.

Feshbach, N. D. (1983). Learning to care: A positive approach to child training and discipline. *Journal of Child Clinical Psychology, 12,* 266–271.

Feshbach, N., Feshbach, S., Fauvre, M., & Campbell, M. (1983). *Learning to care.* New York: Scott, Foresman.

Gagne, R. M. (1970). *The conditions of learning.* New York: Holt, Rinehart & Winston.

Gazda, G. M., Asbury, F. R., Balzer, F. J., Childers, W. C., Desselle, E., & Walters, R. P. (1973). *Human relations development: A manual for educators.* Boston: Allyn and Bacon.

Gazda, G. M., & Brooks, D. J., Jr. (1985). The development of the social/life-skills training movement. *Journal of Group Psychotherapy, Psychodrama, and Sociometry,* Spring, 1–12.

Gesten, E. L., Rains, M. H., Rapkin, B. D., Weissberg, R. P., Fores de Apodaca, R., Cowen, E. L., & Bowen, R. (1982). Training children in social problem-solving competencies: A first and second look. *American Journal of Community Psychology, 10,* 95–115.

Glasser, W. (1969). *Schools without failure.* New York: Harper & Row.

Goodlad, J. I. (1984). *A place called school.* New York: McGraw-Hill.

Gordon, T. *Teacher effectiveness training.* New York: Wyden. 1974.

Gresham, F. M. (1981). Social skills with handicapped children: A review. *Review of Educational Research, 51,* 139–176.

Gresham, F. M. (1982). Misguided mainstreaming: The case for social skills training with handicapped children. *Exceptional Children, 48*, 422–433.

Gresham, F. M. (1984). Social skills assessment and training. In J. E. Ysseldyke (Ed.), *School psychology: The state of the art* (pp. 57–80). National School Psychology Inservice Training network, University of Minnesota, Minneapolis.

Gresham, F. M. (1985). Utility of cognitive-behavioral procedures for social skills training with children: A critical review. *Journal of Abnormal Child Psychology, 13*, 411–423.

Hains, A. A. (1984). A preliminary attempt to teach the use of social problem-solving skills to delinquents. *Child Study Journal, 14*(4), 271–285.

Harter, S. (1982). The perceived competence scale for children. *Child Development, 53*, 87–97.

Harter, S. (1985). Processes underlying the construction, maintenance, and enhancement of the self concept in children. In J. Sulls & A. Greenwald (Eds.), *Psychological Perspectives On the Self* (Vol. 3). Hillsdale, NJ: Lawrence Erlbaum.

Hartup, W. (1980). Peer relations and family relations: Two social worlds. In M. Rutter (Ed.), *Scientific foundations of developmental psychiatry*. London: Heinemann.

Hartup, W. W. (1983). Peer relations. In E. M. Heatherington (Ed.), *Socialization, personality, and social development*. Volume 4 of P. H. Mussen (Editor-in-Chief), *Handbook of child psychology*. New York: Wiley.

Horrocks, J. E., & Buker, M. E. (1951). A study of the friendship fluctuations of preadolescents. *Journal of Genetic Psychology, 78*, 131–144.

Houtz, J., & Feldhusen, J. (1976). The modification of fourth graders' problem solving abilities. *Journal of Psychology, 93*, 229–237.

Jahoda, M. (1953). The meaning of psychological health. *Social Casework, 34*, 349–354.

Jahoda, M. (1958). *Current concepts of positive mental health*. New York: Basic Books.

Janes, C., Hesselbrook, V., Meyers, D., & Penniman, J. (1979). Problem boys in young adulthood: Teachers' rating and 12-year follow-up. *Journal of Youth and Adolescence, 8*, 453–472.

Janes, C. L., Hesselbrook, V. M., & Schectman, J. (1980). Clinic children with poor peer relations: Who refers them and why. *Child Psychiatry and Human Development, 11*, 113–125.

Johnson, D. W., & Johnson, R. T. (1975). *Learning together and alone: Cooperation, competition, and individualization*. Englewood Cliffs, NJ: Prentice-Hall.

Johnson, D. W., & Johnson, R. T. (1986). Mainstreaming and cooperative learning strategies. *Exceptional children, 52*, 553–561.

Johnson, R. J., & Johnson, D. W. (1983). Effects of cooperative, competitive, and individualistic learning experiences on social development. *Exceptional Children*, January, 323–329.

Johnson, W., & Johnson, R. (1979). Conflict in the classroom: Controversy and learning. *Review of Educational Research, 49*, 51–70.

Jones, D. C., Rickel, A. V., & Smith, R. L. (1980). Maternal child rearing practices and social problem solving among preschoolers. *Developmental Psychology, 16*, 241–242.

Kazdin, A. E. (1982). Current developments and research issues in cognitive-behavioral interventions: A commentary. *School Psychology Review, 11*(1), 75–82.

Kendall, P. C., & Braswell, L. (1985). *Cognitive behavioral therapy for impulsive children*. New York: Guilford Press.

Kendall, P. C., & Hollon, S. D. (1979). Cognitive behavioral intervention: Overview and current status. In P. C. Kendall & S. D. Hollon (Eds.), *Cognitive-behavior interventions: Theory, research, and procedures.* New York: Academic Press.

Kendall, P. C., & Hollon, S. D. (1981). *Assessment strategies for cognitive behavioral interventions.* New York: Academic Press.

Kendall, P. C., & Korgeski, G. P. (1979). Assessment and cognitive-behavioral interventions. *Cognitive therapy and Research, 3,* 1–21.

Krasnor, L. R., & Rubin, K. H. (1981). The assessment of social problem-solving skills in young children. In T. Merluzzi, C. Glass, M. Genest (Eds.), *Cognitive assessment.* New York: Guilford Press.

Krasnor, L. R., & Rubin, K. H. (1983). Preschool social problem solving: Attempts and outcomes in naturalistic interactions. *Child Development, 54,* 1545–1558.

Laughlin, F. (1954). *The peer status of sixth- and seventh-grade children.* New York: Bureau of Publication, Teachers College, Columbia University.

LeCroy, C. (Ed.). (1983). *Social Skills Training for Children and Youth.* New York: Haworth Press.

Lochman, J. E., Curry, J. F., Burch, P. R., & Lampron, L. B. (1984). Treatment and generalization effects for cognitive-behavioral and goal-setting interventions with aggressive boys. *Journal of Consulting and Clinical Psychology, 52,* 915–916.

Long, B. (1970). A model for elementary school behavioral science as agent of primary prevention. *American Psychologist, 25,* 571–574.

Mahoney, M. J., & Nezworski, M. T. (1985). Cognitive-behavioral approaches to children's problems. *Journal of Abnormal Child Psychology, 13,* 467–476.

Mannarino, A. P., Durlak, J. A., Christy, M., & Magnussen, M. G. (1982). Evaluation of social competency training in the schools. *Journal of School Psychology, 20,* 11–19.

Marsh, D. T., Serafica, F. C., & Barenboim, C. (1980). Effect of perspective-taking training on interpersonal problem-solving. *Child Development, 51,* 140–145.

Mattox, B. (1975). *Getting it together: Moral dilemmas for the classroom.* San Diego, CA: Pennant Press.

Meyers, J., Parsons, R. D., & Martin, R. (1979). *Mental heatlh consultation in the schools.* San Francisco: Jossey-Bass.

McClure, L., Chinsky, J., & Larcen, S. (1978). Enhnacing social problem-solving performance in an elementary school setting. *Journal of Educational Psychology, 70,* 504–513.

Minuchin, P., Biber, B., Shapiro, E., & Zimules, (1969). *The psychological impact of the school experience.* New York: Basic Books.

Muma, J. R. (1965). Peer evaluation and academic performance. *Personality Guidance Journal, 44,* 405–409.

Muma, J. R. (1968). Peer evaluation and academic achievement in performance classes. *Personality Guidance Journal, 46,* 580–585.

Northway, M. L. (1944). Outsiders: A study of the personality patterns of children least acceptable to their age mates. *Sociometry, 7,* 10–25.

Ojemann, R. (1961). Investigation into the effects of teaching understanding and appreciation of behavior. In G. Caplan (Ed.), *Prevention of mental disorders in children.* New York: Basic Books.

O'Leary, K. D., & Borkovec, T. D. (1978). Conceptual, methodological, and ethical problems of placebo groups in psychotherapy research. *American Psychologist, 33,* 821–830.

Ollendick, T. H., & Hersen, M. (1979). Social skills training for juvenile delinquents. *Behavior Research Therapy*, *17*, 547–554.

Pearl, R. (1985). Cognitive-behavioral interventions for increasing motivation. *Journal of Abnormal Child Psychology*, *13*, 443–454.

Pellegrini, D. S. (1985). Training in social problem-solving. In M. Rutter & L. Hersov (Eds.), *Child and adolescent psychiatry: Modern approaches* (2nd ed.). London: Blackwell.

Pellegrini, D. S., & Urbain, E. S. (1985). An evaluation of cognitive problem-solving training with children. *Journal of Child Psychology and Psychiatry*, *26*, 17–41.

Pitkanen, L. (1974). The effect of simulation exercises on the control of aggressive behavior in children. *Scandinavian Journal of Psychology*, *15*, 169–177.

Porterfield, O. V., & Schlichting, G. F. (1961). Peer status and reading achievement *Journal of Education Research*, *54*, 291–297.

Raths, L., Harmin, M., & Simon, S. (1966). *Values and teaching: Working values in the classroom.* Columbus, OH: Merrill.

Rickel, A., Eshelman, A. K., & Loigman, G. A. (1983). Social problem solving training: A follow-up study of cognitive and behavioral effects. *Journal of Abnormal Child Psychology*, *11*, 15–28.

Robin, A., Schneider, M., & Dolnick, M. (1976). The turtle technique: An extended case study of self control in the classroom. *Psychology in the Schools*, *13*, 449–453.

Roff, M., Sells, S. S., & Golden, M. M. (1972). *Social adjustment and personality development in children.* Minneapolis: University of Minnesota Press.

Rotheram, M. J., Armstrong, M., & Bodraem, C. (1982). Assertiveness training in fourth- and fifth-grade children. *American Journal of Community Psychology*, *10*, 567–582.

Rotter, J. B. (1954). *Social learning and clinical psychology.* Englewood Cliffs, NJ: Prentice-Hall.

Russell, M. L., & Roberts, M. S. (1979). Behaviorally-based decision-making training for children. *Journal of School Psychology*, *17*, 264–269.

Rutter, M. (1983). School effects on pupil progress: Research findings and policy implications. *Child Development*, *54*, 1–29.

Sarason, I. G. (1968). Verbal learning, modeling, and juvenile delinquency. *American Psychology*, *23*, 254–266.

Sarason, I. G., & Ganzer, V. J. (1969). Developing appropriate social behaviors of juvenile delinquents. In J. Krumholtz & C. Thorensen (Eds.), *Behavior counseling cases and techniques.* New York: Holt, Rinehart & Winston.

Sarason, I. G., & Ganzer, V. J. (1973). Modeling and group discussion in the rehabilitation of juvenile delinquents. *Journal of Consulting Psychology*, *20*, 442–449.

Sarason, I. G., & Sarason, B. R. (1981). Teaching cognitive and social skills to high school students. *Journal of Consulting and Clinical Psychology*, *49*(6), 908, 918.

Sarason, S. B. (1971). *The culture of the school and the problem of change.* Boston: Allyn and Bacon.

Schneider, M. (1974). Turtle technique in the classroom. *Teaching Exceptional Children*, *8*, 22–24.

Schneider, M., & Robin, A. (1979). *Turtle Manual.* Unpublished manual, Psychology Department, State University of New York, Stony Brook.

Sharp, K. C. (1981). Impact of interpersonal problem-solving training on preschoolers' social competency. *Journal of Applied Developmental Psychology*, *2*, 129–143.

Sharp, K. C. (1988). Quantity or quality of strategies: Which indicates competency in social problem-solving? ERIC Document 241188, PS 014260, April.

Shure, M. B., & Spivack, G. (1978). *Problem-solving techniques in childbearing.* San Francisco: Jossey-Bass.

Shure, M. B., & Spivack, G. (1979). Interpersonal cognitive problem-solving and primary prevention: Programming pre-school and kindergarten children. *Journal of Clinical Child Psychology, 2,* 89–94.

Sobol, M. P., Earn, B. M., Bennett, D., & Humphries, T. (1983). A categorical analysis of the social attributions of learning-disabled children. *Journal of Abnormal Child Psychology, 11,* 2, 1983, 217–228.

Spivack, G., Platt, J., & Shure, M. (1976). *The problem-solving approach to adjustment.* San Francisco: Jossey-Bass.

Spivack, G., & Shure, M. B. (1974). *Social adjustment in young children.* San Francisco: Jossey-Bass.

Spivack, G., & Spotts, J. (1966). *Devereux Child Behavior Rating Scale manual.* Devon, PA: Devereux Foundation.

Steifvater, K., Kurdek, L. A., & Allik, J. (1986). Effectiveness of a short-term social problem-solving program for popular, rejected, neglected, and average fourth grade children. *Journal of Applied Developmental Psychology, 7,* 33–43.

Stone, G., Hinds, W., & Schmidt, G. (1975). Teaching mental health behaviors to elementary school children. *Professional Psychology, 6,* 34–40.

Strain, P. S., & Odom, S. L. (1986). Peer social initiation? Effective intervention for social skills development of exceptional children. *Exceptional Children, 52,* 543–551.

Suomi, S. J. (1980). Peers, play, and primary prevention. In M. W. Kent & J. E. Rolf (Eds.), *Primary prevention of psychopathology: III. Social competence in children* Hanover, NH: University Press of New England.

Tyne, T. F., & Flynn, J. T. (1979). The remediation of elementary school children's low social status through a teacher-centered consultation program. *Journal of School Psychology, 17,* 244–254.

Urbain, E. S. (1985). *Friendship group manual (elementary grades) (Interpersonal problem-solving training for friendship-making).* St. Paul, MN: Eugene S. Urbain, Wilder Child Guidance Center.

Urbain, E. S. (1980). *Interpersonal problem-solving training and social perspective-taking with impulsive children via modeling, role play, and self-instruction.* Unpublished Doctoral dissertation, University of Minnesota.

Urbain, E. S., & Kendall, P. C. (1980). A review of social-cognitive problem-solving approaches to intervention with children. *Psychological Bulletin, 88,* 109–143.

Van Hasselt, V. B., Hersen, M., Whitehall, M. D., & Bellack, A. S. (1979). Social skill assessment and training for children: An evaluative review. *Behavior Research and Therapy, 17,* 413–437.

Vaughn, S. R., Ridley, C. A., & Bullock, D. D. (1984). Interpersonal problem-solving skills training with aggressive children. *Journal of Applied Developmental Psychology, 5,* 213–223.

Weissberg, R. P., & Caplan, M. (1988). *The evaluation of a social competence promotion program with young, urban adolescents.* Manual submitted for publication.

Weissberg, R. P., Gesten, E., Lieberstein, N., Schmid, K., & Hutton, H. (1980). *The Rochester Social Problem-Solving (SPS) Program: A training manual for teachers of 2nd–4th grade children.* Rochester, NY: Primary Mental Health Project.

Weissberg, R. P., & Gesten, E. L. (1982). Considerations for developing effective school-based social problem-solving (SPS) training programs. *School Psychology Review, 2,* 56–63.

Weissberg, R. P., Cowen, E. L., Lotyczewski, B. S., & Gesten, E. L. (1983). The primary mental health project: Seven consecutive years of program outcome research. *Journal of Consulting and Clinical Psychology, 51,* 100–107.

Weissberg, R. P., Gesten, E. L., Carnrike, C. L., Toro, P. A., Rapkin, B. D., Davidson, E., & Cowen, E. L. (1981a). Social problem-solving skills training: A competence-building intervention with 2nd–4th grade children. *American Journal of Community Psychology, 9,* 411–424.

Weissberg, R. P., Gesten, E. L., Rapkin, B. D., Cowen, E. L., Davidson, E., Flores de Apodaca, R., & McKim, B. (1981b). Evaluation of a social problem-solving training program for suburban and inner-city third-grade children. *Journal of Consulting and Clinical Psychology, 49,* 251–261.

Winer, J. I., Hilpert, P. L., Gesten, E. L., Cowen, E. L., & Schubin, W. E. (1982). The evaluation of a kindergarten social problem solving program. *Journal of Primary Prevention, 2,* 205–216.

Youniss, J. (1980). *Parents and peers in social development.* Chicago: University of Chicago Press.

Ysseldyke, J. E. (Ed.). (1984). *School psychology: The state and the art.* National School Psychology Inservice Training Network, University of Minnesota, Minneapolis.

Zahavi, S., & Asher, S. R. (1978). The effect of verbal instructions on preschool children's aggressive behavior. *Journal of School Psychology, 16,* 146–153.

APPENDIX: SAMPLE INTERPERSONAL COGNITIVE PROBLEM-SOLVING (ICPS) TRAINING ACTIVITIES

Some Practical Problem-Solving Training Tips

Introduce problem-solving concepts in a nonthreatening way (through enjoyable learning activities and exercises) before application to real-life problem situations.

It is important to guide children through the *application* of problem-solving concepts in real-life problem situations if skill generalization is to occur. Problem-solving "dialoguing" with a child in actual problem situations is essential.

There are times when use of the problem-solving dialoguing approach is *not* indicated. For example, if children are very unruly or are fighting, it is necessary to separate them first before asking them to state the problem; or if a child is extremely upset, reflecting feelings and being emotionally supportive may be necessary rather than trying to generate alternatives immediately (Weissburg & Gesten, 1982).

Problem-solving intervention is not a substitute for reasonable behavioral limits and consequences for disruptive behavior. Problem-solving dialogue is best initiated in the initial escalation phase of a conflict (if one can catch the problem early) or after disciplinary consequences have been administered for disruptive behavior (i.e., for verbally processing the situation after a child has calmed down and for discussing alternatives to prevent a recurrence).

Problem-solving interventions work best in a school climate of effective staff organization and supportive interpersonal relationships among school staff. A classroom climate conveying the message that "each child is an important member of the class," as well as positive modeling of reinforcement and compliments by the teacher, are important if children are to apply problem-solving concepts effectively. Children must sense that staff are committed to take the time necessary to discuss real problems as they come up.

Aggressive children often overinterpret other people's actions and intentions as being personally hostile to them; that is, they often feel attacked when this is not necessarily the case (Dodge & Frame, 1982). It may be necessary to acknowledge an aggressive child's feelings and check for distorted interpretations before proceeding with further problem-solving steps.

Do not cognitively overload children with too many problem-solving steps. Introduce feelings identification and consequential and alternative thinking concepts in simple language for preschoolers and young children (e.g., "Tell me a word that says how you feel," "What might happen next if you say or do _____?" "Is there something different you could say or do to make _____ happen?" Teaching means–ends thinking (step-by-step means to a goal) may become more important as children develop more cognitively (late elementary grades and up).

Use multisensory learning aids (key words such as "stop and think," a problem-solving chart, a stop sign, cue cards with pictures representing each problem-solving step, etc.).

Sample Problem-Solving Sequence (for Problem-Solving Dialoguing with a Child)

Stop and think.
Say your feelings and the other person's feelings.
Say what the problem is.
Say what your goal is. What is it you want to happen? (*Note*: Clarify and redirect goal if inappropriate).
Think of different ideas to solve the problem.
  What is something different you could say or do? What might happen next if you do _____?
  Would anyone be unhappy with this idea?
  What else can you think of?
Make a plan. What idea are you going to try first?
  What will you do if your first idea doesn't work?
  (Have a back-up plan).

Problem-Solving Essay

Describe the problem (What happened? What did you do? What did other people do?)

Feelings (How did you feel and why? How did the other person(s) feel and why?)

I felt _____ because

_____

The other people felt _____ because

_____

Consequences (Why was your behavior against the rules? What might happen if this wasn't a rule?)

Choices (List three different things you could do next time that might solve the problem if it happens again.)

1.

2.

3.

Plan: If a situation like this happens again, which idea will you try to solve the problem?

What idea will you try next if this one doesn't work?

PART FOUR
Indirect and Preventive Services

18
COGNITIVE-BEHAVIORAL APPROACHES IN PSYCHOEDUCATIONAL CONSULTATION

JOEL MEYERS
GLENN YELICH
State University of New York at Albany

Psychoeducational consultation has been described as an indirect approach to the delivery of psychological services in which one professional (the consultant) helps another professional (the consultee) provide psychoeducational services to a student (the client) who is the consultee's responsibility (Curtis & Meyers, 1985; Meyers, Parsons, & Martin, 1979). Cognitive-behavioral theory has a number of important implications for the practice of consultation.

Cognitive-behavioral theory is summarized throughout this book, and two points are particularly important for this chapter: (1) Since cognitive events can mediate behavior, a focus on cognitions can be an effective approach to changing behavior, and (2) the individual is an active participant who can exercise control in his or her own learning. Further, this approach implies reciprocal relationships between cognitions, behavior, and the environment.

Cognitive-behavioral theory has important implications for both the process and the content of consultation. The *content* of consultation includes the referral problems discussed in consultation and the approaches recommended by the consultant and considered by the consultee for modifying the referral problem. The *process* of consultation refers to the problem-solving process that occurs between the consultant and consultee, and the nature of the interaction between consultant and consultee. Most of the chapters in this book consider the ways in which cognitive-behavioral approaches can be used to help solve a variety of children's learning and adjustment problems (e.g., impulsivity, depression, anxiety, interpersonal problem solving, effects of mild handicaps, problems with arithmetic and reading). These are each related to the content of consultation. Because these issues are covered thoroughly in the remainder of this book, this chapter will not consider the content of consultation. It will focus, instead, on the implications of cognitive-behavioral theory for the consultation process, to provide ideas indicating how consultants can use a cognitive-behavioral framework in consultation with educators and parents.

In order to frame the context of this discussion for readers who are unfamiliar with psychoeducational consultation, the next section of this chapter will review the rationale and principles behind the consultation model of service delivery. Subsequent to this review, each of the three major theoretical approaches to educational consultation, namely mental health, behavioral, and organizational development, will be considered. A major purpose of this section will be to compare and contrast the use of the cognitive-behavioral perspective with each of these three models.

These introductory sections will be followed by detailed discussions of those theories that illustrate the implications of the cognitive-behavioral approach for the process of psychoeducational consultation.

AN OVERVIEW OF PSYCHOEDUCATIONAL CONSULTATION

Psychoeducational consultation is an alternative system for the delivery of psychological services in schools. The development of a consultation model for the delivery of psychoeducational services is based on a straightforward rationale encompassing the following points (Meyers, Parsons, & Martin, 1979; Parsons & Meyers, 1984).

1. There are too few mental health professionals available to meet the needs of schoolchildren with learning and adjustment problems.
2. Psychoeducational services may be most effective when they are provided in the learning environment by the educational professional (generally the teacher) who has the most regular contact with the student.
3. By intervening in an indirect manner, consultants can maximize their effectiveness and achieve their goal of reducing the numbers of children experiencing learning and adjustment problems in schools. For example, if particular teachers and/or schools tend to refer children with similar problems, consultation may increase the effectiveness with which the educators work with these children, and this in turn might reduce the future development of such problems.

Although many psychologists have contributed to the development of psychoeducational consultation using various theoretical perspectives (e.g., Alpert & Meyers, 1983; Alpert et al., 1982; Bergan, 1977; Caplan, 1970; Conoley, 1981; Curtis & Meyers, 1985, Curtis & Zins, 1981; Fullan, Miles, & Taylor, 1980; Gutkin & Curtis, 1982; Schmuck & Miles, 1971), the following six characteristics have been identified as common across definitions and theories (Meyers, Parsons, & Martin, 1979):

1. It is a helping or problem-solving process.
2. It occurs between a professional help-giver (a consultant) and a help-seeker (a consultee), who has responsibility for the welfare of another person (a client).
3. It is a voluntary relationship.
4. The help-giver and the help-seeker share in solving the problem.
5. The goal is to help solve a current work problem of the help-seeker.
6. The help-seeker profits from the relationship in such a way that future problems may be handled more sensitively and skillfully (p. 4)

In accordance with the first of the six characteristics cited, consultation can be broadly construed as a problem-solving process, which, in turn, consists of a sequence of stages.

Most theoretical models of consultation describe a similar sequence of stages; in fact, Meyers, Parsons, and Martin (1979) describe a series of stages that can be used in consultation regardless of the theoretical model. Although they are described here as discrete stages, in practice they do not necessarily occur in this fixed order. Depending on the problem, a consultant might use more than one stage simultaneously or might move back and forth between stages. The consultation process is best viewed as a dynamic, interactive process, which uses these stages as needed. For the purposes of this discussion, six consultation stages will be described briefly: (1) entry, (2) goal identification, (3) goal definition, (4) intervention planning and implementation, (5) impact assessment, and (6) conclusion of the relationship.

Stage 1: Entry

The consultant initiates consultation by developing an agreement with the organization as well as with the particular consultee(s) who will receive consultative services. Generally, the consultant is likely to be viewed with suspicion and defensiveness because the need for consultation often implies a weakness on the part of the consultee. Therefore, it is important that from the outset the consultant devote energy to establishing a positive and trusting relationship with the consultee. This can be initiated by developing a clear agreement about what will occur during consultation (i.e., a contract). Entry is typically a focus of the first interview with the consultee.

Stage 2: Goal Identification

In addition to establishing a contract and beginning to develop a positive relationship, the first consultation interview often seeks to identify the consultation goal(s), a prerequisite to goal attainment. At this stage the consultant surveys the consultee's perceived needs and interests in an effort to determine jointly the general goals of consultation. Although the focus at this stage is on the work to be done and the goal to be achieved, it is not wise, initially, to use formal data collection procedures. Instead, the consultee has an opportunity to discuss concerns freely in the context of the consultation interview. A major goal at this stage is to determine whether the primary focus of consultation will be at the level of the institution, the educator/consultee, or the student. Given the preventive goals of consultation and the effort to influence the largest possible number of students, the goal is to intervene at the level that provides the greatest leverage for promoting the learning and adjustment of children in school. Thus, other things being equal, the first priority is to intervene at a systemic or organizational level within the school as an institution, the second priority is to offer services focused directly on problems of the consultee or classroom, and the third priority is to offer services focused directly on the referred student (e.g., Meyers, Parsons, & Martin, 1979; Parsons & Meyers, 1984).

Stage 3: Goal Definition

Once it is determined whether consultation should focus on the organization, the consultee, or the student, and once a general goal has been identified as the focus for consultation, it is important to define the consultation goal in concrete detail. Like goal identification, the process of goal definition uses data-gathering procedures; this process, however, involves more narrow, specific, and detailed data, which are needed to develop a clear definition of the consultation goal. A variety of more formal assessment procedures may be used at this stage, and there is a focus on the perceptions and cognitions of the consultee and perhaps on those of the client or other relevant educational personnel as well.

Stage 4: Developing and Implementing the Interventions

Cognitive-behavioral theory suggests that behavior change requires the consultee's active participation, and therefore it can be important to initiate a process in which the consultee's contributions to development of the intervention plan is at least equal to that of the consultant. This can be accomplished by establishing the attitude that there are alternative approaches to the goal. Rather than accepting the first recommendation, the consultee should be encouraged to use brainstorming techniques to seek alternative approaches. In addition to developing the best approach to attaining this particular goal, the brainstorming process will increase the consultee's general skills at developing interventions that may transfer to other situations where the consultee does not have the consultant's support. As the consultee becomes more effective as an independent problem solver through the consultation process, the preventive educational goals of consultation are supported, in that there is an increased likelihood that other children will profit from these emerging skills of the consultee in the future.

Stage 5: Assessing Impact

Assessing impact provides an objective basis for determining when it is necessary to modify interventions that have not been effective, and to provide positive reinforcement when interventions have been effective. Data demonstrating the efficacy of consultation provide a strong empirical basis for continuing the consultative model. This can be important in systems that are suspicious of and resistant to this approach to service delivery. Because consultation interventions may focus on a variety of cognitive and behavioral outcomes, it is important to use assessment procedures focused on each.

Stage 6: Concluding the Relationship

The last stage in the consultation process is to conclude the relationship. One potential pitfall in effective consultation is that the consultee can develop feelings of dependency on the consultant. This can interfere with the educative/preventive goals of consultation, which require the consultee to function independently as a problem solver in the future. It is, therefore, important for the consultant to plan deliberately for and establish a clearly defined point of termination for the consultation relationship. Concluding the relationship can be a renewing experience for the consultee if it is done in an effort to summarize consultation by highlighting the consultee's key accomplishments.

The problem-solving process that takes place within the consultation relationship shares some similarities with certain cognitive-behavioral interventions, such as self-instructional and problem-solving training. These strategies, which are based on the cognitive-behavioral principle of cognition mediating behavior, emphasize the role of self-control via self-talk. Hence, as cognitive-behavioral interventions teach structured problem-solving processes to clients, the process of consultation proceeds according to a similar structured problem-solving approach. In turn, the consultee, like the client in the previously cited example, learns to approach future work problems with a more systemic, efficient problem-solving approach. We will now turn to a consideration of the theoretical models used to conceptualize the consultation process.

THEORETICAL MODELS OF CONSULTATION

Although a variety of approaches to consultation have been presented in the literature (e.g., Conoley, 1981), the three most prominent theoretical models have been mental health consultation, behavioral consultation, and organizational development consultation (e.g., Alpert & Meyers, 1983; Conoley, 1981).

Each of these models is based on different theories of behavior change, which, in turn, means that each model utilizes different techniques and approaches in order to facilitate behavior change. Each theory is reviewed briefly in terms of its implications for the consultation process based on an earlier, more detailed presentation (e.g., Meyers, Alpert, & Fleisher, 1983), and this framework is used to illustrate that cognitive-behavioral approaches have implications for processes occurring within different models of consultation.

Mental Health Consultation

Mental health consultation, which emerged largely from the work of Gerald Caplan (1970), is based on an intrapsychic model of behavior change. This framework suggests that the consultee's underlying feelings must be considered to have a successful impact on the consultee (e.g., the teacher), the referred client (e.g., the student), and future students confronted by this teacher. This intrapsychic perspective is based on four interrelated assumptions (Alpert, 1976):

1. A psychodynamic focus on the consultee can alter the consultee's perceptions.
2. A change in perceptions can result in behavior change.
3. A change in the consultee's behavior will have positive effects on the student's behavior.
4. The consultee's behavior will generalize to future cases.

In addition to intrapsychic factors, mental health consultation considers the impact of socioecological factors in the institution (e.g., Sarason, Levine, Goldenberg, Cherlin, & Bennett, 1966).

This model assumes that a period of time, referred to as the "entry" phase, is necessary to establish the relationship between consultant and consultee. In addition to establishing an effective relationship with the consultee, this period provides an opportunity for the consultant to develop an understanding of the system that will facilitate the development of effective intervention plans. This consultant then uses an understanding of psychodynamic factors affecting the consultee to alter the consultee's perceptions of the problem. This can be done through instruction, role modeling, support and encouragement, and ventilation of feelings (Alpert, 1976). A particular characteristic of mental health consultation is the use of observations and questions to focus on the consultee's feelings in an effort to build the relationship, work through resistance, change the consultee's attitudes and perceptions, and focus the consultee's attention productively on the student's problems. Furthermore, this theoretical model was among the first to describe the potential importance of the collaborative relationship between consultant and consultee (e.g., Caplan, 1970; Meyers, 1973; Meyers, Parsons, & Martin, 1979), which is discussed later in this chapter.

When the model of mental health consultation is compared to cognitive-behavioral theory, a noticeable area of incongruency can be noted regarding the importance placed on the consultee's emotional experience. Within the psychodynamically derived mental health model, affect is theorized as a seminal construct, whereas in a cognitive-behavioral conception, cognition, rather than emotion, is viewed as central to the change process. The role of affect within the mental health approach leads to an emphasis on the consultee's intrapsychic experiences (i.e., unconscious, ego-based transference). By contrast, a cognitive-behavioral perspective recognizes the interactive and mutually dependent roles of cognition, affect, and behavior.

This difference in focus influences practice. For example, the consultant operating from a mental health perspective would consider the initial, rapport-building stages of the consultation relationship as very important; consequently, a great deal of time and energy would be spent at this stage. By contrast, a consultant who was attempting to integrate a cognitive-behavioral perspective into his or her work would anticipate a shorter, more focused entry stage (i.e., with an emphasis on overt behaviors, exploration of cognitions). While recognizing the importance of a "good working alliance" (Deffenbacher, 1985), this consultant would invest relatively more effort in such consultation stages as problem identification and problem definition. There are also numerous similarities between these models, such as an emphasis on collaboration, the use of such techniques as role modeling, and the clarification of cognitions. The important point to underscore here is that a cognitive-behavioral perspective can contribute potentially useful knowledge to consultants who use a mental health orientation.

Behavioral Consultation

Behavioral consultation is based on social learning theory and seeks to understand how antecedents and consequences influence the behaviors of both client and consultee. Human behavior is viewed, further, as resulting from an interaction between the current environment and previously learned behaviors. This frame of reference suggests that the consultant must examine thoroughly the interactions between the client and the environment, between the consultee and the environment, and particularly between the consultee and the client. As in mental health consultation, a basic goal is to facilitate the consultee's development so that he or she becomes more resourceful, self-reliant, and effective in facilitating the present and future learning and adjustment of the student(s).

Intervention in behavioral consultation requires a structured problem-solving process that is similar to the problem-solving stages characteristic of certain interventions (i.e., self-instructional training) derived from cognitive-behavioral theory. This process can be illustrated through five steps. The first step is to observe the behavior, its antecedents, and its consequences in an effort to develop a baseline. The second and third steps are to analyze the data (step 2) and to use this analysis as a basis for setting objectives (step 3). Step 4 is to implement the intervention, and step 5 is to evaluate its efficacy. A variety of behavioral activities can be used to support the consultee through this process; these include modeling, role play, positive reinforcement, stimulus control, and withdrawal of intervention (Meyers, Alpert, & Fleisher, 1983). The consistent use of empirical evaluation based on directly observable behavior is unique to this theoretical model.

It can be argued that cognitive-behavioral theory developed in response to a dissatisfaction with the inability of orthodox behavioral theory to explain behavior and behavior change adequately. The addition of the mediational function of cognition greatly increased the ability of cognitive-behavioral theory to explain and predict behavioral change.

When the behavioral model of consultation is interpreted from a cognitive-behavioral perspective, certain points of continuity and discontinuity become apparent. Behavioral consultation shares many assumptions with a cognitive-behavioral perspective, such as the importance of overt behavior. Consequently, many commonalities will exist between behaviorally derived interventions and those generated from a more cognitive-behavioral perspective, as both would modify the antecedents and consequences of problematic behavior.

The consultant adopting a cognitive-behavioral view, however, will differ from the consultant operating from a strictly behavioral orientation in that they will place a greater emphasis on clients' and consultees' thoughts, beliefs, and attitudes. Consequently, behaviorally trained consultants who are attempting to integrate certain cognitive-behavioral constructions into their work will sometimes try directly to alter cognitive events as a means of effecting behavioral change.

For example, a student who exhibits inattentive, impulsive behavior might be dealt with from a purely behavioral perspective with a contingency contract specifying certain contingencies in response to a targeted behavior. By contrast, the use of a cognitive-behavioral orientation in consultation might result in an intervention that includes a self-talk component for the client (Meichenbaum & Goodman, 1971), which aids in mediating and inhibiting impulsive behavior. Additionally, by attending to the consultee's verbalizations, the cognitive-behaviorally oriented consultant might note certain "irrational" cognitions, (Grieger, 1972), such as, "I can't stand it when Billy doesn't pay attention." In response to this cognitive distortion evidenced by the consultee, the rationale supporting this belief would be collaboratively explored. The expectation would be that after some examination and questioning, consultees might come to modify their expectation of and reaction to off-task behavior exhibited in the future.

Organizational Development Consultation

Like mental health consultation, organizational development consultation considers the influence of socioecological factors as a basis for understanding the function of organizations like schools. Rather than help individuals within the system by changing the consultee's perceptions of the client, the organizational development consultant uses this understanding in an effort to change the system as a whole for the benefit of all those who participate in it. Some of the assumptions underlying school-based organizational development consultation have been summarized by Schmuck (1976):

1. Schools are organizations.
2. Organizations are characterized by roles, norms, and routines that are independent of particular personalities.
3. Change in schools requires attention to this organizational context.
4. Substantial changes in curriculum or instruction imply changes in the roles, norms, and routines that characterize the school.

Organizational development consultation seeks to foster more effective interpersonal communication, to resolve interpersonal and organizational conflict, to promote the development of collective goals, to facilitate effective decision making, and to support organizational efforts to grow and change.

Interventions might teach approaches for effective communication by learning to report both perceptions and feelings to others in the organization. In this context, the organizational consultant can use process observations, surveys, and interviews as a data base for providing feedback to the organization regarding its functioning in terms of roles, communication, leadership, and decision making.

Given that many of the techniques and ideas are applications of social-psychological principles to group dynamics, it is not surprising to note a good deal of congruence when organizational development is considered from a cognitive-behavioral perspective. One similarity is the use of problem-solving techniques in both organizational development and cognitive-behavioral approaches. A more overarching similarity between these two perspectives is the importance placed on the context in which behavior occurs. From a cognitive-behavioral standpoint, cognition is at the center of the person's adaptation to the environment. Organizational development, though acknowledging that individuals construct personal meaning from their interactions with the environment, tends to focus on the importance of intra- and intergroup factors. Hence, although organizational development concepts are useful at a less direct level of consultation, (i.e., service to the organization), cognitive-behavioral conceptions are complementary in that they offer a means by which to consider the individual within the organizational context.

COGNITIVE BEHAVIORAL THEORY AND
THE CONSULTATION PROCESS

Behavioral, organizational, and mental health theories all offer useful perspectives on the process of consultation. A cognitive-behavioral framework, however, affords the practicing consultant some additional techniques and considerations that can be incorporated into the process of consultation. Like the three frameworks of consultation, cognitive-behavioral theories consider the impact of the environment, but this is accomplished by examining the interactive relationships between the person's cognitions, his or her behavior, and the environment. The simultaneous focus on the cognitions and behavior of the individual in an environmental context provides a practical basis for responding to factors that are perceived by educators as real problems. Cognitive-behavioral theory also greatly increases the scope of potential interventions and provides a more accurate conception of the situation by augmenting the number of influence points through this focus on the individual's cognitions and behavior within a systemic context. This provides the consultant with greater flexibility by expanding the number of potential intervention approaches.

Although behavioral theory limits its focus to environmental stimuli such as antecedents and consequences of behavior within a social context, cognitive-behavioral theory considers also the complex cognitive processes individuals use to solve problems. Rather than viewing the individual as a passive respondent to environmental stimuli, the cognitive-behavioral viewpoint considers the complex problem-solving processes that can be applied actively by the individual. Both the mental health and the cognitive-behavioral frames of reference are based on the assumption that the individual's perceptions and cognitions affect behavior. The mental health perspective emphasizes feelings and emotions as the basis for changing perceptions, whereas the cognitive-behavioral perspective emphasizes the individual's thought processes to create this change. The focus on feelings in mental health consultation can be a source of resistance in psychoeducational consultation, which might be less likely to occur when cognitive-behavioral approaches are incorporated in consultation. The cognitive-behavioral emphasis on the individual's thinking processes in problem solving is more compatible with the theory underlying most education, and this may make this theoretical perspective more readily accepted in psychoeducational consultation.

There has been little empirical research on the process of consultation (Parsons & Meyers, 1984). One consistent finding, however, is that collaborative interaction between consultant and consultee relates to successful outome, and it has been argued that collaborative process is effective because it encourages the consultee's active involvement in consultation (e.g., Curtis & Meyers, 1985). This research was stimulated by the literature in mental health consultation, which suggested the importance of a coordinate status between consultant and consultee (Caplan, 1970; Meyers, Parsons, & Martin, 1979), and it provides support for this literature. This research, however, also lends support to cognitive-behavioral theory, which argues that learning, behavior change, and problem solving require active participation by the individual.

A major contention of this chapter is that cognitive-behavioral approaches can be used to expand extant theoretical models of the process of educational consultation. Social-psychological and systemic perspectives are important components of cognitive-behavioral theory with implications for the consultation process. Some of the relevant ideas within these perspectives are considered in the remainder of this chapter.

APPLICATION OF SOCIAL-PSYCHOLOGICAL AND SYSTEMIC MODELS TO THE CONSULTATION PROCESS

> At some point in the consultation process, the consultant attempts to persuade the consultee that the consultant's knowledge and ideas are useful. Thus, consultation can be perceived, at least in part, as persuasion, and the extensive social-psychology literature on attitude change is relevant to this aspect of the consultation process. It is important for consultants to understand the types of persuasion that are most likely to bring positive results and the conditions under which these types of persuasion are most effective. (Meyers, Parsons, & Martin, 1979, p. 45)

The preceding passage indicates that consultation is a process of interpersonal communication and influence. Beyond this point is the fact that in all situations where the provision of mental health services is indirect (including consultation), the service provider (i.e., teacher), not the consultant, will be the person implementing interventions. Therefore, if mental health professionals desire that effective recommendations and/or interventions be carried out by the service provider, it is incumbent that they consider the social-psychological factors that influence their interaction with that individual. This point was recently argued for by Close-Conoley and Gutkin (1986), who maintained that knowledge of social-psychological principles is of seminal importance for all school psychologists. Proceeding from this point, it is the contention of this chapter that social-psychological and systemic conceptions can be usefully incorporated into the interpersonal context that occurs during the process of consultation.

As noted earlier in this chapter, cognitive-behavioral theory suggests that cognitions can influence behavior and that there is a reciprocal relationship between cognitions, behavior, and the environment. Given the reciprocal impact provided by the environment in this model, systemic theories and those that recognize the social context may afford important insight into the determinants of behavior. Social-psychological theory can be particularly relevant to this view of cognitive-behavioral theory, because social psychology conceptualizes the relationship between various social/environmental variables and certain attitudes that can characterize the individual's cognitive frame of reference. Further, consultation approaches based on social-psychological theories of behavior change are particularly compatible with cognitive-behavioral theory in that both theoretical viewpoints emphasize the effects of the individual's perceptions on behavior. Several theories from social-psychological and systemic frameworks have implications for the cognitive-behavioral approach to the consultation process. These include (1) social power, (2) cognitive dissonance, (3) attribution, and (4) systemic theory.

Social Power

French and Raven (1959) identified five types of power that may form the basis for exercising control in social situations: legitimate power, coercive power, reward power, expert power, and referent power. Later, a sixth type, informational power, was presented (Raven, 1965). Martin has argued that expert power and referent power may be relevant to the consultation process (Martin, 1978; Meyers, Parsons, & Martin, 1979), and it has been suggested, further, that informational power may be relevant to consultation (Parsons & Meyers, 1984).

Expert power exists when one person is viewed as having the particular expertise needed to solve another person's problem, and *referent power* is the ability to influence other persons based on the degree to which they identify with or see themselves as having similar characteristics to the first person. *Informational power* occurs when the information provided by one person is viewed as relevant and practical by a second person. This differs from expert power, which is based on the person's characteristics (experience, dress, advanced degree, etc.), in that informational power is based on what the person says. Reward power, coercive power, and legitimate power are not appropriate for a collaborative or a cognitive-behavioral approach to consultation process, because these models would place too much direct control in the hands of the consultant, which might inhibit the consultee's active participation. The other three approaches to social power (expert, referent, and informational) can be appropriate to the cognitive-behavioral and collaborative views of consultation process because these approaches do leave room for the consultee's active involvement.

The consultation literature has devoted more attention to the concept of referent power than to either expert or informational power. The substantial literature demonstrating the impact of collaborative techniques uses approaches that derive from the concept of referent power (e.g., Curtis & Meyers, 1985; Parsons & Meyers, 1984). Expert power and informational power, however, can each facilitate social influence as well. Expert power can be enhanced when the consultant develops a small number of content areas of expertise beyond his or her general training, limits consultation to those cases where he or she possesses expertise, and works with those consultees who attribute relevant expertise to the consultant.

Parsons and Meyers (1984) suggest that consultation may be most effective when there is an appropriate balance between expert and referent power. When there is an imbalance, the consultant may seek to increase the weak source of power and deemphasize the stronger source. These factors are consistent with a cognitive-behavioral perspective in that each of these sources of social influence derives from the cognitive perceptions of the consultee, which can be influenced by the consultant through careful attention to each of these sources of power.

Cognitive-Dissonance Theory

Cognitive-dissonance theory (Brehm & Cohen, 1962; Festinger, 1957; Wicklund & Brehm, 1976) is another social-psychological theory with implications for the consultation process. Because it describes the conditions needed to change the consultee's attitudes, cognitions, and behaviors, this viewpoint is consistent with cognitive-behavioral theory.

It is beyond the scope of this chapter to provide a comprehensive review of cognitive-dissonance theory, which can be obtained elsewhere (Festinger, 1957; Wicklund & Brehm, 1976). Nevertheless, there are some basic ideas that must be understood before considering their application to consultation. Our discussion of these factors is based on Hughes's (1983) presentation. Two cognitions held by an individual can be related in three ways: they can be consonant, dissonant, or irrelevant. Two cognitions are *consonant* when one cognition is consistent with the other. For example, knowing that a teacher teaches social skills (cognition 1) is consistent with the teacher's belief that it is important for children to develop social skills (cognition 2). Two cognitions are *dissonant* when one cognition is incompatible with the second. Knowing that a teacher teaches social skills (cognition 1) is inconsistent with a teacher's belief that schools should only teach the 3 Rs. Finally, two cognitions are *irrelevant* when the first has nothing to do with the second, as is true of most cognitions. The teacher's knowledge that he or she teaches social skills has nothing to do with the teacher's cognition that he or she dislikes sushi.

When a person holds two cognitions that are dissonant, a state of dissonance is created, which produces tension. This tension provides motivation to reduce the dissonance by changing one or both of the cognitions. The amount of this tension depends on the importance of the cognitions and on the proportion of dissonant to consonant cognitions currently held by the individual. Dissonance is at its peak when the importance of the dissonant cognitions is greatest and when there is a large number of dissonant cognitions relative to the number of consonant cognitions. Attempts at dissonance reduction are most likely to be made when there is a greater degree of tension resulting from dissonance. Dissonance can be reduced by adding consonant elements, by changing dissonant elements so they become consonant, by eliminating dissonant elements, and by minimizing the importance of one or more dissonant cognitions (Hughes, 1983).

The individual's approach to dissonance reduction is determined on the basis of how likely it is to succeed. Thus, for example, the individual might try to change the cognition that is most easily modified. When one of the two cognitions is tied directly to behavior, it will be particularly difficult to change. For example, when a teacher has implemented a new social skills curriculum, it is difficult for the teacher to deny that social skills are taught in his or her classroom. Rather than seek to modify the cognition that is tied directly to such a behavior, dissonance reduction is more likely to focus on changing the second cognition, with attitude change as a frequent result.

The application of dissonance theory to the practice of psychology has been reviewed by Brehm (1976), and its application to the consultation process has been discussed by Hughes (1982). Dissonance theory is particularly applicable to the consultation process when the consultant wants the consultee to implement an intervention that is inconsistent with the consultee's attitudes. When the consultee is convinced to try such a counterattitudinal behavior, this may stimulate dissonance; then the consultee will be motivated to reduce dissonance by changing toward attitudes that are more consistent with the new teaching behavior. These attitudes would support and maintain the new behavior, thereby contributing to the long-term efficacy and potential generalization of consultation effects to other similar cases. According to Hughes (1983), three components of cognitive-dissonance theory are most relevant to consultation: (1) choice, (2) justification, and (3) effort.

Maximizing choice is an important consultation strategy, which can help to produce dissonance when two cognitions are discrepant. When the consultee does not perceive a choice regarding a behavioral change that is discrepant with an important attitude, there is little dissonance arousal. Dissonance does not occur under this circumstance because there is no feeling of responsibility for the behavior; and when dissonance arousal does not occur, there is no motivation for attitude change. This principle is congruent with the literature suggesting that consultation must be a voluntary, nonauthoritarian, and collaborative relationship between professional colleagues (e.g., Caplan, 1970; Meyers, Parsons, & Martin, 1979; Schein, 1969). These authors suggest that the consultee must contribute ideas and suggest modifications to the consultant's recommendations, and must be free to accept or reject the consultant's ideas. This choice increases the consultee's feeling of responsibility for behavioral change resulting from consultation. On the basis of these principles, Hughes (1983) suggested that those teacher/consultees offered a high degree of choice will report consultation as more useful and will implement recommendations more frequently than those offered a low degree of choice.

Keeping justification minimal is another process technique that can be used to maximize dissonance in order to increase the probability of attitude change resulting from consultation, whereas strong persuasive efforts may have the opposite effects. More powerful efforts to convince the consultee to engage in counterattitudinal behavior (i.e., strong justification for the behavior change) generally stimulate important cognitions in the consultee that support the commitment to the behavioral change. Although this may seem like a good way to change the consultee's attitude, it is more likely to have the effect of reducing the dissonance aroused initially by the proposed behavior change. Given the reduced dissonance, there would be less motivation for an attitude change.

Therefore, it may be important to avoid strong persuasive arguments by minimizing justification for the behavior change in order to maximize dissonance. At the same time, however, the consultant must use just enough justification to ensure the consultee's cooperation in trying the recommendation. Thus, Hughs (1983) suggests that consultants encourage behavior change while avoiding the temptation of overemphasizing the positive consequence of following their recommendations. Instead, consultants should be tentative when they describe the potential effects of consultation. This principle resulted in the following hypotheses by Hughes (1983): "Teacher-consultees given high justifications (e.g., payment or a promise of success) for trying a new approach with a child will show less attitude change in the direction of support of the new approach than teacher-consultees given low justification for trying a new approach" (p. 354).

Making consultation effortful is another factor from cognitive-dissonance theory that has been applied to the consultation process by Hughes (1983). The more effort required of the consultee, the greater the probability of high levels of dissonance, and this should result in attempts at dissonance reduction. The anticipation of great effort, however, reduces the likelihood that the consultee will actually implement the recommendation. Thus, although the consultant must ensure that the consultee expects that consultation will require considerable hard work, time, inconvenience, and so forth, the consultant must not make this seem so difficult as to inhibit follow-through on the recommendations. This principle has resulted in a third hypothesis by Hughes (1983). Teacher/consultees who are required to use more effort to engage in consultation are more likely to perceive consultation as effective. These teacher/consultees will report that they perceive consultation as more useful and that they implement a new approach more frequently as a result of consultation.

In summary, the most effective consultation process will use minimum justification and will require maximum effort, while still ensuring that the consultee is willing to implement the behavioral recommendation. An effective consultation process also requires the consultant to provide maximum freedom of choice for the consultee. This combination of principles increases the probability that the consultee will actually engage in a behavior change that is counterattitudinal for the consultee. This will stimulate dissonance, and the consultee's efforts to reduce dissonance will increase the probability of attitudinal change necessary if long-term and generalized change is to result from consultation. Although this theory is consistent with collaborative notions about the consultation process, some of its implications for practice are not necessarily intuitive and are not obviously consistent with the consultation literature. At times, for example, a consultant is tempted to provide substantial justification in order to minimize the effort required or to minimize the consultee's choice simply to convince the consultee to engage in the recommended behavior change. It is important for consultants to realize that although this may achieve the desired behavior change in the short run, it will not result in the dissonance reduction and attitudinal change needed for long-term, generalizable results in consultation.

Attribution Theory

Attribution "theory" is something of a misnomer, given that a number of writers in the area of attribution maintain that there is no unified theory of attribution (Harvey & Weary, 1981). Rather, there exist a number of different theoretical approaches to attribution, each of which is limited to somewhat circumscribed contexts. Given space considerations, this section will consider attribution theory as a "set of ideas coming out of research in social psychology which attempts to describe how persons explain their own behavior and the behavior of others in their social environment," (Martin, 1983, p. 35).

Attributions are, by definition, extant in all areas of an individual's life where some interpretation of causation is made. Attributions are cognitive processes that are motivated by the individual's desire to predict and control the environment, and are based on the ability to understand cause–effect relationships (Brehm, 1976). Attributions facilitate judgments regarding why an event was unsuccessful, as well as predictions regarding future success. In essence, attributions can be thought of as hypotheses constructed to explain how and why others and we ourselves behave as we do.

Despite the theoretical diversity alluded to before, certain basic tenets of attributional processes have been identified (Harvey & Weary, 1985). Chief among these tenets are the following:

1. Attribution is a pervasive activity. The individual may engage in attribution spontaneously and/or without conscious recognition.
2. Because of the number and complexity of the factors on which they are based, attributions are not always accurate. Hence, "attributional bias" often exists within an individual's attributional process. Such attributional bias may serve an adaptive function, such as protecting one's self-esteem.
3. Following from the preceding conception of subjective interpretations of reality, attributional conceptions of behavior maintain that people, by and large, behave according to their perceptions and understandings.
4. Attributions serve the needs of adaptation in the sense that they are constructed in such a manner as to facilitate people's feelings of control.

Given that attribution is such a pervasive activity, the application of this approach to the process of consultation is relevant. A cogent point made by Martin (1983), is that each participant in the consultative enterprise (consultant, consultee, client) will construct his or her own attributional system to "explain" events taking place within the social environment. The following comprehensive system of categorization (Frieze, 1980) is considered in an effort to provide a structure for this discussion of attributions.

Frieze contends that the classification of causal attributions can be made on the following three dimensions: (1) internality, (2) stability, and (3) intentionality. *Internality* is concerned with whether the cause of the event is attributed to the individual (i.e., a focus on a trait or characteristic of the person whose behavior is in question as the primary causal agent) or to outside events (i.e., a focus on the environment or situation as the primary causal agent.) *Stability* refers to the degree to which causal factors remain constant or change over time. Whereas ability is a relatively stable factor, for example, effort may be unstable. *Intentionality* is concerned with the degree to which the individual has control over the causal factor. For example, effort would be an intentional causal factor, whereas ability would be considered unintentional in this scheme.

A guiding principle that appears to be at work as the individual assigns attributions to self and others is the need for individuals to maintain the perception of personal control. One result of this dynamic is that individuals tend to assign internal, intentional, and stable attributions (often in the form of personality traits) when explaining the behavior of others, whereas they use external attributions to describe their own behavior ("It depends on the situation") (Nisbett, Caputo, Legant, & Marocek, 1973). This tendency for observers to utilize internal attributions to explain others' behavior and, hence, to underestimate the impact of situational factors, has been termed "fundamental attribution error." Such attributional bias can influence the process of consultation.

Consultation can be conceived of as two sets of interacting pairs: the client–consultee pair and the consultee–consultant pair (Martin, 1983). Within the first dyad, attribution theory predicts that the consultee would attribute the cause of the client's behavior to internal factors. For example, the attribution of "emotional disturbance" would relieve the consultee of having to engage in any critical self-observation as to whether he or she was doing anything that was exacerbating the situation. A clear implication of this finding is that consultants need to be aware that teachers generally will construct internal attributions to explain students' misbehavior or failure to achieve at expected levels (e.g., Medway, 1979). For the consultant, attributions such as "lazy," "disturbed," and "environmentally deprived" have the effect of minimizing the number of potential interventions that can be considered in consultation. Relative to the process of consultation, consultees who demonstrate such attributions may need to be shown how the client's behavior varies according to the situational context. This can be accomplished by having the consultee engage in systemic behavioral observation to provide a more objective measure of the target behavior. The consultant can also facilitate this change in perception by questioning the consultee regarding exceptions or situations where the client has demonstrated "different" behavior.

When the client's attributional system is considered within the client–consultee pair, it would be expected that causal explanations would center on the surroundings or the situation (i.e., that the client would blame the teacher or other students). Although this observation has only limited application to the consultation process, it does represent potentially important information for the consultant to keep in mind when interacting with the client (as in direct service to the child) or when helping the consultee diagnose and intervene with the client (as in client-centered consultation).

A similar consideration of the attributional processes that occur within the consultee–consultant dyad would predict that the consultant would exhibit a bias toward identifying internal, stable, and intentional traits or dispositions of the consultee as contributing to the referral problem. For example, such attributions as a lack of consultee knowledge, skill, objectivity, or confidence (Meyers, Parsons, & Martin, 1979) might be used by consultants in their understanding of the consultation situation. Whereas these factors may accurately explain the consultee's problem, the consultant's use of these explanations may be an example of attributional bias. It is, therefore, important that consultants maintain an objective view of their own attributional processes to mitigate the potential difficulties with the consultation that can result from such bias.

Another manifestation of attributional bias within the consultee–consultant dyad is the process by which consultants explain the outcome of consultation. A review of two studies will help to clarify and demonstrate this point.

Martin and Curtis (1981) distributed questionnaires to 164 school psychologists and requested that they provide rationales for two consultative experiences, one particularly successful and the other particularly unsuccessful. The responses were coded into the following four major categories: (1) behaviors or characteristics of the consultant, (2) behaviors or characteristics of the consultee, (3) nature of the relationship between the consultant and the consultee, and (4) nature of the intervention recommended. The most striking results from this study were that consultants blame consultees for failure much more than they do themselves, and blame consultees for causing failure much more than they give them credit for contributing to successful outcomes.

An update and replication of this study was undertaken by Smith and Lyon (1986). Responses were obtained from 243 school psychologists who used the consultation model of service delivery. In the case of "successful" outcomes of consultation, most consultants attributed the success to the consultees (42%), secondarily to themselves (22%), and finally to the consultant–consultee relationship (14%). Interestingly, few attributions of success were given for effective interventions, external factors, or client behaviors (18% combined). In order to derive implications for the process of consultation, a review of the specific reasons given within the three major categories may be useful.

Within the "consultee responsible for success" condition, the following three rationales were given most frequently by consultants: (1) cooperation and motivation (36%), (2) flexibility and openness to new ideas (21%), and (3) follow-through and consistency (19%). When consultants attributed success to themselves, they did so on the basis of credibility (57%) and interpersonal skills (25%). Finally, when successful outcomes were attributed to the consultant–

consultee relationship, the most frequently cited reasons were either mutual cooperation (44%) or effective communication (34%).

With the caveat in mind that these attributions have been developed from the consultants' point of view, and therefore suffer from some degree of attributional bias, some tentative observations regarding the process of successful consultation can be made. First, consultants are well advised to establish an adequate level of credibility before engaging in consultation. In this regard, the concepts of social power may prove useful. Second, the utilization of effective interpersonal communication skills on the part of the consultant is important. Weissenburger *et al.* (1982) determined that consultee-reported satisfaction was highly correlated with the consultant being facilitative (empathic, understanding, collaborative, etc.). Although the Weissenburger *et al.* study did not investigate causal attributions per se, when considered in conjunction with the Smith and Lyon (1986) results, specialized training of consultants in human relationship and communication skills appears warranted.

A third general observation that can be made is the overriding importance of a collaborative relationship, wherein responsibility is shared equally by consultant and consultee. Only when consultee feel themselves to be equal partners in the consultative enterprise will they manifest such qualities as cooperation, motivation, flexibility, and follow-through. The importance of this point is highlighted by the fact that specific ideas regarding effective interventions were far down on the list of reasons for successful consultation. This implies that the process by which, and the context within which, interventions are developed (the *process* of consultation) is more important than the particular interventions that are used (the *content* of consultation).

When unsuccessful consultation took place, the school psychologists in the Smith and Lyons sample demonstrated the following pattern of attributions; consultee responsible for the failure (77%), consultant responsible (6%), other factors responsible (17% combined). Within the "consultee responsible" classification, attributions fell primarily into four categories: (1) lack of cooperation and motivation (26%), (2) inflexibility and resistance to new ideas (25%), (3) lack of follow-through and consistency (15%), and (4) inability to acknowledge the existence of a problem (14%).

When considering these results relative to the process of consultation, several implications emerge. The most overarching observation is that the very nature of these above attributions is internal, stable, and intentional. Hence, although they allow consultants to explain the failure of consultation in a tidy manner, they also absolve consultants from the responsibility of looking at their own responsibility within the interaction. This point is made by Martin (1983):

First, he [the consultant] attributes the failure of the client exclusively to a lack of skill, lack of knowledge, or to a lack of professional judgement on the part of the consultee. Then, if the consultee fails to act on this analysis, the consultant attributes the failure exclusively to the consultee, usually in the form of a defensiveness explanation. The consultant does not see the part he played in the reaction. (p. 40).

Clearly, the consultant who uses such constructions as "resistance" is closing down a number of potential points of intervention. By contrast, the consultant who understands that the process of attributing meanings is a seminal activity, unique to each individual, will be able to construct more meaningful explanations for consultee behavior than such linear-causal explanations as "defensiveness." The guiding principle at work in this process is for consultants to join actively with consultees and appreciate their point of view prior to any attempt at dissuasion.

This point can be made more clearly by considering the attributional process of the consultee within the consultant–consultee dyad. It is anticipated that the consultee would make attributions, particularly in the case of consultation failure, to the most salient environmental event within the context of consultation. Clearly, the most salient environmental event is the behavior of the consultant. Martin (1983) uses the example of the consultee attributing the cause of a consultation failure to the fact that the "consultant is insensitive to the difficulty of dealing with behavior like Johnny's in a classroom situation" (p. 37). Hence, consultants, according to attribution theory, need not only to engage consultees in a collaborative effort, but also to demonstrate to consultees that they truly "understand" and "empathize" with the consultees' difficulties.

Systemic Theory

Recently, there has been rapid growth in literature pertaining to the use of a "systemic" perspective to conceptualize behavior in school settings (Pfeiffer & Tittler, 1983; Worden, 1981). The systemic perspective is philosophically consistent with the belief that behavior is a "product" of the situational context, which includes child, task, teacher, classroom, school, and family dynamics (Havelock, 1973), and since it considers the interaction among these factors it is consistent with cognitive-behavioral theory.

Worden (1981) uses the analogy of a home heating system to describe the dynamic quality of systemic theory. Each of the component parts of the heating system can be considered as a subsystem that interacts to maintain a dynamic balance in the overall system. In the example of the heating system, this balance is the temperature setting of the thermostat, whereas in human systems the balance is obviously more complex and ambiguous. The cybernetic principles of the system, such as monitoring and ongoing readjustment, translate into a situation where there is a constant interaction and influence of the component parts of the system on one another, so that a change in one part of the system must, by definition, affect all other parts of the system.

"Circular causality" is one of the most important contributions that systemic theory has made to the conceptualization of behavior and behavior change (e.g., Selvini-Palazzoli, Cecchin, Prata, & Boscolo, 1978). The "goal" of all systems is to maintain some degree of homeostatic balance, and this balance can be upset when a teacher experiences classroom problems, or even through the presence of a consultant. When a systemic imbalance does occur, a "symptom" such as acting out may become evident. This symptom serves the dual purpose of representing an attempted solution while also allowing the system to maintain some degree of equilibrium. Thus, equilibrium is a dynamic concept where there is no set point, and where change is continual.

The systemic perspective can be useful to the school consultant because both the family and the school are systems with important impacts on the child and on the teacher (Wendt & Zake, 1984). An awareness of the mutual interaction of these subsystems can facilitate a more effective consultation process (Pfeiffer & Tittler, 1983). In particular, the school consultant needs to be aware of the role that the teacher holds in the system's context. In addition to being an important component of the child's environment, the teacher is influenced by systemic factors and by the child's behavior. From this perspective, (Fine & Holt, 1983), a common pitfall of the consultation process is encountered when the consultant becomes "triangulated" in the system. Triangulation, in this context, refers to the case of a consultant who becomes aligned with one of two conflicting parties—for example, a consultant who advocates for a child and who is "used" by the parents against the teacher, while, in turn, the teacher seeks to have the consultant support his or her agenda with the parents. This is a common problem in consultation because the consultant must "join" the system while still maintaining distance in order to provide an objective perception of the systemic/organizational dynamics.

Two major interventions derived from a systemic perspective with implications for the consultation process are reframing and paradoxical instructions (Weeks & L'Abate, 1982). *Reframing* is an intervention based on the idea that a change in the conceptual or emotional viewpoint from which a situation is perceived can result in a new way of perceiving that experience (Watzlawick, Weakland, & Fisch, 1974). Reframing achieves this change in perception by giving the behavior a different explanation. The philosophical perspective underlying this intervention is the belief that there is no single reality. Rather, we each construct our own realities by the explanations we supply. The technique of reframing offers a way to step outside of the current dilemma by developing a different explanation, which results in alternative solutions when the system has been stuck in an unproductive dilemma. Reframing is consistent with cognitive-behavioral theory in that each individual's subjective experience of reality is what influences that person's reactions to the environment.

Reframing can take a number of forms, although generally it is of either a positive or a negative nature. An example of positive reframing is offered by Fine and Holt (1983) who described Billy, a child who refused to turn in his assignments and was falling behind academically. This led to conflict with the teacher, which only seemed to perpetuate the child's negative behavior, which was reframed for the teacher as an enactment of a "bad child" role in the family structure. Billy's role as the "bad child" was explained as being rooted in parental expectations and maintained by the systemic need for a symptom bearer. Prior to reframing, the teacher in this case had categorized Billy as a "bad" child and responded punitively. With the change in perspective gained from positive reframing, the teacher could alter her expectations and respond to Billy in a more appropriate and productive manner. Some examples of the changes resulting from this new perspective might be encouraging Billy in areas of interest and/or ability, conferencing with parents regarding their own expectations, and attempting to achieve more of a match between home and school expectations and roles.

Another form of reframing is to give behavior an especially negative or exaggerated explanation. In the process of consultation, the use of negative or defiance-based reframing with consultees is generally not recommended, as it serves to induce resistance. Rather, as the work of Kolko and Milan (1986) exemplifies, the consultee and consultant can work cooperatively to use negative reframing with resistant and potentially resistant clients, but this relates more to the content than to the process of consultation.

The use of paradoxical instructions is another systemically derived intervention. Paradoxical instructions can take a number of different forms, but basically they encourage an individual to continue engaging in a problematic behavior. There is no agreed-on theoretical rationale for the effectiveness of paradoxical injunctions. One explanation is that they arouse a reactance reaction (Hughes & Falk, 1981), described in detail in the section of this chapter focused on resistance. Haley (1979), believes that paradoxical instructions are effective because they place an individual in a double bind. In the example of a consultee, the instruction to continue utilizing a particular procedure, such as time out, requires that the consultee comply and give up power in the system. By contrast, if consultees wish to maintain power, they cannot continue to use time-out, but must substitute other management techniques (Haley, 1979). Paradoxical injunctions, moreover, may be most effective when combined with other systemically derived interventions, particularly reframing (Ascher & Turner, 1980). An example of the combination of these techniques is included later in this chapter as an illustration of dealing with consultee resistance via systemically derived interventions.

The use of systematically derived interventions to address issues of consultation content can lead to resistance on the part of the teacher/consultee (e.g., Clavell, Frentz, & Kelley, 1986; Kolko & Milan, 1983), thereby making the application of these techniques to consultation content an issue of process. In order to mimimize this consultee reaction, the consultant can "reframe" the intervention in conjunction with the following guidelines (Kolko & Milan, 1983). Paradoxical procedures must be described clearly while presenting a compelling rationale. The rationale for this procedure must include an understandable analysis of the behavior and the contingencies of reinforcement maintaining the behavior. It can be important to build in contingencies that provide reinforcement for any behavioral gains achieved by the child, and to emphasize to the consultee the importance of consistency. Resistance to these interventions can also be reduced by describing, in advance, possible undesirable effects, and by indicating that the regular, mutual involvement of the consultee and the client (i.e., the teacher and the child) is an important component of the intervention.

Several sources suggest that systemically derived interventions, such as reframing and paradoxical injunctions, can be used to reduce consultee resistance (Fine, 1984; Hughes & Falk, 1981). Reframing with the consultee can be an effective process technique to increase the probability that the consultee will change. As Fine and Holt (1983), note, schools are rule-oriented systems wherein students are given ready-made classifications such as "good," "bad," "trouble-maker," and "underachiever." These stereotypes imply that students have a quality that resides within them. An example given by McDaniel (1981), is the statement, "The child *is* angry." The language of this statement supports the conception that the cause of the behavior can be found *within* the child, and this reduces the teacher's motivation to change. By contrast, the statement, "The child *acts* angrily," denotes a more systemic description of behavior and allows for more flexibility in the construction of potential interventions. Reframing can be used to overcome such problems and increase the probability of productive change by the consultee.

For example, Fine (1984) describes a teacher who was reluctant to allow a mildly retarded student into the classroom. The teacher's cognition was reframed by the consultant, who suggested that the consultee might have a genuine concern for the effects of this placement on the quality of other students' instructional experience. This reframing recognized the teacher's concerns and allowed him to "move on" and begin working with the mainstreamed student in a more appropriate manner.

Reframing can be used in conjunction with a paradoxical instruction (Hughes & Falk, 1981). In this example, reframing was used with one teacher, who encouraged and maintained the dependency of a socially immature child in her class, by describing the child's behavior as indicative of an important need stemming from a history of neglect. The paradoxical instruction to the teacher, which followed, was that she should do even *more* tasks for the child, thus supporting the dependency needs to an even greater extent. The reframing gave the consultee a rationale, or frame of reference, that allowed the paradoxical directive to be more effective.

Numerous ethical issues need to be sorted out regarding the manipulative quality of some systemic interventions that may run counter to the collaborative nature of the consultative enterprise. Some of these questions are as follows:

1. Is there a need for informed consent? If so, at all levels of consultation? Given that informing the individual regarding a paradoxical instruction may undo the bind, and hence make the intervention ineffective, should informed consent still be pursued?
2. Is the application of systemically derived interventions consistent with the

collaborative model of consultation? Are these interventions deceitful and manipulative?

3. How does the consultant feel about the issue of credibility? In other words, if a paradoxical technique works, the consultee may likely believe that the consultant is inept, a perception that, in the context of an ongoing professional relationship, may lead to professional disregard at one level or personal distrust at another (Brown & Slee, 1986; Hughes & Falk, 1981).

Resistance to Consultation

Anyone who has worked as a consultant in educational settings has experienced resistance within the consultation relationship. Resistance occurs for a variety of reasons, ranging from consultant ineptness to being a function of the consultee. The common effect of resistance, regardless of its etiology, is to inhibit effective consultation (e.g., Parsons & Meyers, 1984). Resistance to consultation often can be overcome through the application of social-psychological principles that are consistent with cognitive-behavioral theory; some of these have been noted in the earlier discussions on attribution theory and systemic theory. The term "resistance" has negative connotations, which imply that something is wrong with the consultee who makes the mistake of not accepting the consultant's viewpoint. It may be more productive, however, to assume that resistance reflects a problem in the relationship that is not the fault of one party in particular. Regardless of who is right and who is at fault when resistance occurs, the consultant needs to know how to respond, and two useful approaches consistent with cognitive-behavioral theory derive from the social-psychology literature: (1) conflict resolution theory (Deutsch, 1973) and (2) psychological-reactance theory (Brehm, 1966).

Conflict Resolution Theory

According to Deutsch (1973), interactions in which both parties act in a cooperative manner are those in which conflict (or, for the purposes of this discussion, resistance) is most likely to be overcome. In contrast, he found that there was a lesser probability of resolving conflict in competitive interactions. He describes a cooperative interchange as one in which both parties assume that there will be a positive outcome occurring simply because they are interacting with another person. A competitive interaction is one characterized by suspicion, in which each person assumes that a negative outcome is likely because he or she is interacting with another person. Cooperative styles of interaction might be characterized by egalitarian and trusting relationships might be characterized by egalitarian and trusting relationships in which there is open and honest comunication. Competitive styles are characterized by authoritarian, aggressive, and exploitive relationships in which one person attempts to control the second person. Whereas cooperative interactions are characterized by positive and optimistic views of human behavior, competitive interactions are characterized by negative and pessimistic views of human behavior.

Parsons and Meyers (1984) have suggested that four particular relationship dynamics from conflict resolution theory may be applicable to the resolution of resistance in consultation. First, when a competitive consultee works with a competitive consultant, conflict resolution (i.e., the reduction of resistance) is least likely to occur; likely outcomes instead are rejection, verbal attack, and aggressiveness. Second, when a cooperative consultee interacts with a competitive consultant, conflict resolution is still unlikely. Third, when a competitive consultee interacts with a consultant using a cooperative style, conflict resolution and the reduction of resistance are likely to occur over time. Finally, when a consultee and consultant interact where each has a cooperative style, conflict resolution is most likely to occur in a timely manner. This theory suggests, therefore, that a consultant engaged in a relationship characterized by resistance should make a concerted effort to implement a cooperative mode of consultation. This might be accomplished by the consultant using greater levels of empathy; egalitarian, nonauthoritarian, and noncoercive modes of interaction; and open, honest communication (Parsons & Meyers, 1984).

Psychological-Reactance Theory

Reactance is a social-psychological theory that conceptualizes the interpersonal phenomenon of "resistance." In the wide variety of resistant behaviors, the common element appears to be the individual's perception that going along with the suggested behavior change would restrict his or her free will. The assumption that individuals act in order to maintain behavioral freedom is the foundation of reactance theory.

As originally postulated by J. W. Brehm (1966), reactance theory maintained that individuals would experience psychological reactance whenever they perceived that any of their "free behaviors" were either threatened or eliminated. The free behaviors mentioned here are a theoretical set of behaviors in which the individuals knows he or she may engage, and for which he or she also possesses the prerequisite knowledge and skills. In practice, free behaviors are not restricted to observable behaviors but also include cognitions, emotions, and attitudes.

The psychological reactance that is aroused is considered to be a motivational condition, in which the individual seeks to maintain or restore the threatened or eliminated free behavior. Brehm conjectured that the magnitude of the individual's reactance reaction would be predicated on the following three factors: (1) the perceived importance of the threatened freedom, (2) the proportion of the freedoms eliminated or threatened with elimination, and (3) the subjective evaluation of threat. Maximum reactance is activated by the actual loss of a freedom.

How each individual reacts to and expresses his or her experience of reactance is dependent on a large number of factors. At one extreme, the individual may seek to restore the threatened freedom by taking direct action. If direct action is impossible, as when the freedom has already been eliminated, the individual may use indirect methods, which has also been termed "reestablishing freedom by implication." This might be accomplished by such techniques as engaging in another behavior of the same class, disobeying the other individuals' next request, or observing someone else restoring his or her own freedom.

In certain situations where both direct and indirect methods of response are not available, the individual may suppress his or her reaction and, it is conjectured, the reactance will diminish over time. A fourth and final expression of reactance is aggression, where direct physical action is taken against the social agent perceived to be responsible for the loss of freedom.

The process of consultation is rife with opportunities for reactance reactions because the goal of consultation is to change the attitudes or behaviors of the consultee, a change that may be viewed as a restriction of freedom. Reactance reactions will usually be experienced by the consultant as "resistance." The application of reactance theory to the therapeutic context was undertaken by S. Brehm (1976) and was applied to consultation by Hughes and Falk (1981). There are two basic areas of potential application of reactance theory to consultation: (1) the minimization/suppression of reaction and (2) the utilization of reactance.

The *minimization and suppression of reactance* is a direct approach to reducing resistance to consultation. The need to maintain a collaborative, joint decision-making model in consultation is supported by reactance theory. Grabitz-Gniech (1971) determined that if an individual commits to a joint decision-making process, the likelihood of a reactance reaction is reduced. Hence, the consultant should emphasize the collaborative nature of the consultation process.

Consistent with the collaborative model, S. Brehm (1976) cautions against the use of such terms as "must," "should," and "have to," all of which can be perceived by consultees as a threat to their freedom. Statements such as, "It's your decision," "It's up to you," and, "It's important that both of us feel comfortable with our decision," emphasize the responsibility of the consultee and the joint nature of the consultative process. Along with the verbal content of communications, S. Brehm (1976) emphasizes that nonverbal aspects of interaction can be interpreted as conveying strong social pressure for agreement. It is, therefore, important to convey the collaborative nature of the relationship through nonverbal as well as verbal communications.

Consistent with the collaborative orientation described here, Brock (1965), determined that the more intent an individual is on persuading another, and the more anticipation there is for future persuasive attempts, the greater likelihood there is for ineffective communication and resistance. The implications for the consultant are clear. There should not be a great investment in a particular point of view, and it should be clear that a current persuasive communication is independent of future interactions, which will not necessarily seek to persuade the consultee. This is similar to the finding from cognitive-dissonance theory suggesting that the consultant should strive to keep justifications for behavior change minimal. Consultants who prompt a reactance reaction as a result of the fervor of their persuasive attempts may wish to change their approach, recognizing that a variety of approaches can be used to solve a particular problem. It has been determined that the earlier in a communicational sequence a reactance-arousing statement is made, the more freedoms are perceived to be threatened and the more easily reactance is aroused (Wicklund, Slattum, & Solomon, 1970). Therefore, the consultant may want to minimize overt persuasive attempts, especially in the early stages of consultation, when it is appropriate to gather data and avoid making premature interpretations.

When persuasive attempts are thought to be necessary, they can be framed as circumscribed suggestions, which will not be needed in the future (i.e., "This situation will probably never come up again"). Understanding of the need for this temporally constrained framing stems from the work of Pellak and Heller (1971), who demonstrated that the implication of future persuasive attempts tends to result in increased reactance. The cognitive process at work is something akin to, "If I let you influence me this time, I might establish a pattern for future influence attempts." In practice, the goal of consultation is to allow the consultee to be more self-sufficient in the future. Hence, this aspect of the relationship can be highlighted and communicated by the consultant. For consultees who are not demonstrating a reactance reaction, consultants can emphasize their continued availability and interest in collaborating in future consultative enterprises with the consultees.

The importance of assessment and data gathering regarding consultees' beliefs is emphasized in the final two approaches to reactance minimization/ suppression. A study by Wicklund and Brehm (1968) determined that the more competent an individual feels on an issue, the more likelihood there is of arousing a reactance reaction if there is a perception that personal freedoms are being threatened. By contrast, the individual who feels incompetent or unsure of a behavior is much less likely to respond with reactance to a directive communication. In practice, this interaction means that an assessment of consultees' level of comfort with a particular course of action needs to be made, and consultants should gauge their level of directiveness accordingly. This is not meant to imply that consultants interacting with inexperienced consultees should take unilateral control of the consultation process, but, rather, that consultants in such situations may offer more direct suggestions and encouragement.

A final application of reactance theory to consultant efforts to minimize the possibility of consultee resistance is offered by the work of Wicklund (1974). The gist of Wicklund's work is that individuals who receive a communication strongly advocating a position with which they already agree demonstrate a reactance reaction. By contrast, those individuals who receive initial exposure to positions contrary to the one they hold do not experience the same degree of reactance. One implication for consultants is that an assessment of consultees' current position and biases regarding the consultation situation should be made. If consultees' beliefs are in accord with those of the consultant, they should not immediately be endorsed as appropriate; rather, alternative approaches may be introduced. This opportunity for consultees to demonstrate their freedom helps to ensure that the originally endorsed approach will not arouse resistance.

Using reactance is an approach that may be helpful when resistance occurs despite the use of techniques to minimize and suppress reactance. This section will present a variety of techniques for dealing with consultee resistance from a reactance-theory perspective. One of the most provocative ways of using reactance is to use what are commonly called "paradoxes." The literature on the theory and application of paradoxes is burgeoning, particularly with regard to family systems theory (see the discussion earlier in this chapter, in the section on systemic theory), and paradox can be conceptualized from the perspective of reactance theory.

Paradoxical techniques are implemented by suggesting to individuals that they continue to engage in problematic behavior; for example, the insomniac is urged to stay awake. From the perspective of reactance theory, paradoxical injunctions are effective because they threaten the individual's freedom *not* to engage in the symptomatic behavior (Brehm, 1976). Hence, when instructed to engage in a behavior in which they are already engaging, individuals may experience a reactance reaction and cease the behavior in order to demonstrate their freedom.

A similar dynamic may occur in the phenomenon referred to as "baseline curing." Certain individuals exhibit a reduction in target behaviors after they begin to count these behaviors to establish a baseline (i.e., Thoresen & Mahoney, 1974). Reactance theory suggests that as the individual attends to the target behavior, the behavior is perceived as a threat to the person's freedom not to engage in it, or as a threat to the person's freedom to engage in alternative behaviors.

Brehm and Mann (1975) determined that reactance can sometimes be circumvented by removing the perceived source of social pressure and allowing the individual who is the target of the influence more time to adjust. This "sleeper effect" works because the termination of influence attempts decreases the perception of social pressure and the perceived threat to freedom. In turn, the individual experiences less reactance and can respond to behavioral alternatives in a more "objective" manner. In consultation, this finding implies that a consultant who is stuck in a seemingly unproductive consultation may wish to renegotiate and discontinue consultation temporarily. If the consultant checks back with the consultee after a period of time, there may be a reduction in resistance.

Reactance may be aroused in consultees by the mere consideration of alternative behaviors, or "new freedoms." The consideration of these new, attractive freedoms may result in the perception of a threat to engage in the old behaviors, and a consequent retreat to them (Brehm & Rosen, 1971). One of the most effective ways to cope with this sort of reactance is to assure consultees that they have the freedom to engage in the old behavior.

For example, a consultee who has sought out consultation because of difficulties with classroom management may begin to experience reactance relative to his or her ability to engage in their previous, albeit ineffective, classroom management style. This reactance might develop as the consultee considers new, different approaches to exercising control in the classroom. Given that the consultee might revert to the old, problematic style of management as a result of a reactance reaction, the consultant might encourage the consultee to "go slow" and actually continue to use the original method of management. In turn, reactance theory would predict that the consultee would then feel free to attempt the new methods of control.

A somewhat more confrontational technique for dealing with this situation involves structuring events so that the consultee must make a decision. S. Brehm (1976) conjectures that although some reactance will result from this approach, most likely consultees will be committed to the choice as long as they perceive some responsibility for the choice.

Many of these techniques may prove helpful to the consultant in dealing with resistance stemming from reactance reactions. In general, the approach suggested by reactance theory supports the philosophy of consultation as a mutual, collaborative effort where both individuals take responsibility and ownership for the process. One exception to this statement is the use of paradoxical injunctions, which have an arguably manipulative quality. Taken as a whole, however, reactance theory can be usefully applied to dealing with resistance in consultative relationships.

SUMMARY AND SUGGESTED APPLICATIONS

As this review of social-psychological and systemic theories demonstrates, perspectives with a cognitive-behavioral orientation are particularly amenable to application with the consultation process. A number of cogent factors appear to contribute to the "fit" between psychoeducational consultation and the cognitive-behavioral perspective.

Consultation, in its most general terms, can be considered a process of interpersonal communication and influence. Another seminal component of consultation is that it is an indirect model of service provision, wherein the consultee has the responsibility for implementing any interventions. By considering the cognitive processes by which the consultee is mediating and giving meaning to the environment, the consultant is in a much stronger position to engage in consultation that will result in meaningful and effective interventions.

Another factor contributing to the fit between cognitive-behavioral theory and psychoeducational consultation is that many of the techniques associated with consultation practice are also used in cognitive-behavioral approaches.

Some examples of common techniques include modeling, role playing, positive reinforcement, and altering expectations.

A major aspect of congruence between the two approaches is the importance and priority given to collaborative consultation. This viewpoint was presented, first, as a pragmatic technique by authors such as Caplan (1970) with little theoretical or empirical basis. Recently, the consultation literature has begun to provide some empirical support for this assumption (e.g., Curtis & Meyers, 1985). This chapter has demonstrated, moreover, that a variety of theoretical models consistent with cognitive-behavioral theory provide support for a cooperative, nonhierarchical style—that is, cognitive-dissonance, attribution, social power, conflict resolution, and reactance theories. In each instance, these models suggest that the consultee must be an active participant in the consultation process, who, along with the consultant, makes an important contribution to the consultation process.

Cognitive-behavioral approaches may be particularly applicable to consultation in educational settings because the underlying philosophy is easily understood by educators and is consistent with much educational practice. Like behavioral theory, cognitive-behaviorism focuses explicitly on the observable classroom problem and relies on reinforcement principles that are used frequently by classroom teachers. By also focusing on cognition, the cognitive-behavioral approach is broadened in a way that is perfectly consistent with schools. The traditional focus of schools on the 3 Rs represents an emphasis on cognitive goals. Further, the cognitive approach to social skills as a basis for improving social/emotional behavior is really an educational approach to psychological problems of social and emotional behavior. It is more consistent with the experience of most educators to remediate children's problem behaviors by teaching them cognitive skills rather than dealing with children's internal personality conflicts or using counseling strategies for which they have had no training.

Despite the potential intuitive appeal of this approach for many teachers, it must be acknowledged that it does emphasize the individual as an active learner who must exercise control in the learning process. This aspect of cognitive-behavioral theory is not consistent with educational practice in many schools, where there may be a passive learning process in which the teacher provides active input and the student is a passive respondent. Using these approaches as a guide to the consultation process may help to model the utility of a learning model in which the learner is actively involved.

In summary, the consultation process will be most effective if consultants use a collaborative process that is informed by social-psychological and systemic theories like those described in this chapter. Although each of these approaches can be used to minimize resistance to consultation, two theories, in particular (reactance and conflict resolution), are likely to facilitate this goal. Attribution theory and cognitive dissonance provide pragmatic models that suggest approaches to facilitate a maximally effective consultation process. It is noted, however, that paradoxical instruction, an approach derived from both systemic and reactance theory, may not be consistent with the collaborative principles supported by the remaining theoretical work cited in this chapter. Paradoxical instruction has a manipulative quality that may not be consistent with collaborative interaction between professional colleagues. Further research on the efficacy of this approach is needed, along with careful theoretical study of the approach to determine how it fits with other cognitive-behavioral approaches to the consultation process.

REFERENCES

Alpert, J. L. (1976). Conceptual bases of mental health consultation in the schools. *Professional Psychology, 7*, 619–626.

Alpert, J. L., & Meyers, J. (Eds.). (1983). *Training in consultation: Perspectives from mental health, behavioral, and organizational consultation.* Springfield, IL: Thomas.

Alpert, J. L., & Associates. (1982). *Psychological consultation in educational settings.* San Francisco: Jossey-Bass.

Ascher, L. M., & Turner, R. M. (1980). A comparison of two methods for the administration of paradoxical intention. *Behavior Resources Therapy, 18*, 121–126.

Bergan, J. R. (1977). *Behavior consultation.* Columbus, OH: Merrill.

Brehm, J. W. (1966). *A theory of psychological reactance.* New York: Academic Press.

Brehm, J. W., & Cohen, A. R. (1962). *Explorations in cognitive dissonance.* New York: Wiley.

Brehm, J. W., & Mann, M. (1975). The effect of importance of freedom and attraction to group members on influence produced by group pressure. *Journal of Personality and Social Psychology, 31*, 816–824.

Brehm, J. W., & Rosen, E. (1971). Attractiveness of old alternatives when a new, attractive alternative is introduced. *Journal of Personality and Social Psychology, 20*, 261–266.

Brehm, S. S. (1976). *The application of social psychology to clinical practice.* New York: Halstead.

Brock, T. C. (1965). Communicator–recipient similarity and decision change. *Journal of Personality and Social Psychology, 1*, 650–654.

Brown, J. E., & Slee, P. T. (1986). Paradoxical strategies: The ethics of intervention. *Professional Psychology: Research and Practice, 17*, 487–491.

Caplan, G. (1970). *The theory and practice of mental health consultation.* New York: Basic Books.

Clavell, T. A., Frentz, C. E., & Kelley, M. L. (1986). Acceptability of paradoxical interventions: Some nonparadoxical findings. *Professional Psychology: Research and Practice, 17*, 519–523.

Close-Conoley, J., & Gutkin, T. B. (1986). Educating school psychologists for the real world. *School Psychology Review, 15*(4), 457–465.

Conoley, J. (Ed.). (1981). *Consultation in schools.* New York: Academic Press.

Curtis, M. J., & Meyers, J. (1985). School-based consultation: Guidelines for effective practice. In J. Grimes & A. Thomas (Eds.), *Best practices in school psychology* (pp. 79–94). Washington, DC: National Association of School Psychologists.

Curtis, M. J., & Zins, J. F. (1981). *The theory and practice of school consultation.* Springfield, IL: Thomas.

Deffenbacher, J. L. (1985). A cognitive-behavioral response and a modest proposal. *Counseling Psychologist, 13*(2), 261–269.

Deutsch, M. (1973). *The resolution of conflict: Constructive and destructive processes.* New Haven, CT: Yale University Press.

Festinger, L. (1957). *A theory of cognitive dissonance.* Evanston, IL: Row, Peterson.

Fine, M. J. (1984). Integrating strategic and structural components in school-based intervention: Some cautions for consultants. *Techniques, 1,* 44–52.

Fine, M. J., & Holt, P. (1983). Intervening with school problems: A family systems perspective. *Psychology in the Schools, 20,* 85–92.

French, J. R., Jr., & Raven, B. (1959). The basis of social power. In D. Cartwright (Ed.), *Studies in social power* (pp. 150–167). Ann Arbor: Institute of Social Research, University of Michigan.

Frieze, I. H. (1980). Beliefs about success and failure in the classroom. In J. H. McMillan (Ed.), *The social psychology of school learning* (pp. 39–78). New York: Academic Press.

Fullan, M., Miles, M. B., & Taylor, G. (1980). Organization development in schools: The state of the art. *Review of Educational Research, 50,* 121–183.

Grabitz-Gnietch, G. (1971). Some restrictive conditions for the occurrence of psychological reactance. *Journal of Personality and Social Psychology, 19,* 188–196.

Grieger, R. M. (1972). Teacher attitudes as a variable in behavior modification consultation. *Journal of School Psychology, 10*(3), 279–287.

Gutkin, T. B., & Curtis, M. J. (1982). School-based consultation: Theory and techniques. In C. R. Reynolds & T. B. Gutkin (Eds.), *The handbook of school psychology* (pp. 796–828). New York: Wiley.

Haley, J. (1979). *Problem-solving therapy.* San Francisco: Jossey-Bass.

Harvey, J. H., & Weary, G. (1981). *Perspectives on attributional processes.* Dubuque, IA: Brown.

Harvey, J. H., & Weary, G. (1985). *Attribution: Basic issues and applications.* Orlando, FL: Academic Press.

Havelock, R. (1973). *The change agent's guide to innovation in education.* Englewood Cliffs, NJ: Educational Technology Publications.

Hughes, J. N. (1983). The application of cognitive dissonance theory to consultation. *Journal of School Psychology, 21,* 349–357.

Hughes, J. N., & Falk, R. S. (1981). Resistance, reactance and consultation. *Journal of School Psychology, 19,* 134–142.

Kolko, D. J., & Milan, M. A. (1986). Reframing and paradoxical instruction to overcome "resistance" in the treatment of delinquent youths: A multiple baseline analysis. *Journal of Consulting and Clinical Psychology, 51,* 655–660.

Martin, R. P. (1978). Expert and referent power: A framework for understanding and maximizing consultation effectiveness. *Journal of School Psychology, 16,* 49–55.

Martin, R. P. (1983). Consultant, consultee, and client explanations of each others' behavior in consultation. *School Psychology Review, 12*(1), 35–41.

Martin, R. P., & Curtis, M. (1981). Consultants' perceptions of causality for success and failure in consultation. *Professional Psychology, 71,* 671–676.

McDaniel, S. (1981). Treating school problems in family therapy. *Elementary School Guidance and Counseling, 15,* 214–222.

Medway, F. J. (1979). Causal attributions for school-related problems: Teacher perceptions and teacher feedback. *Journal of Educational Psychology*, *71*, 809–818.

Meichenbaum, D. H., & Goodman, J. (1971). Training impulsive children to talk to themselves: A means of developing self-control. *Journal of Abnormal Psychology*, *77*, 115–126.

Meyers, J. (1973). A consultation model for school psychological services. *Journal of School Psychology*, *11*, 5–15.

Meyers, J., Alpert, J. L., & Fleisher, B. (1983). Models of consultation. In J. L. Alpert & J. Meyers (Eds.), *Training in consultation* (pp. 5–16). Springfield, IL: Thomas.

Meyers, J., Parsons, R. D., & Martin, R. (1979). *Mental health consultation in the schools*. San Francisco: Jossey-Bass.

Nisbett, R. E., Caputo, C. G., Legant, P., & Marocek, J. (1973). Behavior as seen by the actor and as seen by the observer. *Journal of Personality and Social Psychology*, *27*, 154–164.

Parsons, R. D., & Meyers, J. (1984). *Developing consultation skills*. San Francisco: Jossey-Bass.

Pellak, M. S., & Heller, J. F. (1971). Interactive effects of committment to future interaction and threat to attributional freedom. *Journal of Personality and Social Psychology*, *17*, 325–331.

Pfeiffer, S. I., & Tittler, B. I. (1983). Utilizing the multi-disciplinary team to facilitate a school–family systems orientation. *The School Psychology Review*, *12*, 168–173.

Raven, B. H. (1965). Social influence on power. In I. D. Steiner & M. Fishbein (Eds.), *Current studies in social psychology*. New York: Holt, Rinehart & Winston.

Sarason, S. B., Levine, M., Goldenberg, I. I., Cherlin, D. L., & Bennett, E. M. (1966). *Psychology in community settings*. New York: Wiley.

Schein, E. H. (1969). *Process consultation*. Reading, MA: Addison-Wesley.

Schmuck, R. A. (1976). Process consultation and organizational development. *Professional Psychology*, *7*, 626–631.

Schmuck, R. A., & Miles, M. (Eds.). (1971). *Organization development in the schools*. Palo Alto, CA: National Press Books.

Selvini-Palazzoli, M., Cecchin, G., Prata, G., & Boscolo, L. (1978). *Paradox and counterparadox*. New York: Jason Aronson.

Smith, D. K., & Lyon, M. A. (1986). School psychologists' attributions for success and failure in consultations with parents and teachers. *Professional Psychology*, *17*, 205–209.

Thoresen, C. E., & Mahoney, M. J. (1974). *Behavioral self-control*. New York: Holt, Rinehart & Winston.

Watzlawick, P., Weakland, J., & Fisch, R. (1974). *Change*. New York: Norton.

Weeks, G. R., & L'Abate, L. (1982). *Paradoxical psychotherapy: Theory and practice with individuals, couples and families*. New York: Brunner-Mazel.

Weissenburger, J. W., Fine, M. J., & Poggio, J. P. (1982). The relationship of selected consultant/teacher characteristics to consultation outcomes. *Journal of School Psychology*, *20*, 263–270.

Wendt, R. N., & Zake, J. (1984). Family systems theory and school psychology: Implications for training and practice. *Psychology in the Schools*, *21*, 204–210.

Wicklund, R. A. (1974). *Freedom and reactance*. Hillsdale, NJ: Lawrence Erlbaum.

Wicklund, R. A., & Brehm, J. W. (1968). Attitude change as a function of felt competence and threat to attitudinal freedom. *Journal of Experimental Social Psychology*, *4*, 64–75.

Wicklund, R. A., & Brehm, J. W. (1976). *Perspectives on cognitive dissonance.* Hillsdale, NJ: Lawrence Erlbaum.

Wicklund, R. A., Slattum, V., & Solomon, E. (1970). Effects of implied pressure toward commitment on ratings of choice alternatives. *Journal of Experimental Social Psychology, 6,* 449–457.

Worden, M. (1981). Classroom behavior as a function of the family system. *School Counselor, 28,* 178–188.

19
COGNITIVE-BEHAVIORAL
APPROACHES AND PREVENTION
IN THE SCHOOLS

JANE CLOSE CONOLEY
University of Nebraska

To prevent children from having mental health and behavioral difficulties, researchers have expended considerable effort to understand the causes and the correlates of disabling conditions. Although there has been some success, there has also been significant dissatisfaction with psychology's progress in creating enabling environments for children, and in psychologically inoculating them from mental disorder. This chapter reviews cognitive-behavioral efforts to prevent children's problems.

A broadened focus, from children alone to the significant others who surround them, is particularly important when considering children and prevention. Children are undoubtedly active agents in creating their environments, but they are also vulnerable to the influence of other people and to their physical, social, and emotional contexts. Detailed analyses of causes of dysfunction and health reveal a complex, multivariable situation that suggests a need for prevention programs that target children, their caregivers, and their environments. Cowen's (1984) call for the construction of a generative base (i.e., identification of the causal links involved in specific disorders, early manifestations of the disorder, and potentially helpful intervention approaches) prior to prevention efforts is a necessary precursor to deciding intervention targets and timetables.

The purview of this chapter is cognitive-behavioral approaches to the primary and secondary prevention of children's mental health problems. Other intervention strategies are, for the most part, not considered. Cognitive-behavioral approaches have held out significant promise for those interested in remediation as well as for those interested in prevention. For example, if people's cognitive appraisal of life events (rather than the events per se) is of primary importance, then changing children's ways of thinking about the situations they confront suggests an avenue to highly generalized improvements in childhood behavior and emotional reactions. In addition, if social decision-making skills can be taught to children in one setting and generalized to many others, the potential benefit to children is enormous.

PREVENTION

Definition

Primary prevention of mental health difficulties refers to initiatives to improve the life situations of the masses of people such that mental health problems are made less likely to appear. Caplan (1964) described this primary level as well as secondary and tertiary prevention levels. Secondary prevention targets vulnerable or impaired individuals with help either to remove them from an at-risk status or to improve their functioning to optimal levels. Tertiary prevention efforts are aimed at preventing further deterioration of people who are already quite impaired. Improvement, however, is not expected.

Several researchers and conceptualizers have argued that the secondary and tertiary levels are not representative of true preventive efforts (Cowen, 1973, 1983; Felner, Jason, Moritsugu, & Farber, 1983; Zax & Spector, 1974). These writers see all but primary prevention efforts as reinforcing traditional mental health perspectives and service delivery options.

Implementation

Primary prevention interventions are targeted at groups that may or may not be known to be at risk for particular dysfunctions. The interventions have a before-the-fact quality; that is, the programs are initiated before any problems are noted. Experience has shown that these primary prevention efforts must be built on solid research bases concerning specific causal links related to specific behaviors to be prevented. Commonsense notions about what people need to be invulnerable to mental health problems have not always proved true. For example, the idea that people act rationally—that is, will make good decisions if given correct information—has reflected a disappointingly incomplete understanding of human behavior (Chassin, Presson, & Sherman, 1985; Cowen, 1984).

Mounting primary prevention efforts has been difficult. By the 1970s the impact of life-style on physical health was widely recognized (7 out of 10 leading causes of death in the United States have crucial behavioral determinants), but the analogy to mental health was not widely accepted (Goldston, 1986; Heffernan & Albee, 1985). The Vermont Conferences on Primary Prevention (e.g., Albee & Joffe, 1977; Bond & Rosen, 1980; Forgays, 1978; Kent & Rolf, 1979) have provided consistent prods to mental health agencies and researchers to include preventive initiatives in their agendas. Although important and supportive research has been accomplished in such fields as competence and competency building, learned helplessness, maternal self-concept and perception of the newborn, the preventive potential of self-help groups, environmental influences on behavior, marital disruption as a psychopathological stressor, community dysfunctions or disintegration as factors in mental disorder, promotion of self-esteem, and measurement and assessment of the effects of critical life events and life transitions, a coordinated policy to study and also implement preventive interventions has been elusive (Goldston, 1986).

Potential Target Levels

Primary prevention programs aim both at reducing the possibility of dysfunction and at enhancing the quality of life. For example, when considering the options for primary prevention with children, Rosenberg and Reppucci (1985) identify four ecological target levels with examples of known dysfunctional events. At the individual level, children are born with different temperaments and physical strengths and vulnerabilities—differences that make children more or less likely to be well parented, easy to manage, and teachable. Children may suffer a history of abuse, parental rejection, or inappropriate expectations from their parents.

At the familial level, children may be a part of ineffective interactions among family members, may suffer the effects of conflictual spousal relationships, or may behave in ways that increase the probability of abuse from their parents. At the community level, children may experience isolation from helpful supports, family unemployment, and other instances of unmanageable stress. Finally, at the societal level, children are embedded in cultures that may sanction physical punishment, be unsupportive of education, or be uninvolved in facilitating family functioning.

These already well-known stressors can be chosen as primary prevention targets, as can activities that are competency-enhancing. For example, the teaching of parenting skills, social problem solving, provision of child development information, training in coping strategies useful in reducing and managing stress, and training in skills in finding employment are additional possibilities for primary prevention programs.

Many programs are a combination of approaches. Preventing abusive behavior by parents has become an increasingly urgent item on the national agenda. Typical programs have made use of media campaigns, information provision, crisis lines, and referral services. More comprehensive programs have also provided home visits by nurses for the first 2 years of a baby's life; some rooming-in of the baby with the new mother while still in the hospital; and training of new parents in home safety, money management, use of leisure time, nutrition, and job finding (Gray, 1983; Gray, Cutler, Dean, & Kempe, 1976; Gray & Kaplan, 1980; Klaus & Kennell, 1976; Lutzker, Wesch, & Rice, 1984; Olds, 1984).

School Programs

School-based prevention programs have been both child-focused and more broadly ecologically based (Durlak, 1985). Examples of child-focused programs include affective education, social problem-solving/coping skills, and prevention of academic problems (Baskin & Hess, 1980; Blechman, Kotanchick, & Taylor, 1981; Blechman, Taylor, & Schrader, 1981; Boike, 1986; Durlak, 1983; Hansford & Hattie, 1982; Jason, Durlak, & Holton-Walker, 1984; Medway & Smith, 1978; Rickel, Eshelman, & Loigman, 1983; Sharp, 1981).

Although the results of these child-focused interventions clearly challenge researchers to continue refinement, a recent meta-analysis of 40 primary prevention strategies indicates that the approaches differ in their effectiveness (Baker, Swisher, Nadenichek, & Popowicz, 1984). The overall effect size of studies using cognitive coping skills as the intervention was only about .26 (a small effect, according to Cohen, 1969). In contrast, communication skills training had an effect size of about 3.90 (a large effect). The overall effect size for primary prevention studies was about .55 (a medium effect). This .55 effect size suggests that a person receiving primary preventive interventions whose score on a variable was that of the mean of the control group would improve on that variable .55 standard deviations above the mean. This would translate into a change from the 50th percentile on some hypothetical variable to the 73rd percentile.

Obviously, however, the improvements vary according to the type of preventive intervention received. Career maturity enhancement, communication skills training, deliberate psychological education programs, and a combination of deliberate psychological education and moral education programs show large effect sizes. Values clarification programs have medium effect sizes. Cognitive coping skills training programs, moral education programs (alone), substance abuse prevention programs, and programs blending values clarification with other strategies are viewed as showing low effect sizes (see Baker et al., 1984, for a list of studies and specific effect sizes).

Ecological interventions with children in schools include classroom organization, interdependent learning, peer tutoring, parent programs, teacher programs, and program implementation research. These last three areas are badly neglected in terms of research, whereas the first three seem neglected by practitioners (Allen, 1976; Gump, 1980; Harris & Sherman, 1973; Jason, Frasure, & Ferone, 1981; Stallings, 1975; Turk, Meeks, & Turk, 1982).

Ecological interventions appear very promising. For example, interventions involving interdependent learning or peer tutoring have been associated with improved attitudes toward school, better peer relations, and other social and academic gains for both tutors and tutees (Hightower & Avery, 1986). Classroom structures have been prescriptively described, with open classrooms facilitating the achievement of high-SES and high-IQ students while worsening the achievement of low-IQ students. Increased structure has been associated with gains in math and reading, whereas less structure has facilitated growth in independence, cooperation, and initiation, as well as reduced absenteeism. Overall, Stallings (1975) reports that about 40% of children's achievement can be accounted for by classroom instructional procedures (and 30% by their entry abilities).

The earliest primary prevention program at the elementary school level, the St. Louis Project of 1947 (Glidewell, Gildea, & Kaufman, 1973), involved parents, but more recent work at the elementary level has not included parents. This is in sharp contrast to preschool programs, which have frequently and successfully included parental components (Gray & Wandersman, 1980; Lazar & Darlington, 1982).

Analogously, only minor explorations have been made in the area of teacher interventions for primary prevention (Durlak, 1985). This is a serious oversight. There is increasing evidence that work with parents helps children adjust. In fact, some research suggests that direct work with parents may be more effective than direct interventions with maladapting children (Epstein, Wing, Koeske, Andrasik, & Ossip, 1981; Griest et al., 1982). It may be that direct work with teachers would be as fruitful in terms of improving the coping abilities of children.

An additional oversight has been a lack of attention to implementation realities. It is disheartening to consider that carefully conceptualized prevention programs may never be correctly implemented at classroom or building levels. Such may be the case, however, indicating a crucial need to identify elements that affect the implementation process (Berman & McLaughlin, 1976; Fullan & Pomfret, 1977).

Conclusions

Preventive psychology is an area of promise and problem.

> Primary prevention is a glittering, diffuse, thoroughly abstract term. Its aura is so exalted that some put it on the same plane as the Nobel Prize. It offers a sharp contrast to all that mental health has done, a shadowy, but nevertheless grand, alternative. It is terribly "major" in the lingo of childhood games I have known, something to be approached with massive giant steps. (Cowen, 1980, p. 1)

Lorion (1983) cites the reality, however, that only small steps are possible given the developmental changes characteristic of children and the necessity to develop particular research bases for each intervention (i.e., generative base):

> In the absence of knowledge of a disorder's causes and/or of the individual, familial, and environmental conditions for its manifestations, the initiation of a primary prevention effort appears premature. Similarly, if ignorant of the preliminary manifestations of target disorders, unable to systematically detect their

presence, or incapable of altering their evolution, one is unprepared to attack a problem at the secondary level. Finally, if we are unaware of how a specific skill develops and is maintained in the everyday environment, enhancement efforts may need to be deferred. (p. 265)

A critical analysis of prevention efforts will, therefore, suggest both hopeful beginnings of programs and strategies, and the enormity of the challenge. Preventing childhood problems *is* "terribly major," yet disquieting evidence of what is unknown or simply too expensive to implement is quite sobering.

SCHOOL-BASED COGNITIVE-BEHAVIORAL PREVENTION

Recent years have seen prevention programs and research both refine long-standing areas of interest and introduce new programs in response to societal pressures. The school has remained a prime environment to introduce prevention programs (Allen, Chinsky, Larsen, Lochman, & Sellinger, 1976; Bower, 1965; Cowen, 1973). The advent of cognitive-behavioral approaches may be particularly attractive to school personnel because of the intuitive relationship between academic goals and those of cognitive training.

Social problem solving continues to attract attention, especially in terms of relating skills in problem solving or decision making to adjustment. Programs to combat teenage pregnancy, substance abuse by children and youth, divorce support groups for children and parents, and programs to provide skills to children to avoid or report physical and sexual abuse are newer additions to the prevention armamentarium.

Each of the prevention approaches reviewed in this chapter contains interventions reflecting core assertions of cognitive-behavioral therapy (Mahoney, 1977; Mahoney & Nezworski, 1985). These are:

1. Humans respond to cognitive representations of their environments rather than to the environments per se.
2. The cognitive representations are functionally related to the processes and parameters of learning.
3. Most human learning is cognitively mediated.
4. Thoughts, feelings, and behaviors are causally interactive.

A framework, commonly used in prevention research, may be a useful device to organize what is currently known or being attempted in the cognitive-behavioral area for prevention. When considering how children might avoid emotional, behavioral, learning, or adjustment problems, the challenge can be divided into interventions directed at the agent (those things or people that cause problems for children), the environment (places where children spend their time and where they can experience either health-producing or debilitating effects), and the host (the children themselves).

For each of the intervention areas, attention to agent, environment, and host will be highlighted. This analysis suggests gaps in preventive efforts with children. The next three sections cover social problem solving, social skills training, and rational-emotive therapy. These three approaches have much in common and form the building blocks of applications in substance abuse, pregnancy, suicide, and injury prevention.

Social Problem Solving

Social problem solving (SPS) is the most mature of the cognitive-behavioral intervention approaches. Based on Meichenbaum's pioneering work with impulsive children (Asarnow & Meichenbaum, 1979; Meichenbaum & Burland, 1979; Meichenbaum & Goodman, 1969), SPS has attracted proponents primarily because of its promise of a "portable" reinforcement system. Efforts with SPS are aimed at hosts, that is, children themselves. Dismayed with the generalization problems so frequently encountered after apparently successful behavioral remediation, researchers and practitioners have seen SPS as a way for children to mediate their own behavioral programs and thus achieve social competence, that is, "those coordinated sets of behaviors that help people adapt effectively within the contexts of their social environment" (Kirschenbaum & Ordman, 1984, p. 381).

Certainly, behaviors that facilitate successful adaptation to the social environment are prime targets for prevention-minded professionals. Such adaptation, often termed "adjustment" in the research literature, is the sine qua non of prevention. The consistent success of SPS training in improving cognitive skills in dealing with analogue problems is an exciting finding. The inconsistency with which SPS is related to adjustment is a serious concern (Olsen & Work, 1986).

Because the SPS training literature is critically evaluated in the excellent chapter by Urbain and Savage (Chapter 17, this volume), it is not reviewed herein. As Urbain and Savage conclude, researchers have been successful in improving children's performance on tests of social problem solving. The goal of improved behavioral adjustment, however, has been more elusive.

Work in mathematics may be instructive to SPS researchers (Silver & Thompson, 1984). Problem solving is a major focus of math teachers. Mathematics educator researchers (e.g., Dodson, 1970; Hollander, 1979; Kilpatrick & Wirszup, 1976; Peacock, 1980; Robinson, 1973; Talton, 1973) have identified characteristics or skills associated with successful math problem solving. Some of these are: (1) grasps the structure of the problem; (2) visualizes and interprets quantitative or spatial facts and relationships; (3) exhibits flexibility of mental processes; (4) generalizes on the basis of a few examples; (5) strives for clarity, simplicity, economy, and rationality of solutions; (6) possesses a generalized memory for mathematical relationships, schemes of arguments and proofs, structural characteristics, and so on; (7) recognizes irrelevant information; and (8) estimates answers.

Although these are math skills, they include some skills analogous to those needed in social situations. For example, grasping the implications of a problem, being flexible in solution generation, generalizing from a few experiences, forecasting consequences of actions, and ignoring irrelevant information all seem crucial to high-level social functioning.

Efforts to improve or create these skills in mathematics students have shown that heuristic teaching methods are effective in promoting the skills if the methods are grounded in math concepts. For example, children taught to make tables, draw diagrams, estimate answers before solving the problem, and judge the reasonableness of the answer improve in math performance (deBono, 1976, 1977; Feuerstein, 1980; Marcucci, 1980). These grounded methods were far more effective than more general approaches that emphasized divergent thinking (e.g., Covington & Crutchfield, 1965; Olton et al., 1967; Jerman, 1971; Treffinger, 1969).

Apparently, children (and perhaps adults) learn how to do tasks within a context. They do not easily learn, nor do they require, general principles applicable across many situations (Tharp & Gallimore, 1985). As Ryle (1971) has suggested, "Rules like birds must live before they are stuffed" (p. 221). The teaching of only general skills may be a serious waste of time and may account for some of the variability in the research findings concerning SPS. Researchers and practitioners using SPS might examine the Spivack and Shure methods in terms of the combination of competency and skill training. This combination may ground the problem-solving process in a content domain of social skills.

Social Skills Training

A related and overlapping literature that holds promise as a prevention area is that of social skills training (Adkins, 1970, 1974; Argyle, Tower, & Bryant, 1974; Carroll & Elliott, 1984; Elardo & Cooper, 1977; Goldstein, Sprafkin, Gershaw, & Klein, 1980; Guerney, 1977; Hawley & Hawley, 1975; McGinnis & Goldstein, 1984; Stephens, 1978). In fact, Goldstein and Pentz (1984) call specifically for social skills training programs to follow "both the spirit and much of the substance of community psychology" (p. 321) by emphasizing preventive applications.

Almost all social skills training packages include modeling, instructions, performance feedback, and role playing. The research literature overwhelmingly supports the efficacy of these four elements in teaching, even to very skill deficient children, new skills (e.g., starting a conversation, giving feedback, accepting criticism, finishing work, dealing with anger, negotiating). The importance of these skills is supported by research in the area of, for example, aggressive or delinquent youngsters (Freedman, Rosenthal, Donahoe, Schbundy, & McFall, 1978; Spence, 1981). Aggressive and nonaggressive children differ on a wide array of interpersonal, planning, anger management, and psychological skills. These differences suggest the potential efficacy of training offered to children who are at risk for serious delinquency problems.

The relation of cognitive-behavioral training (CBT) to social skills training is unclear. Although clearly efficacious programs (Goldstein, 1981) include cognitive components, especially coaching and modeling (Hobbs, Moguin, Tyroler, & Lahey, 1980; Lahey & Strauss, 1982), Gresham (1985) has questioned whether CBT induces more generalization of social skills training than do merely operant techniques. Obviously, the generalization of the skills is the test of the usefulness of social skills training as a primary prevention strategy.

Efforts at improving generalization by teaching problem-solving skills and coping strategies (Mahoney, 1974; Walker & Buckley, 1972) and providing *in vivo* treatment (Drum & Figler, 1973; Goldstein, Heller, & Sechrest, 1966) have been somewhat promising, but the bulk of the research literature in social skills training has not successfully attended to the generalization problem (see Goldstein & Pentz, 1984, for review).

Gresham (1985) has provided an interesting outcome variable framework relevant to research efforts and evaluation of social skills training. He distinguishes among three types of outcome measures:

1. Type I measures are socially valid markers of whether or not skills are being utilized in a child's life space.
2. Type II measures are empirically related to Type I measures but are not socially valid in and of themselves (e.g., observations of children's friendship patterns).
3. Type III measures are the least socially valid (of these three), show poor reliability, and have low or insignificant correlations with Types I and II measures.

To be judged successful, social skills training must produce effects on Type I measures—for example, peer acceptance, teacher and parent judgments, or psychological referral rates. Unfortunately, much of the work in social skills training and in CBT relies on Type III measures as criterion variables—for example, behavior in role plays, tests of social problem solving, or perspective taking (e.g., Russel & Roberts, 1979).

Awaiting empirical validation are some promising directions for social skills trainers to pursue. These include: (1) allowing subjects to choose the skills they learn or teaching a skill initially that is likely to yield immediate, real-world rewards for the trainee; (2) using trainers who can create prescriptively appropriate relationships with trainees (e.g., low empathy and high directiveness with aggressive boys) (Edelman & Goldstein, 1984); (3) holding *in vivo* training during times that allow children to escape less reinforcing activities; (4) adding the teaching of prosocial values and aggression inhibitors to the basic package of social skills training (Spatz-Norton, 1984; Zimmerman, 1984); (5) targeting teachers and parents for special training along with children (Goldstein, Apter, & Harootunian, 1984); and (6) selection of target skills that do not reflect simple skill deficits but distinguish more finely among degrees of deficiency, the interpersonal and environmental contexts in which the deficiency manifests itself, and the particular nature (i.e., knowledge, behavior, or self-feedback) of the deficit (Goldstein & Pentz, 1984; Ladd & Mize, 1983).

Goldstein and Glick (1987) present a social skills approach to reducing aggressive behavior that combines social skills and moral education (i.e., behavioral, affective, and cognitive components). Baker *et al.* (1984) noted that large effect sizes of such combination approaches. It may be that social skills programs are not enhanced with the addition of, for example, only decision-making skills, but require attention to affective issues and a grounding in moral values.

Rational-Emotive Therapy

Ellis's rational-emotive therapy (RET; Ellis, 1973; Ellis & Harper, 1975) and Maultsby's rational behavior therapy (RBT; 1971) are closely related to SPS and social skills training. Because RET and RBT are so similar, the following discussion uses RET to indicate both approaches. RET's concern with the identification of self-defeating (irrational) thoughts, and conviction that people are disturbed more by their appraisals of events than by the events themselves, place it clearly within the province of cognitive-behavioral therapy. RET has been used extensively with youth (e.g., Beckmeyer, 1974; Bernard & Joyce, 1984; DiGiuseppe, 1975; Hauck, 1967; Knaus, 1974; Knaus & Boker, 1975; Maultsby, 1975; McMullin & Casey, 1974; Moleski & Tosi, 1976; Roush, 1984; Tosi, 1974; Tosi & Moleski, 1973; Young, 1974, 1975).

Of particular note has been the success of RET approaches in increasing grade-point averages and attendance, and decreasing disruptiveness and the discipline–referral–recidivism rates of high school students (Block, 1978; Warren, Smith, & Velten, 1984; Zelie, Stone, & Lehr, 1980). These variables are Type I measures and relate to the successful adjustment of individuals to their school environment. RET in schools has been delivered via small counseling groups or as an alternative to the usual discipline response after a teacher referral. A group format increases the usefulness of RET as a preventive intervention, as does the likelihood that RET could be incorporated into the usual procedures of a school program. RET has usually been offered to students on a weekly or twice per week basis for a class period over the course of 3 to 12 weeks (Cangelosi, Gressard, & Mines, 1980; Maultsby, Knipping, & Carpenter, 1974). Optimal time frames and intensity for RET training have not been well researched but certainly deserve attention, especially if large-scale preventive programs are envisioned.

Analysis

Several observations may be pertinent to the use of social problem solving, social skills training, and rational-emotive therapy by prevention-minded professionals. First, most of the work in this area has focused on the host—that is, the child—to the exclusion of environmental and agent considerations. Second, even this focus on the child has been rather narrow in that developmental considerations and other person variables (sex, ethnicity, preexisting skills, causal attributional style, motivation for change) have not been part of experimental designs. Finally, despite evidence that time may be a factor in seeing generalized effects of training, most research work still relies on brief posttesting periods with measures that may lack social validity.

These criticisms do not apply equally to all the available research. The ICPS work of Shure and Spivack has included training efforts with both teachers and parents. In this way, the child's environment has been changed and possible agent problems addressed. Spivack has identified the training of significant caregivers as the important difference between his and others' less successful work (Bales, 1985). In like manner, the application of RET in the schools has necessitated different adult responses to children's difficulties. Such adult changes may account for the success of the technique with children.

There is growing evidence that these techniques must be used prescriptively. For example, the experience of Weissberg *et al.* (1981a, 1981b) shows that social class may interact with the success of SPS programs. Olsen and Work (1986) suggest that children's empathy levels affect their success in applying SPS: Those who are initially highest in empathy benefit most from training. Little is known about how developmental levels and basic cognitive-processing strengths and deficits of the host interact with successful cognitive-behavioral interventions (Eastman & Rasbury, 1981). It seems obvious, however, that more effective training models could be established if these variables were taken into consideration. For example, because children's friendships change over time (e.g., from parallel play partner to confidante), the kinds of skills taught at different ages should be different (Kendall, 1985). In like manner, the severity of the problem being addressed, the host's preexisting skills and competencies, self-perceived efficacy, causal attribution for success and failure, motivation for change, and the quality of the child's school and home environments are all variables that are likely to contribute to treatment by subject interactions (Abikoff, 1985; Meichenbaum & Asarnow, 1979; Whalen, Henker, & Hinshaw, 1985).

Although attention to all these considerations is difficult under any circumstances, the need to individualize implies that SPS, social skills training, and perhaps even RET are not panaceas for preventive work. Mahoney and Nezworski (1985) categorize rationalistic versus developmental approaches in cognitive-behavior therapy. Their distinctions are valuable in the context of this discussion as they argue that teaching skills is probably not enough. The teaching must be done with a thorough knowledge of the inner person being taught. They assert that attention to the impact of early experience on individual differences in cognitive style, the role of affective processes in adaptation, the role of the family and other social systems on the acquisition of cognitive patterns, and the role of self-identity processes in psychological change and maintenance are crucial to the continued health of the cognitive-behavioral approaches to change.

The significant issues raised by Mahoney and Nezworski (1985) and others suggest that attention beyond the host is crucial. Well-trained teachers and parents could presumably accomplish the individualization of cognitive-behavioral programs that researchers find impossible to do because of internal validity concerns. The future of the SPS, social skills training, and RET as preventive interventions may depend on the application of the techniques to and by members of children's daily environments.

SPECIFIC APPLICATIONS OF COGNITIVE-BEHAVIORAL METHODS FOR PREVENTION

There are many examples of applying cognitive-behavioral methods to preventing children's problems. For example, work is being done for children of divorce, pregnancy and drug prevention, prevention of abuse and injury, and suicide prevention for children. Again, in most of this work, the host is the major target, but some notable exceptions exist. Several of these areas are reviewed below.

Pregnancy Prevention

Forty percent of young women will become pregnant while they are teenagers. Eighty percent of teenage males and 70% of teenage females report having had sexual intercourse (Brody, 1986; Marecek, 1987). The social and personal costs of teenage pregnancy are enormous. Not only do many young pregnant women drop out of school, and thus become candidates for substandard employment or income assistance programs, but infants born to young mothers are more likely to exhibit a host of physiological problems. Even with about 40% of the 1.1 million teenage pregnancies ending every year in abortion (Dryfoos & Bourque-Scholl, 1981; Interdivisional Committee on Adolescent Abortion, 1987), it is clear that many infants are being born into environments characterized by economic hardship and deficit parenting skills. Pregnancy prevention programs are either generic sex education programs or more focused programs aimed specifically at pregnancy prevention and counseling.

Sex Education

The core goal of any sex education program is to improve a young person's ability to make informed choices (Calderone, 1975; Gilgun & Gordon, 1983; Gordon, Scales, & Everly, 1979; Passmore, 1980; World Health Organization, 1975). Passmore wrote that "sex education is to teach children to act more responsibly, to think about what they are doing" (p. 30). With this definition in mind, the (potentially) central role of cognitive-behavioral strategies is clear.

Juhasz (1983) argues convincingly that sex education curricula should reflect information from Piaget, Erikson, and social learning theory. Although Juhasz does not provide evidence concerning training so conceptualized, her line of reasoning is reflective of Mahoney and Nezworski's (1985) call for increased developmental stage sophistication on the part of researchers and practitioners of cognitive-behavioral therapy.

Most American parents are favorable to schools providing sex education as a regular curriculum area. Many parents and most adolescents would like sex education courses to cover controversial topics such as abortion, masturbation, contraception, homosexuality, and values (Roberts, Klein, & Gagnon, 1978; Scales, 1981).

Despite this apparent mandate, the experience of school personnel is that sex education programs are predictably polarizing (Hazard & Einstein, 1983; Wayne, 1982). Exemplary programs do exist, however, and strategies to enhance program acceptability have been developed (Harris, Baird, Clyburn, & Mara, 1983; Rogers, Merriam, & Munson, 1983). Cognitive-behaviorists can note that successful programs have emphasized means–end thinking and a change in young people's understanding of themselves and others. For example, one favorable change has been from seeing others as sexual conquests or symbols of status to an understanding of the dignity and worth of individuals.

Despite the importance of sex education programs and the potential to develop excellent ones, most new teachers are unprepared to teach sex education (Thompson, 1983). A change in teacher preparation programs to include sex education training might facilitate a positive change in children's school environment.

Pregnancy Prevention

The role of cognitive-behavioral interventions is very striking in pregnancy prevention programming. Contraceptive failure has been associated with various cognitive and behavioral skill deficits (Campbell & Barnlund, 1977; Cvetkovich, Grote, Lieberman, & Miller, 1978; Dembo & Lundell, 1979).

Successful programs provide both decision-making skills and training in assertiveness, interpersonal competencies, and communication skills (Blyth, Gilchrist, & Schinke, 1981; Schinke, Blyth, & Gilchrist, 1981). These researchers point out that even teenagers who have made a decision to avoid intercourse may lack the assertiveness skills to say, "No," or the communication skills to explain their decision persuasively to others.

The Blyth *et al.* (1981) and Schinke *et al.* (1981) programs consisted of 14 one-hour sessions emphasizing modeling, role play, coaching, feedback, and social reinforcement. Positive results were obtained on knowledge, decision-making skills, student evaluation of the programs, and follow-up measures of students' intentions to delay pregnancy, and on their use of contraception.

Substance Abuse Prevention

Rates of tobacco, alcohol, and drug use are unacceptably high among teenagers (MacDonald, 1984). The use of these agents is associated with health, school, and behavioral problems in young people (Hawkins, Lishner, & Catalano, 1985). For example, even though about 1 million arrests take place yearly for driving under the influence of alcohol (U.S. Department of Commerce, 1984), alcohol is still involved in 50% to 55% of all fatal accidents, 18% to 25% of injury-producing crashes, and 5% to 8% of property damage crashes (Fell, 1983). Further, early use of these substances predicts later abuse (Kellam, Simon, & Ensminger, 1983; Yamaguchi & Kandel, 1984). The area of substance abuse prevention is clearly a high-priority prevention target and matches recent descriptions of modern psychology as being particularly concerned with prevention, health enhancement, life-style change, and interdisciplinary approaches (Matarazzo, 1982).

Substance abuse programs have begun to shift away from mere information about the dangers and problems associated with use of the agents to an emphasis on lifelong decision making (St. Pierre & Miller, 1985–1986). New programs use cognitive-behavioral strategies to improve decision making; skills in dealing with peer pressure; and skills in clarifying values associated with health, behavior, conformity, etc. (Engs, 1981; Glynn, Leukefeld, & Ludford, 1983).

Apparently the skills of teachers are important in this area, as some researchers have found that teachers not specifically trained in substance abuse issues were ineffective in improving the decision-making skills of 12- to 15-year-olds with respect to the use of harmful substances (Newman, Mohr, Badger, & Gillespie, 1984). Analogously, the skills of those who serve alcoholic beverages have been found to affect the drinking behavior of individuals. Russ and Geller (1986) report on a program to teach servers to discriminate among drinkers on the basis of level of intoxication and age. Their program also taught various skills—for example, reducing the flow of alcohol to the intoxicated patron, providing alternative drinks or food to the patron, asking who was driving, checking identification, explaining tavern policies regarding serving drinks to intoxicated individuals, putting less alcohol in a drink, and seeking support from management and peers for monitoring intoxication levels.

Some of these same skills might be taught to adolescents to monitor the drinking behaviors of their friends. The server program had positive preliminary effects on changing server behavior and reducing blood alcohol levels of patrons served by trained servers. This program deserves attention as an effort to change the environment in which alcohol abuse occurs.

Very little evaluative information appears to be available concerning the effects of drug education programs. Historically, most programs affected people's reported knowledge and attitudes toward dangerous substances but did nothing to lessen use. Schinke and Gilchrist (1985) report on a successful school-based program that emphasized problem-solving skills, self-instruction, interpersonal communication, knowledge about substances, and peer testimonials. Two-year follow-up results were encouraging.

Substance abuse is clearly an area that demands multimodal action involving educational, legal, and social interventions with hosts, agents, and environments. One disconcerting finding has been, for example, that a large percentage of the alcohol consumed by underage minors is provided to them by parents. It is already well known that drug abusing teens tend to come from families in which alcohol, prescription drugs, and/or illicit drugs are abused. In addition, schools are primary sites for the purchase of drugs. Yet, the overwhelming amount of literature in the area concerns interventions with the child host alone. Such a narrow focus may explain the disappointing results.

Prevention of Child Injury

Accidents are the number one killer of children under 18 years of age (Gratz, 1979; Wright, Schaefer, & Solomons, 1979). In fact, more children die in accidents than as a result of the next six leading causes combined. One out of every three medical interventions with children deals with child injury, whether due to accidents or to abuse by adults.

Accidental Injury

The host characteristics of accident victims have been determined (Peterson & Mori, 1985). Those children most likely to be involved in accidents are boys, aggressive children, children from single-parent families, children of teenage mothers, and children from large families. Toddlers are most likely to be injured by poisons, preschoolers by drownings, and school-aged children through pedestrian accidents.

Agents involved in hurting children are automobiles, swimming or bath water, fire or hot surfaces, poisons, falls, and dangerous adults. Environments in which children are most frequently injured include the home (especially in the absence of adult supervision); automobiles (especially in the absence of seatbelt use); and family situations characterized by illness, relocation, the birth of a sibling, or economic hardship (Peterson & Mori, 1985).

This information is, of course, crucial to designing programs that target particular ages and populations of children. These data also speak to the need for cooperative efforts among many disciplines. For example, interventions concerning the agents that injure children may require legislation, education, and persuasion and are likely to involve psychologists at policymaking (rather than individual) levels (DeLeon, VandenBos, & Kraut, 1984).

Successful cognitive-behavioral programs have been reported to deal with pedestrian safety (Yeaton & Bailey, 1978), reactions to fire (Jones, Kazdin, & Haney, 1981), and the correct way to recognize and report emergencies (Rosenbaum, Creedon, & Drabman, 1981). Galambos and Garbarino (1983) report on a successful program to train latchkey children to respond to emergencies, deal with strangers, and contact their parents. Their intervention focused on teaching problem solving, self-reinforcement, and discrimination among stimuli. This work is especially noteworthy as it targeted children who were in high-risk environments, that is, unsupervised home situations. Of course, as Zigler

(1982) has pointed out, there would be less need for such programming if high-quality, low-cost day care were made available to parents. While child-oriented professionals await a change in the political climate, the schools provide a base from which to offer programs that have been shown to lessen accidental injury to children.

Physical and Sexual Abuse

Although the prevalence and incidence of child abuse has become a national scandal (Finkelhor, 1979; National Center on Child Abuse and Neglect, 1982), surprisingly little research has been done in the area, despite the large number of programs currently in use to teach children skills for preventing abuse. The history of such efforts may help to explain the lack of research evidence on effectiveness. Hazzard and Angert (1986) cite rape crisis centers and social service agencies as the original providers of information and intervention on abuse. These were locally funded efforts; abuse prevention programs did not receive federal funding until 1980. This grass-roots history naturally led to an emphasis on service rather than evaluation. Research was not reported in academic journals but, rather, exists in hard-to-access program reports—or not at all.

Most programs focus on elementary school children and usually have the goal of increasing children's information about abuse. Only a few programs report targeting skills development (Downer, 1984; Finkelhor, 1986; Poche, Brouwer, & Swearingen, 1981). Such a knowledge focus is ironic because those who have already been abused seem to be least prepared to avoid it in the future. Merely knowing about abuse is not a sufficient inoculation against its occurrence (Toal, 1985).

The skill programs teach assertiveness, communication, and specific behavioral skills to avoid abuse (e.g., run away from a stranger, scream if someone tries to grab you, seek the help of a mother with children or a grandmother if you are lost), while also providing a cognitive context for the child to use in understanding abuse. This context usually involves teaching children their rights to privacy, differences between good and bad touching, their right to report abuse and keep reporting if not believed the first time, and their blamelessness for abusive events. As staggering as the abuse problem is, evaluation of skills is difficult because abuse is a relatively low frequency event and because ethical concerns make analogue evaluations impossible.

Suicide Prevention

Although the need for an array of suicide prevention activities in schools is clear, almost no information is available concerning the outcomes of existing programs. Suicide is the second leading cause of death among adolescents and the eighth among children 5 through 14 years old. Given the historical underreporting of suicide, the actual rates may be much higher, with some suicides reported as accidental deaths (Greuling & DeBlassie, 1980; National Center for Health Statistics, 1986). In fact, some experts suggest the true child rate of suicide could be anywhere between 7 and 100 suicides per 100,000 rather than the more widely quoted rate of 1.6 suicides per 100,000 (McGuire & Ely, 1984).

The predictors of suicidal behavior in children and adolescents are known, and some of these may be amenable to cognitive-behavioral interventions. For example, the loss or threatened loss of a love object, a history of discord between child and parents, physical or sexual abuse, substance abuse, poverty, suicidal parents or siblings, social isolation, academic problems, and mistaken cognitions concerning death may all contribute to a child's decision to engage in suicidally dangerous behavior (Hawton, 1982). There are research reports concerning the effectiveness of cognitive-behavioral strategies with at least six out of those nine predictors (Dodge, Murphy, & Bushbaum, 1984; Kendall, 1985; Meichenbaum, Bream, & Cohen, 1983; Milich & Dodge, 1984; Stevens & Pihl, 1982; Whalen, Henker, & Hinshaw, 1985; Wong, 1985).

Because the predictors of suicidal behavior are well known, school-based professionals could identify vulnerable children, who could then be offered services for depression, substance abuse problems, physical and sexual abuse prevention, social isolation, communication skills training, and so on. Screening programs to target vulnerable children are already well researched and have had significant success in reducing later maladjustment (Cowen, 1982; Lorion, Work, & Hightower, 1984).

Work with vulnerable children seems the most efficacious in terms of suicide prevention. Suicidal children give many clues to their disturbance but often spend their days in schools with no well-developed personal counseling services available. In recent years, school personnel have reacted to child and adolescent suicides with crisis intervention teams and teacher/parent education efforts. Longitudinal research could ascertain the relative effectiveness of prescriptively targeted counseling versus these crisis intervention attempts on overall suicide rates among already vulnerable children.

INTERVENTIONS WITH TEACHERS

Most of the reviewed studies up to now have been concerned with improving children's skills. As important as this approach is, a narrow focus on the host alone is both practically and theoretically unsound. Children's behavior is the product of reciprocal influences among their unique temperaments, learning histories, and social and physical environments (Bandura, 1978). The adults who care for children have important effects on the entire spectrum of childhood behaviors. In addition, as Albee (1968, 1982) predicted, there are many more needy people than there are persons available to provide care. The next logical steps are both to teach child caregivers important skills, thus increasing the reach of professionals, and to attend to the mental health needs of caregivers.

Attending to the mental health needs of caregivers is explored in the following section. Teacher wellness may be an important aspect of comprehensive preventive services to children.

Stress Reduction

The incidence among teachers of emotional maladjustment, especially anxiety, has been the focus of several national studies (e.g., National Education Association [NEA], 1967; New York State United Teachers, 1980). Since 1938 a sizable minority of teachers have described themselves as seriously worried and nervous, and as working under considerable strain (Leach, 1984). An NEA survey revealed that 78% of U.S. teachers experience moderate to considerable levels of stress (Coates & Thoresen, 1976). Similarly, the Chicago teachers' union reported that 56% of members responding to a survey reported a physical illness they related to their occupational distress, and 25% blamed job stress for mental disorders (cited in Sparks & Hammond, 1981).

The correlates of teachers' perceptions of their situations are disturbing. Between 7 and 10 million suburban and 13 and 22 million urban teachers report feeling "burned out." Only about 59% of teachers last more than 4 years in teaching, and only about 60% say they intend to remain teachers until retirement (Farber, 1984). Burned-out teachers see themselves as more negative toward students (Schwab, 1983); suffer physical symptoms including fatigue, headaches, weight loss, gastrointestinal problems, skin rashes, and high blood pressure; and report psychological manifestations including feelings of helplessness, paranoia, mood swings, and irritability (Eskridge & Coker, 1985). Estimates suggest that one-third of all teacher sick days are related to stress (Block, 1978).

Teacher stress has been related to less effective teaching and discipline strategies and to higher levels of student anxiety (Coates & Thoresen, 1976; Doyal & Forsyth, 1973). In addition, stressed teachers seem to have poor rapport with and show less warmth toward students (Kracht & Casey, 1968; Petrusich, 1966).

The sources of teacher stress are diverse. They are reported to include student violence, lack of administrative support and appreciation, coping with student apathy, poor staff communication, time pressures, unprofessional behavior of colleagues, low salaries, and stressors from family or nonwork environments (Eskridge & Coker, 1985; Johnson, Gold, & Vicker, 1982; New York State United Teachers, 1980; Raschke, Dedrick, Strathe, & Hawkes, 1985; Woodhouse, Hall, & Wooster, 1985).

Stress reduction programs are common, and most rely heavily on cognitive-behavioral principles (e.g., Forman, 1982; Forman & Forman, 1980; Friedman, Lehrer, & Stevens, 1983; Gmelch, 1983; Jaremko, 1984; Moracco & McFadden, 1982; Sparks, 1983; Tolman & Sheldon, 1985). Most of the programs emphasize individual strategies. These programs may show only short-term improvements, however, because the structural or organizational causes of stress remain even when teachers learn to relax, set realistic goals, seek peer support, engage in exercise programs, or reinforce themselves (Blase, 1984).

Tunnecliffe, Leach, and Tunnecliffe (1986) provided a test of the relative effectiveness over time of a collaborative behavioral consultation (CBC) treatment versus relaxation training on perceived stress levels among 21 Australian teachers. They conceptualized the CBC as attending to systemic and environmental stressors as well as providing teachers with individual problem-solving skills. In contrast, relaxation training was presented as an individualistic, clinical approach to stress. Consonant with their predictions, CBC was most effective in reducing teacher stress both immediately following treatment and at a 3-month follow-up. The authors' credit CBC's success to its focus on joint problem solving of organizational problems, an increased commitment to carrying out solutions because teachers were part of the decision-making process, and the effect CBC had on increasing the collegiality in the experimental school.

If comprehensive programming for teacher wellness were to occur, it would undoubtedly have to include attention to host skills and environmental and agent manipulations. Conners (1983) provides a fascinating assessment of one source of teacher stress—the actual physical environment of the school building. He points out that such physical features as availability of activity areas, floor plan, building and room orientation, color, density, seating arrangements, privacy areas, and noise level have all been related to teachers' stress levels. Changes in any of these factors would be a bit far afield from common cognitive-behavioral strategies, but would validate the importance of individuals' perceptions of their personal contexts as vitally important to their high-level functioning.

Analysis

There is a dearth of evaluative literature on the long-term effects of stress reduction programs for teachers. Most measurement is of the Type III variety and is collected immediately after training (Gresham, 1985). The evaluation of programs that benefit teachers directly is an important research priority in an ecological approach to the prevention of childhood difficulties. As such, it deserves serious attention from researchers as well as practitioners. This research situation is analogous to the one still prevalent in teacher consultation research. That is, although a primary purpose of teacher consultation is to have an effect on the daily activities of consultees, very little research actually documents that effect. Most interventions aimed at teachers are hoped to improve both teacher and student circumstances. This hope may be futile, however, if carefully designed research efforts are not implemented to discover and build on the generative bases for teacher and student dysfunction.

Reducing teacher stress is, of course, only one avenue to promoting children's mental health. Earlier in this chapter, efforts to improve teacher skills were mentioned in reference to social problem-solving curricula. Most efforts at improving teacher skills and knowledge are implemented via in-service training, although the effectiveness of in-service training approaches is notoriously suspect in terms of facilitating behavioral change among participants. Even the most carefully prepared in-service program is unlikely to help teachers use new skills. The factors that enhance implementation of knowledge must be studied. Such study may suggest that one-shot in-services without follow-up consultation are useless or that districts should design year-long systematic study of only a few topics instead of the cafeteria-style programming that is now so common. Whatever the results, implementation studies are just as crucial as are tests of new cognitive-behavioral interventions. If no one uses the "truth," not much has changed for children.

SUMMARY AND CONCLUSIONS

This chapter has defined prevention, reviewed cognitive-behavioral research with children with an emphasis on preventive applications, and noted the disappointingly sparse information available about preventive interventions with teachers. Despite mixed research findings, a broad analysis of what is currently extant in cognitive-behavioral therapy with children suggests a very exciting future.

Although no one strategy provides perfect inoculation of children against future difficulties, there are increasingly strong suggestions that combination approaches are very promising. Cognitive-behavioral therapy can be a part of a comprehensive prevention program that attends to hosts, environments, and agents. Cognitive-behavioral applications seem most feasible with hosts and with members of children's environments, especially teachers and parents. Affecting harmful agents may be most difficult for psychological intervention, especially if interventions are conceptualized at only individual or small-group levels. Some thoughts on a school-based preventive orientation follow.

Host

All children should receive training in decision making, problem solving, assertiveness, empathy, and social skills as part of their regular curricula from kindergarten onward. This training should be adjusted for their social class and entry skills. As they enter kindergarten, children identified as vulnerable deserve special attention, whether or not they are eligible for special education. This screening may be quite comprehensive or as simple as noting the children who do not hand in work.

As children progress through school, their special circumstances should be tracked. Children who experience trauma such as abuse, divorce, poverty, injury, and so on could be identified and involved in special support programs. Children who attempt suicide or engage in reckless behavior also need immediate attention.

At each age, predictable presses should be anticipated and appropriately grounded training offered. This would include instruction on how to make friends, study for tests, prepare large assignments, avoid drugs, manage emergencies when home alone, avoid or report abuse, prevent pregnancy, and prepare for relationships and parenthood. These programs would be offered, not as one-shot classes, but as pervasive components of the curriculum. All teachers would be prepared in sex education, substance abuse prevention, and the teaching of social skills and decision making.

Environment

Children live in homes, schools, and neighborhoods. They must be taught skills to manage successfully in all their environments (study skills, cooperation, locking doors, asking for help). They deserve environments free of dangerous physical objects and abusive or unskilled people. Children's environments are enhanced through parent training, high-quality teacher preparation programs, facilitative classroom structures and procedures, and accessible mental health services for them and their families. Optimal environments are the result of a convergence of action from many systems at all levels.

For example, although we know we can teach children safer pedestrian behavior, we also need legislation regarding drunk driving, speed limits, seatbelt use, and the like. Similarly, although we can teach parents skills that are useful in raising children and structuring leisure time, parents also benefit from social service policies that promote family competence and from national priorities to provide high-quality child care (Edelman, 1981).

The skills needed to operate beyond the individual level and to apply cognitive-behavioral interventions with legislators as well as clients are not well known to all psychologists. They should be well known to school and community psychologists, however, and must be routinely practiced.

Agent

The agents that harm children are controlled primarily through macrosystem interventions. Laws regarding drinking ages and the enforcement of school building safety standards are not in the cognitive-behavioral arena. There are, however, important social policy and consultation roles available to cognitive-behaviorists (Burchard, 1986). For example, school principals who want to mount effective substance abuse or pregnancy prevention programs might be well served by consultants who understand both system realities (e.g., the effects of community standards on acceptable curriculum, the political leverage of various community groups, the preparation needs of teachers) and the way people learn to monitor and change their behavior. Experts in functional analysis are vital resources for legislators who want to understand the factors that maintain poverty, violence, illiteracy, and abuse in a country as resource-rich as the United States.

Harmful agents, the people and things that endanger children, are best handled by removing them from a child's environment. This however, remains a very great challenge.

The New School Psychologist

Clearly, a new kind of psychologist is called for when prevention is the important school system goal. Cowen *et al.* (1975) have called for a "quarterback"—a psychologist who manages people and programs that anticipate and meet the needs of children. This psychologist is an expert about children: who they are, where they live, what they need, and what can go wrong. He or she is a family and school systems expert because to fail to know families and schools is to fail to know children.

The activities of the new school psychologist are quite varied in terms of roles, functions, and operational levels. This new clinician works from micro- to macrosystem levels to piece together comprehensive, coordinated service packages for children and families. He or she is part of many teams and plans interventions for children on the basis of their particular needs and their special potentials. Children identified as vulnerable or at risk in the school environment absorb a good portion of this psychologist's time, but some planning is always in process concerning prevention and enhancement programs for children, their teachers, and their parents.

To make the ideal prevention program work, there must be enough of these new psychologists to keep ahead of the unrelenting press of clinical cases, so that some can be assigned to go out and learn how to stop the casualties, rather than everyone waiting for the next crisis to explode.

The impact of a preventive mindset on the activities and priorities of the school psychologist would be profound, indeed. Traditional norm-referenced testing would become an optional, and perhaps infrequently used, choice. Children would be known by their strengths and weaknesses, not by shorthand descriptions of their problems. Psychologists' recommendations would be tied to the daily behavior of teachers and parents and would be based on well-tested cognitive-behavioral principles.

Psychologists would become far more active in teacher and parent consultation. If 40% of children's achievement is explained by teacher instructional behavior (Stallings, 1975), then teachers and psychologists belong together, working to produce optimal instructional environments for children (Ysseldyke & Christenson, 1986). And if another 30% of achievement is explained by entry skills, then parents are prime targets for intervention as well (Conoley, 1987; Hansen, 1986).

Prevention sounds perfect. It is clearly what most of psychology should be about. Unfortunately, prevention is harder than most thought it would be, and most psychologists (despite some frustration with existing remedial technologies) are socialized as healers, not preventers. Preventing problems is not only a massive logistical problem (i.e., getting services to people), but a difficult theoretical problem (i.e., developing the generative base—the causal links involved in dysfunctions). But some problems are well understood already, and others can be dissected. The school remains the place to reach children. Schools are not perfect platforms for primary and secondary prevention programs but, along with day-care centers, could be sites for a revolution in psychological service delivery if psychologists would have the will to make it happen.

REFERENCES

Abikoff, H. (1985). Efficacy of cognitive training in hyperactive children: A critical review. *Clinical Psychology Review, 5*, 479–512.

Adkins, W. R. (1970). Life skills: Structured counseling for the disadvantaged. *Personnel and Guidance Journal, 49*, 108–116.

Adkins, W. R. (1974). Life coping skills: A fifth curriculum. *Teachers College Record, 75*, 507–526.

Albee, G. W. (1968). Conceptual model and manpower requirements in psychology. *American Psychologist, 23*, 317–320.

Albee, G. W. (1982). Preventing psychopathology and promoting human potential. *American Psychologist, 37*, 1043–1050.

Albee, G. W., & Joffe, J. M. (Eds.) (1977). *The issues: An overview of primary prevention.* Hanover, NH: University Press of New England.

Allen, G. J., Chinsky, J. M., Larsen, S. W., Lochman, J. E., & Selinger, H. V. (1976). *Community psychology and the schools: A behaviorally oriented multilevel preventive approach.* Hillsdale, NJ: Lawrence Erlbaum.

Allen, V. L. (1976). *Children as teachers: Theory and research on tutoring.* New York: Academic Press.

Argyle, M., Tower, P., & Bryant, B. (1974). Explorations in the treatment of personality disorders and neuroses by social skill training. *British Journal of Medical Psychology, 47*, 63–72.

Asarnow, J. R., & Meichenbaum, D. (1979). Verbal rehearsal and serial recall: The medication training of kindergarten children. *Child Development, 50*, 1173–1177.

Baker, S. B., Swisher, J. D., Nadenichek, P. E., & Popowicz, C. L. (1984). Measured effects of primary prevention strategies. *Personnel and Guidance Journal, 63*, 459–463.

Bales, J. (1985). Prevention: NIMH funds five approaches to excellence in prevention. *APA Monitor, 16*, 16–18.

Bandura, A. (1978). The self-system in reciprocal determinism. *American Psychologist, 33*, 344–358.

Baskin, E. J., & Hess, R. D. (1980). Does affective education work? A review of seven programs. *Journal of School Psychology, 18*, 40–50.

Beckmeyer, G. H. (1974). Rational counseling with youthful offenders. *American Journal of Correction, 6*, 34.

Berman, P., & McLaughlin, M. W. (1976). Implementation of educational innovation. *Educational Forum, 40*, 345–370.

Bernard, M. E., & Joyce, M. R. (1984). *Rational emotive therapy with children and adolescents.* New York: Wiley.

Bernhardt, G. R., & Praeger, S. G. (1985). Preventing child suicide: The elementary school death education puppet show. *Journal of Counseling and Development, 63,* 311–312.

Blase, J. J. (1984). A data based model of how teachers cope with work stress. *Journal of Educational Administration, 22,* 173–191.

Blechman, E. A., Kotanchick, N. L., & Taylor, C. J. (1981). Families and school together: Early behavioral intervention with high risk children. *Behavior therapy, 12,* 308–319.

Blechman, E. A., Taylor, C. J., & Schrader, S. M. (1981). Family problem solving versus home notes as early intervention for high-risk children. *Journal of Consulting and Clinical Psychology, 49,* 919–926.

Block, A. M. (1978). Combat neurosis in inner-city schools. *American Journal of Psychiatry, 135,* 1189–1192.

Blyth, B. J., Gilchrist, L. D., & Schinke, S. P. (1981). Pregnancy prevention groups for adolescents. *Social Work, 26,* 503–504.

Boike, M. F. (1986). *Classroom coping skills program.* Paper presented at the Annual Meeting of the American Psychological Association, Washington, DC, August.

Bond, L. A., Rosen, J. C. (Eds.). (1980). *Competence and coping during adulthood.* Hanover, NH: University Press of New England.

Bower, E. M. (1965). Primary prevention of mental and emotional disorders: A conceptual framework and action possibilities. In N. M. Lambert (Ed.), *The protection and promotion of mental health in schools* (pp. 1–9). Public Health Service Publication 1226. Bethesda, MD: U.S. Department of Health, Education and Welfare.

Brody, J. (1986). Personal health. *The New York Times,* April 30, p. C12.

Burchard, J. D. (1986). *Prevention, social policy, and the applied behavior analyst.* Paper presented at the Annual Meeting of the American Psychological Association, Washington DC, August.

Calderone, M. S. (Ed.). (1975). *Sexuality and human values.* Chicago: Association Press/Follett.

Campbell, B. K., & Barnlund, D. C. (1977). Communication patterns and problems of pregnancy. *American Journal of Orthopsychiatry, 97,* 134–139.

Cangelosi, A., Gressard, C. F., & Mines, R. A. (1980). The effects of a rational thinking group on self-concepts of adolescents. *School Counselor,* 357–361.

Caplan, G. (1964). *Principles of preventive psychiatry.* New York: Basic Books.

Carroll, J., & Elliott, S. N. (Eds.). (1984). Social competence and social skills. [Special issue]. *School Psychology Review, 13.*

Chassin, L. A., Presson, C. C., & Sherman, S. J. (1985). Stepping backward in order to step forward. *Journal of Consulting and Clinical Psychology, 53,* 612–622.

Coates, T. J., & Thoresen, C. E. (1976). Teacher anxiety: A review with recommendations. *Review of Educational Research, 46,* 159–184.

Cohen, J. (1969). *Statistical power analysis for the behavioral sciences.* New York: Academic Press.

Conners, D. A. (1983). The school environment: A link to understanding stress. *Theory into Practice, 22,* 16–20.

Conoley, J. C. (1987). Schools and families: Theoretical and practical bridges. *Professional School Psychology, 2,* 191–203.

Covington, M. V., & Crutchfield, R. S. (1965). Facilitation of creative problem solving. *Programmed Instruction, 4,* 3–5.

Cowen, E. L. (1973). Social and community interventions. *Annual Review of Psychology*, *24*, 423–472.

Cowen, E. L. (1977). Baby-steps toward primary prevention. *American Journal of Community Psychology*, *5*, 1–22.

Cowen, E. L. (1980). The wooing of primary prevention. *American Journal of Community Psychology*, *8*, 258–284.

Cowen, E. L. (1982). Primary prevention research: Barriers, needs and opportunities. *Journal of Prevention*, *2*, 131–137.

Cowen, E. L. (1983). Primary prevention in mental health: Past, present, and future. In F. D. Felner, L. A. Jason, J. N. Mortisugu, & S. S. Farber (Eds.), *Preventive psychology: Theory, research, and practice* (pp. 11–25). New York: Pergamon Press.

Cowen, E. (1984). Training for primary prevention in mental health. *American Journal of Community Psychology*, *12*, 253–259.

Cowen, E. L., Trost, M. A., Lorion, R. P., Dorr, D., Izzo, L. D., & Isaacson, R. V. (1975). *New ways in school mental health: Early detection and prevention of school maladaption*. New York: Human Science Press.

Cvetkovich, G., Grote, B., Lieberman, J., & Miller, W. (1978). Sex role development and teenage fertility-related behavior. *Adolescence*, *13*, 231–236.

deBono, E. (1976). *Teaching thinking*. London: Maurice Temple Smith.

deBono, E. (1977). *Lateral thinking: A textbook of creativity*. Harmondsworth, England: Penguin.

DeLeon, F., VandenBos, G. R., & Kraut, A. G. (1984). Federal legislation recognizing psychology. *American Psychologist*, *39*, 933–946.

Dembo, M. H., & Lundell, B. (1979). Factors affecting adolescent contraception practices: Implications for sex education. *Adolescence*, *14*, 657–664.

DiGiuseppe, R. (1975). The use of behavior modification to establish rational self-statements in children. *Rational Living*, *10*, 18–19.

Dodge, K. A., Murphy, R. R., & Bushbaum, K. (1984). The assessment of intention-cue skills in children: Implications for developmental psychopathology. *Child Development*, *55*, 163–173.

Dodson, J. W. (1970). *Characteristics of successful insightful problem solvers*. Unpublished doctoral dissertation, University of Georgia.

Downer, A. (1984). *Evaluation of talking about touching: Personal safety curriculum*. Summary Report. Seattle, WA: Committee for Children.

Doyal, G. T., & Forsyth, R. A. (1973). Relationship between teacher and student anxiety levels. *Psychology in the Schools*, *10*, 231–233.

Drum, D. J., & Figler, H. E. (1973). *Outreach in counseling*. New York: Intex Educational Publications.

Dryfoos, J., & Bourque-Scholl, N. (1981). *Factbook on teenage pregnancy*. New York: Alan Guttmacher Institute.

Durlak, J. A. (1983). Social problem-solving as a primary prevention strategy. In R. D. Felner, L. A. Jason, J. N. Moritsugu, & S. S. Farber (Eds.), *Preventive psychology: Theory, research, and practice* (pp. 31–48). New York: Pergamon Press.

Durlak, J. A. (1985). Primary prevention of school adjustment problems. *Journal of Consulting and Clinical Psychology*, *53*, 623–630.

Eastman, B. G., & Rasbury, W. C. (1981). Cognitive self-instruction for the control of impulsive classroom behavior: Ensuring the treatment package. *Journal of Abnormal Child Psychology*, *9*, 381–387.

Edelman, E., & Goldstein, A. P. (1984). Prescriptive relationship levels for juvenile delinquents in a psychotherapy analog. *Aggressive Behavior, 10*, 269–278.

Edelman, M. W. (1981). Who is for children? *American Psychologist, 36*, 109–116.

Elardo, P. T., & Cooper, M. (1977). *AWARE: Activities for social development.* Reading, MA: Addison-Wesley.

Ellis, A. (1973). *Humanistic psychotherapy: The rational-emotive approach.* New York: Julian Press.

Ellis, A., & Harper, R. A. (1975). *A new guide to rational living.* Englewood Cliffs, NJ: Prentice-Hall.

Engs, R. C. (1981). Responsibility and alcohol. *Health Education, 12*, 20–22.

Epstein, L. H., Wing, R. R., Koeske, R., Andrasik, F., & Ossip, D. J. (1981). Child and parent weight loss in family-based behavior modification programs. *Journal of Consulting and Clinical Psychology, 49*, 674–685.

Eskridge, D. H., & Coker, D. R. (1985). Teacher stress: Symptoms, causes, and management techniques. *The Clearing House, 58*, 387–390.

Farber, B. A. (1984). Teacher burnout: Assumptions, myths, and issues. *Teachers College Record, 86*, 321–338.

Fell, J. C. (1983). Tracking the alcohol involvement problem in U.S. highway crashes. In *Twenty-seventh Annual Proceedings, American Association for Automotive Medicine* (pp. 23–42). San Antonio, TX: American Association for Automotive Medicine.

Felner, R. D., Jason, L. A., Moritsugu, J. N., & Farber, S. S. (Eds.). (1983). *Preventive psychology: Theory, research and practice.* New York: Pergamon Press.

Feuerstein, R. (1980). *Instrumental enrichment.* Baltimore, MD: University Park Press.

Finkelhor, D. (1979). *Sexually victimized children.* New York: Free Press.

Finkelhor, D. (1986). *A sourcebook on child sexual abuse.* Beverly Hills, CA: Sage Publications.

Forgays, D. G. (Ed.). (1978). *Environmental influences and strategies in primary prevention.* Hanover, NH: University Press of New England.

Forman, S. G. (1982). Stress management for teachers: A cognitive behavioral program. *Journal of School Psychology, 20*, 180–187.

Forman, S. G., & Forman, B. D. (1980). Rational emotive staff development. *Psychology in the Schools, 17*, 90–96.

Freedman, B. J., Rosenthal, R., Donahoe, C. P., Schbundy, D. G., & McFall, R. M. (1978). A social behavioral analysis of skill deficits in delinquent and nondelinquent adolescent boys. *Journal of Consulting and Clinical Psychology, 46*, 1448–1462.

Friedman, G. H., Lehrer, B. E., & Stevens, J. P. (1983). The effectiveness of self-directed and lecture/discussion stress management approaches and the locus of control of teachers. *American Educational Research Journal, 20*, 563–580.

Fullan, M., & Pomfret, A. (1977). Research on curriculum and instruction implementation. *Review of Educational Research, 47*, 335–397.

Galambos, N. L., & Garbarino, J. (1983). Identifying the missing links in the study of latchkey children. *Children Today, 12*(2–4), 40–41.

Gilgun, J., & Gordon, S. (1983). The role of values in sex education programs. *Journal of Research and Development in Education, 16*, 27–33.

Glidewell, J. C., Gildea, M. C., & Kaufman, M. K. (1973). The preventive and therapeutic effects of two school mental health programs. *American Journal of Community Mental Health, 1*, 295–329.

Glynn, T. J., Leukefeld, C. G., & Ludford, J. P. (Eds.). (1983). *Preventing adolescent drug abuse: Intervention strategies.* Research Monograph No. 47. Rockville, MD: National Institute on Drug Abuse.

Gmelch, W. H. (1983). Stress for success: How to optimize your performance. *Theory into Practice, 22,* 7–14.

Goldstein, A. P. (1981). *Psychological skill training.* New York: Pergamon Press.

Goldstein, A. P., Apter, S. J., & Harootunian, B. (1984). *School violence.* Englewood Cliffs, NJ: Prentice-Hall.

Goldstein, A. P., & Glick, B. (1987). *Aggression replacement training.* Champaign, IL: Research Press.

Goldstein, A. P., Heller, K., & Sechrest, L. B. (1966). *Psychotherapy and the psychology of behavior change.* New York: Wiley.

Goldstein, A. P., & Pentz, M. A. (1984). Psychological skills training and the aggressive adolescent. *School Psychology Review, 13,* 311–323.

Goldstein, A. P., Sprafkin, R. P., Gershaw, N. J., & Klein, P. (1980). *Skillstreaming the adolescent.* Urbana, IL: Research Press.

Goldston, S. E. (1986). Primary prevention: Historical perspectives and a blueprint for action. *American Psychologist, 41,* 453–460.

Gordon, S., Scales, P., & Everly, K. (1979). *The sexual adolescent: Communicating with teenagers about sex* (2nd ed.). North Scituate, MA: Duxbury Press.

Gratz, R. R. (1979). Accidental injury in childhood: A literature review on pediatric trauma. *Journal of Trauma, 19,* 551–555.

Gray, E. B. (1983). *Final report: Collaborative research on community and minority group action to prevent child abuse and neglect: Vol. 1. Perinatal interventions.* Chicago: National Committee for Prevention of Child Abuse.

Gray, J., Cutler, C., Dean, J., & Kempe, C. H. (1976). Perinatal assessment of mother-baby interaction. In R. E. Helfer & C. H. Kempe (Eds.), *Child abuse and neglect: The family and the community* (pp. 377–392). Chicago: University of Chicago Press.

Gray, J., & Kaplan, B. (1980). The lay health visitor program: An eighteen month experience. In C. H. Kempe & R. E. Helfer (Eds.), *The battered child* (pp. 363–378). Chicago: University of Chicago Press.

Gray, S. W., & Wandersman, L. P. (1980). The methodology of home-based intervention studies: Problems and promising strategies. *Child Development, 51,* 993–1009.

Gresham, F. (1985). Utility of cognitive-behavioral procedures for social skills training with children: A critical review. *Journal of Abnormal Child Psychology, 13,* 411–423.

Greuling, J. W., & DeBlassie, R. R. (1980). Adolescent suicide. *Adolescence, 15,* 591–601.

Griest, D. L., Forehand, R., Rogers, T., Breiner, J., Furey, W., & Williams, C. A. (1982). The effects of parent enhancement therapy on the treatment outcome and generalization of a parent training program. *Behavior Research and Therapy, 20,* 429–436.

Guerney, B. G., Jr. (1977). *Relationship enhancement.* San Francisco: Jossey-Bass.

Gump, P. V. (1980). The school as a social situation. *Annual Review of Psychology, 31,* 553–582.

Hansen, D. A. (1986). Family–school articulations: The effects of interaction rule mismatch. *American Educational Research Journal, 23,* 643–659.

Hansford, B. C., & Hattie, J. A. (1982). The relationship between self and achievement/ performance measures. *Review of Educational Research, 52*, 123–142.

Harris, D., Baird, G., Clyburn, S. A., & Mara, J. R. (1983). Developing a teenage pregnancy program the community will accept. *Health Education, 14*, 17–20.

Harris, V. W., & Sherman, J. A. (1973). Effects of peer tutoring and consequences on the math performance of elementary school classroom students. *Journal of Applied Behavior Analysis, 6*, 587–597.

Hauck, P. (1967). *The rational management of children.* New York: Libra.

Hawkins, J. D., Lishner, D. M., & Catalano, R. F., Jr. (1985). Childhood predictors and the prevention of adolescent substance abuse. In R. Battjes & C. Jones (Eds.), *Etiology of drug abuse: Implications for prevention* (pp. 75–126). Washington, DC: U.S. Government Printing Office.

Hawley, R. C., & Hawley, I. L. (1975). *Developing human potential: A handbook of activities for personal and social growth.* Amherst, MA: Education Research Associates.

Hawton, K. (1982). Attempted suicide in children and adolescents. *Journal of Child Psychology and Psychiatry, 23*, 497–503.

Hazard, W. R., & Einstein, V. (1983). Legal aspects of sex education: Implications for school administrators. *Journal of Research and Development in Education, 16*(2), 34–40.

Hazzard, A., & Angert, L. (1986). *Child sexual abuse prevention: Previous research and future directions.* Paper presented at the Annual Meeting of the American Psychological Association, Washington, DC, August.

Heffernan, J. A., & Albee, G. W. (1985). Prevention perspectives from Vermont to Washington. *American Psychologist, 40*, 202–204.

Hightower, A. D., & Avery, R. R. (1986) *The study buddy program.* Paper presented at the Annual Meeting of the American Psychological Association, Washington, DC, August.

Hobbs, S. S., Moguin, L. E., Tyroler, M., & Lahey, B. B. (1980). Cognitive behavior therapy with children: Has clinical utility been demonstrated? *Psychological Bulletin, 87*, 147–165.

Hollander, S. K. (1979). *Strategies of selected sixth graders reading and working verbal arithmetic practice as they affect outcomes in instruction in problem solving.* Unpublished doctoral dissertation, Ohio State University.

Interdivisional Committee on Adolescent Abortion. (1987). Adolescent abortion: Psychological and legal issues. *American Psychologist, 42*, 73–78.

Jaremko, M. E. (1984). Stress inoculation training: A generic approach for the prevention of stress-related disorders. *Personnel and Guidance Journal, 63*, 544–550.

Jason, L. A., Durlak, J. A., & Holton-Walker, E. (1984). Prevention of child problems in the schools. In M. C. Roberts & L. Peterson (Eds.), *Prevention of problems in childhood: Psychological research and applications* (pp. 311–341). New York: Wiley.

Jason, L. A., Frasure, S., & Ferone, L. (1981). Establishing supervising behaviors in eighth graders and peer-tutoring behaviors in first graders. *Child Study Journal, 11*, 201–219.

Jerman, M. E. (1971). *Problem solving in arithmetic as a transfer from a productive thinking program.* Unpublished doctoral dissertation, Stanford University.

Johnson, A. B., Gold, V., & Vicker, L. L. (1982). Stress and teachers of the learning disabled, behavior disordered, and educable mentally retarded. *Psychology in the Schools, 19*, 552–557.

Jones, R. T., Kazdin, A. E., & Haney, J. I. (1981). Social validation and training of emergency fire safety skills for potential injury prevention and life saving. *Journal of Applied Behavior Analysis, 14*, 249–260.

Juhasz, A. M. (1983). Sex education: Today's myth—tomorrow's reality. *Health Education, 14*, 16–18.

Kellam, S. G., Simon, M. B., & Ensminger, M. E. (1983). Antecedents in first grade of teenage substance use and psychological well-being. In D. F. Ricks & B. S. Dohrenwend (Eds.), *Origins of psychopathology* (pp. 17–42). Cambridge, MA: Harvard University Press.

Kendall, P. C. (1985). Toward a cognitive-behavioral model of child psychopathology and a critique of related interventions. *Journal of Abnormal Child Psychology, 13*, 357–372.

Kent, M. W., & Rolf, J. E. (Eds.). (1979). *Social competence in children.* Hanover, NH: University Press of New England.

Kilpatrick, J., & Wirszup, I. (Eds.). (1976). *The psychology of mathematical abilities in school children.* Chicago: University of Chicago Press.

Kirschenbaum, D. S., & Ordman, A. M. (1984). Preventive interventions for children: Cognitive behavioral perspectives. In A. W. Meyers & W. E. Craighead (Eds.), *Cognitive-behavioral therapy with children* (pp. 377–409). New York: Plenum Press.

Klaus, M. H., & Kennell, J. H. (1976). *Maternal-infant bonding.* St. Louis, MO: Mosby.

Knaus, W. (1974). *Rational-emotive education: A manual for elementary school teachers.* New York: Institute for Rational Living.

Knaus, W., & Boker, S. (1975). The effect of rational-emotive education lessons on anxiety and self-concept in sixth-grade children. *Rational Living, 11*, 7–10.

Kracht, C. R., & Casey, I. P. (1968). Attitudes, anxieties, and student teaching performance. *Peabody Journal of Education, 45*, 214–217.

Ladd, G. W., & Mize, J. (1983). A cognitive-social learning model of social-skill training. *Psychological Review, 90*, 127–157.

Lahey, B. B., & Strauss, C. C. (1982). Some considerations in evaluating the clinical utility of cognitive behavior therapy with children. *School Psychology Review, 11*, 67–74.

Lazar, I., & Darlington, R. (1982). Lasting effects of early education: A report from the consortium for longitudinal studies. *Monograph of the Society for Research in Child Development, 47,*(2–3, Serial No. 195).

Leach, D. J. (1984). A model of teacher stress and its implications for management. *Journal of Educational Administration, 22*, 157–172.

Lorion, R. P. (1983). Evaluating preventive interventions: Guidelines for the serious social change agent. In R. D. Felner, L. Jason, J. Moritsugu, & S. S. Farber (Eds.), *Preventive psychology: Theory, research, and practice in community intervention* (pp. 251–268). New York: Pergamon Press.

Lorion, R. P., Work, W. C., & Hightower, A. D. (1984). A school-based, multilevel preventive intervention: Issues in program development and evaluation. *Personnel and Guidance Journal, 63*, 480–484.

Lutzker, J. R., Wesch, D., & Rice, J. M. (1984). A review of "Project 12-Ways": An ecobehavioral approach to the treatment and prevention of child abuse and neglect. *Advances in Behavior Research and Therapy, 6*, 63–73.

MacDonald, D. I. (1984). *Drugs, drinking, and adolescents.* Chicago: Yearbook Medical Publishers.

Mahoney, M. J. (1974). *Cognition and behavior modification.* Cambridge, MA.: Ballinger Publishing Company.

Mahoney, M. J. (1977). Reflections on the cognitive learning trend in psychotherapy. *American Psychologist, 32,* 5–13.

Mahoney, M. J., & Nezworski, M. T. (1985). Cognitive-behavioral approaches to children's problems. *Journal of Abnormal Child Psychology, 13,* 467–476.

Marcucci, R. G. (1980). *A meta-analysis of research methods of teaching mathematical problem solving.* Unpublished doctoral dissertation, University of Iowa.

Marecek, J. (1987). Counseling adolescents with problem pregnancies. *American Psychologist, 42,* 89–93.

Matarazzo, J. D. (1982). Behavioral health's challenge to academic, scientific, and professional psychology. *American Psychology, 37,* 1–14.

Maultsby, M. C. (1971). *Handbook of rational self counseling.* Lexington: University of Kentucky.

Maultsby, M. C. (1975). Rational behavior therapy for acting-out adolescents. *Social Casework, 56,* 35–43.

Maultsby, M. C., Knipping, P., & Carpenter, L. (1974). Teaching self-help in the classroom with rational self-counseling. *Journal of School Health, 44,* 445–448.

McGinnis, E., & Goldstein, A. P. (1984). *Skillstreaming the elementary school child.* Champaign, IL: Research Press.

McGuire, D. J., & Ely, M. (1984). Childhood suicide. *Child Welfare, 18,* 17–26.

McMullin, R., & Casey, B. (1974). *Talk sense to yourself.* Denver, CO: Creative Social Designs.

Medway, F. J., & Smith, R. C., Jr. (1978). An examination of contemporary elementary school affective education programs. *Psychology in the Schools, 15,* 260–269.

Meichenbaum, D. H., & Asarnow, J. (1979). Cognitive-behavioral modification and metacognitive development: Implications for the classroom. In P. C. Kendall & S. D. Hollon (Eds.), *Cognitive-behavioral interventions: Theory, research, and procedures* (pp. 103–139). New York: Academic Press.

Meichenbaum, D. H., Bream, L. A., & Cohen, G. S. (1983). A cognitive-behavioral perspective of child psychopathology: Implications for assessment and training. In R. J. McMahon & R. D. Peters (Eds.), *Childhood disorders: Behavioral developmental approaches* (pp. 36–52). New York: Brunner/Mazel.

Meichenbaum, D. H. & Burland, S. (1979). Cognitive behavior modification with children. *School Psychology Digest, 8,* 426–433.

Meichenbaum, D. H., & Goodman, J. (1969). Reflection–impulsivity and verbal control of motor behavior. *Child Development, 40,* 785–797.

Milich, R., & Dodge, K. A. (1984). Social information process in child psychiatric populations. *Journal of Abnormal Child Psychology, 12,* 471–490.

Moleski, R., & Tosi, S. (1976). Comparative psychotherapy: Rational-emotive therapy versus systematic desensitization in the treatment of stuttering. *Journal of Consulting and Clinical Psychology, 44,* 309–311.

Moracco, J. C., & McFadden, H. (1982). The counselor's role in reducing teacher stress. *Personnel and Guidance Journal, 61,* 549–552.

National Center for Health Statistics (1986). Types of injuries and impairments due to injuries, United States. *Vital and Health Statistics,* Series 10, No. 159, Department of Health and Human Services Publication No. (PHS) 87-01587, U.S. Public Health Service. Washington, DC: U.S. Government Printing Office.

National Center on Child Abuse and Neglect. (1982). *Profile of child sexual abuse.* Rockville, MD: Clearinghouse on Child Abuse and Neglect Information.

National Education Association (1967). Teachers' problems. *Research Bulletin, 45,* 116–117.

Newman, I. M., Mohe, P., Badger, B., & Gillespie, T. S. (1984). Effects of teacher preparation and student age on an alcohol and drug education curriculum. *Journal of Drug Education, 14,* 23–36.

New York State United Teachers. (1980). Disruptive children greatest source of stress. *American Teacher, 64,* 17.

Olds, D. L. (1984). *Final report: Prenatal/early infancy project.* Washington, DC: Maternal and Child Health Research, National Institute of Health.

Olsen, K. H., & Work, W. C. (1986). *Refinements in the curriculum and evaluation of a social problem solving program.* Paper presented at the Annual Meeting of the American Psychological Association, Washington, DC, August.

Olton, R. M., Wardrop, J. L., Covington, M. V., Goodwin, W. L., Crutchfield, R. S., Klausmeier, J. J., & Ronda, T. (1967). *The development of productive thinking skills in fifth-grade children.* Technical Report No. 34. Madison: University of Wisconsin Center for Cognitive Learning.

Passmore, J. (1980). A philosophical essay: Sex education. *The New Republic, 183*(14), 27–32.

Peacock, A. A. (1980). Analysis of process sequence traces observed in mathematical problem solving (Doctoral dissertation, University of Oregon). *Dissertation Abstracts International, 40,* 9876A. (University Microfilms No. 80-85, 793).

Peterson, L., & Mori, L. (1985). Prevention of child injury: An overview of targets, methods, and tactics for psychologists. *Journal of Consulting and Clinical Psychology, 53,* 586–595.

Petrusich, M. M. (1966). Separation anxiety as a factor in the student teaching experience. *Peabody Journal of Education, 14,* 353–356.

Piaget, J. (1923). *Language and thought of the child.* London: Routledge & Kegan Paul.

Poche, C., Brouwer, R., & Swearingen, M. (1981). Teaching self-protection to young children. *Journal of Applied Behavior Analysis, 14,* 169–176.

Raschke, D. B., Dedrick, C. V., Strathe, M. I., & Hawkes, R. R. (1985). Teacher stress: The elementary teacher's perspective. *Elementary School Journal, 85,* 559–564.

Rickel, A. U., Eshelman, A. K., & Loigman, G. A. (1983). Social problem solving training: A follow-up study of cognitive and behavioral effects. *American Journal of Community Psychology, 11,* 15–28.

Roberts, E., Klein, D., & Gagnon, J. (1978). *Family life—and sexual learning.* Cambridge, MA: Project on Human Sexual Development.

Robinson, M. L. (1973). *An investigation of problem-solving behavior and cognitive and affective characteristics of good and poor problem solvers in sixth grade mathematics.* Unpublished doctoral dissertation, State University of New York at Buffalo.

Rogers, V., Merriam, K., & Munson, M. (1983). Sex education: Curriculum issues. *Journal of Research and Development in Education, 16,* 45–52.

Rosenbaum, M. S., Creedon, D. L., & Drabman, R. S. (1981). Training preschool children to identify emergency situations and make emergency phone calls. *Behavior Therapy, 12,* 425–435.

Rosenberg, M. S., & Reppucci, N. D. (1985). Primary prevention of child abuse. *Journal of Consulting and Clinical Psychology*, *53*, 576–585.

Roush, D. W. (1984). Rational-emotive therapy and youth: Some new techniques for counselors. *Personnel and Guidance Journal*, January, pp. 223–227.

Russ, N. W., & Geller, E. S. (1986). *Evaluation of a server intervention program for preventing drunk driving*. Final Report No. DD-3, Department of Psychology Virginia Polytechnic Institute and State University, Blacksburg.

Russel, M. L., & Roberts, M. S. (1979). Behaviorally-based decision-making training for children. *Journal of School Psychology*, *17*, 264–269.

Ryle, G. (Ed.). (1971). *Collected papers* (Vol. 2). New York: Barnes & Noble.

Scales, P. (1981). Arguments against sex education: Fact vs. fiction. *Children Today*, *10*(5), 22–25.

Schinke, S. P., Blyth, B. J., & Gilchrist, L. D. (1981). Cognitive-behavioral prevention of adolescent pregnancy. *Journal of Counseling Psychology*, *28*, 451–454.

Schinke, S. P., & Gilchrist, L. D. (1985). Preventing substance abuse with children and adolescents. *Journal of Consulting and Clinical Psychology*, *53*, 596–602.

Schwab, R. L. (1983). Teacher burnout: Moving beyond psychobabble. *Theory into Practice*, *22*, 22–26.

Sharp, K. C. (1981). Impact of interpersonal problem-solving training on preschoolers' social competency. *Journal of Applied Developmental Psychology*, *2*, 129–143.

Silver, E. A., & Thompson, A. G. (1984). Research perspectives on problem solving in elementary school mathematics. *Elementary School Journal*, *84*, 529–545.

Sparks, D. (1983). Practical solutions for teacher stress. *Theory into Practice*, *22*, 33–42.

Sparks, D., & Hammond, J. (1981). *Managing teacher stress and burnout*. ERIC Document Reproduction Service No. ED200522. Washington, DC: ERIC Clearinghouse.

Spatz-Norton, C. (1984). *The effect of self-statement and structured learning training of empathy upon aggressive behavior and pro-social conflict resolution in aggressive elementary school aged males*. Unpublished master's thesis, Syracuse University.

Spence, S. H. (1981). Differences in social skills performance between institutionalized juvenile male offenders and a comparable group of boys without offense records. *British Journal of Clinical Psychology*, *20*, 163–171.

Stallings, J. (1975). Implementation and child effects of teaching practices in follow through classroom. *Monograph of the Society for Research in Child Development*, *40*(7-8, Serial No. 163).

Stephens, T. M. (1978). *Social skills in the classroom*. Columbus, OH: Cedars Press.

Stevens, R., & Pihl, R. O. (1982). The remediation of the student at-risk for failure. *Journal of Clinical Psychology*, *38*, 298–301.

St. Pierre, R., & Miller, D. N. (1985/86). Future directions for school-based alcohol education. *Health Education*, *17*, 11–13.

Talton, C. F. (1973). *An investigation of selected mental, mathematical, reading, and personality assessments as predictors of high achievement in sixth-grade mathematical problem solving*. Unpublished doctoral dissertation, Northwestern State University of Louisiana.

Tharp, R., & Gallimore, R. (1985). The logical status of metacognitive training. *Journal of Abnormal Child Psychology*, *13*, 455–466.

Thompson, D. N. (1983). Sex education curricula in teacher education institutions: A survey. *Journal of Research and Development in Education*, *16*(2), 41–44.

Toal, S. D. (1985). *Children's safety and protection training project: Three interrelated analysis.* Stockton, CA: Total Consultation Services.

Tolman, R., & Sheldon, D. R. (1985). Coping with stress: A multimodal approach. *Social Work,* March–April, 151–158.

Tosi, D. (1974). *Youth: Toward personal growth—A rational-emotive approach.* Columbus, OH: Merrill.

Tosi, D., & Moleski, R. (1973). Rational-emotive counseling: Implications for self-directed behavior change. *Focus on Guidance, 6,* 1–11.

Treffinger, D. J. (1969). *The effects of programmed instruction on productive thinking, verbal creativity, and problem solving in grades 4, 5, 6, and 7.* Unpublished doctoral dissertation, Cornell University.

Tunnecliffe, M. R., Leach, D. J., & Tunnecliffe, L. P. (1986). Relative efficacy of using behavioral consultation as an approach to teacher stress management. *Journal of School Psychology, 24,* 123–132.

Turk, D. C., Meeks, S., & Turk, L. M. (1982). Factors contributing to teacher stress: Implications for research, prevention, and remediation. *Behavioral Counseling Quarterly, 2,* 2–25.

U.S. Department of Commerce. (1984). *Statistical abstracts of the United States, 1984.* Washington, DC: U.S. Government Printing Office.

Walker, H. M., & Buckley, N. K. (1972). Programming generalization and maintenance of treatment effects across time and across settings. *Journal of Applied Behavior Analysis, 5,* 209–224.

Warren, R., Smith, G., & Velten, E. (1984). Rational-emotive therapy and the reduction of interpersonal anxiety in junior high school students. *Adolescents, 19,* 893–902.

Wayne, J. E. (1982). Sex education: The principle and the principal. *Education, 102*(1), 60–64.

Weissberg, R. P., Gesten, E. L., Carnilce, C. L., Toro, P. A., Rapkin, B. D., Davisdon, E., & Cowen, E. L. (1981a). Social problem-solving skills training: A competence building intervention with 2nd–4th grade children. *American Journal of Community Psychology, 9,* 411–424.

Weissberg, R. P., Gesten, E. L., Rapkin, B. D., Cowen, E. L., Davidson, E., Flores de Apondaca, R., & McKim, B. J. (1981b). The evaluation of a social problem-solving training program for suburban and inner city third grade children. *Journal of Consulting and Clinical Psychology, 49,* 251–261.

Whalen, C. K., Henker, B., & Hinshaw, S. P. (1985). Cognitive-behavioral therapies for hyperactive children: Premises, problems, and prospects. *Journal of Abnormal Child Psychology, 13,* 391–410.

Wong, B. Y. L. (1985). Issues in cognitive-behavioral interventions in academic areas. *Journal of Abnormal Child Psychology, 13,* 425–442.

Woodhouse, D. A., Hall, E., & Wooster, A. D. (1985). Taking control of stress in teaching. *British Journal of Educational Psychology, 55,* 119–123.

World Health Organization. (1975). *Education and treatment in human sexuality: The training of health professionals.* Technical Report No. 572. Washington, DC: WHO Publications.

Wright, L., Schaefer, A. B., & Solomons, G. (1979). *Encyclopedia of pediatric psychology.* Baltimore, MD: University Park Press.

Yamaguchi, K., & Kandel, D. B. (1984). Patterns of drug use from adolescence to young adulthood: Predictors of progression. *American Journal of Public Health, 74,* 673–681.

Yeaton, W., & Bailey, J. S. (1978). Teaching pedestrian safety skills to young children: An analysis and one year followup. *Journal of Applied Behavior Analysis, 11*, 315–329.

Young, H. (1974). *A rational counseling primer.* New York: Institute for Rational Living.

Young, H. (1975). Rational casework with adolescents. *Journal of School Social Work, 1*, 15–20.

Ysseldyke, J., & Christenson, S. (1986). *The instructional environment scale.* Austin, TX: Pro-Ed.

Zax, M., & Spector, G. A. (1974). *An introduction to community psychology.* New York: Wiley.

Zelie, K., Stone, C. I., & Lehr, E. (1980). Cognitive-behavioral intervention in school discipline: A preliminary study. *Personnel and Guidance Journal, 59*, 80–83.

Zigler, E. (1982). *Current social policy issues related to children and families.* Paper presented at the Annual Meeting of the American Psychological Association, Washington, DC, August.

Zimmerman, D. (1984). *Enhancing perspective-taking and moral reasoning via structured learning therapy and moral education with aggressive adolescents.* Unpublished master's thesis, Syracuse University.

INDEX